ADVANCED TOPICS IN ENVIRONMENTAL HEALTH AND AIR POLLUTION CASE STUDIES

Edited by **Anca Maria Moldoveanu**

Advanced Topics in Environmental Health and Air Pollution Case Studies
Edited by Anca Maria Moldoveanu

Published by InTech

Janeza Trdine 9, 51000 Rijeka, Croatia

Publishing Process Manager Ivana Lorkovic

Technical Editor Teodora Smiljanic

Cover Designer InTech Design Team

Additional hard copies can be obtained from orders@intechopen.com

Advanced Topics in Environmental Health and Air Pollution Case Studies,
Edited by Anca Maria Moldoveanu
p. cm.
ISBN 978-953-307-525-9

For EU product safety concerns:
IN TECH d.o.o., Prolaz Marije Krucifikse Kozulić 3, 51000 Rijeka, Croatia,
info@intechopen.com or visit our website at intechopen.com.

Meet the editor

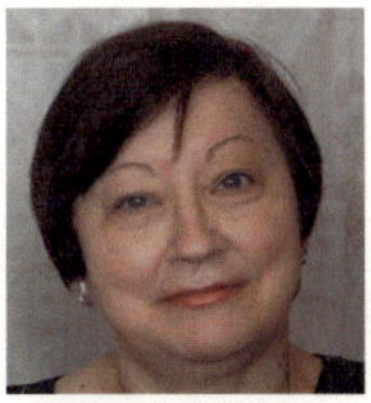

Dr. Anca Maria Moldoveanu
Details of Education: Medical Doctor Degree, University of Medicine and Pharmacy Timisoara 1981, PhD in Medicine, University of Medicine and Pharmacy Bucharest, 1997, Certificates from London School of Hygiene and Tropical Medicine (1996, 1997), Michigan State University (2005, 2006), World Health Organization (1995, 1996).
Career to date: Specialist in Hygiene and Environmental Medicine since 1988. Specialist with the highest degree in Hygiene and Environmental Medicine since 1993. Appointments held: Clinical Hospital "Coltea" Bucharest, Romania, 1981 -1984 as medical doctor; Institute of Hygiene and Public Health Bucharest, Romania, 1985 -1991 with full time job as specialist in Hygiene and Environmental Medicine; National Institute of Public Health, Bucharest, part time job 1991 onward; University of Medicine and Pharmacy "Carol Davila" Bucharest, chair of hygiene and medical ecology – full time job since 1991: assistant professor (1991-1997), lecturer (1997 – 2005), associate professor (2005 onward), head of the chair of hygiene and medical ecology.
Publications: 4 book, 3 chapters in books, 66 articles and 38 communications in scientific events in Romania and abroad.

Contents

Preface

One of the greatest environmental problems is air pollution. This book provides an overview on air pollution as well as its impact on human health.

Beginning with the assessment of what the minimum risk that can be estimated from a study is and trying to find a link between pollution and human health, the book describes the effects of air pollutants on human physiology. Air pollutants can influence inflammation biomarkers, can influence the pathogenesis of chronic cough, can influence reactive oxygen species (ROS) and can induce autonomic nervous system interactions that modulate cardiac oxidative stress and cardiac electrophysiological changes, can have impact on morbidity and mortality related to the cardio-vascular system, can participate in the onset and exacerbation of upper respiratory diseases, can lead to the exacerbation of asthma and allergic diseases. Multiple ways of assessing the relation between environment and human health were described. For example, the Neural Network approach was used to model the relations between the environment, meteorological data and health effects and to investigate cardio-respiratory hospitalisations. Possible air pollutants were investigated in outdoor spaces as well as in indoor spaces like residential homes or primary schools.

The book also presents how the urban environment can influence and modify the impact of various pollutants on human health. Specific pollution situations are described in different cities like Moscow, São Paulo, Rijeka, Bucharest, Lisbon, Mexico, Trabzon-Turkey as well as in different countries like Japan, China, Korea, Israel, South Africa, Brazil, Chile and Poland and the pollutants involved were: particulate matter, sulphur dioxide, nitrogen oxides, ozone, carbon monoxide, formaldehyde, benz(a)pyrene, asbestos, allergens, and biological contaminants.

Several chapters present how indoor air quality may affect the health of children and elderly people.

One study presents the relation between odor perception and air pollution and the fact that different aspects of odor perception are altered to varying degrees.

The book is the result of the effort of many experts, from many countries and from different parts of the world and it shows that the interest in environmental health is growing.

I wish to offer special thanks to the team from InTech Open Access Publisher for their exceptional assistance.

Assoc. Prof. Anca Maria Moldoveanu MD, PhD,
University of Medicine and Pharmacy "Carol Davila" Bucharest
Romania

Part 1

Environment and Health - New Approach

1

What is the Minimum Risk that can be Estimated from an Epidemiology Study?

Mark J. Nicolich[1] and John F. Gamble[2]
[1]*Cogimet, Lambertville, NJ*
[2]*Somerset, NJ*
USA

1. Introduction

Risk is commonly thought of as related to the chance of suffering a loss. In the following discussion we formally define risk and show that epidemiology and risk assessment are related to the probability that a specified event occurs. The risk will be in the form of a *relative risk* where the probability of an event occurring under specified conditions is expressed as a multiplier for the probability of the event occurring at some defined 'background level.'

The goal of the paper is to determine if there is a smallest relative risk that can be determined. That is, is there a risk level at which we can say 'An estimated risk less than X cannot be considered different from background level no matter what estimation methods are used or what the estimated statistical significance level is.' We are assuming the estimated risk level is based on data from an epidemiological study such as the health effects of ambient air pollution or arsenic in the public drinking water. We assume that there is a True Risk Level that applies to a defined population and we wish to estimate it based on the data from an epidemiology study. We assume the data are statistically analyzed either by simple ratios of the observed data or by model-based Bayesian or Classical statistical methods. There are specific epidemiological and statistical considerations that are needed to develop the formal estimate of the true risk as diagramed in Figure 1.

Figure 1 indicates the flow is from a true, but unknown, risk to a final estimate of the risk. It could have been shown as a flow from the initial hypothesis, through the design of the experiment, the analysis of the data, and the final estimate of the true risk. Either structure can be used, but we have chosen the method shown in Figure 1.

In practice the statistical and epidemiological considerations are not separate and distinct steps in the estimation process, but are shown and discussed separately for convenience. The following sections will cover:

- Basic Conclusions,
- Meaning of relative risk (RR),
- Epidemiological considerations in estimating a RR,
- Statistical considerations in estimating a RR,
- Discussion of how to answer the question "what is the smallest relative risk that can be determined"?
- Conclusion and summary,
- An appendix of quotes from knowledgeable researchers in the field

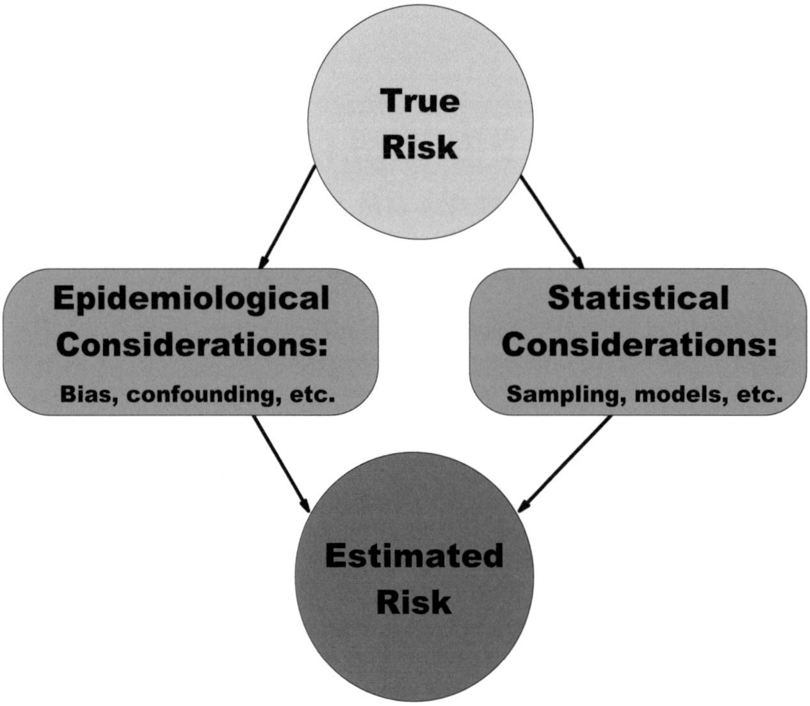

Fig. 1. Considerations needed to develop the point estimate and the significance level of an estimated risk.

2. Basic conclusions

There is no minimum estimable risk in the sense that there is no minimum measure of length. To accurately and precisely measure risk, or length, one needs a tool that is accurate and precise enough for the measurement being made. For example, a meterstick is inadequate for measuring length to a precision of 0.1 mm. When measuring risk in epidemiology, precision and accuracy depend on many factors including the degree to which the experimental data and analysis are free of the errors associated with experimental design flaws (i.e. confounding, bias, reliability, measurement error and misclassification, potential alternate risk factors), and statistical analysis errors (i.e. sampling error, violations of model assumptions, model shopping, multiple subgroup analyses, reliance on significance levels or *p*-values). Indeed, it is theoretically possible to correctly estimate significant risks near 1.000001 if there were no confounding, no biases, no measurement error, exact model specifications, etc. But it is unlikely, if not impossible, these conditions ever exist for an epidemiology study.

While there is no 'lower bound' to an estimable risk, and while many experienced researchers have made opinions about approximate lower bounds, a practical lower limit does exist. To believe an estimated risk the researchers must demonstrate that they have carefully considered the array of possible errors that can arise from the tools and techniques used. As important as these demonstrations are, the difficulty of actually performing these demonstrations leaves many questions about the 'true risk,'and at some point the demonstration may become infeasible or meaningless and leave the realm of conventional science. As exposures approach background levels and apparent risks approach 1.0, the estimates enter the realm of 'trans-science.'When a problem is in the area of trans-science, risk assessment tools of standard science are, by definition, not useful. The most useful outcome possible may be the understanding that the problem belongs to the area of trans-science.

Epidemiology has provided society with many benefits by providing clues to the causes of infectious diseases and identifying factors that contribute to the start and development of non-communicable diseases. Causal knowledge allows quick and effective preventive measures to lessen or halt the diseases without a full understanding of the underlying mechanism. As the RR to be estimated becomes smaller the need for the analyses to be free of errors becomes greater and at some point it becomes impossible to reduce the error further.

3. Meaning of Relative Risk

We will consider epidemiologically based risk as measured by the relative risk (RR). By definition, RR is the ratio of disease frequency in exposed individuals divided by the disease frequency in unexposed individuals (or controls). RR can be thought of as the multiplier of the probability of an event occurring in a special situation relative to the probability of the event occurring in a baseline situation. For example, if the probability of developing lung cancer among smokers was 15% and among non-smokers was 3%, then the relative risk of cancer associated with smoking would be 5. Smokers would be five times as likely as non-smokers to develop lung cancer

Related to the concept of a RR is the idea of Association. Association is measured by absolute differences in rates of disease and by ratios of disease frequency.

- The difference measure of association is the absolute difference in disease frequency between exposed and unexposed. It is an estimate, in the absence of bias, of the absolute amount of disease caused by or attributable to exposure. This absolute difference is proportional to the prevalence of exposure, and so is not especially useful in assessing causality
- The ratio measure is the ratio of disease frequency between exposed and unexposed. It is an estimate of the proportional increase or excess of disease in exposed relative to unexposed and is unaffected by prevalence of exposure. The ratio measure of an association is used when determining whether there is a plausible evidence for a causal association between exposure and disease, or the etiology of disease. The evidence for a causal association is strengthened when there is a strong association, or when the relative risk (RR) is high. The larger the RR the greater the likelihood that an association is causal. Associations may be misleading, because other factors can cause apparent, but spurious, associations that are not true associations. The larger the RR the more unlikely it is that unrelated factors (e.g., bias, confounding) could overcome a true association. However, a RR cannot be used as the sole proof of causality.

The RR is derived from study designs where the study population is selected on the basis of exposure (e.g. cohort study), or disease (e.g. case-control design) and may have different names depending on the context:

- In a cohort mortality study the RR is called a standardized mortality ratio (SMR).
- In a cohort incidence study the RR is called a standardized incidence ratio (SIR).
- In a morbidity cohort or cross-sectional study the RR may be called a prevalence ratio.
- In a case-control study the RR is called an odds ratio (OR).

In a case-control study design the study population is selected on the basis of disease, and the strength of association is based on the odds of exposure (odds ratio or OR), which is the ratio of the proportion of exposed among cases divided by the proportion of exposed among non-cases. The OR is based on the assumption that the disease is rare. [There are methods for estimating risk ratios and confidence intervals from adjusted odds ratios (Greenland 2004, and King and Zeng, 2010).] In everyday applications the OR is used in a way similar to a RR for assessing causality. Differences include the fact that the risk is for exposure, not disease, as in the cohort-based RR. And there are usually differences in some of the confounders. For example, recall bias is likely to be a problem in a case-control study because cases are more likely than non-cases to remember more or exaggerate exposures related to their disease. This is not a likely confounder in a cohort study since the exposure data should be collected blind to disease status.

A weak association means the proportional excess of disease in the exposed relative to unexposed (RR) is small in magnitude, or less than about 2-fold. As associations becomes increasingly weak the importance of spurious factors (e.g., confounding, bias) increases until a point is reached where they overcome (become larger) than the effect of interest. Or in other words, as the power of the signal decreases it will eventually be unintelligible when it is overwhelmed by the noise level in the system.

In epidemiology practice 'weak' and 'strong' relate only to ratio associations and not to the difference measure of association (Rothman and Poole 1988). The strength of association for a particular agent varies over time because the estimated effect depends on the "time-specific distribution of its causal complements in the population" (Rothman and Greenland 2005), which varies over time and between populations.

Strength of association is a major guideline in determining causality (Hill 1965). But there is no agreed upon value for an association to be considered weak or strong. A less than two-fold increased risk has been generally accepted as a 'weak' association. For example, in litigation the court accepts a causal association if the connection between exposure and disease is 'more likely than not.' In epidemiology an *etiological fraction* or *attributable risk* (AR) can be calculated to estimate what proportion of a disease is attributable to exposure to a risk factor when that risk factor is believed to be a cause of the disease. The formula for this calculation expressed as a percent (x 100) is:

$$AR = 100 \cdot \frac{RR - 1}{RR} \tag{1}$$

If the RR for a risk factor of interest = 2.0, then 50% of the disease is attributed to that risk factor. Therefore RR must be greater than 2.0 for the exposure to 'have more likely than not' caused the disease in a particular individual.

4. Epidimiological considerations

In this section we consider areas dealing with study design, confounding, biases, measurement error, misclassification, reliability, and the effects of multiple risk factors.

Epidemiology is an observational, not an experimental science. Because humans are the study subjects it is not possible to manipulate or control exposure. Exposure often consists of the exposures experienced at work, as in occupational epidemiology. The investigators (and the study subjects) lack the capability of producing a specific intensity of exposure. The duration and intensity of exposure cannot be controlled, and only the population can be defined. So there is a distribution of exposures of different intensity and duration among the study population. This is in contrast to the experimental design of animal studies where a desired exposure intensity and duration are produced for a selected number of animals selected at random from the same population.

In epidemiology, estimates of uncertainty are limited by real world limitations. The investigator in an industrial exposure study can increase the size of the study population by including more work sites (or cases with disease), but the total size of the study population is often limited.The investigator has no control regarding intensity and duration of exposures in the workplace, and exposures are generally not to a pure substance but to a mixture of different chemicals that varies over time. Also the investigator has no control on the presence of potential lifestyle confounders (e.g., smoking, obesity, alcohol, age, sex). It is possible to statistically account for confounders, but adjustments will be incomplete because a) the risk associated with each confounder is an imprecise estimate; and b) because there are some unknown confounders for which no statistical adjustment is possible. Note that we use the term 'account for confounders' or 'adjust for confounders' instead of the more popular 'correct for confounders' because an additional term in a statistical model can not *correct* for the presence of confounders, but can only apply a term that might account for the confounder if the adjustment term is adequate.

All estimates of associations in epidemiology are uncertain because of "unknown levels of systematic error from measurement, uncorrected confounding, selection bias, and other biases" that "may even dwarf the random sampling error" (Phillips 2003). The significance of random sampling error is estimated via *p*-values or confidence intervals. But statistical uncertainty tells us nothing about hidden uncertainties with regard to bias and confounding.

Measurement error is a major problem in evaluating causality in epidemiology. Rothman and Greenland (2005) argue that measurement error includes all errors, which range from statistical error to uncertainty problems relating to study design (such as subject selection and retention) through uncontrolled confounding and all other forms of bias. The "true risk"is unknown and is always an estimate because every study has some type of error. "The real issue is to quantify the errors. As there is no precise cutoff with respect to how much error can be tolerated before a study must be considered invalid, there is no alternative to the quantification of study errors to the extent possible." Whether or not one is assessing causality via a set of guidelines such as those of Hill, (Hill, 1965) one must estimate the "total error that afflicts the study" to obtain a reliable estimate of risk. This part of the project further defines and explains this goal of quantifying study errors but excludes consideration of statistical errors.

What are the guidelines for estimating reliability? A minimally reliable RR must be the same order of magnitude or greater than the maximum risks from unknown confounding and bias. The magnitude of the unknown confounding should be less than the minimum known confounding, assuming the investigator is rigorous in the design of the study.

Taking statistical significance into account, guidelines for reliability of a RR are outlined in Table 1.

4.1 Minimal reliable RR

There are several points that define a minimal reliable RR (MRRR).

	Confounding	Observational Study Results	Experimental (clinical) Study Results
Statistically significant	NOT controlled	Unreliable	Unreliable
	Controlled	Possible Real Effect	More likely Real Effect
Not statistically Significant; RR > Minimal RR from hidden uncertainties	NOT Controlled	More Unreliable	More Unreliable
	Controlled	Possible Real Effect; Not significant because of small n?	Unreliable
Not Statistically Significant; RR < minimal RR from hidden uncertainties	NOT controlled	Very Unreliable- likely no relation	Very likely no association
	Controlled	Likely No association	Very likely no association

Table 1. Guidelines for Reliability of a RR

4.1.1 Point 1: There is no single number for a minimal reliable risk that pertains to all studies

The strength of association and magnitude of the uncertainty (and therefore the MRRR) can vary from study to study because of the influence from several sources such as: study population, the causal components of the disease, the frequency and magnitude of the biases, measurement error, etc. MRRR is not dependent on sample size, and is therefore independent of statistical uncertainty or the *p*-value.

As an example of this point, Maldonado et al. (2003) conducted sensitivity analyses on four studies investigating relationships between occupational exposures to glycol ether and congenital malformations. They specifically examined methodological errors that produced biased results that could have incorrectly increased RRs from 24% to 300%. Unfortunately, "without information that can be used to judge the plausibility of different error-producing scenarios, we cannot know the true impact of error on study results....currently available evidence does not refute the [alternative hypothesis] conjecture that elevated OR estimates are due to error." (Maldonado, et al. 2003)

Study Example 1: (Cordier, Bergeret et al. 1997)

This is a case-control study of glycol ether and congenital malformations with multiple positive associations that were substantively modified by adjustments for potential biases. They reported

- Overall OR = 1.4 (1.1-1.9) for all malformations combined.
- Elevated ORs ranging from 1.3 to 2.0 for all eight major categories of malformations
- Elevated ORs ranging from 1.2 to 2.6 for 17/18 subcategories of malformations
- Most likely causal association was for cleft lip with an OR of 2.51 and monotonic E-R trend with ORs of 1.0, 1.5, 2.2, and 2.9 with increasing exposures from no to certain exposure.

These results were consistent with previous studies showing similar associations. Are these risks greater than a MRRR? Are the risks strong enough to support a causal association and greater than hidden uncertainties such as bias? Sensitivity analyses address these questions.

- Potential selection bias from unreported abortion rates differing between exposed and controls could produce errors estimated to range from 0.85 to 1.17. A 3% difference was calculated to produce a spurious OR of about 1.1.
- Potential selection bias from case non-response may have produced error factors ranging from 0.68 to 1.61. If 50% of identified cases were not included in the study the error factor was calculated to be 1.03.
- Potential selection bias may occur if controls are selected differently than cases and are from different populations, as was the case in this study. They suggest the error factor might range from 0.50 to 2.0, and the original authors needed to assess effects of this bias.
- Potential information bias due to exposure measurement error was inadequately presented so the magnitude of the error factor could not be reliably estimated. Maldonado et al. (2003) suggested information bias might produce error factors ranging from 1.4 to 2.3 for exposure misclassification effects related to cleft lip.
- Potential biases in combination are estimated by multiplication of the error factors, which in this case was an error factor of 2.47 (= 1.1 x 1.03 x1.09 x 2). With crude ORs of 2.51 (for cleft lip) and an error factor of 2.47, the corrected OR is 2.51/2.47, or 1.02. Cordier et al. (1997) adjusted for other biases and estimated an error factor of 1.24 (which changed the crude OR of 2.51 to 2.03). Combining the error factors of Maldonado et al. (2003) and Cordier et al. (1997) (2.47 x 1.24 = 3.06) changes the original crude OR of 2.51 to an adjusted OR of 0.82.

Similar sensitivity analyses of three reproductive studies are summarized in Table 2.

Types of Bias	(Cordier, Bergeret et al. 1997) Error Factor	(Shaw, Velie et al. 1999) Error Factor	(Cordier, Szabova et al. 2001) Error Factor
Due to losses	1.1	0.91	1.03
Case non-response	1.03	0.89	0.96
Non-random Control selection	2.0	0.50	2.0
Exposure measurement error	1.09	0.63	1.83
Subtotal of scenarios	2.46	0.26	3.62
Confounding	Largely unknown	Largely unknown	Largely unknown
Author adjustments	1.24	None	None
EF: Bias in combination	2.46 x 1.24 =3.06	0.26	3.62
Adjusted ORs	2.50 / 3.06 → 0.82	0.93 / 0.26 →3.58	3.4 / 3.62 → 0.94

Table 2. Summary of potential error factors (EF) due to bias and confounding in three studies of occupational exposure to glycol ethers and congenital malformations. Based on plausible scenarios (Maldonado, Delzell et al. 2003)

These combined biases are quite large and indicate a MRRR in these studies is far from 1.0. Reproductive studies of this type tend to have large error factors, and the minimal interpretable RRs for these 3 studies should be at least >3, <0.2 and > 3.6 before assessing associations of glycol ether and congenital malformations in these studies. Maldonado, et al. (2003) indicate that because there is a lack of investigation and information available to estimate the extent of the biases, results of these studies are basically uninterpretable.

4.1.2 Point 2: If the estimated RR is smaller than the estimated bias of one of the confounders, then the estimated RR is not reliable and there is a low probability that a causal association exists

Or in more general terms, if the estimated uncertainty or noise is greater than the estimated RR a causal association is unlikely and undetectable.

This is the situation for the results outlined in Table 2, which are based on scenarios whose plausibility is basically unknown. Until the extent of the biases is measured with more reliability, determination of a causal association will remain speculative because of the large size of the potential biases in both positive and negative directions.

There are several examples of studies where the strength of the associations is quite low and the question has arisen as to whether it is possible to measure such associations. These include dozens of studies examining associations between ambient concentrations of air pollutants (especially PM) and acute mortality and morbidity. These are mostly time-series studies where daily concentrations of pollutants in a city are correlated with the daily number of some health effect such as deaths, hospitalizations or asthma cases. Associations in these studies are quite weak with relative risks often around the null value of 1.0. For example, associations with mortality range from negative (<1.0) to a high of about 1.05. That is, the statistical model suggests that as PM concentrations increase by some amount (e.g.10 $\mu g/m^3$) there is 5% increase in mortality or morbidity. For a RR of 0.95 the model suggests a decrease in disease of 5% for every unit increase in exposure.

The primary known confounders in these studies are weather and co-pollutants. Can adequate adjustments be made of these confounders? Are the effects of these confounders greater than the effect of the pollutant of interest? If the answers are no and yes to each question respectively, it is probable the results are spurious and the PM effect cannot be distinguished from the confounding effect.

Lumley and Sheppard (Lumley and Sheppard, 2000) assessed the magnitude of biases in a time-series study of asthma admissions and ambient PM concentrations in Seattle, WA. In the original study the estimated RR was 1.03 per 10 $\mu g/m^3$ increase in PM. They then changed the exposure data (PM concentrations) to different time periods so no association would be expected (RR = 1.0). Deficits or increases in RRs under these conditions would indicate the magnitude of uncontrolled bias. Exposure data from 1 and 2 years in the future produced negligible bias. Exposure data 3 and 4 years in the future produced RRs larger than effect estimates from the real data. The authors concluded "the bias is small in absolute terms but of the same order as the estimated health impacts." Results from these types of studies where RRs are on the order of 1.03 may be measurements of bias not of effects. If so, the observed RR is spurious and can produce an incorrect and misleading interpretation.

The HEI Health Effects Committee (2003) reviewed a selected number of time-series studies after it was discovered that there were errors in the calculation of risk ratios and confidence intervals in these air pollution studies. They indicated there is *no* satisfactory way to adjust for weather and other time-varying confounders such as co-pollutants (HEI 2003).They concluded "no strictly data-based (i.e., statistical) method can exist to insure that the amount of residual confounding due to that variable is small. This means that no matter what statistical method one uses...it is always logically possible that even if the true effect of pollution is null, the estimated effect is far from null due to confounding bias." Because the associations are so weak in these studies the effects that are being attributed to air pollution may "actually be due to...other factors, including weather (typically temperature and relative humidity), as well as unmeasured factors that also vary with time."

The Lumley and Sheppard paper suggests a minimal RR for a causal association in time-series studies must be greater than about 1.05 or the RR said to be associated with air pollution may, in actuality, be produced by unmeasured factors. A RR <1.05 should be considered too weak an association to interpret in the context of time-series air pollution studies, no matter how significant the *p*-value. And the RR may need to be even greater than that since there is no objective method to adjust for confounding from weather or time-related factors. Since weather may have a larger effect on health than PM we may be in an untenable situation with risk factors (e.g., weather, co-pollutants) having potentially greater effects than the exposure of interest.

Exposure misclassification is another unresolved problem in time-series studies. All cases in a time-series study are considered exposed to the same concentration of pollution in the ambient air. Ambient ozone does not permeate into homes, so cases may have 1% or less actual exposure than measured ozone exposure, and minimal estimated risk may be much higher than 1.05. The effect of this exposure misclassification error in this type of study should be studied and adjusted for.

4.1.3 Point 3: There are two kinds of uncertainty associated with relative risks and confounding: Known risk called RR (kc) and unknown risk called RR (uc)

Epidemiology is an observational science so there is natural variation or background uncertainty inherent in every study. Sometimes some of the effects of this uncertainty can be estimated. For example, a heavy smoker is at about a 20-fold greater risk of lung cancer than a non-smoker.

Issues of hidden uncertainty (e.g., bias, confounding) may be more important than frequentist statistical significance (Sterne and Smith 2001; Phillips 2003) and are important concerns that must be considered when evaluating possible etiological agents.

Statistical inferences (e.g., *p*-values) are based on the assumption that the statistical model is correct. However, statistical models can *never* account for all factors. Incompletely accounted for factors are subsumed under the general rubric of bias and confounding. If these factors are not accounted for in comparisons between exposed and non-exposed populations, results may be rendered invalid or unreliable.

Confounding occurs when effects of two agents are not separated and they are counted as one effect. As a result, a difference in disease rates is not due to the exposure of interest alone, but is due to effects of exposure plus other factors such as smoking, diet, etc. By definition a confounder must (1) cause the disease (or be associated with a causal risk factor); (2) be correlated with exposure, either positively or negatively; and (3) not be affected by the exposure.

Confounding arises due to a lack of comparability between exposed and unexposed groups. If both exposed and non-exposed are all non-smokers, smoking cannot be a confounder

because smoking is not associated with exposure and exposed/unexposed groups are comparable with respect to the prevalence of smoking. Confounding is an issue that must always be addressed in assessing issues of causality (McNamee 2003).
Strictly speaking there will always be differences between exposed and unexposed groups, but sometimes the differences are small and unimportant. What is important is the magnitude and direction of confounding effects on the estimated relative risk. The degree of confounding is measured as the ratio of the measured confounded RR divided by the true unconfounded RR. For a single dichotomous confounder, the degree of confounding depends on 1) the strength of the association between confounder and disease (RR); and 2) the percentage (p) of subjects in the exposed (p_1) and unexposed (p_0) groups. It is calculated from the formula:

$$\frac{confounded\,RR}{true\,RR} = \frac{(100 - p_1) + RR \bullet p_1}{(100 - p_0) + RR \bullet p_0} \tag{2}$$

For example, a confounded RR will be 1.4 times the true RR if the strength of association for the confounder is 5 and the prevalence of the confounder in exposed and unexposed populations are 50% and 30% respectively. The statistical significance between p_1 and p_0 should not be used to assess the potential importance of confounding. If there were 40 subjects in each group in this example, the difference between 50 and 30% is not significant at the 5% level. But a 1.4-fold difference between confounded and true RR is important. Table 3 illustrates the degree of confounding that can occur for a strength of association = 5 (McNamee 2003).

Unexposed	Exposed Group: prevalence of confounder (p_1)								
p_0	10%	20%	30%	40%	50%	60%	70%	80%	90%
10%		1.3	1.6	1.9	2.1	2.4	2.7	3.0	3.3
20%	0.8		1.2	1.4	1.7	1.9	2.1	2.3	2.6
30%	0.6	0.8		1.2	1.4	1.5	1.7	1.9	2.1
40%	0.5	0.7	0.8		1.2	1.3	1.5	1.6	1.8
50%	0.5	0.6	0.7	0.9		1.1	1.3	1.4	1.5
60%	0.4	0.5	0.6	0.8	0.9		1.1	1.2	1.4
70%	0.4	0.5	0.6	0.7	0.8	0.9		1.1	1.2
80%	0.3	0.4	0.5	0.6	0.7	0.8	0.9		1.1
90%	0.3	0.4	0.5	0.6	0.7	0.7	0.8	0.9	

Table 3. Degree of confounding due to differences in prevalence between exposed and unexposed when the true risk=5

The degree of confounding is affected more by differences in prevalence of a confounding factor than by strength of the associations, especially above RRs of 5 or so. For example, at prevalences of 60 vs. 40% in exposed and unexposed, the degree of confounding at RR of 2, 5, 10, 15, and 20 are 1.14, 1.31, 1.39, 1.42, and 1.44 respectively.

4.1.4 Point 4: Reliance on *p*-values is an ill-founded strategy. The veracity of a research finding is not dependent on a *p*-value and vice-versa

Too commonly results are considered conclusive on the basis of a *p*-value less than 0.05. This is an 'ill-founded strategy' because of the high rate of non-replication (lack of confirmation) from a "single study assessed by formal statistical significance' (Ioannidis 2005).Others have made the same point (Sterne and Davey Smith 2001; Wacholder, Chanock, et al. 2004). The probability that a finding is actually true when based simply on achieving statistical significance is called the positive predictive value, PPV (Ioannidis 2005). The formula for calculating PPV is

$$\text{PPV (Positive Predicted Value)} = (1\text{-}\beta)R \;/\; ((1\text{-}\beta)R + \alpha) \qquad (3)$$

where
β = Type II error rate, usually 0.20
α = Type I error rate, usually 0.05
R = ratio of the number of 'true relationships' to 'no relationships' among tested hypotheses.
That is, the higher the PPV the greater the chance the estimated RR is an accurate estimate of the true risk. If was assume $\beta = 0.20$, $\alpha = 0.05$, and R=1.0 (half the hypotheses that were tested were found to be statistically significant), the probability of a statistically significant RR being true is estimated to be 0.89. If R = 0.06 (as when 3 of 53 of the hypotheses being tested was statistically significant), then PPV < 0.5 and chances are better than even that the results are not true.

But bias and repeated independent testing by different investigators may further reduce the probability of a true (replicable) result. One definition of bias is 'the combination of various design, data, analysis and presentation factors that tend to produce research findings when they should not be produced' (Ioannidis 2005). This definition is analogous to publication bias *in situ (PBIS)* (Phillips 2004). It can involve manipulation of the analysis and cherry picking of the reported results. In the presence of this kind of bias the probability of a true finding is further reduced and can be estimated from the formula

$$\text{PPV} = ([1\text{-}\beta]\, R + u\beta R) \;/\; (([1\text{-}\beta]\, R + [1\text{-}\alpha]u + \alpha + u\beta R) \qquad (4)$$

where u = the proportion of probed analyses that would not have been "research findings" but nevertheless end up presented and reported as such.'

For example, in air pollution studies of PM thousands of models may be investigated, only a small percentage of which are reported. Assuming both R and u are 0.5 (not unusual in studies with many test models), there is less than a 50-50 chance that a finding is actually true (PPV = 0.46).

On the basis of the above considerations, Ioannidis (2005) proposes several corollaries about the probability that a research finding is true or not.

Corollary 1: The smaller the study, the less likely the findings are true.

Sample size is related to power, and PPV 'for a true research finding decreases as power decreases towards $1 - \beta = 0.05$.'

Corollary 2: The smaller the RR (the weaker the association) the less likely the findings are to be true.

Findings are more likely to be true for strong risk factors such as effects of smoking on cancer or cardiovascular disease (RR 3-20) than for small RRs such as genetic risk factors for multi-genetic diseases (RR 1.1-1.5). Modern epidemiology increasingly targets smaller effect sizes as most risk factors with large RRs have been studied. As a result the proportion of true findings is expected to decrease. Similarly, if the majority of RRs are very small (e.g., RR < 1.05 as in genetic, nutritional and air pollution epidemiology), 'this field is likely to be plagued by almost ubiquitous false positive claims...[and are] largely utopian endeavors.'

Corollary 3: 'The greater the number and the lesser the selection of tested relationships' the more likely the findings will be spurious.

The higher the probability that the pre-study hypothesis is true, the more likely results of a study testing that hypothesis will be true and vice-versa. For example, meta-analyses and studies attempting to confirm hypotheses are more likely to produce true findings than hypothesis-generating studies.

Corollary 4: Increased flexibility in design, definitions, outcomes, and analytical modes increases the likelihood of spurious findings.

Adherence to common standards and protocol is likely to decrease the probability of false findings. Flexibility (e.g., multifarious outcomes such as scales for schizophrenia; experimental analytical methods such as artificial intelligence methods; reporting only 'best' results) 'increases the potential for transforming what would be "negative" results into "positive" results, i.e., bias, μ.' But cherry-picking the data and manipulating outcomes and analyses reported remains a 'common problem' even within the most stringent research designs such as randomized trials (Chan, Hrobjartsson, et al. 2004).

Corollary 5: 'The greater the financial and other interests and prejudices...[of the investigator] the less likely the research findings are to be true.'

These factors increase bias and may be common and widespread. Examples cited included prejudice because of belief in a particular theory or commitment to their own previous findings; university-based studies conducted for no other reason than to increase qualifications for promotion or tenure; peer reviews written to suppress findings that refute the reviewer's research findings. And there is evidence that expert opinion is 'extremely unreliable' (Antman, Lau et al. 1992).

Corollary 6: 'The hotter a scientific field (with more scientific teams involved), the less likely the research findings are to be true.'

For example in molecular genetics there is competition between laboratories to be the first to publish positive associations (e.g., race to describe DNA). This can lead to each lab pursuing and publishing their most impressive 'positive' results, or 'negative' results to contradict positive results from another lab. This is called the 'Proteus phenomenon,' where there are rapidly alternating findings followed by extremely opposite refutations (Ioannidis and Trikalinos 2005).

Based on this reasoning, it is difficult to exceed a 50% probability that results are likely to be true. Considering effects of power, ratio of true to non-true relationships, and bias in various settings and study designs, Ioannidis (Ioannidis 2005) conducted simulations to estimate PPV. These are summarized in the Table 4.

This analysis indicates the majority of modern biomedical research operates where the pre- and post-probability of true findings is very low. In a 'null field' where true positive associations are unlikely to occur (or where RRs are very low), one 'would ideally expect all observed effect sizes to vary by chance around the null in the absence of bias. The extent that observed findings deviate from what is expected by chance alone would be simply a pure measure of the prevailing bias.' For example, suppose 60 nutrients had been examined for causing a specific cancer and RRs were in the range 1.2-1.4 comparing high to low exposed groups. 'Then the claimed effect sizes are simply measuring nothing else but the net bias that has been involved in the generation of this scientific literature.'

1-β	R	μ	Practical Example	PPV
0.80	1:1	0.10	Adequately powered randomized control trial with little bias and 1:1 pre-study odds	0.85
0.95	2:1	0.30	Confirmatory meta-analysis of good quality randomized control trials	0.85
0.80	1:3	0.40	Meta-analysis of small inconclusive studies	0.41
0.20	1:5	0.20	Underpowered, but well-performed phase I/II randomized control trials	0.23
0.20	1:5	0.80	Underpowered, poorly performed phase I/II randomized control trials	0.17
0.80	1:10	0.30	Adequately powered exploratory epidemiological study	0.20
0.20	1:10	0.30	Underpowered exploratory epidemiological study	0.12
0.20	1:1000	0.80	Discovery-oriented exploratory research with massive testing	0.0010
0.20	1:1000	0.20	As in previous example, but with more limited bias (more standardized)	0.0015

Table 4. Positive predictive Value (PPV) of research findings for various combinations of power (1-β), ratio of true to not-true relationships (R), and bias (μ) (Ioannidis 2005)

4.1.5 Point 5: Multiple exposures are a special case of confounding. Research studies investigating a single exposure in observational studies can lead to biased estimates of risk because there is no accounting for exposure to other risk factors that are always present

Exposure measurement errors and confounding are problem areas when studying effects of exposure to multiple chemical agents, and become more difficult when exposure to physical, biological, and psychological stressors are considered. In many epidemiology studies, exposure is limited to one, or at most two, agents in any analysis even though in most situations humans are exposed to chemical mixtures instead of a single chemical (Feron et al., 2002) as well as a wide variety of other stressors. Biological considerations have shown that exposure to some mixtures of chemical compounds can result in lower toxicity (antagonism) or higher toxicity (synergism) than expected based on knowledge of the potency of the individual components (Calabrese, 1991). There are many examples of these antagonistic and synergistic interactions in the literature (Chang et al., 2005).

A classic description of a set of confounders occurs when there are several risk factors, each of which engenders the same response as the agent under analysis and whose magnitudes co-vary. Confounding effects can be accounted for if it is known that these risk factors are present in the environment and their interaction patterns are known. Since it is rare that the presence and interaction patterns are well known, observed risk may be an under- or overestimate of the 'true risk." This problem is clearly exacerbated when the underlying risk is near unity.

4.2 Summary of the epidemiologically based points

It is difficult to account for all the pitfalls associated with designing an epidemiology study where potential risk is very low. The following quote (Ioannidis 2005) suggests the magnitude of the difficulties inherent in the air pollution field:

'For fields with very low PPV, the few true relationships would not distort this overall picture much. Even if a few relationships are true, the shape of the distribution of the observed effects would still yield a clear measure of the biases involved in the field. This concept totally reverses the way we view scientific results. Traditionally, investigators have viewed large and highly significant effects with excitement, as signs of important discoveries. Too large and too highly significant effects may actually be more likely to be signs of large bias in most fields of modern research. They could lead investigators to careful critical thinking about what might have gone wrong with their data, analyses, and results.'

Ioannidis (2005) suggest several steps be taken to improve post-study probability of reporting true findings and avoiding spurious interpretations:

i. Look at the totality of the evidence.
ii. Enhanced research standards and curtailment of prejudices may help. Part of this process is through 'developing and adhering to a protocol' in a fashion similar to that followed in randomized clinical trials.
iii. Improve your 'understanding of the range of R values-- the pre-study odds—where research efforts operate….[I]nvestigators should consider what they believe the chances are that they are testing a true rather than a non-true relationship.'
iv. Don't rely on significance as the primary basis for interpreting results. '[S]tatistical significance testing in the report of a single study gives only a partial picture, without knowing how much testing has been done outside the report and in the relevant field at large…[U]sually it is impossible to decipher how much data dredging…has preceded a reported research finding.'

5. Statistical considerations

Statistical considerations are not independent or exclusive from epidemiological considerations. The distinction provides a possible separation between the strictly epidemiological steps of study planning and sample selection and the statistical steps of data analysis. Both areas come into play in the critical interpretation and reporting steps of the study. In this section we will concentrate mainly on the ideas of violation of model assumptions, model shopping and multiple subgroup analyses, and reliance on significance levels or *p*-values.

5.1 Violation of model assumptions

Relative risks from epidemiological studies often are derived from complex statistical models based on statistical assumptions that are not always clearly understood by non-statisticians but which need to be met to reduce potential errors. The choice of a final model in the model-building process is important because when the RR is small one cannot always verify whether the estimated risks are consistent with the graphic or tabular data. If statistical assumptions are not met the validity of the results is uncertain. We would like to be sure that an appropriate statistical model has been chosen and important assumptions have been met for applying the model to the data.

There is a wide array of concerns relating to the final model choice. Among them is the form of the model including questions such as:

- Is the risk assumed to be linear with exposure?
- Does the model admit to or allow for a threshold or a ceiling?
- Are confounders accounted for?

Other important concerns include

- Have the distributional assumptions of the model been met? For example, do counts follow a Poisson distribution, or are they better described by a negative binomial, or are the residuals normally distributed?
- Are observations independent of each other? Are the residuals free of any auto-correlation?
- Has the appropriate model estimation technique been applied, such as least squares, GAM, GLM?

5.2 Model shopping

The widespread availability of statistical and computing technology is an important factor contributing to the potential for estimating RR with unrealistic precision. It is now easy to routinely engage in sophisticated optimizations across a large number of models and/or variables to identify associations of potential scientific interest. Even with a single risk factor and a single response, it has become standard practice to consider a potentially large number of models in an effort to adjust for differences among the exposed and the unexposed (Peng, et al., 2006). This phenomenon is often called 'model-shopping.' It is an underlying assumption that the significance level of an estimate is developed from a model that was specified *before* statistical analyses were performed. In practice, models often are modified in ways that violate this basic assumption of a completely pre-specified model in order to maximize model efficacy (or maximize the ability to produce a desired result). These violations include such acts as choosing different forms of background effects, selecting smoothing parameters, or choosing different lags for explanatory variables. Such 'model shopping' produces a spuriously inflated significance level, or narrowed confidence interval, that often overstates the significance of the predictors unless there is some adjustment. Hodges (1987) pointed out that reporting only the 'best' model result and essentially ignoring the uncertainties associated with model assumptions may lead to overconfident predictions and policy decisions that are riskier and more uncertain than one thinks they are.

The degree of overstating is related to the number of models tested. Chatfield commented "It is indeed strange that we [statisticians] often admit model uncertainty by searching for the best model but then ignore this uncertainty by making inferences and predictions as if certain that the best fitting model is actually true" (Chatfield 1995).

Bayesian model averaging (BMA) is one method that can help eliminate the concern of multiple models and provide more realistic estimates of uncertainty of relative risks (Clyde

2000). BMA works on the principal that it is possible to calculate the Bayes probability that a model is the correct model for a given data set. After considering all possible models one can estimate a common parameter of interest and its standard deviation and take into account multiple testing. The parameter of interest in many of our examples that follow is the risk associated with an increase in PM concentration.

A cruder method to deal with problems of multiple model testing is to change the criteria for significance, as for example from $p < 0.05$ to $p < 0.005$. This method was suggested by the HEI Health Review Committee (2003) for revised analyses of ACS and Six Cities cohort studies (Krewski, Burnett et al. 2000).

Neither of these methods (BMA or changing the level at which significance is declared) has been universally applied, so the concern remains about minimizing the reported error in a RR associated with multiple testing. Note Hill's advice when interpreting for causality: don't over-emphasize statistical significance tests, as systematic error is often greater than random error. He questions the usefulness of statistical significance in situations where differences are negligible. What could be worse than when the "glitter of the *t* table diverts attention from the inadequacies of the fare" (Hill 1965).

5.3 Multiple subgroup analyses

Closely related to the phenomenon of model shopping is the analysis of subgroups of the original sample. Subgroups are often formed by 'interesting observations' seen during the initial analyses and can be useful and lead to important discoveries. "Nearly everything that has been learned in epidemiology has been derived from the analysis of subgroups. This is an incisive, effective technique to which we owe our sustenance." (Stallones, 1987). When subgroups are not selected *a priori* and are not part of the initial sample size determination, results from sub-group analyses must be looked on with caution and replications in a different experiment or sample are needed before any conclusions can be made.

5.4 Over-reliance on significance levels

It is a common misconception that the precision of a small RR depends on the significance level or *p*-value of an estimated RR. It is not true that the *p*-value or confidence interval "can provide a number that by itself reflects a probability of reaching erroneous conclusions." (Goodman 1999a)

The *p*-value is an informal index for measuring the difference between results of a study and the null hypothesis of no effect. A *p*-value of 0.05 does *not* mean that the null hypothesis has a probability of 5% of 'being true' (or that there is a 95% chance of no effect). This interpretation is incorrect because the study data alone cannot provide the probability that the null hypothesis is true. Tests based on probability (such as *p*-value and 95% confidence intervals) cannot provide "any valuable evidence of the truth or falsehood of a hypothesis" (Neyman and Pearson 1933; Goodman 1999a). The *p*-value *only* tells whether the results are statistically significant (Goodman 1999a).

The strength of evidence for an effect estimate with a *p*-value of 0.05 is actually much weaker than the number 0.05 suggests. Goodman (Goodman 1999b) suggests using the Bayes Factor in lieu of the *p*-value. The Bayes Factor, related to the likelihood ratio, is an index for evaluating evidence outside of individual study results that can be used for assessing the likelihood that a relationship is true. The Bayes Factor compares the predictive value of the null and alternative hypotheses based on the weight of evidence. It can help keep chance (statistical evidence) distinct from conclusions, while being part of a calculus that formally links them (Goodman 1999b).

"We must expect that most truly new research findings in observational research will be unexpected and an unexpected result may well appear aberrant. To distinguish between those exceptional subgroups that have epidemiological significance and those that do not may be difficult. Statistical treatment is of little use in addressing the problem. A probability statement is of value in assessing the magnitude of an association in relation to the number of persons in the study; that is, it may help us restrain our enthusiasm over large difference in small groups. However, a *p*-value of 0.01 in an observational study does not mean that a difference as great or greater than the one observed will occur no more often than 1 in 100 trials. By and large, statistical significance is a meaningless term in observational research. This is true for many reasons, but mainly because a *p*-value does not know any epidemiology; it was born into a world of tossing pennies and urns full of black and white balls, and it never read a book about disease. It can't tell the difference between truth and bias, and it worships sample size more than truth" (Stallones, 1987).

6. Discussion

What should be done when an estimated RR is small, and consideration of epidemiological and statistical concepts do not provide a clear answer to the question of whether the estimated RR is too small to be accurately estimated? Two possible approaches are discussed in this section. The first is a technical solution that involves gathering more data and testing the statistical model; the second is a more philosophical approach. They are not mutually exclusive ways to approach this difficulty, and they are not always practical or satisfactory.

6.1 A Direct method

A direct method to demonstrate that a RR has been accurately estimated is to demonstrate that the same risk is seen in a similar, but disjoint, population using the same model used to develop the initial estimate. A statistical model developed to estimate an RR can be thought of as a descriptive model because it describes the data at hand. It was crafted to be 'the best' at estimating the RR, and by extension for describing the data set. However, when a descriptive model is going to be used to predict future effects that will accrue because of a change in exposure, thinking and application of the model must also change. Chatfield (1995) noted, "...model builders should adopt a more pragmatic approach in which they search not for a true model, but rather a *parsimonious* model giving an adequate approximation to the data at hand and then concentrate on determining the model's *accuracy* and *usefulness*, rather than testing it [for significance]."

For example, a descriptive time-series regression model in a mortality study of air-pollution can be used to describe relationships in a specific city for the previous 10 years say. For prediction of pollution effects, use the same model with the same coefficients to predict one year (or more) into the future. Then determine the accuracy and precision of the predicted measurements. A kind of sensitivity analysis could be done by developing two time-series models on the past data: one with an air pollution term in the model and one without the air pollution term. Then see if either can accurately predict the future data, and if the model with the air pollution term has a better fit to the "new data."

This type of validation would be a major demonstration that the estimated risk was useful both as a descriptor and a predictor.
However, in many situations this method is not feasible. In a cohort study all the 'cases' have usually been identified and there are no more cases to use in the second, confirmatory, study. Or the study population may be too small to divide it for both descriptive and predictive purposes. A similar problem occurs with case-control studies. In air pollution time-series studies there are technical difficulties that preclude using the exact coefficients from past data in a new data set, although there is some hope that this problem can be overcome. In the time-series example, it is not sufficient to develop a model in a different location and show the form of the model is the same. This procedure only demonstrates that the model is descriptive for another data set; the goal is to show the model is predictive because it may be used to set policy for future exposures.

6.2 Trans-science

Weinberg (1972) coined the term *trans-science* to describe the realm of scientific questions of facts that are properly formulated, but cannot be answered by science. The answers transcend science, usually because of the impracticality of expending the required time and money. Such questions include the shape of an exposure response curve at very low levels of exposure, or probabilities of extremely improbable events such as failures in complex systems like nuclear reactors and dams. His point is that we will never know, with a reasonable expenditure of resources, what the precise risks are at low (often environmental) levels. He discusses the Science Republic (the realm of scientists), and the Political Republic (the realm of politicians).These two are joined in the Republic of Trans-Science, the character of which depends on place and time. A major difficulty is to draw the line between matters of science and matters of trans-science, and is a crucially important role of the scientist. This is a difficult task, but often it is beneficial to draw the line and declare a question to be in the realm of trans-science. Then it can be dealt with on moral or aesthetic grounds, rather than having a scientific debate that has no hope of resolution. He concludes with the upbeat idea that the most science can do is to inject some intellectual discipline into the Republic of Trans-science and hope that politics in an open society will keep it democratic.
In a paper that deals with a topic similar to the current one about estimating minimum risk, Weinberg (1985) proposes a method for dealing with trans-science questions that are concerned with setting limits on an exposure response curve. He calls the trans-science problem of setting an environmental standard based on incomplete information 'The Regulator's Dilemma' and suggests initiating a branch of science called Regulatory Science. In this new branch of science the norms of scientific proof would be less demanding than in standard science. Instead of asking science for answers to questions that are unanswerable, the regulators should be content with less far-reaching and seemingly less precise answers. He suggests that where ranges of uncertainty can be well established, then regulations can be based on the uncertainty. Where the ranges of uncertainty are so wide as to be meaningless, then ask the question so that the regulation does not depend on answers to an unanswerable question.
Weinberg (1985) provides an idea on how to provide some assurance of public safety despite uncertainty in the estimation of the risk. The idea, called *de minimis*, is to set the

permissible exposure level at some fraction above the natural background level irrespective of the possible risk. The idea is that for almost all environmental hazards, or putative hazards, there is a natural background level, such as for cosmic radiation or exposure to the suite of pollutants regulated by the National Ambient Air Quality Standards. A *de minimis* standard would be at some level above background level, for example 1.0 or 1.5 standard deviations above the mean. The idea is that man has lived with the natural exposure, and if it was harmful man would not have survived. So, an increase that is small relative to natural background should be acceptable.

7. Conclusion

Theoretically, there is no relative risk that is too small to be estimated. The relative risk is a construct or a concept, not a physical reality. Since it is a mathematically defined concept it can be mathematically estimated to any degree of precision. However, we have shown in this paper that (1) there are many assumptions that must be met to make certain that the RR estimate is accurate and precise; and (2) the significance level or uncertainty associated with the RR estimate has its own set of assumptions that must be met. So, while there may be no theoretical minimum RR that can be estimated, in practice there is a minimum risk and varies depending on uncertainties present in the context of each study.

An analogy in the physical world of estimating a RR is to measure the length of an object. A meterstick is precise enough to determine the width of a table to see if it will fit through a doorway, but a meterstick is not precise enough to measure the diameter of a shaft in an automobile engine with a tolerance of ±1.0 mm. To measure the shaft diameter one would use a micrometer. The micrometer while sufficiently precise to measure the shaft is not adequate to determine the size of a dust mite, usually in the range of 200 to 300 µm. The analogy can be carried through to the size of molecules, to the wavelength of visible light, and to the diameter of an electron. The conclusion is that while all the tasks involve measuring length and there is no practical 'minimum length', different tools and considerations are needed depending on the object to be measured and the precision required.

The analogy carries over to the estimation of a RR. There is less concern about detailed assumptions when estimating a RR of lung cancer among pack-a-day smokers with estimated RRs ranging from 10 to 25. But there is greater concern about meeting detailed assumptions when estimating the RR of mortality from a 10 $\mu g/m^3$ increase in PM air pollution where RRs may be as low as 1.004 (or 3 to 4 orders of magnitude smaller than that of lung cancer and smoking), and concluding the association is causal.

What is to be done when an estimated RR is small and in the controversial range? Two suggestions were provided: (1) verify the estimated risk with new data; and (2) regulate on exposure not on the response as done in the regulatory arena when the consequences of exposure are controversial. In many cases neither of these solutions will be considered acceptable, putting us back into the realm of uncertainty.

Epidemiology has provided society with many benefits by providing clues to the causes of infectious diseases and identifying factors that contribute to the start and development of non-communicable diseases (Wynder, 1987). Causal knowledge allows quick and effective preventive measures to lessen or halt diseases without a full understanding of the underlying mechanism. Some examples of interventions fruitfully undertaken without a full understanding of mechanisms include tobacco-related diseases, radiation and leukemia, and UV light and skin cancer. In these cases RRs were quite high, with magnitudes exceeding 10 -fold increases at reasonably low exposures.

However, when it comes to weaker associations, errors in the estimation of the risk can produce a false positive association when in fact no association exists, and vice-versa (Wynder, 1987). Epidemiological data may have the required quality to address a research hypothesis and estimate risk if thought, planning and care are taken in the design of the study with consideration of how cases and controls are selected or the cohort is defined, when possible biases and confounders have been avoided or properly considered, when problems of subgroup analysis are clearly understood, and when the protocol is carefully and accurately carried out. It is likely a correct interpretation may be possible if all available evidence is subjected to a careful review of the biological plausibility of the initial hypothesis, if the criteria discussed above are implemented, and if the data analyses are correctly carried out without pre-conceived bias. There are times, however, that such care is not given to epidemiological studies and their interpretations. There is a great concern that in the "rush to publish," often as a preliminary report, false associations are reported which do not do justice to the factor being incriminated as harmful, nor to public safety if a risk in fact does not exist, nor to the science of epidemiology.

Most of the problems in epidemiology, as they relate to reliable and interpretable estimations of small RRs, can be avoided if researchers pay attention and carefully consider issues relating to study design, confounding, the many forms of bias, reliability, measurement error and misclassification, multiple agents, sampling error, violation of model assumptions, model shopping, multiple subgroup analyses, and over-reliance on significance levels or *p*-values.

We agree with Wynder (1987) that epidemiology is able to correctly interpret relatively small relative risks, but only if the best epidemiological methodology is applied and only if the data are fully evaluated by examining all judgment criteria, especially those of biological plausibility. As RRs become smaller, the need for close adherence to these basic principles becomes greater. If these ideas are applied, a conclusion of no risk should reassure society. And when a risk is reported as positive, appropriate preventive measures to reduce avoidable illness can be used to successfully reach the ultimate goal of epidemiology and preventive medicine.

8. Appendix

8.1 Quotes from knowledgeable researchers in the field

There are many references from experienced health scientists as to what a reasonable minimum relative risk should be. Gary Taubes (1995) in his 1995 Science article had collected a number of quotes, not all of which could be independently verified. The following is a collection of some of Taubes' quotes and other comments from various sources, presented in almost alphabetical order.

"As a general rule of thumb, we are looking for a relative risk of 3 or more before accepting a paper for publication."

Marcia Angell, editor of the New England Journal of Medicine, reported in Taubes 1995.
"If it's a 1.5 relative risk and it's only one study and even a very good one, you scratch your chin and say maybe."

John Bailar, reported in Taubes 1995
"Relative risks of less than 2.0 may readily reflect some unperceived bias or confounding factor, those over 5.0 are unlikely to do so."

Breslow and Day, 1980, Statistical methods in cancer research, Vol. 1, The analysis of case control studies. Published by the World Health Organization, International Agency for Research on Cancer, Sci. Pub. No. 32, Lyon, p. 36.
"Epidemiological studies, in general are probably not able, realistically, to identify with any confidence any relative risks lower than 1.3 (that is a 30% increase in risk) in that context, the 1.5 [reported relative risk of developing breast cancer after abortion] is a modest elevation compared to some other risk factors that we know cause disease."

Dr. Eugenia Calle, Director of Analytic Epidemiology, American Cancer Society, Washington Post - Oct 27,1994
" ... when relative risk lies between 1 and 2 ... problems of interpretation may become acute, and it may be extremely difficult to disentangle the various contributions of biased information, confounding of two or more factors, and cause and effect."

Richard Doll, F.R.S. and Richard Peto "The Causes of Cancer," Oxford-New York, Oxford University Press, 1981, p. 1219.
"An association is generally considered weak if the odds ratio [relative risk] is under 3.0 and particularly when it is under 2.0, as is the case in the relationship of ETS and lung cancer."

Dr. Geoffrey Kabat, Senior Epidemiologist, Albert Einstein College of Medicine, from E.L. Wynder & G.C. Kabat, Environmental Tobacco Smoke and Lung Cancer: A Critical Assessment, I.SAB.7.1 at 6 (JA 7,216),
http://www.forces.org/evidence/epafraud/files/osteen.htm, accessed 26 Dec 2007
"In epidemiologic research, [increases in risk of less than 100 percent] are considered small and are usually difficult to interpret. Such increases may be due to chance, statistical bias, or the effects of confounding factors that are sometimes not evident." "It is not size of the RR alone (but we have to agree at some point low is too low say 1.03 relative risk) but the results of other studies addressing the same issue and concerns about biological plausibility have to be factored in. Even though the size of the RR or OR is not necessarily determinative it is easy to cite a number of experts in the field who favor the notion that RR less than 2 should be- if not dismissed- at least looked at with a very skeptical eye."

National Cancer Institute, "Abortion and Possible Risk for Breast Cancer: Analysis and Inconsistencies," October 26, 1994 press release
"Differences in risk of 50% (Relative risk of 1.5) are small in epidemiological terms and severely challenge our ability to distinguish whether it reflects cause and effects or whether it simply reflects bias."

Lynn Rosenberg, Boston University School of Medicine quoted in Press Release U.S. National Cancer Institute Oct 26,1994
"Any scientist worth his qualifications knows that a RR of less than two or even three is unreliable and too shaky to place much reliance upon."

John K. Sutherland quoted from "The Week That Was", April 22, 2006,
"My basic rule is if the relative risk isn't at least 3 or 4, forget it."

Robert Temple, director of drug evaluation at the Food and Drug Administration, reported in Taubes 1995

"With epidemiology you can tell a little thing from a big thing. What's very hard to do is to tell a little thing from nothing at all."

Michael Thun, VP of Epidemiology and Surveillance Research at the American Cancer society reported in Taubes 1995

9. References

Antman, E. M., J. Lau, et al. (1992). "A comparison of results of meta-analyses of randomized control trials and recommendations of clinical experts. Treatments of myocardial infarction." JAMA 268: 240-248.

Calabrese, 1991 E.J. Calabrese, Multiple Chemical Interactions, Lewis Publishers, Chelsea, MI, USA (1991).

Chan, A. W., A. Hrobjartsson, et al. (2004). "Empirical evidence for selective reporting of outcomes in randomized trials: comparison of protocols to published articles." JAMA 291: 2457-2465.

Chang et al., 2005, "The effects of simultaneous exposure to methyl ehyl ketone and toluene on urinary biomarkers of occupational N,N-dimethylformamide exposure.", Tox Letters, Vol 155(3), 15 March 2005, Pages 385-395

Chatfield, C. (1995). "Model uncertainty, data mining and statistical inference." J Roy Stat Soc (Ser A) 158: 419-466.

Clyde, M. (2000). "Model uncertainty and health effect studies for particulate matter." Environmetrics 11: 745-763.

Cordier, S., A. Bergeret, et al. (1997). "Congenital malformations and maternal occupational exposure to glycol ethers." Epidemiology 8: 355-363.

Cordier, S., E. Szabova, et al. (2001). "Congenital malformations and maternal exposure to glycol ethers in the Slovak Republic." Epidemiology 12: 592-593.

Feron, VJ,. Cassee, J.P. Groten, P.W. van Vliet and J.A. van Zorge, (2002) "International issues on human health effects of exposure to chemical mixtures", Environ. Health Persp. 110 (2002), pp. 893–899.

Goodman, S. (1999a). "Toward Evidence-Based Medical Statistics. 1: The P Value Fallacy." Ann Intern Med 130: 995-1004.

Goodman, S. (1999b). "Toward Evidence-Based Medical Statistics. 2: The Bayes Factor." Ann Intern Med 130: 1005-1013.

Greenland, S. (2004). "Model-based estimation of relative risks and other epidemiologic measures in studies of common outcomes and in case-control studies." Am J Epid 160: 301-305.

HEI (2003). Revised analyses of time-series studies of air pollution and health. Special Report: Revised analyses of the National Morbidity, Mortality, and Air Pollution Study. Boston, MA, Health Effects Institute.

Hill, A. (1965). "The environment and disease: association or causation?" Proc R Soc Med 58: 295-300.

Hodges, J. (1987). "Uncertainty Policy Analysis and Statistics." Stat Sci 2: 259-291.

Ioannidis, J. P. A. (2005). "Why most published research findings are false." PLoS Med 2(8): e124.

Ioannidis, J. P. A. and T. A. Trikalinos (2005). "Early extreme contradictory estimates may appear in published research: The Proteus phenomenon in molecular genetics research and randomized trials." J Clin Epidemiol 58: 543-549.

King, Gary, and Langche Zeng. "Inference in Case Control Studies." In Encyclopedia of Biopharmaceutical Statistics, edited by Shein-Chung Chow. 3rd ed. New York: Marcel Dekker, 2010.

Krewski, D., R. T. Burnett, et al. (2000). Reanalysis of the Harvard Six Cities Study and the American Cancer Society Study of Particulate Air Pollution and Mortality. Special Report. Cambridge, MA, Health Effects Institute.

Lumley, T. and L. Sheppard (2000). "Assessing seasonal confounding and model selection bias in air pollution epidemiology using positive and negative control analyses." Environmetrics 11(6): 705-717.

Maldonado, G., E. Delzell, et al. (2003). "Occupational exposure to glycol ethers and human congenital malformations." Int Arch Occup Environ Health 76: 405-423.

McNamee, R. (2003). "Confounding and confounders." Occup Environ Med 60: 227-234.

Neyman, J. and E. Pearson (1933). "On the Problem of the most efficient tests of statistical hypotheses." Philosophical Transactions of the Royal Society. Series A 231: 289-337.

Peng, RD, Dominici, F and Zeger SL, (2006) "Reproducible Epidemiologic Research," Am J Epid 163: 783-789.

Phillips, C. (2003). "Quantifying and reporting uncertainty from systematic errors." Epidemiology 14: 459-466.

Phillips, C. (2004). "Publication bias *in situ*." BMC Medical research Methodology; online at http://www.biomedcentral.com/1471-22884/20. 4: 20.

Rothman, K. J. and C. Poole (1988). "A strengthening programme for weak associations." Int J Epidemiol 17((Suppl 4)): 955-959.

Rothman, K. J. and S. Greenland (2005). "Causation and causal inference in epidemiology." AJPH 95((Supplement 1)): S144-S150.

Shaw, G. M., E. M. Velie, et al. (1999). "Maternal occupational and hobby chemical exposures as risk factors for neural tube defects " Epidemiology 10:124-129 (erratum appears in Epidemiology 10:777).

Stalones, RA. (1987). "The use and abuse of subgroup analysis in epidemiological research." Preventive Medicine 16:183-194.

Sterne, J. A. and G. Davey Smith (2001). "Sifting the evidence-what's wrong with significance tests." BMJ 322: 226-231.

Taubes, G. (1995) "Epidemiology faces its limits." Science 269(5221):164-9.

Wacholder, S., S. Chanock, et al. (2004). "Assessing the probability that a positive report is false: an approach for molecular epidemiology studies." J Natl Cancer Inst 96: 434-442.

Weinberg, A. (1972) "Science and Trans-Science," Minerva 10:209-222.

Weinberg, A. (1985) "The regulator's dilemma." Issues in Science and Technology 2:59-72.

Wynder, E., "Workshop on Guidelines to the Epidemiology of Weak Associations." Preventive Medicine 16:139-212; 1987

2

Effect of Short-Term Exposure to Near Highway Pollutants in Motor Vehicle Exhaust on Inflammation Sensitive Biomarkers

Ori Rogowski, Eran Leshem-Rubinow, Itzhak Shapira and Arie Steinvil
Tel Aviv Sourasky Medical Center and the Sackler Faculty of Medicine,
Tel Aviv University,
Israel

1. Introduction

Urban atmospheric air pollution is considered a significant challenge for environmental Health (Brunekreef & Holgate, 2002; World Health Organization [WHO], 2003). Growing epidemiological evidence has supported the association between air pollution and cardiovascular morbidity and mortality (Brook et al., 2010). The biological mechanisms underlying these associations remain obscure (Kaufman 2010). One possible explanation to this association is that air pollution has been shown to cause pulmonary inflammation which is further associated with the production of local inflammatory mediators (Nurkiewicz et al., 2008; Nurkiewicz et al., 2009; Kido et al., 2011). These mediators in turn enter the systemic circulation and could contribute to the acceleration of atherothrombotic disease (Seaton et al., 1999; Ghio et al., 2000; Peters et al., 2001b; van Eeden & Hogg, 2002; Pope et al., 2004). Animal models of accelerated atherosclerosis following exposure to air pollution, strongly support this potential mechanism (Sun et al., 2005; Niwa et al., 2008). Low grade systemic inflammation has repeatedly been shown to be a contributing factor in the etiopathogenesis of atherothrombotic disease (Libby 2002; Danesh et al., 2005; Libby, 2006). A hint to the link between air pollution and systemic inflammation arises from studies demonstrating some type of correlation between inflammatory biomarkers, and the amount of outdoor atmospheric particles and volatile gases (Schwartz, 2001; Ghio et al., 2003; Liao et al., 2005; Diez Roux et al., 2006; Steinvil et al., 2008).

Exposure to combustion-derived air pollution is associated as well to an early (1-2 h) and sustained (24 h) rise in cardiovascular morbidity and mortality (Peters et al., 2001a; Peters et al., 2004). Toxicological diesel exposure studies have demonstrated a selective and persistent impairment of endothelium-dependent vasodilatation that occurs in the presence of mild systemic inflammation (Mills et al., 2007; Tornqvist et al., 2007), coronary vasoconstriction (Cherng et al., 2009), as well as an increase in ex-vivo thrombus formation and in- vivo platelet activation (Lucking et al., 2008). Less attention has however been given to measuring pollutants and exposures near heavily-trafficked highways. The most widely reported pollutants in vehicular exhaust include carbon monoxide, nitrogen and sulfur oxides, unburned hydrocarbons (from fuel and crankcase oil), particulate matter, polycyclic aromatic hydrocarbons, and other organic compounds that derive from combustion (Brugge et al., 2007). While several recent studies have shown that sharp pollutant gradients exist near highways, most reports did not however examine this effect on the inflammatory response in over 400 meters (Brugge et al., 2007).

2. Methods

In the present analysis we have investigated the relationship between commonly measured combustion derived air pollutants and inflammatory biomarkers in apparently healthy individuals residing at a 1000 meter radius from a traffic air pollution monitoring station.

2.1 Population

In the present study we analyzed the data collected as part of the Tel-Aviv Medical Center Inflammation Survey (TAMCIS), a registered data bank of the Israeli Ministry of Justice (Rogowski et al., 2006). This is a relatively large survey comprising of apparently healthy individuals attending a center for periodic health examinations. In our study, patients attending the Tel-Aviv Sourasky Medical Center, Tel-Aviv, Israel for a routine health examination between September 2002 and August 2010 were invited to participate in the TAMCIS. All individuals enrolled were recruited during their routine annual health check-up and gave their written consent in accordance with the guidelines of the Institutional Ethics Committee. A total of 15,605 subjects gave their informed consent (9,881 males, 5,724 females). 2,773 subjects were later excluded from the analysis due to known inflammatory disease (arthritis, inflammatory bowel disease, psoriasis, etc.), pregnancy, steroidal or nonsteroidal treatment (except for aspirin at a dose of ≤ 325 mg/dl), acute infection or invasive procedures (surgery, catheterization, etc.) during the last 6 months. An additional 12,387 subjects were further excluded for living more than 1000 meter away from the nearest traffic-related air pollution monitoring station. Following these exclusions the study group comprised of 445 individuals (262 males and 183 females). All distance calculations between the traffic-related air pollution monitoring stations and the specific household addresses of all TAMCIS participants were performed by the Survey of Israel, a national authority for mapping, cadastre, geodesy and geoinformation.

2.2 Laboratory methods

As part of the survey, we employed a set of analyzes to assess the levels of the inflammation sensitive biomarkers of the acute phase: Fibrinogen was quantified by the method of Clauss (Clauss, 1957) and a Sysmex 6000 (Sysmex Corporation, Hyaga, Japan) autoanalyzer while the high sensitivity C-reactive protein (hs-CRP) was measured using a Behring BN II Nephelometer (DADE Behring, Marburg, Germany) (Rifai et al., 1999). The erythrocyte sedimentation rate (ESR) was determined by using the method of Westergren(International Council for Standardization in Haematology [ICSH], 1993).

2.3 Definition of atherothrombotic risk factors

Results of the routine health check-up were assessed employing certain definitions in order to recognize atherothrombotic risk factors in individuals. These included diabetes mellitus which was defined as a fasting blood glucose concentration of ≥ 126 mg/dl (7.0 mmol/L) or the intake of insulin or oral hypoglycemic medications. Hypertension was defined as a blood pressure of >140/90 mm Hg on two separate measurements or the use of antihypertensive medications. Dyslipidemia was defined as the low density lipoprotein cholesterol (LDL-C) or non-high density lipoprotein cholesterol (non-HDL-C) concentrations, for individuals displaying elevated triglyceride concentrations of > 200 mg/dl (2.26 mmol/L), above the recommended levels according to the risk profile defined by the updated adult treatment panel III (ATP III) recommendations or the use of lipid lowering medications(National Cholesterol Education Program/Adult Treatment Panel III [NCEP/ATPIII], 2001). The diagnosis of the metabolic syndrome was based on the joint interim statement of the International Diabetes Federation Task Force on Epidemiology and Prevention; National Heart, Lung, and Blood Institute; American Heart Association; World Heart Federation; International Atherosclerosis Society; and International Association for the Study of Obesity (Alberti et al., 2009). In short, Elevated waist circumference was defined as ≥94 cm (37 inches) in men and ≥80 (31.5 inches) in women as recommended for europid and middle east; Elevated triglycerides (TG) were defined as ≥150 mg/dl (1.7 mmol/l) or on drug treatment for elevated triglycerides; Reduced HDL-C was defined as <40 mg/dL (1.0 mmol/l) in men and <50 mg/dl (1.3 mmol/l) in women or on drug treatment for reduced HDL-C; Elevated blood pressure was defined as ≥130 mm Hg systolic blood pressure or ≥85 mm Hg diastolic blood pressure or on antihypertensive drug treatment in a patient with a history of hypertension; Elevated fasting glucose was defined as ≥100 mg/dl (5.55 mmol/l). Smokers were defined as individuals who smoked at least 5 cigarettes per day while past smokers had quit smoking for at least 30 days prior to examination.

2.4 Air pollution and weather data

Air pollution and weather data were downloaded online from the Israeli Ministry of Environmental Protection web page. Major air pollutants and the weather data are routinely measured every half hour by the same traffic-related air pollution monitoring stations, which are adjacent to specific heavy traffic sites. The Israeli Ministry of Environmental Protection has deployed seven of such stations thorough out Israel. These stations routinely measure several major pollutants including nitrogen oxides (NO, NO_2, NOx) and carbon monoxide (CO). Since only one traffic-related air monitoring station measured PM_{10} (particles less than 10 microns in aerodynamic diameter) and sulfur dioxide (SO_2) the number of individuals included in a 1 km radius was too small for statistical power. Thus we have only analyzed the effect of the former pollutants on the inflammatory variables. The analytical monitors in each station are fully automated and U.S. Environmental Protection Agency (EPA) approved. They also include a daily automated calibration system. Once a year, the stations conduct quality control and quality assurance tests. Nitrogen dioxide was measured by Chemiluminescence NO-NO_2-NO_x analyzer (*Thermo Environmental Instruments Inc. USA*, Model 42C) and Carbon monoxide by Gas Filter Correlation (GFC) CO Analyzer (*Thermo Environmental Instruments Inc. USA, Model 48C).*

2.5 Statistical analysis

All data was summarized and displayed as mean, standard deviation (SD), and quartiles for the continuous variables and as number of patients plus the percentage in each group for categorical variables. Since High Sensitivity C-Reactive Protein (hs-CRP), ESR and the triglyceride concentrations displayed irregular distributions, we used a logarithmic transformation which converted the distributions to normal ones for all statistical procedures. Therefore all results of hs-CRP, ESR or triglyceride concentrations are expressed as back transformed geometrical mean and standard deviation. The One-Way Kolmogorov-Smirnov test was used to assess the distributions.

In contrast to many other studies that evaluated air pollution, we did not divide the different air pollutants into tiles or commonly used cut-off points, rather we treated them as continuous variables. In order to quantify the contribution of each air pollutant to the variability of the different inflammation sensitive biomarkers we performed linear regression models using the forward stepwise method, where the inflammatory biomarkers were regarded as the dependent variable and many possible and known confounding parameters in addition to the air pollution as the independent variables. These confounders include parameters with known or suspected influences on inflammatory sensitive biomarkers and in addition to each air pollution, included gender, age, waist circumference, BMI, complete lipid profile including low-density lipoprotein (LDL), high-density lipoprotein (HDL), and triglycerides, diastolic and systolic blood pressure measurements, glucose concentration, alcohol consumption, sport intensity, medications including aspirin, beta blockers, calcium channel blockers, angiotensin converting enzyme inhibitors, angiotensin II receptor blockers, statins, fibrates and oral contraceptives or hormonal replacement therapy for women, cardiovascular risk factors including diabetes mellitus, current and past smoking status and family history of coronary heart disease or personal history of proven atherothrombotic event (myocardial infarction, cerebrovascular event or peripheral artery disease).

In addition, in order to control for seasonal variation and for the differences in climate between the years the models included the same day's climate parameters (temperature and relative humidity), the season and the year of measurement. Single pollutant linear regression models were fitted for the inflammatory variables and air pollution parameters with the appropriate meteorological parameters with various lag days ranging from the day of blood withdrawal to as much as three days lag. In all linear regression models we tested the distribution of the residuals for normality. The results of the linear regression models are presented as the mean change plus the 95% confidence interval for one standard deviation (SD) increase in the air pollutant. According to the logarithmic transformation of hs-CRP and ESR, the expected change in the linear model for hs-CRP and ESR reflects relative change and is presented as percent of change, rather than absolute change. All above analyses were considered significant at $p<0.05$ (two tailed). The SPSS statistical package was used to perform all statistical evaluation (SSPS Inc., Chicago, IL, USA).

3. Results

We have presently analyzed a total of 445 individuals (262 males and 183 females) at the respective mean (SD) age of 44 (13). The characteristic age, BMI, blood pressure, lipid profile as well as alcohol consumption and sport intensity are presented in Table 1, while the respective percentage of individuals with different cardiovascular risk factors and relevant medications in Table 2. Table 3 presents the distribution of the different air pollutants and weather parameters collected.

	Mean	S.D	25th percentile	Median	75th percentile
Age (years)	45	13	34	45	55
Waist (cm)	88	13	79	89	97
BMI (kg/m²)	26	4	23	25	28
Systolic BP (mmHg)	121	17	110	120	130
Diastolic BP (mmHg)	76	9	70	75	80
Glucose (mg/dL)	93	17	84	90	97
HDL Cholesterol (mg/dL)	58	17	46	55	68
LDL Cholesterol (mg/dL)	119	32	95	117	139
Triglycerides (mg/dL)	103	2	70	105	143
Alcohol consumption (glass/week)	1.4	2.9	0	0	2
Sport intensity (hours/week)	2.3	3.1	0	2	3.5
hsCRP (mg/L)	1.4	3.0	0.7	1.3	2.9
Fibrinogen (mg/dL)	292	59	246	289	330
ESR (mm/hr)	10	2	6	12	19

BMI – Body Mass Index; HDL – High Density Lipoprotein; LDL – Low Density Lipoprotein; hsCRP – High-Sensitivity C-Reactive Protein.

Table 1. Baseline topometric and laboratory data of the study population.

	N	%
Current smoker	98	22.0
Past Smoker	96	21.6
Diabetes Mellitus	21	4.7
Hypertension	97	21.8
Dyslipidemia	124	27.9
Family History of CHD	68	15.3
Aspirin	35	7.9
Beta blockers	29	6.5
Calcium channel blockers	12	2.7
ACE Inhibitors / ARB's	17	3.8
Statins	48	10.8
Fibrates	5	1.1
Oral hypoglycemics	11	2.5
Insulin	2	0.4

ACE – Angiotensin Converting Enzyme; ARB – Angiotensin II Receptor Blocker; CHD – Coronary Heart Disease.

Table 2. Baseline characteristics and medications use of the study population.

	Mean	S.D.	25th percentile	Median	75th percentile
Temperature (°C)	21.1	5.3	16.6	20.9	26.6
Relative Humidity (%)	65.4	10.0	59.9	67.1	72.5
NO_2 (PPB)	29.9	9.3	23.0	27.7	35.4
NO (PPB)	50.6	41.6	21.3	38.6	64.8
NO_X (PPB)	63.2	47.4	32.2	46.8	81.9
CO (PPM)	0.8	0.4	0.6	0.8	1.0

PPB - Parts Per Billion; PPM - Parts Per Million.

Table 3. Air pollution and meteorology parameters

We systematically evaluated the contribution of each air pollution parameter to the variability of the inflammatory biomarker following adjustment for weather conditions at the same day, seasonal influence and many known and possible contributors. The results are displayed in Table 4 through 6 for hs-CRP, fibrinogen and ESR. It is evident that, in our study group, a statistically significant increase was noted in hs-CRP following exposure to NO_2 and NO at the day of measurement alone. This affect was only marginally significant with regard to CO and NOx. Fibrinogen however, showed a statistically significant decrease following same day exposure to NO and CO as well as following exposure of a 3 day lag. The ESR however, was not significantly affected by any air pollutant in our study.

		Partial correlation	Relative (95% CI) change (%) for 1 SD increase	P Value
NO_2	*Same day*	*0.280*	*38% (19% – 59%) §*	*<0.001*
	Previous day	0.119	13% (-1% - 30%)	0.080
	2 days ago	0.073	8% (-6% - 23%)	0.283
	3 days ago	0.052	5% (-7% - 18%)	0.441
NO	*Same day*	*0.193*	*22% (7% – 39%) §*	*0.004*
	Previous day	0.077	9% (-6% - 26%)	0.261
	2 days ago	0.086	8% (-4% - 23%)	0.205
	3 days ago	0.080	7% (-4% - 18%)	0.232
NO_X	Same day	0.113	13% (-2% - 31%)	0.097
	Previous day	-0.022	-3% (-18% - 15%)	0.743
	2 days ago	-0.016	-2% (-14% - 13%)	0.814
	3 days ago	0.030	3% (-9% - 16%)	0.655
CO	Same day	0.120	12% (-1% - 28%)	0.077
	Previous day	0.114	12% (-2% - 29%)	0.095
	2 days ago	0.051	4% (-7% - 17%)	0.449
	3 days ago	0.074	6% (-5% - 18%)	0.269

Table 4. Partial correlation and mean (95% CI) change in hs-CRP for one SD increase in each air pollutant

		Partial correlation	Mean (95% CI) change (%) for 1 SD increase	P Value
NO_2	Same day	0.047	3.1 (-5.8 – 12.0)	0.494
	Previous day	0.092	5.6 (-2.6 – 13.9)	0.182
	2 days ago	0.054	3.2 (-4.7 – 11.1)	0.054
	3 days ago	-0.087	-4.8 (-12.1 – 2.5)	0.197
NO	Same day	-0.141	-8.3 (-16.1 – -0.4)	0.040
	Previous day	-0.105	-6.6 (-15.1 – 1.8)	0.127
	2 days ago	-0.074	-4.1 (-11.4 – 3.3)	0.279
	3 days ago	-0.160	-7.6 (-13.8 – -1.4)	0.018
NO_X	Same day	-0.006	-0.4 (-8.9 – 8.1)	0.925
	Previous day	0.020	1.5 (-8.6 – 11.6)	0.768
	2 days ago	0.010	0.6 (-7.4 – 8.7)	0.882
	3 days ago	-0.038	-2.1 (-9.4 – 5.3)	0.577
CO	Same day	-0.151	-8.4 (-15.8 – -0.9)	0.028
	Previous day	-0.123	-7.4 (-15.4 – 0.7)	0.075
	2 days ago	-0.116	-5.8 (-12.5 – 0.9)	0.090
	3 days ago	-0.166	-8.0 (-14.4 – -1.7)	0.014

Table 5. Partial correlation and mean (95% CI) change in fibrinogen for one SD increase in each air pollutant

		Partial correlation	Relative (95% CI) change (%) for 1 SD increase	P Value
NO_2	Same day	0.085	7% (-4% - 20%)	0.231
	Previous day	0.015	1% (-9% - 12%)	0.838
	2 days ago	-0.088	-6% (-15% - 4%)	0.215
	3 days ago	-0.032	-2% (-11% - 7%)	0.641
NO	Same day	-0.049	-4% (-13% - 7%)	0.484
	Previous day	-0.091	-7% (-17% - 4%)	0.200
	2 days ago	-0.085	-6% (-14% - 4%)	0.228
	3 days ago	-0.039	-2% (-10% - 6%)	0.572
NO_X	Same day	0.016	1% (-9% - 13%)	0.820
	Previous day	-0.011	-1% (-13% - 13%)	0.873
	2 days ago	-0.001	0% (-10% - 11%)	0.993
	3 days ago	0.049	3% (-6% - 14%)	0.480
CO	Same day	-0.084	-6% (-14% - 4%)	0.236
	Previous day	-0.035	-3% (-12% - 8%)	0.624
	2 days ago	-0.085	-5% (-13% - 3%)	0.230
	3 days ago	0.008	0% (-7% - 9%)	0.911

Table 6. Partial correlation and mean (95% CI) change in ESR for one SD increase in each air pollutant

4. Discussion

In the present analysis we present statistically significant associations between the short term exposure to traffic-related air pollutants and several inflammatory biomarkers including hs-CRP, and quantitative fibrinogen. The effect was documented in individuals residing within a 1000 meter radius of a traffic-related air pollution monitoring station, intentionally positioned in proximity to specific heavy traffic sites. We believe our results support the hypothesis of a direct influence of this short term exposure to traffic-related air pollutants and an eventual heightened inflammatory response that might trigger clinical events (Brook et al., 2010).

Notably, we found CRP to be increased by ~40% following a one SD increase in NO_2, and by ~20% following a one SD increase in NO. Similar, albeit smaller and marginally significant increments, were noted for both NO_x and CO, implying that an analysis in a larger sample size might have shown more consistent results. This rise in CRP was noted for the same day exposure alone, supporting the notion of its role as an acute phase reactant (Steel & Whitehead, 1994). In their toxicological studies in men with and without prior myocardial infarction, who were exposed to dilute diesel exhaust (300 µg per cubic meter) or filtered air for 1 hour during periods of rest and moderate exercise in a controlled-exposure facility, both Mills and Tornqvist did not show increments in serum C-reactive protein concentrations 6 or 24 hours by exposure to diesel exhaust or filtered air (Mills et al., 2007; Tornqvist et al., 2007). Lucking et al (Lucking et al., 2008) has shown similar results when reporting his toxicological study in which no changes in plasma TNF-a, IL-6, C-reactive protein, and soluble ICAM-1 concentrations were observed. These measurements were obtained however, only 6 hours following both diesel exhaust and filtered air exposures. Tornqvist et al, did in fact show a 24 hour significant rise in IL-6 following diesel exhaust exposure (Tornqvist et al., 2007). IL-6 is widely known as a direct inducer of CRP production in the liver hepatocytes (Steel & Whitehead 1994). Thus, our environmental real-life 1000 meter radius traffic-related exposure findings can be supported by his toxicological findings. Interestingly, following exposure to CO and NO, fibrinogen concentrations decreased both in same day as well in 3 days following exposure. Previous environmental air pollution epidemiological studies have shown conflicting trends. Although some have demonstrated increased levels of fibrinogen, other studies measuring the same factors have failed to show any association with particulate exposure. Schwartz et al (Schwartz, 2001) found a significant negative association between the previous day fibrinogen concentration and NO_2, as did Seaton et al (Seaton et al., 1999) for the previous three days average of PM_{10}. In contrast, Pekkanen et al. (Pekkanen et al., 2000) reported a positive significant correlation between fibrinogen concentration and NO_2 or CO in London, with three days lag. In a large epidemiological study we have previously reported that mainly NO_2, SO_2 and CO affected fibrinogen in several lag days, with maximal effect for a lag of four days (Steinvil et al., 2008). Finally, Baccarelli et al (Baccarelli et al., 2007) reported no consistent relations between air pollution and fibrinogen in 1218 normal subjects from the Lombardia Region, Italy. Thus, Even though both fibrinogen (Danesh et al., 2005) and air pollution (Maitre et al., 2006) have been independently shown to be positively correlated with cardiovascular morbidity and mortality, most epidemiological studies report mainly negative correlations between the air pollutants measured and fibrinogen concentrations. Unfortunately enough, the direct affect of diesel exhaust exposure on fibrinogen concentration was not reported in most of the recent human toxicological studies (Carlsten et al., 2007; Mills et al., 2007;

Tornqvist et al., 2007; Lucking et al., 2008). As far as we know the only toxicological report was by Bloomberg et al (Blomberg et al., 2005) were no effect was found on fibrinogen concentrations. Due to the scarcity of data fibrinogen role as an acute phase reactant following diesel exhaust exposure cannot be evaluated. Fibrinogen however, can be viewed both as an inflammatory acute phase reactant, as well as a marker for thrombus formation. Its consumption, and therefore decrease in concentration following thrombus formation has been proposed to increase the diagnostic accuracy of venous thromboembolism (Kucher et al., 2003). Lucking et al (Lucking et al., 2008) has established that diesel exhaust inhalation increased thrombus formation under low and high shear conditions. The concept of fibrinogen consumption due to increased thrombus formation, subsequently leading to a decrease in its concentration following exposure to air pollutants, is therefore a subject for future toxicological studies.

Among the possible reasons for the previous conflicting results, in similar studies are: the lack of consistent air pollution measurement methodology, the lack of systematic examination of the time relationship between air pollution variables and markers of inflammation, and the fact that not all studies were controlled for multiple possible confounders. These confounders include parameters with known influences on the inflammatory response such as age (Larbi et al., 2004), gender (Zeltser et al., 2004), body mass index (BMI) and waist circumference (Santos et al., 2005), exercise (Petersen & Pedersen, 2005), the presence of hyperlipidemia (Pirro et al., 2004), hypertension (Tsioufis et al., 2006), alcohol consumption (Imhof et al., 2001), smoking habits (Yasue et al., 2006), glucose concentrations (Kerner et al., 2005), as well as the intake of medications with a potential pro- and anti-inflammatory effect (Kushner et al., 2006). In addition there are many possible confounders regarding air pollution, mainly meteorological parameters (temperature, humidity and precipitants) which may also be related to cardiovascular events (Danet et al., 1999) as well as wind speed (Brugge et al., 2007). Finally there are seasonal confounders that are closely associated with both cardiovascular morbidity and mortality, and air pollution (Nawrot et al., 2006). In order to attain more accurate results we accordingly controlled for all these possible confounders. Other than the effect possible confounders could have, there were some reports about enhanced sensitivity to the effect of air pollution in specific subgroups including asthmatic (Barck et al., 2002), elderly persons (Le Tertre et al., 2002), individuals with history of heart failure or arrhythmia (Mann et al., 2002), females (Chen et al., 2005), naturally higher fibrinogen concentrations (Prescott et al., 2000), history of cardiorespiratory hospitalization (Zanobetti & Schwartz, 2005) or myocardial infarction (von Klot et al., 2005). This enhanced sensitivity was also suggested in diabetic, obese and hypertensive individuals who display an association to systemic inflammation as evident by CRP, IL-6 and WBC levels (Dubowsky et al., 2006).

We acknowledge several limitations of the present study. First, we did not account for the effect indoor pollutants could have on our study population and their possible influence on the results. Second, we did not account for time spent outdoors, which depends on the work status and occupation type of each individual in the study. Third, as gender has been known to have a significant role in inflammation (Zeltser et al., 2004) and air pollution research (Chen et al., 2005) this might have stumped our results. Finally, we note that most previous studies have shown a significant decrease in combustion derived air pollutants in distances of above 400 meters (Brugge et al., 2007). Thus, and in spite of our multiple adjustments, the possibility exist the associations we present are of chance. We therefore encourage repeating this analysis in future studies.

5. Conclusion

We have found significant associations between inflammation sensitive biomarkers and between combustion derived air pollutants, in individuals residing in a 1000 meter radius from a traffic-related air pollution monitoring station, positioned in proximity to heavy traffic sites. While our significant results suggest a positive correlation with CRP and a negative correlation with fibrinogen and several air pollutants, our results showed be cautiously interpreted due to the study limitations.

6. References

Alberti, KG., Eckel, RH., Grundy, SM., Zimmet, PZ., Cleeman, JI., Donato, KA., Fruchart, JC., James, WP., Loria, CM., & Smith, SC. Jr. (2009). "Harmonizing the metabolic syndrome: a joint interim statement of the International Diabetes Federation Task Force on Epidemiology and Prevention; National Heart, Lung, and Blood Institute; American Heart Association; World Heart Federation; International Atherosclerosis Society; and International Association for the Study of Obesity." Circulation 120(16): 1640-5.

Baccarelli, A., Zanobetti, A., Martinelli, I., Grillo, P., Hou, L., Giacomini, S., Bonzini, M., Lanzani, G., Mannucci, PM., & Bertazzi, PA. et al. (2007). "Effects of exposure to air pollution on blood coagulation." J Thromb Haemost 5(2): 252-60.

Barck, C., Sandstrom, T., Lundahl, J., Hallden, G., Svartengren, M., Strand, V., Rak, S., & Bylin, G. (2002). "Ambient level of NO2 augments the inflammatory response to inhaled allergen in asthmatics." Respir Med 96(11): 907-17.

Blomberg, A., Tornqvist, H., Desmyter, L., Deneys, V., & Hermans, C. (2005). "Exposure to diesel exhaust nanoparticles does not induce blood hypercoagulability in an at-risk population." J Thromb Haemost 3(9): 2103-5.

Brook, RD., Rajagopalan, S., Pope, CA. 3rd, Brook, JR., Bhatnagar, A., Diez-Roux, AV., Holguin, F., Hong, Y., Luepker, RV., & Mittleman, MA. et al. (2010). "Particulate matter air pollution and cardiovascular disease: An update to the scientific statement from the American Heart Association." Circulation 121(21): 2331-78.

Brugge, D., Durant, JL., & Rioux, C. (2007). "Near-highway pollutants in motor vehicle exhaust: a review of epidemiologic evidence of cardiac and pulmonary health risks." Environ Health 6: 23.

Brunekreef, B., & Holgate, ST. (2002). "Air pollution and health." Lancet 360(9341): 1233-42.

Carlsten, C., Kaufman, JD., Peretz, A., Trenga, CA., Sheppard, L., & Sullivan, JH. (2007). "Coagulation markers in healthy human subjects exposed to diesel exhaust." Thromb Res 120(6): 849-55.

Chen, LH., Knutsen, SF., Shavlik, D., Beeson, WL., Petersen, F., Ghamsary, M., & Abbey, D. (2005). "The association between fatal coronary heart disease and ambient particulate air pollution: Are females at greater risk?" Environ Health Perspect 113(12): 1723-9.

Cherng, TW., Campen, MJ., Knuckles, TL., Gonzalez Bosc, L., & Kanagy, NL. (2009). "Impairment of coronary endothelial cell ET(B) receptor function after short-term inhalation exposure to whole diesel emissions." Am J Physiol Regul Integr Comp Physiol 297(3): R640-7.

Clauss, A. (1957). "Gerinnungsphysiologische Schnellmethode zur Bestimmung des Fibrinogens." Acta Haematol Basel 17: 237-246.

Danesh, J., Lewington, S., Thompson, SG., Lowe, GD., Collins, R., Kostis, JB., Wilson, AC., Folsom, AR., Wu, K., & Benderly, M. et al. (2005). "Plasma fibrinogen level and the risk of major cardiovascular diseases and nonvascular mortality: an individual participant meta-analysis." Jama 294(14): 1799-809.

Danet, S., Richard, F., Montaye, M., Beauchant, S., Lemaire, B., Graux, C., Cottel, D., Marecaux, N., & Amouyel, P. (1999). "Unhealthy effects of atmospheric temperature and pressure on the occurrence of myocardial infarction and coronary deaths. A 10-year survey: the Lille-World Health Organization MONICA project (Monitoring trends and determinants in cardiovascular disease)." Circulation 100(1): E1-7.

Diez Roux, AV., Auchincloss, AH., Astor, B., Barr, RG., Cushman, M., Dvonch, T., Jacobs, DR. Jr., Kaufman, J., Lin, X., & Samson, P. (2006). "Recent exposure to particulate matter and C-reactive protein concentration in the multi-ethnic study of atherosclerosis." Am J Epidemiol 164(5): 437-48.

Dubowsky, SD., Suh, H., Schwartz, J., Coull, BA., & Gold, DR. (2006). "Diabetes, obesity, and hypertension may enhance associations between air pollution and markers of systemic inflammation." Environ Health Perspect 114(7): 992-8.

Ghio, AJ., Kim, C., & Devlin, RB. (2000). "Concentrated ambient air particles induce mild pulmonary inflammation in healthy human volunteers." Am J Respir Crit Care Med 162(3 Pt 1): 981-8.

Ghio, AJ., Hall, A., Bassett, MA., Cascio, WE., & Devlin, RB. (2003). "Exposure to concentrated ambient air particles alters hematologic indices in humans." Inhal Toxicol 15(14): 1465-78.

ICSH (1993). "ICSH recommendations for measurement of erythrocyte sedimentation rate. International Council for Standardization in Haematology (Expert Panel on Blood Rheology)." J Clin Pathol 46(3): 198-203.

Imhof, A., Froehlich, M., Brenner, H., Boeing, H., Pepys, MB., & Koenig, W. (2001). "Effect of alcohol consumption on systemic markers of inflammation." Lancet 357(9258): 763-7.

Kaufman, JD. (2010). "Does Air Pollution Accelerate Progression of Atherosclerosis?" J Am Coll Cardiol 56(22): 1809-1811.

Kerner, A., Avizohar, O., Sella, R., Bartha, P., Zinder, O., Markiewicz, W., Levy, Y., Brook, GJ., & Aronson, D. (2005). "Association between elevated liver enzymes and C-reactive protein: possible hepatic contribution to systemic inflammation in the metabolic syndrome." Arterioscler Thromb Vasc Biol 25(1): 193-7.

Kido, T., Tamagawa, E., Bai, N., Suda, K., Yang, HH., Li, Y., Chiang, G., Yatera, K., Mukae, H., & Sin, DD. et al. (2011). "Particulate matter induces translocation of IL-6 from the lung to the systemic circulation." Am J Respir Cell Mol Biol 44(2): 197-204.

Kucher, N., Kohler, HP., Dornhofer, T., Wallmann, D., & Lammle, B. (2003). "Accuracy of D-dimer/fibrinogen ratio to predict pulmonary embolism: a prospective diagnostic study." J Thromb Haemost 1(4): 708-13.

Kushner, I., Rzewnicki, D., & Samols, D. (2006). "What does minor elevation of C-reactive protein signify?" Am J Med 119(2): 166 e17-28.

Larbi, A., Dupuis, G., Douziech, N., Khalil, A., & Fulop, T. Jr. (2004). "Low-grade inflammation with aging has consequences for T-lymphocyte signaling." Ann N Y Acad Sci 1030: 125-33.

Le Tertre, A., Medina, S., Samoli, E., Forsberg, B., Michelozzi, P., Boumghar, A., Vonk, JM., Bellini, A., Atkinson, R., & Ayres, JG. et al. (2002). "Short-term effects of particulate air pollution on cardiovascular diseases in eight European cities." J Epidemiol Community Health 56(10): 773-9.

Liao, D., Heiss, G., Chinchilli, VM., Duan, Y., Folsom, AR., Lin, HM., & Salomaa, V. (2005). "Association of criteria pollutants with plasma hemostatic/inflammatory markers: a population-based study." J Expo Anal Environ Epidemiol 15(4): 319-28.

Libby, P. (2002). "Inflammation in atherosclerosis." Nature 420(6917): 868-74.

Libby, P. (2006). "Inflammation and cardiovascular disease mechanisms." Am J Clin Nutr 83(2): 456S-460S.

Lucking, AJ., Lundback, M., Mills, NL., Faratian, D., Barath, SL., Pourazar, J., Cassee, FR., Donaldson, K., Boon, NA., & Badimon, JJ. et al. (2008). "Diesel exhaust inhalation increases thrombus formation in man." Eur Heart J 29(24): 3043-51.

Maitre, A., Bonneterre, V., Huillard, L., Sabatier, P., & de Gaudemaris, R. (2006). "Impact of urban atmospheric pollution on coronary disease." Eur Heart J 27(19): 2275-84.

Mann, JK., Tager, IB., Lurmann, F., Segal, M., Quesenberry, CP. Jr., Lugg, MM., Shan, J., & Van Den Eeden, SK. (2002). "Air pollution and hospital admissions for ischemic heart disease in persons with congestive heart failure or arrhythmia." Environ Health Perspect 110(12): 1247-52.

Mills, NL., Tornqvist, H., Gonzalez, MC., Vink, E., Robinson, SD., Soderberg, S., Boon, NA., Donaldson, K., Sandstrom, T., & Blomberg, A. et al. (2007). "Ischemic and thrombotic effects of dilute diesel-exhaust inhalation in men with coronary heart disease." N Engl J Med 357(11): 1075-82.

Nawrot, TS., Nemmar, A., & Nemery, B. (2006). "Air pollution: To the heart of the matter." Eur Heart J 27(19): 2269-71.

NCEP/ATPIII (2001). "Executive Summary of The Third Report of The National Cholesterol Education Program (NCEP) Expert Panel on Detection, Evaluation, And Treatment of High Blood Cholesterol In Adults (Adult Treatment Panel III)." Jama 285(19): 2486-97.

Niwa, Y., Hiura, Y., Sawamura, H., & Iwai, N. (2008). "Inhalation exposure to carbon black induces inflammatory response in rats." Circ J 72(1): 144-9.

Nurkiewicz, TR., Porter, DW., Hubbs, AF., Cumpston, JL., Chen, BT., Frazer, DG., & Castranova, V. (2008). "Nanoparticle inhalation augments particle-dependent systemic microvascular dysfunction." Part Fibre Toxicol 5: 1.

Nurkiewicz, TR., Porter, DW., Hubbs, AF., Stone, S., Chen, BT., Frazer, DG., Boegehold, MA., & Castranova, V. (2009). "Pulmonary nanoparticle exposure disrupts systemic microvascular nitric oxide signaling." Toxicol Sci 110(1): 191-203.

Pekkanen, J., Brunner, EJ., Anderson, HR., Tiittanen, P., & Atkinson, RW. (2000). "Daily concentrations of air pollution and plasma fibrinogen in London." Occup Environ Med 57(12): 818-22.

Peters, A., Dockery, DW., Muller, JE., & Mittleman, MA. (2001a). "Increased particulate air pollution and the triggering of myocardial infarction." Circulation 103(23): 2810-5.

Peters, A., Frohlich, M., Doring, A., Immervoll, T., Wichmann, HE., Hutchinson, WL., Pepys, MB., & Koenig, W. (2001b). "Particulate air pollution is associated with an acute phase response in men; results from the MONICA-Augsburg Study." Eur Heart J 22(14): 1198-204.

Peters, A., von Klot, S., Heier, M., Trentinaglia, I., Hormann, A., Wichmann, HE., & Lowel, H. (2004). "Exposure to traffic and the onset of myocardial infarction." N Engl J Med 351(17): 1721-30.

Petersen, AM., & Pedersen, BK. (2005). "The anti-inflammatory effect of exercise." J Appl Physiol 98(4): 1154-62.

Pirro, M., Schillaci, G., Savarese, G., Gemelli, F., Vaudo, G., Siepi, D., Bagaglia, F., & Mannarino, E. (2004). "Low-grade systemic inflammation impairs arterial stiffness in newly diagnosed hypercholesterolaemia." Eur J Clin Invest 34(5): 335-41.

Pope, CA. 3rd, Hansen, ML., Long, RW., Nielsen, KR., Eatough, NL., Wilson, WE., & Eatough, DJ. (2004). "Ambient particulate air pollution, heart rate variability, and blood markers of inflammation in a panel of elderly subjects." Environ Health Perspect 112(3): 339-45.

Prescott, GJ., Lee, RJ., Cohen, GR., Elton, RA., Lee, AJ., Fowkes, FG., & Agius, RM. (2000). "Investigation of factors which might indicate susceptibility to particulate air pollution." Occup Environ Med 57(1): 53-7.

Rifai, N., Tracy, RP., & Ridker, PM. (1999). "Clinical efficacy of an automated high-sensitivity C-reactive protein assay." Clin Chem 45(12): 2136-41.

Rogowski, O., Shapira, I., Ben Assayag, E., Bornstein, NM., Toker, S., Melamed, S., Shirom, A., & Berliner, S. (2006). "Lack of significant effect of low doses of aspirin on the concentrations of C-reactive protein in a group of individuals with atherothrombotic risk factors and vascular events." Blood Coagul Fibrinolysis 17(1): 19-22.

Santos, AC., Lopes, C., Guimaraes, JT., & Barros, H. (2005). "Central obesity as a major determinant of increased high-sensitivity C-reactive protein in metabolic syndrome." Int J Obes (Lond) 29(12): 1452-6.

Schwartz, J. (2001). "Air pollution and blood markers of cardiovascular risk." Environ Health Perspect 109 Suppl 3: 405-9.

Seaton, A., Soutar, A., Crawford, V., Elton, R., McNerlan, S., Cherrie, J., Watt, M., Agius, R., & Stout, R. (1999). "Particulate air pollution and the blood." Thorax 54(11): 1027-32.

Steel, DM., & Whitehead, AS. (1994). "The major acute phase reactants: C-reactive protein, serum amyloid P component and serum amyloid A protein." Immunol Today 15(2): 81-8.

Steinvil, A., Kordova-Biezuner, L., Shapira, I., Berliner, S., & Rogowski, O. (2008). "Short-term exposure to air pollution and inflammation-sensitive biomarkers." Environ Res 106(1): 51-61.

Sun, Q., Wang, A., Jin, X., Natanzon, A., Duquaine, D., Brook, RD., Aguinaldo, JG., Fayad, ZA., Fuster, V., & Lippmann, M. et al. (2005). "Long-term air pollution exposure and acceleration of atherosclerosis and vascular inflammation in an animal model." Jama 294(23): 3003-10.

Tornqvist, H., Mills, NL., Gonzalez, M., Miller, MR., Robinson, SD., Megson, IL., Macnee, W., Donaldson, K., Soderberg, S., & Newby, DE. et al. (2007). "Persistent endothelial dysfunction in humans after diesel exhaust inhalation." Am J Respir Crit Care Med 176(4): 395-400.

Tsioufis, C., Dimitriadis, K., Taxiarchou, E., Vasiliadou, C., Chartzoulakis, G., Tousoulis, D., Manolis, A., Stefanadis, C., & Kallikazaros, I. (2006). "Diverse associations of microalbuminuria with C-reactive protein, interleukin-18 and soluble CD 40 ligand in male essential hypertensive subjects." Am J Hypertens 19(5): 462-6.

van Eeden, SF., & Hogg, JC. (2002). "Systemic inflammatory response induced by particulate matter air pollution: the importance of bone-marrow stimulation." J Toxicol Environ Health A 65(20): 1597-613.

von Klot, S., Peters, A., Aalto, P., Bellander, T., Berglind, N., D'Ippoliti, D., Elosua, R., Hormann, A., Kulmala, M., & Lanki, T. et al. (2005). "Ambient air pollution is associated with increased risk of hospital cardiac readmissions of myocardial infarction survivors in five European cities." Circulation 112(20): 3073-9.

WHO (2003). Working Group of Health Aspects of Air Pollution with Particulate Matter, Ozone and Nitrogen Dioxide. Bonn, Germany.

Yasue, H., Hirai, N., Mizuno, Y., Harada, E., Itoh, T., Yoshimura, M., Kugiyama, K., & Ogawa, H. (2006). "Low-grade inflammation, thrombogenicity, and atherogenic lipid profile in cigarette smokers." Circ J 70(1): 8-13.

Zanobetti, A., & Schwartz, J. (2005). "The effect of particulate air pollution on emergency admissions for myocardial infarction: a multicity case-crossover analysis." Environ Health Perspect 113(8): 978-82.

Zeltser, D., Rogowski, O., Berliner, S., Mardi, T., Justo, D., Serov, J., Rozenblat, M., Avitzour, D., & Shapira, I. (2004). "Sex differences in the expression of haemorheological determinants in individuals with atherothrombotic risk factors and in apparently healthy people." Heart 90(3): 277-81.

3

Application of Neural Net Model to Estimate the Cardiovascular and Respiratory Diseases by Air Pollution Data in Urban Area

A. Pelliccioni and R. Cotroneo
Inail-Dipia,
Monteporzio Catone,
Italy

1. Introduction

One of the major environmental problems is air pollution that has important effects on human health. According to the World Health Organization (WHO), air pollution is the eighth cause of death and is the main environmental risk factor in Europe.
Air pollution depends by number and diversity of emission sources and concomitant risk factors that took into account meteorology that plays an inferential action on adverse effects of pollution in term of space-time.
Such situations are very important especially for the Mediterranean coastal countries (like Italy) and for urban sites that are affected by the microclimatic conditions that could lead to atmospheric stagnation events.
In recent years, a broad number of scientific studies have shown that the linkage between urban settlements with high population density and large industrial centers resulted worsening of air pollution due to the impact resulting from intensive traffic, from domestic heating and from industrial and energy plants. Severe cases of pollution, which have had important impacts on the population, have occurred in urban or industrial areas and this in conjunction with unfavorable atmospheric dispersion and dilution of air pollutants. Air pollution is a set of pollutants, many of which are correlated to each other. In this work, we will focus only on the particulate matter (PM10) and ground-level ozone (O3) [Gariazzo et al., 2007],that in general have been identified as two of the most important air pollutants for Europe [Jol and Kielland, 1997]; [Brunekreef and Holgate, 2002].
Particulate Matters (PM) are tiny particles of solid or liquid suspended. They range in size from 0.1 nanometers to 100 micrometers in diameter. PM10 can be either primary or secondary, in nature. In general, primary particles are emitted directly into the atmosphere by natural and anthropogenic sources, whereas secondary particles are formed in the atmosphere from chemical and physical reactions of SO2, NOx, NH3 and VOC. The PM10 composition depends on the source of emission. The PM10, being rich in biologically active substances, contains inside carcinogens substances (polycyclic aromatic hydrocarbons, volatile organic compounds), elemental carbon, heavy metals, mineral dust, fragments of soil, sulfates and nitrates that can have an irritating action, ammonium. In the atmosphere, particulate concentrations depend on both natural sources (soil erosion, marine aerosol,

production of biogenic aerosols plant fragments, pollen, spores , volcanic emissions -fire- and long distance transport sand) and anthropogenic sources (motors, heating, industry, power plants, etc.).In urban areas, the most important anthropogenic factors, leading to increase in PM10, are linked to road traffic and heating, as well as those related to possible industrial plants (refineries, cement plants, power plants, incinerators, etc...).
The territorial distribution of the emission sources of PM10 is an important aspect in order to have a complete analysis of the PM pollutant. They are analyzed through the inventory of emissions at local scale (province).The Table 1 shows in the short period the disaggregation of emissions as regards sectors of Transport, Industry and Domestic. In particular, the table shows the percentage of each sector of the total actual emissions. These percentages represent quantitatively the potential for absorption of the respective sectors.

	Tons	**%**
Transport	3263.20	48%
Industry	887.73	13%
Domestic sectors and Commercial	14151.91	17%
Agriculture and forests	16.07	0,23%
Energy	1004.10	15%
Other	541.94	8%
Total	**6864.95**	**100%**

Table 1. Emission sources of PM10 (tons) in Rome (2000) - (Source: www.**sinanet.apat**.it)

In Rome the traffic's contribution is around 48%. The portion of the PM10 produced by civil heating represents a share ranging from 20% to 30% of the total. The item "Other" were collected PM10 emissions are not considered in the inventory. These emissions, produced by raw materials handling, construction activities, smoke and fireworks, together represent approximately 10% of total emissions of PM10.
Ozone is a well known secondary air pollutant, results from complex chemical reactions such as nitrogen oxides (NOx) and volatile organic compounds (VOCs) and is a very reactive gas and presents concentration levels which are strongly dependent both from the micro-meteorological conditions and the seasonal effects.
Its presence as a layer in stratosphere serves as a screen (called ozone shield) to block harmful ultraviolet radiation from reaching the earth's surface. At ground level it is formed by the combination of hydrocarbons and nitrogen oxides (NOx) at the presence of sunlight and is the main ingredient of smog.
In the air, the persistence time of ozone is a few hours in the presence of other pollutants, whereas clean air could remain to several months.This means that the highest concentrations levels of ozone are often in rural areas near cities or industrial areas.
In addition, the Ozone:

- is absent in the cold months and short (no sunshine duration)
- smell is noticeable at a concentration 0.008 and 0.02 parts per million (ppm)
- is an irritant at a concentration of 0.10 to 0.15 ppm
- is harmful mainly for people with respiratory and cardiac diseases.

The relationship between the various factors and daily occurrence of pathologies related to cardio-respiratory apparatus is a task not easy and immediate to solve. In recent years, a great number of environmental and epidemiological publications [World Health Organisation, 2006, 2003, 2001] have confirmed that the linkage between urban sites with high population density and great industrial centers resulted in the deterioration of air pollution due to the impact resulting by auto-vehicular traffic, the domestic heating and by the industrial and energy plants. High levels of air pollution concentrations have had major impacts on the population. They have occurred in urban or industrial areas and this in conjunction with not favorable situations of atmospheric dispersion and of dilution of pollutants. It is to underline that the impact of the fine and total particulate matter on health are related to the air quality by means of pollutants across during the time of work. In particular, PM10 and O3 have been associated with pulmonary function decrements in exposed populations. Inhalation of fine, airborne particulate matter has serious chronic human health effects and is a major cause of premature death, whereas high levels of ozone concern their effects on human health related with respiratory problems, above all for children during the peak episodes [World Health Organisation, 2003]. These symptoms can last for a few hours after exposure to ozone and may even become painful. Furthermore, these effects could cease once the person is no longer exposed to elevated levels of pollutant. This paper is a contribution in the field of air pollution due to particulate matter and ozone concentrations. In particular, the objective of this pilot study was to determine a way of assessing exposure to outdoor pollution. In the short term (the data used covered a period of two years: 2005 and 2006) their impact assessment on population (especially on children, the patients, pregnant women and elderly and on people who suffer from chronic cardio-respiratory diseases) in terms of morbidity and mortality by cardio-pulmonary diseases [Murray & Mittleman, 2007] in the urban area of Rome.

Our aim is to analyze the annual trend of morbidity and mortality in hospital for cardio-respiratory diseases due to PM10 and ozone by using neural net (NN) techniques [Bishop, 1995], which are important tools to forecast because it can work as universal approximators of non-linear functions. The NN capacity to learn non-linear functions is an important issue in our problem. Moreover, neural network does not require assumptions about the input variable distribution or absence of correlations between such variables. Consequently, NN can be used in evaluating cardio-respiratory diseases due to environmental systems [Rojas, 1996] and can capture without many of the usual limiting assumptions of other traditional advanced statistical methods, which make not particularly appropriate.

Thus it will be possible to increase the knowledge of levels of concentration of pollution in urban areas and inform the public about environmental risks on human health.

By applying NN to the field of environmental epidemiology [World Health Organisation, 2004] we want to:

- examine the most injurious pollutants to human health and their mechanisms of dispersion
- identify the factors and mechanisms of epidemic diffusion
- model the cardiovascular and respiratory diseases by means the use of air pollution data coming from urban monitoring station
- formulate a methodological suggestion to apply to Neural Net to predict the human health impact due to the different pollutants

2. Material and methods

2.1 Data collection

In short-term, data of the hospital discharge records Hospital Discharge Records (HDR) were analyzed for the calendar years 2005 and 2006 in Rome, to measure the effects on population health due to exposure to physical, chemical and biological agents outside the human body. In public health, the HDRs are the tool of information gathering for every patient discharged from public and private hospitals throughout the territory. They provide relevant information about the diagnosis. This information is collected in a special database (EPICS) by Agency of Public Health (ASP) of Lazio, that contain list the variables to be reported, their descriptions and reporting format, and other information associated with data submission.

The minimum data set for each reported discharge include the following data elements:

- Patient's Address: City, State and Zip Code
- Patient's age (0-14; 15-64, over 65; the class's distribution allows you to observe with greater precision the effects of pollution on cardio-respiratory)
- Patient's Sex
- Admission and dismissal date: admissions were examined from 01 January 2005 to17 December 31, 2005
- Type of care: acute hospital admissions in ordinary regime (until 60 days), i.e. taking 19 into account the rules for implementing the treatment
- Admission type: at home, death, dismissal protection, voluntary dismissal, transfer to another inpatient, transfer
- Days in hospital
- Source of admission
- Patient's Status
- Principal Diagnosis Codes (ICD9CM -390-459: Circulatory system diseases ;460-519: Respiratory Diseases) Local Health Units of Residence: were analyzed only hospitalized residents in Rome
- Mode of arrival at hospital: general practitioners, first aid physicians, specialist doctor, transferred from another hospital, transferred from the first aid of the same hospital (including voluntary presentation of the patient), transferred from another regime of inpatient of the same hospital, transferred from first aid of another hospital. The mode of arrival at hospital determines which part of the cardio-pulmonary disease is attributable to the characteristics of patients - and which part is attributable to the quality of care.

Instead, the data used on primary pollutants and meteorological variables cover the 2005 and 2006 period and coming from monitoring stations of the ARPAL (Environmental Protection Agency of Lazio Region) positioned in Rome, which have had for each year at least 50% valid data (taking count of EoI - Exchange of Information).

In Table 2, it is described the network of the main monitoring stations of the pollutants of Rome. The urban monitoring stations are used to measure the concentration level of pollution influenced mainly by emissions from traffic. They are located in high risk areas such as roads with high traffic exhibition (Decision 2001/752/EC).

The background station is located within Villa ADA's park , in other words, in an area not directly affected by urban emission sources. It is used to monitor the natural level of pollution in urban areas. Villa Ada monitoring station is particularly important to measure the concentration levels of ozone. In the same monitoring station, we have available a set of meteorological variables such as solar radiation, temperature and humidity, and the main primary pollutant variables (NO, NO2, CO).

Monitoring Station	Activation Date	Type Station	Type Area
Corso Francia	01/01/1993	Traffic	Urban Area
Cinecittà	13/01/1998	Traffic	Urbana Area
Largo Arenula	01/01/1993	Traffic	Urban Area
Largo Magna Grecia	01/01/1993	Traffic	Urban Area
Villa Ada	01/04/1994	Background	Urban Area

Table 2. Air quality monitoring station of Lazio (Source: BRACE's database - http://www.brace.sinanet.apat.it/)

As can be seen from Table 2, five monitoring stations have been taken into consideration: four traffic stations and one station of background. In this case, we considered at hourly time steps concentrations of primary pollutants and meteorological variables coming from monitoring stations. This study utilises a significant number of pollutants (ozone and main relevant primary and secondary pollutants) and main meteorological variables in order to maintain parsimony [Occam's razor] and keep the resulting models simple enough for meaningful comparison.

Our environmental dataset examines about 90,000 hourly pattern data, coming from 5 monitoring stations, and is composed by pollutants variables and conventional meteorological variables:

- observed pollutants variables:
  - Carbon monoxide (mg/m^3)- CO-
  - Nitrogen Oxide (μg/m3) -NO-
  - Nitrogen Dioxide (μg/m3) -NO2-
  - Mono-Nitrogen Oxides ($\mu g/m^3$) -NOx-
  - Ozone (μg/m3) - O3 -
  - Pm10 (μg/m3) - PM10
- meteorological variables:
  - Temperature (C°) – T;
  - Global Solar Radiation ($W\backslash m^2$) – GSR;
  - Relative Humidity - RH (%)
  - Pressure (mbar)–P-
  - Rain (mm).

It was decided that this study would use a conservative number of pollutant (concentrations of ozone, PM10 and other relevant pollutants) and meteorological variables, according to parsimony principle, and keep the NN models simple enough for meaningful comparison. We observed that global radiation were analysed to investigate the ozone correlation with photochemical reactions.

Moreover, we observe that our environmental time series contain information at different scales, some of which are periodic, such as day and hour that represent seasonality and

diurnal variation. These variables were treated in term of cosine and sine. In this way, it is possible to take into account the effects of seasonality and diurnal variation.
Before conducting any analysis, previously all data were standardised (pollutants and meteorological conditions).

2.2 Pre-processing

Table 3 and Table 4 show the general statistics calculated by the pollutants and meteorological parameter analysed in this study for 2005 and 2006. The descriptive statistics are a necessary passage to establish some properties of the distribution of our dataset. We examine the following statistical characteristics of the distribution of hourly data: mean, standard deviation, skewness (SK) that shows the direction and measures the asymmetry of the distribution of our variables, kurtosis, that refers to the peak of a frequency curve, maximum, minimum and variation filed values calculated on the chemical and meteorological parameters.
O3's concentrations present a significant variability between 2005 and 2006 (0.98 and 0.97 respectively). The concentration values of NO2 are within a range (0 to 250.19 mg/m^3).
As regard to acute events exceeding the recommended limits for NO2 and O3 concentrations, which was fixed at 180 μg/m^3 for ozone (hourly information threshold for human health protection) and 200 μg/m^3 1-hour mean for NO2 [DM25/11/1994]. A first indication of their occurrence can be deducted from the maximum value for each time series. In particular, it is noted that NO2 and O3 concentrations exceeding the level of attention.

- The CO has kurtosis's values greater than the critical value, 3, and its distribution is highly asymmetrical, with a value of sk near to 3
- The NO2 has kurtosis's values below the critical value, 3, and with a value of sk near to zero
- Kurtosis's ozone does not exceed the critical value for 2005 and 2006, while there is a positive asymmetry (sk is equal to 1 for two years)
- The NO and NOx kurtosis values are higher than the critical value, 3, and their distributions are highly asymmetrical, with a value of sk near to 3
- The kurtosis of PM10 exceeds the critical value in two years, whereas there is a discrete positive asymmetric (sk is approximately 1) for 2005. For 2006 it is noted that the kurtosis value is less than the critical value, while there is a slight positive asymmetry.

The analysis of meteorological data provides support interpretive information of descriptive statistics calculated on data from pollution, because air pollution is also strongly influenced by meteorological factors [Seinfeld and Pandis, 1998].
On a local scale, air pollution depends by meteorological variables such as temperature, humidity, solar radiation, cloudiness and rain. This means that the distribution of pollutants is not only dependent on the spread of its emissions, but is also affected by various meteorological drivers [Giorgi and Meleux, 2007].
As known, global radiation was analyzed to investigate the ozone correlation between and photochemical reactions. In fact, when solar radiation is high, Table 3 and Table 4 temperature becomes a key variable between the meteorological data. Remarkably, NO2 and atmospheric pressure show low values. Finally, relative humidity appears as input of minor relevance; this does not mean that they do not influence the pollutant values.
Finally, the analysis of epidemiological data shows that for cardio-respiratory admission, kurtosis does not exceed the critical value for 2005 and 2006, moreover the skewness is approximately zero.

At the end, in our environmental time series, we observed that missing values depend on different working periods of the monitoring stations or occasional malfunctions of the instruments. In this analysis, missing values were not taken into account.

2005		Mean	Sd	Skewness	Kurtosis	N	Missing	Min	Max	CV (%)
CO	(mg/m³)	1.06	0.82	2.99	16.70	40795	3005	0.00	12.16	0.77
NO2	(µg/m³)	63.42	31.85	0.53	0.26	40773	3027	0.45	249.84	0.50
NO	(µg/m³)	47.85	67.62	2.95	13.11	40784	3016	0.00	860.07	1.41
Nox	(µg/m³)	136.76	126.82	2.40	9.41	40806	2994	0.50	1365.47	0.93
O3	(µg/m³)	35.99	35.30	1.12	0.75	24300	19500	0.00	220.54	0.98
PM10	(µg/m³)	36.33	17.15	1.52	5.06	23478	20322	0.00	202.49	0.47
Rain	(mm)	0.09	0.64	14.19	290.46	8494	35306	0.00	20.00	6.88
Press	(mbar)	1016.14	6.80	-0.42	0.95	17396	26404	986.47	1035.81	0.01
GSR	(W/m2)	133.56	230.59	1.88	2.44	34394	9406	0.00	1031.11	1.73
Temp	(C°)	14.37	8.12	0.10	-0.70	43145	655	-5.90	41.61	0.57
RH	(%)	70.21	19.49	-0.32	-0.83	43143	657	0.05	99.14	0.28
Cardiac Admission		172.48	50.30	-0.60	-.29	365	0	3	286	29.16
Respiratory Admission		78.74	25.51	0.07	-0.14	365	0	1	149	32.40

Table 3. General statistics (2005)

2006		Mean	Sd	Skewness	Kurtosis	N	Missing	Min	Max	CV (%)
CO	(mg/m³)	0.99	0.75	2.68	12.46	36322	7478	0.00	11.34	0.75
NO2	(µg/m³)	69.80	35.47	0.49	0.15	40385	3415	0.00	250.19	0.51
NO	(µg/m³)	50.50	71.78	2.85	12.95	40392	3408	0.00	1228.35	1.42
Nox	(µg/m³)	147.18	134.82	2.25	8.17	40400	3400	0.00	1734.78	0.92
O3	(µg/m³)	36.63	35.41	1.04	0.63	15248	28552	0.00	227.59	0.97
PM10	(µg/m³)	39.83	17.35	0.80	0.35	33102	10698	0.18	104.90	0.44
Rain	(mm)	0.60	5.53	18.11	435.33	8697	35103	0.00	182.00	9.17
Press	(mbar)	1017.51	6.06	-0.07	0.45	17401	26399	996.00	1040.00	0.01
GSR	(W/m2)	138.38	230.18	1.78	2.08	34853	8947	0.00	1005.00	1.66
Temp	(C°)	15.64	7.79	0.26	-0.56	42813	987	0.00	44.00	0.50
RH	(%)	70.25	19.92	-0.37	-0.79	34794	9006	1.00	99.00	0.28
Cardiac Admission		167.78	48.21	-0.60	-0.31	364	1	7	259	28.73
Respiratory Admission		72.89	21.09	-0.08	-0.04	364	1	6	134	28.93

Table 4. General statistics (2006)

The size of the archive data that you have allows for an analysis of correlation between the variables available with the aim of identifying those most related. The correlation matrix of Pearson calculated over the entire set of hourly data is shown in Table 5 that describe:

- CO is both very marked positive correlations with NOx and NO2

- NO2 is anti-correlated with O3
- O3 presents positive correlation values with temperature and solar radiation, negative values, with relative humidity and cardio-respiratory admissions
- PM10 presents positive correlation values with air pollutants, excepted O3, HR and low positive values with cardio-respiratory admissions. Negative values with meteorological variables.

	PM10	*CO*	*NO2*	*NOX*	*O3*	*Rain*	*T*	*UR*	*GSR*	Cardiac	Respiratory
PM10	1										
CO	0.76	1									
NO2	0.67	0.79	1								
NOX	0.72	0.93	0.78	1							
O3	-0.42	-0.71	-0.57	-0.76	1						
Rain	-0.14	-0.05	0.00	-0.03	-0.06	1					
T	-0.21	-0.45	-0.33	-0.49	0.64	-0.08	1				
RH	0.14	0.40	0.13	0.34	-0.59	0.25	-0.39	1			
GSR	-0.30	-0.56	-0.40	-0.60	0.79	-0.20	0.74	-0.61	1		
Cardiac	0.05	0.28	0.34	0.21	-0.16	-0.01	-0.16	0.05	-0.04	1	
Respiratory	0.19	0.41	0.36	0.33	-0.32	0.00	-0.46	0.16	-0.29	0.73	1

Table 5. Correlation Matrix

The analysis of stratified data by day allow you to see what shape it takes the distribution of different variables at each day and verify the existence of particular trends in the time series associated with these layers of time (see Fig.1 and Fig.3). In particular, in Fig.1 and Fig.3, it is possible to observe a not linear relation between averages of CO's daily distributions and their skewness (Sk), of the CO's daily distributions and averages of O3's daily distributions and their skewness (Sk). These relations allow explaining in a good manner the latent factors that are not manifest variables. For this reason, we included these indices as input for NN, because the greatest advantage of a neural network is its ability to model a complex non-linear relationship between independent and dependent variables [Gardner, 1999], [Gardner, 2000], [Abdul-Wahab, 2002].

In particular for CO, it can observed the following:

- CO is less than 1 mg/m3 the Sk's values are very higher up to 10
- CO is greater than 2 mg/m3 the Sk's values are low (from 2 to 0),therefore daily distributions are symmetric
- CO is greater than 2 mg/m3 the Sk's values are approximately zero.

Fig. 1 explains very well the significant positive asymmetry of CO distribution.

For this study, we calculated the daily distributions (PDF) of each pollutant (760 PDFs for each variable), for confirming the hypothesis of a concentration trends related to changes in the day. In Table 6 and Fig.2 we synthesized these PDFs through their mean, standard deviation and skewness that are able to capture environmental performance. If a daily distribution presents a negative asymmetry, it means that its values will be below of alert values for the exposure of population.

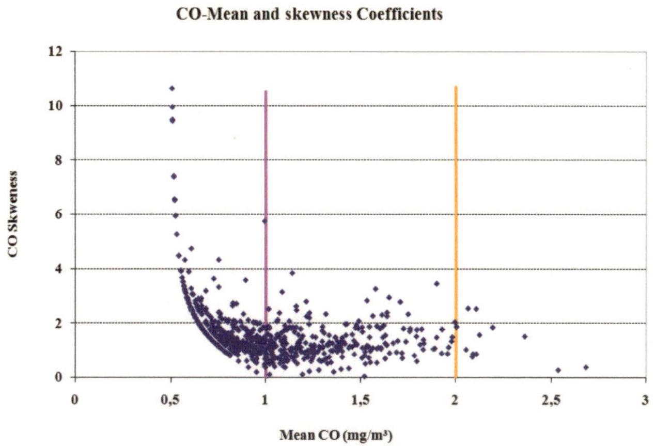

Fig. 1. Relation between Mean(CO) and Skenewss(CO)

Table 6 and Fig.2 show that when the daily average value of the PDF of CO is between 0.5 and 1.0 mg /mc, the skewness is 1.95 and contains 58.2% of data, whereas in the second class the skewness is 1.26 and contain 40.2% of overall data and the third class only 1.6%. In particular, Fig.2 shows that CO presents a decreasing skewness, but not too much variable.

CO Range	Mean	Standard Deviation	Skewness
CO(0.5.-1.0)	0.77	0.48	1.95
CO(1.0-2.0)	1.31	0.92	1.26
CO(2.0-3.0)	2.20	1.55	1.34

Table 6. General statistics of daily distributions of CO

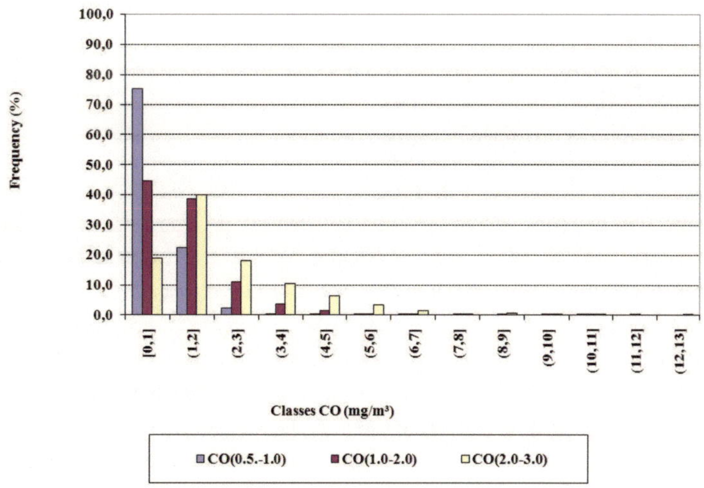

Fig. 2. Distribution of CO for different classes

For ozone (see Fig.3), you can see the following:

- O3 is less than 30 µg/m3, the Sk's values are very higher up to 8
- O3 is greater than 30 µg/m3 and less than 60 µg/m3 the Sk decreases.
- O3 is greater than 60 µg/m3, the Sk's values are decreases further (from 2 to -2).

Fig.3 shows that first function of SK is inefficient and then it is very efficient. This trend resembles the potential of the neural network.

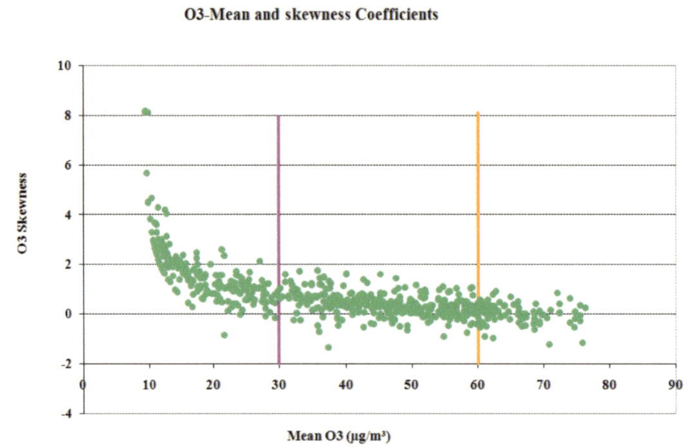

Fig. 3. Relation between Mean(O3) and Skenewss(O3)

In Table 7 and Fig.4, the values of the third class of ozone are those associated with exposure, whereas the values of the first class, with 1.88 skewnees, have no great relevance to the exposure.

O3 Range	Mean	Standard Deviation	Skewness
O3(0.0-30.0)	17.65	1.40	1.88
O3(30.0-60.0)	47.42	0.45	0.36
O3(60.0-120.0)	72.25	0.39	-0.03

Table 7. General statistics of daily distributions of O3

By modulating the time-series of daily values of CO, O3, NO, NO2, NOx and PM10 based on the profile average weekly (or typical week) , calculated as the average concentrations for each day of the week. The Fig.5 and Fig.6 show the weekly evolution of the concentrations of CO, O3, NO, NO2, NOx and PM10 that are characterized by "critical" days, typically Thursday and Friday, by minimum values at the weekend, excepted for ozone, due to the physiological decrease in traffic volumes and the reduction of industrial activity and by an increase in the levels of pollutant concentration by the resumption of work activities during the week.

For the weekly cycle of ozone we observe an increasing of O3 levels over the weekend, whereas the situation is reversed on working days. This effect known as "weekend" [European Environment Agency, 1989] can be explained by the low level of NOx and volatile organic compounds during the Saturday and Sunday(Fig.5 and Fig.6), taking into account the meteorological conditions. During weekend, elevated ozone levels are caused by NOx emissions. Under stagnant meteorological conditions, week-day morning's become NOx saturated due to the morning rush hour.

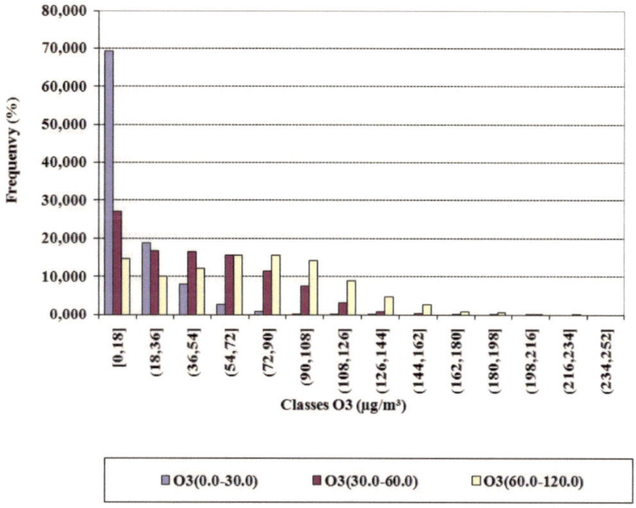

Fig. 4. Distribution of O3 for different classes

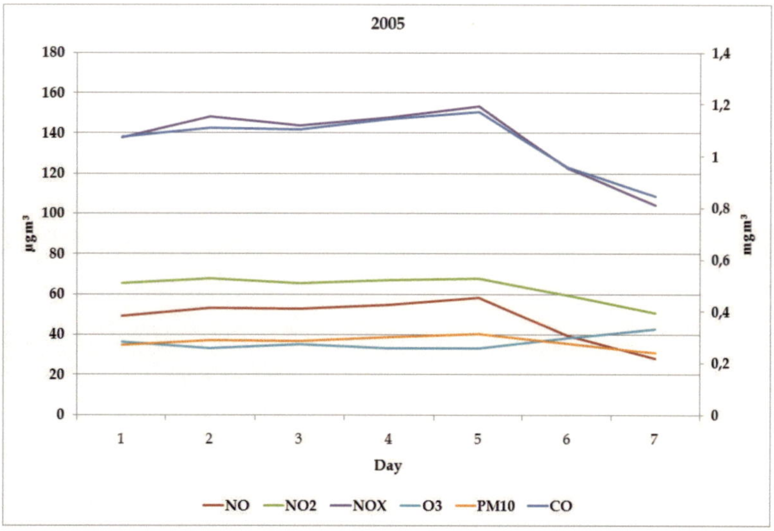

Fig. 5. Weekly cycles for CO, O3, NO, NO2, NOx and PM10 concentrations (2005)

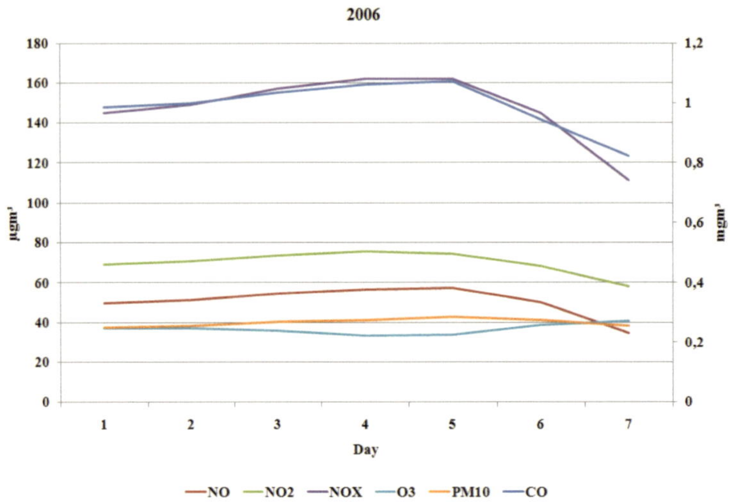

Fig. 6. Weekly cycles for CO, O3, NO, NO2, NOx and PM10 concentrations (2006)

In terms of weekly cycle, for respiratory disease we observed a decrease approximately 40% of admissions at the weekend and equal to nearly 50%for cardiovascular admissions. This reduction is probably due to the fact that in general the hospitalizations, except in urgent cases, are scheduled on weekdays (Fig. 7-8).

For deaths from respiratory disease, there were no significant differences, whereas for cardiac deaths there is a moderate decrease in the weekend, which is almost completely irrelevant when considering only deaths sent from the hospital emergency room.

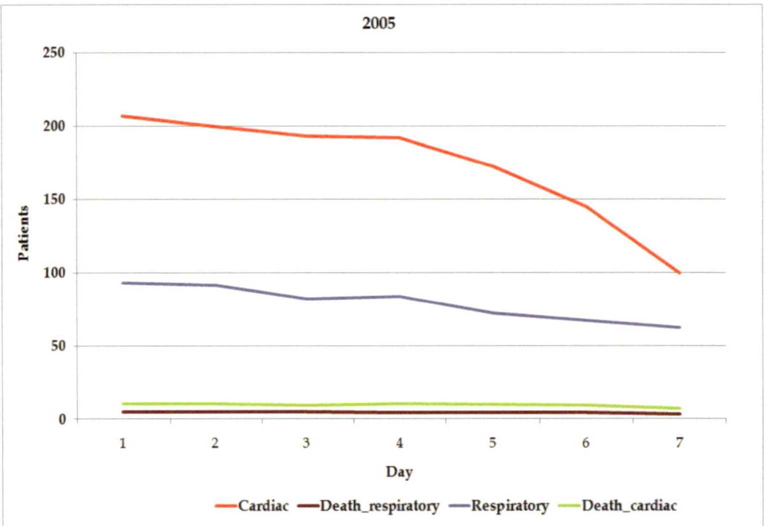

Fig. 7. Weekly cycles for cardio-respiratory admissions (2005)

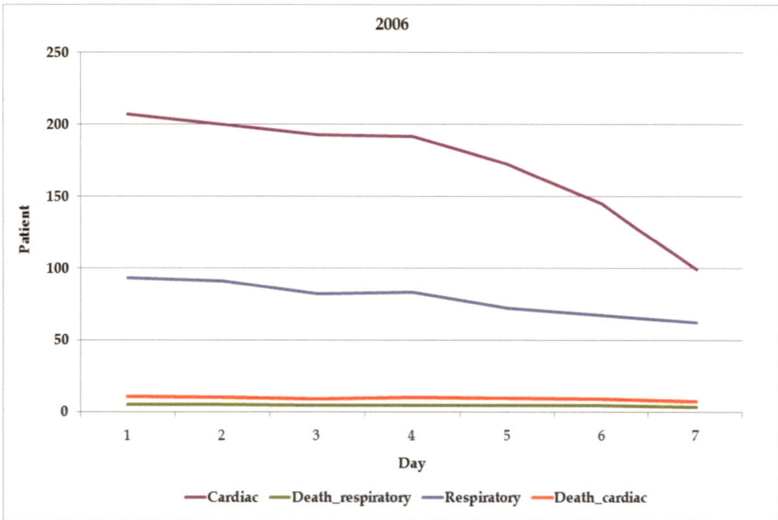

Fig. 8. Weekly cycles for cardio-respiratory admissions (2006)

3. Methodologies

Some preliminary retrospectives analysis were carried out on hourly environmental time series [Battaglia, 2007] (pollutants and meteorological variables) and on daily time series related to admissions for cardio-respiratory disease, identifying and examining graphically their trends. Such time series constitute a summary of the "history" of the phenomenon under study. Thus we proceeded first to examine the fundamental characteristics of the series.
Then by a spectral analysis we proceeded to detect the most relevant periodic components for the explanation of the variability of the series. The Fourier analysis is based on the decomposition of the original time series in a sum of periodic functions at different frequency:

$$Y_t = \sum_{k=0}^{n/2} (a_k \cos w_k t + b_k \sin w_k t) \quad \text{con } t = 1,2 \ldots n \tag{1}$$

where Y_t is the observation at t time and w_k, a_k e b_k are respectively the frequencies and the Fourier coefficients.
The spectral analysis consents to highlight what are the frequencies (and hence the periodicity) more important. The periodogram, in fact, measures the intensity of k-frequency within the range of values and hence the importance that assume each period p_k.
Based on the results coming from the preliminary analysis of these series, was designed and developed a simulation model of interpretation implemented by neural network. The greatest advantage of a neural network is its ability to model a complex non-linear relationship [Gardner & Dorling, 1999, 2000]; [Abdul-Wahab & Al-Alawi, 2002], such as those in the environmental systems, without a priori assumptions on its nature [BuHamra et al, 2003], by means of an accurate choice of the variables of the system and of the meaningful patterns, and data distribution.
For transfer function, the most suitable architectures are considered to be the Multi Layer Perceptron (MLP) [Abdi, 1994], [MacQueen, 1967], [Fausett, 1994]; [Bishop, 1995], [Ripley

1996] with an error-back-propagation supervised learning rule [Rojas, 1996]. This net architecture is able to reproduce non linear models, without any a priori assumptions, by means of an accurate choice of the variables of the system and of the meaningful patterns. A learning algorithm is an adaptive method by which a network of computing units self-organises to reproduce the desired model. This is done with learning algorithms that present some examples of the desired input-output mapping to the network. A correction step (the error-backpropagation rule) is performed iteratively until the network learns to produce the desired response.

"Backpropagation nets" can be interpreted in statistical terms as variations of maximum likelihood estimation and is a feed-forward neural network type and generally uses back-propagation algorithm to develop a model to illustrate relationships between inputs and desired output for training data (see Fig.9)

Multi Layer Perceptron (MLP) is also the most popular architecture for NNs and is used to identify models for the prediction of cardio-respiratory diseases.

The selection of appropriate network architecture depends on the number of parameters, the network weights, the selection of an appropriate training algorithm and the type of transfer functions used.

As architecture we used a 3-layer perceptron model with a single hidden layer, 10 hidden neurons and with sigmoid activation function (see equation 2) that approximates nonlinearities.

$$F(P) = \frac{1}{1 + e^{-(p-s)}} \tag{2}$$

where P is the activation potential and S is the activation threshold.

The model optimisation mechanism takes place through the automatic update of the weights. The update of weights among neurons is guided by the following function (see equation 2 and 3):

$$\Delta w_{ij} = -\eta \frac{\partial E}{\partial w_{ij}} \tag{3}$$

where η is the learning rate (a characteristic parameter for updating) and the network output error is defined as:

$$E = \frac{1}{2} \sum_{j=1,npatt} (y_j - \overline{y}_j) \quad (4)$$

where E provides a quantification of the overall difference over all the examples and for all the reproduced variables.

The first input layer contains the input variables of the net, pollutants and meteorological variables. The second layer consists of the neurons of the hidden layer. The third layer is the output layer, which consists of the target of the forecasting model.

The number of neurons of the hidden layer is one of the parameters to be chosen in the NN model architecture, the well known multi-layer perceptron. We tested different numbers of neurons in the hidden layer (8, 10 and 12 hidden neurons), but the best performance of perceptron network was obtained by 10 neurons. The choice of 10 hidden neurons is based on two considerations: maximizing the hidden neurons to increment the NN parameters and simultaneously minimizing this number in relation with the main situations linked to the input patterns. Moreover, we utilise different methods to optimize the weight values of hidden layers, in the manner that the errors of the network's output could be minimized.

During the training phase, one of the most important parameters of selection is the choice of the function of correction related to each weight between the different layers of NN. In fact, the inner weights to the NN have to be determined by minimizing a well defined function (namely Error Function -EF) that usually coincides with the sum of error square. The best solution for the weights derives from the search of the minimum of EF in the space of total weights. This work is very complex and is the target of the NN training. There is no way to find absolute minimum for the NN's weights and the performances of NN are highly dependent by the way to find this "local" minimum. We try three different way to find the best solution.

In according with Table 8, we utilized different methods: Conjugate gradient (CG), the Quasi-Newton or Broyden-Fletcher-Goldfarb-Shanno (BFGS) and the popular Gradient Descent (GD) [StatSoft, Inc. , 2006]

While the first two are based on the second order approximations for search of the minimum of EF, the last method is a first order of approximations and can be used to find a local minimum in very fast way.

In particular, Conjugate Descent is a training algorithm that proceeds by a series of line searches through error space. After search directions are selected to be conjugates (non-interfering). It is a good generic algorithm with generally fast convergence.

The Quasi-Newton method is a powerful second order training algorithm with very fast convergence but require a high computational complexity due to memorize the Hessian matrix.

The comparison of different performances of these three methods is out of aim of the work and results will be not shown here. For ours data set, we selected the CG as better method of work respect to the BFGS or GD ones.

As second important choice to be considered is the activation function. We tested mainly the two main functions that are usually used: the logistic (LOGISTIC) and Hyperbolic tangent (TANH).

As schematized in figure 9, each layer uses a linear combination activation function. The inputs are fully connected to the first hidden layer, each hidden layer is fully connected to the next, and the last hidden layer is fully connected to the outputs.

In our study, we observed that the input and the hidden layer contain multiple units whereas the output layer only has a single unit.

The nature of the functional relationship between inputs and outputs is learnt during a supervised training process directly from the data. In our case, Neural Net model takes into account the influence of the pollutant and meteorological variables and latent variables such as source emission factors, turbulence conditions, local topology, reactions rate.

A great advantage of Neural Networks is that it can be trained to generalize accurately when it is presented a new data.

As above, by testing the best choice of NN parameters, we found that the Multi Layer Perceptron (MLP) model with a single hidden layer that was able to explain about the total 90% of the variance of the phenomena investigated, with 10 hidden neurons and with conventional sigmoid activation function (logistic) for the hidden units.

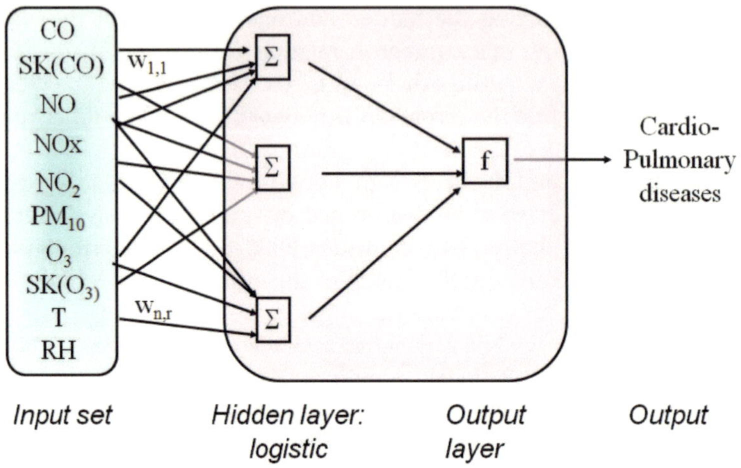

Fig. 9. MLP architecture

NEURAL NETWORK MODEL	MLP 6-10-1
Hidden neurons	8-10-12
ALGORITHM	CG-BFGS-GD
EPOCH	3000
ERROR FUNCTION	Sum of Square
HIDDEN ACTIVATION FUNCTION	LOGISTIC-TANH
OUTPUT ACTIVATION FUNCTION	IDENTITY
NETWORK RANDOMIZED	NORMAL

Table 8. Neural Networks architecture

The nature of the functional relationship between inputs and outputs is learnt during a supervised training process directly from the data. Neural Networks can be trained to accurately generalize when presented with new, unseen data. Often, especially in the atmospheric sciences, successfully modeling the average behavior of a system is not the main goal. It is important sometimes that the model can also interpret infrequent outliers, which are often of great importance, as for the health related with exposure.

In this work, we face also the question of the best variables of input to be used and the optimum selection of patterns for having results that represent the health response to the different pollutants and to meteorological factors.

At the end, to compare NN result we analysed the results coming from autoregressive model that assess the linear nature of the relationship between the dependent and independent datasets. The main disadvantages consist in transformation of non-linear relations are into linearity and the existence of multicollinearity.

4. Results and discussion

4.1 Pollutants and meteorological trends

Based on the analysis of the time series of PM10 concentration levels coming from the monitoring stations of the city of Rome, is observed that in 2005, there were about 20% of exceedances of the daily maximum value (50µg/m³) of PM10 (approximately 72 days). The maximum annual value was equal to 39.4 µg/m³ just below the limit value for the protection of human health (40µg/m³).

Elevated levels of PM10 concentrations have occurred during the winter and late autumn, especially in December and January, where we can observe frequent thermal inversion conditions (in the evening and in the night), high traffic volumes, intensive use domestic heating systems, whereas during the summer season there is a low concentration of the pollutant due to favourable meteorological conditions that allow a major dispersion in the atmosphere (see Fig.10). On average, in January and March, there have been no less than 16 days of exceedances over the threshold. The concentrations over 50µg/m³ during the summer season, however, depend on factors other than those that led to the overcoming of this limit during the winter season.

Moreover, we observe that the number of days with PM10's values greater than 75µg/m³ (equal to the value limit for the protection of human health plus 25µg/m³) was equal to 10 days where the most of exceedances is found in the winter season. The distribution of values between 50 and 75µg/m³ notice a predominance of winter season with a dozen of exceedances.

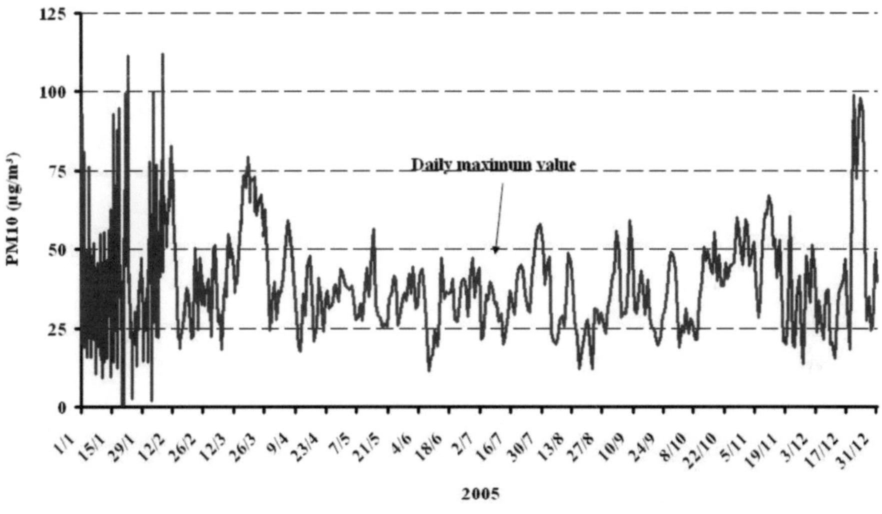

Fig. 10. PM10 trend (2005)

For 2006, PM10 exceeds about 23% of exceedances of the daily maximum value (50µg/m³) of PM10 (approximately 83 days). The maximum annual value was equal to 39.64 µg/m³ just below the limit value for the protection of human health (40µg/m³).

Elevated levels of PM10 concentrations have occurred during the winter and late autumn, especially in December, January and February, whereas during the summer season there is a low concentration of the pollutant (see Fig.11). The concentrations over 50µg/m³ during the summer season, however, depend on factors other than those that led to the overcoming of this limit during the winter season.

Moreover, we observe that the number of days with PM10's values greater than 75µg/m³ (equal to the value limit for the protection of human health plus 25µg/ m³) was equal to 12 days. The distribution of values between 50 and 75µg/m³ notice a predominance of winter season with 71 days of exceedances.

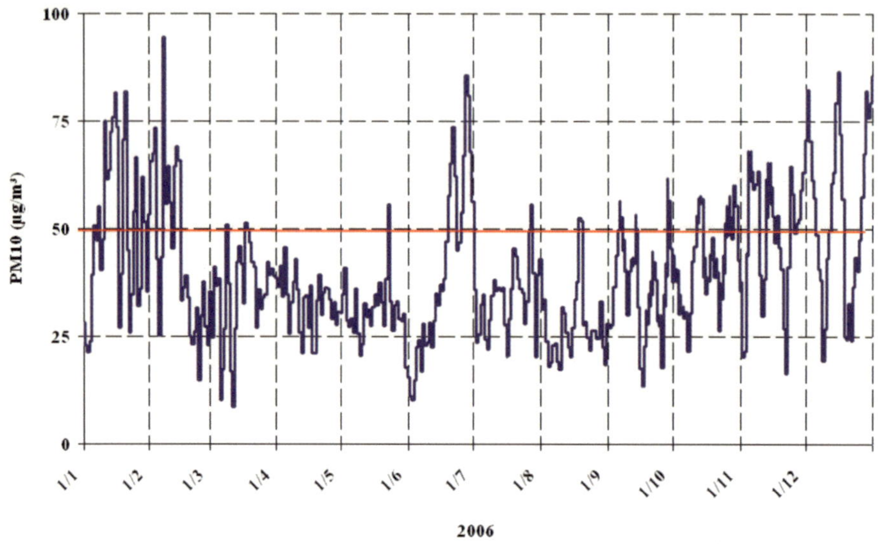

Fig. 11. PM10 trend (2006)

For 2005, O3 shows the peak maximum equivalent to 221µg/m³, exceeding the limit value of 200µg/m³, especially in summer (June-September) is characterized by a greater number of Days, where it is most noticeable the action of solar radiation and the increase of temperature. In addition, for 2005 we can observe that the number of days exceeding the information threshold (180µg/m³) is 11 (Fig.12).

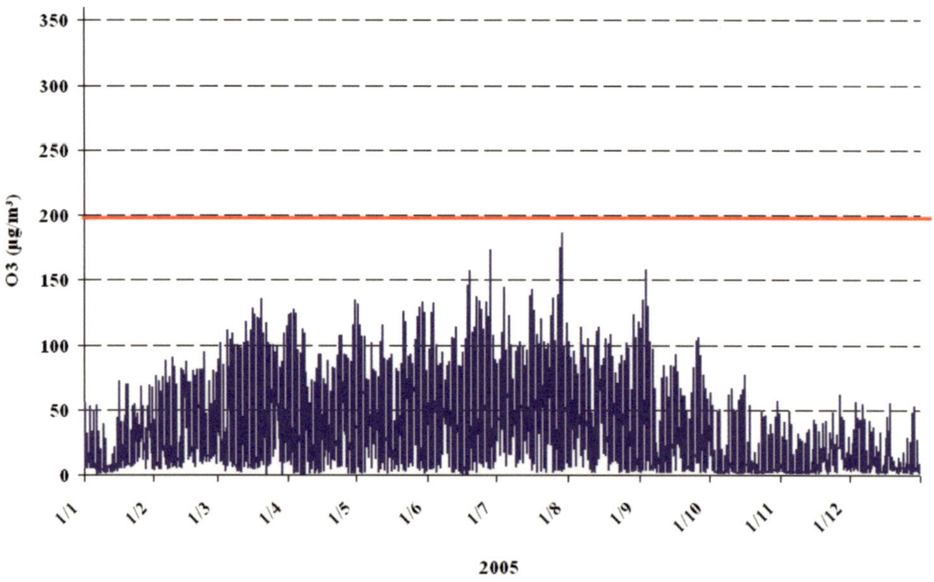

Fig. 12. O3 trend (2005)

For 2006, O3 shows the peak maximum equivalent to 228μg/m³, exceeding the limit value of 200μg/m³, especially in summer (June-September) is characterized by a greater number of days where it is most noticeable the action of solar radiation and the increase of temperature. As known, O3 levels have the highest peak concentrations in summer, on the contrary NO and NO2, have characterized by a summer minimum and a maximum in winter (Fig.13).

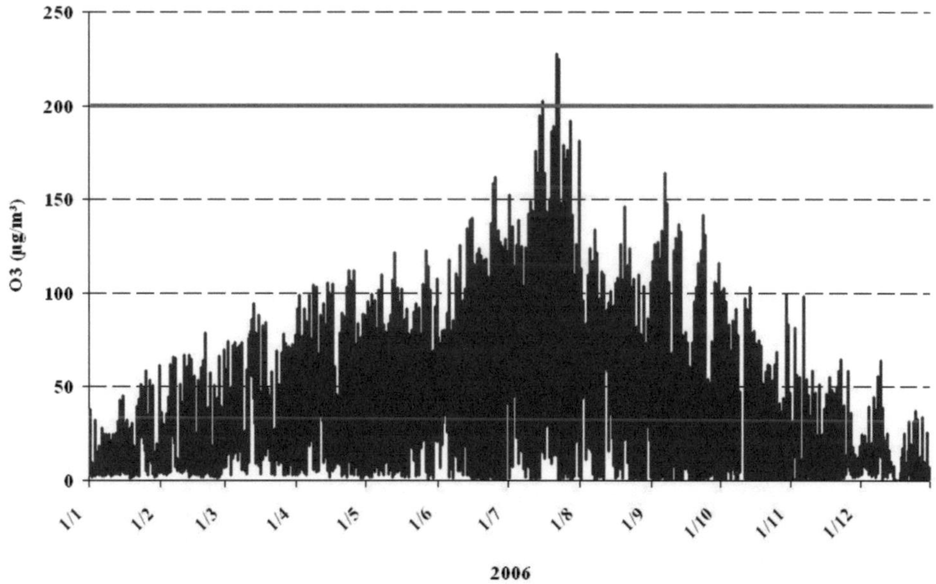

Fig. 13. O3 trend (2006)

Finally, the Fourier analysis has identified a periodicity of PM10 on 2 and 6 days for 2005 and 2 and 12 days for 2006 (see Fig.14 and 15).

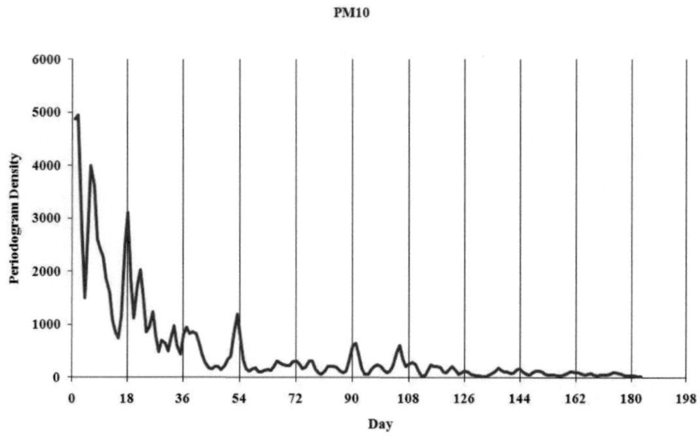

Fig. 14. Fourier analysis for PM10 (2005)

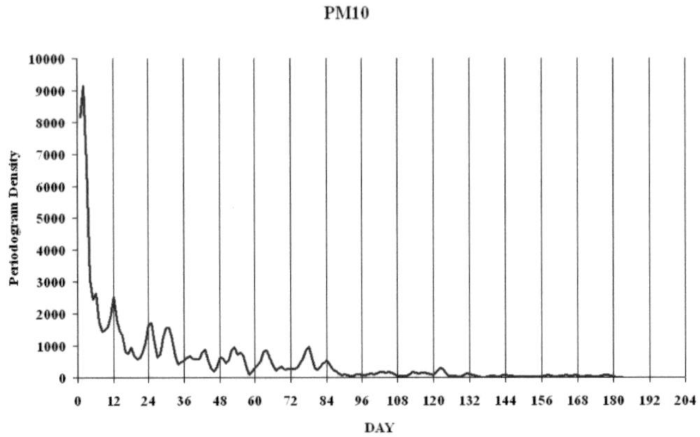

Fig. 15. Fourier analysis for PM10 (2006)

For 2005 and 2006 the spectral analysis of ozone (see Fig.16 and 17), carried out by periodogram, shows a peak at 3 hours and 684 hours (approximately 28 days).

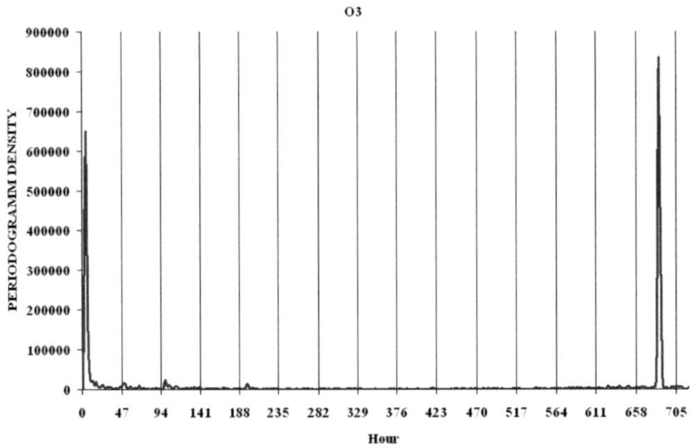

Fig. 16. Fourier analysis for O3 (2005)

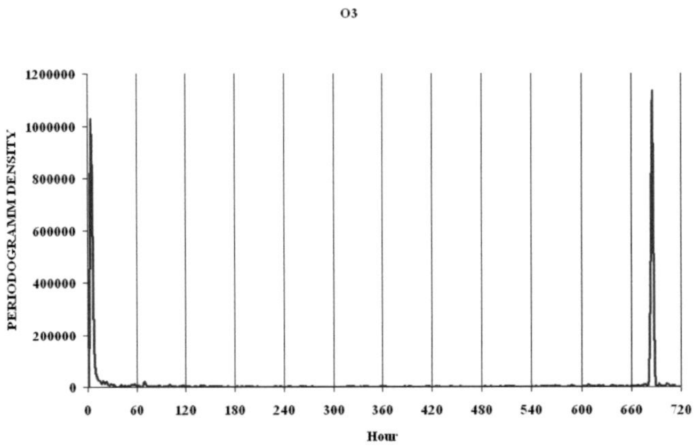

Fig. 17. Fourier analysis for O3 (2006)

4.2 Epidemiological analisys

It is to be noted that epidemiological data refer cases to hospital admissions rather than sick or dead the whole city of Rome, so there is an under-estimation of the morbidity and mortality.

For 2005, the analysis of hospitalizations related to cardio-respiratory disease, shows a peak at the end of March. A meaningful number of hospitalizations are found in the first four months of the year and later a decrease for those related to respiratory disease until the summer season, with a recovery by the cold season (autumn-winter).

The admissions for cardiac disease are the trends in absolute terms, ranging from 100-250 patients for almost all of 2005. Patients with respiratory disease are also the trends in absolute terms, ranging from 0-150 patients (Fig.18).

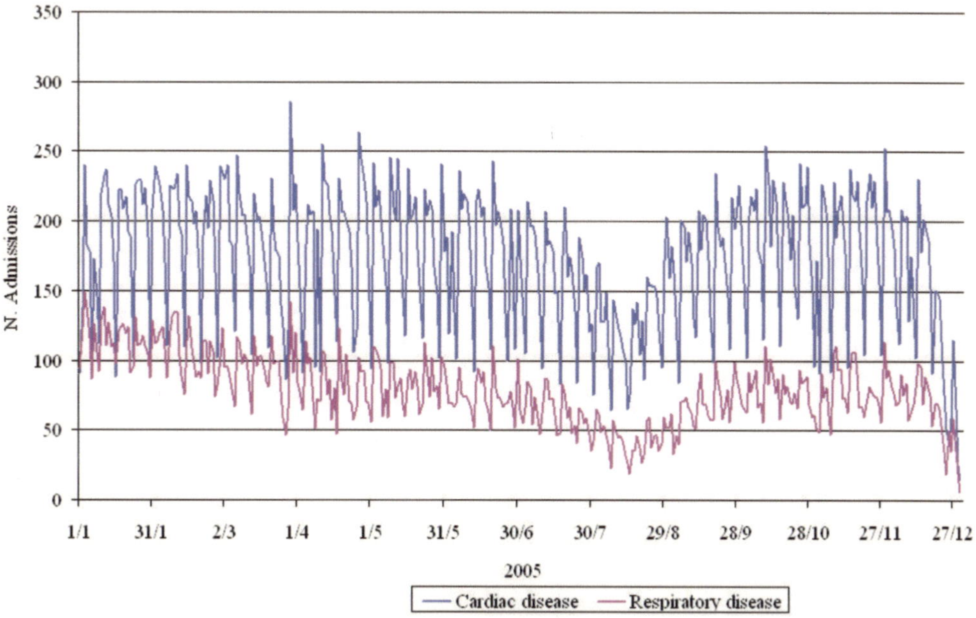

Fig. 18. Cardio-respiratory disease trend - 2005- (Source: Elaboration on EPICS Database of Public Health Agency of Lazio)

For 2006, the analysis of hospitalizations related to cardio-respiratory disease, shows a peak at the end of April. A meaningful number of hospitalizations are found in the first four months of the year and later a decrease until the summer season, with a recovery by the cold season (autumn-winter) (Fig. 19).

The admissions for cardiac disease are the trends in absolute terms, ranging from 100-250 patients for almost all of 2006. Patients with respiratory disease are also the trends in absolute terms, ranging from 0-150 patients (Fig.18).

For 2005 and 2006, deaths for cardio-respiratory disease, which constitute a very small percentage of total admissions (about 5.5%), are higher in colder months. The deaths from respiratory disease do not exceed 15 units (see Fig.20 and 21).

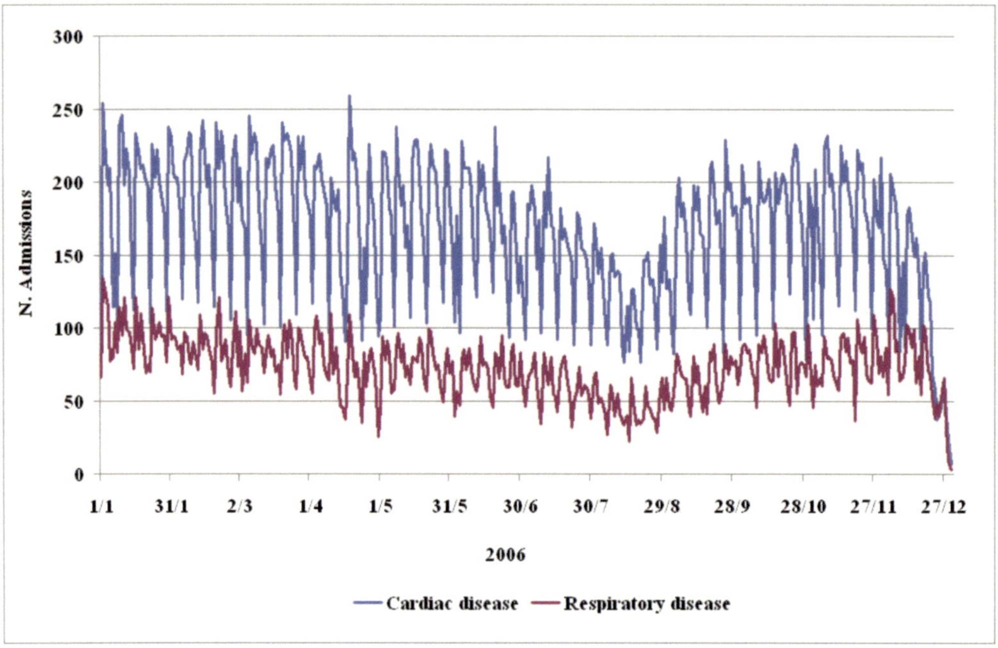

Fig. 19. Cardio-respiratory disease trend – 2006- (Source: Elaboration on EPICS Database of Public Health Agency of Lazio)

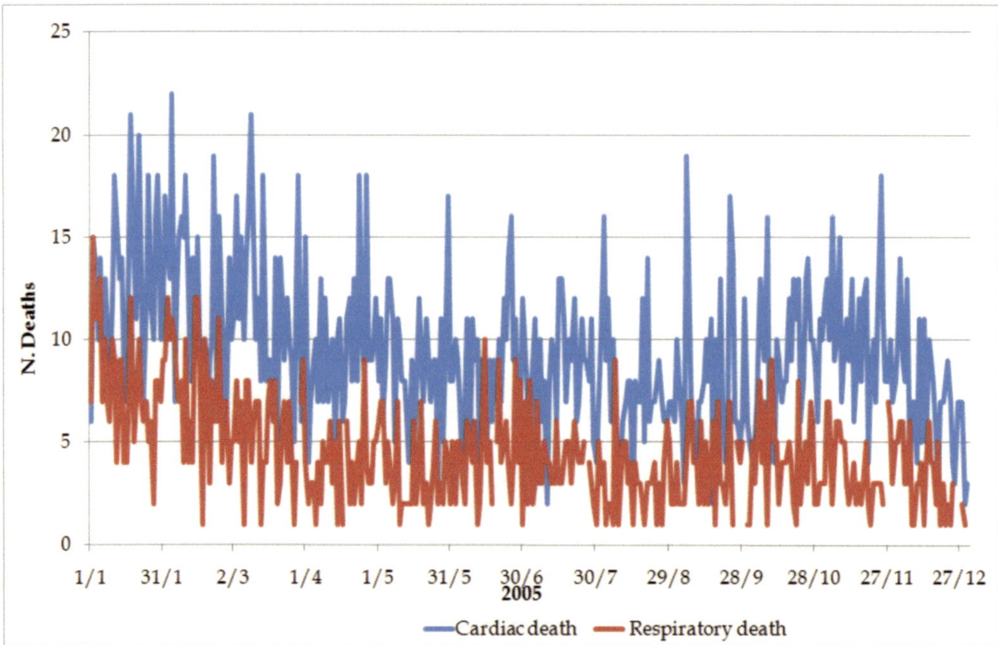

Fig. 20. Cardio-respiratory death trend – 2005- (Source: Elaboration on EPICS Database of Public Health Agency of Lazio)

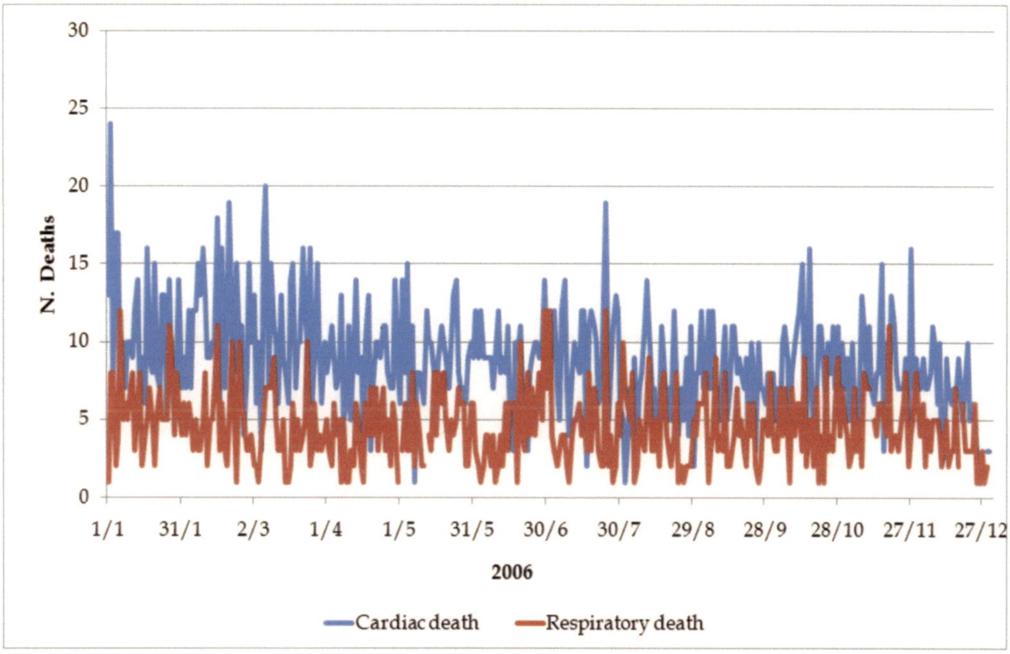

Fig. 21. Cardio-respiratory death trend - 2006- (Source: Elaboration on EPICS Database of Public Health Agency of Lazio)

For 2005 and 2006 the spectral analysis carried out by periodogram, shows a peak at two days for respiratory diseases and cardiac disease for 3 days (see Fig.22-25).

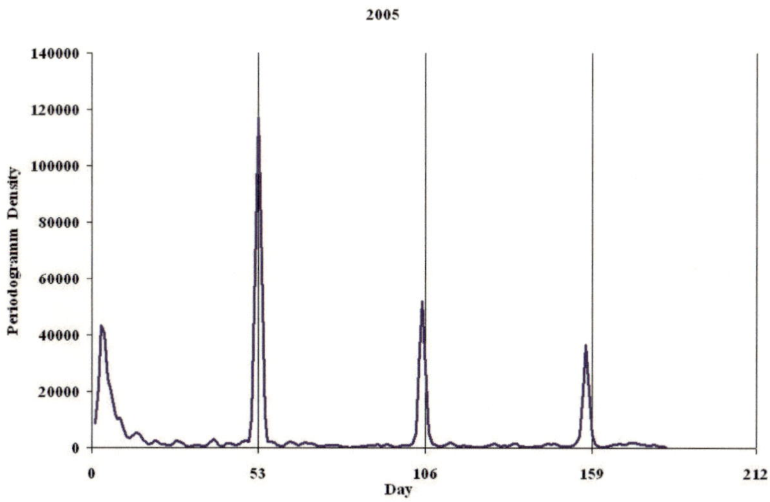

Fig. 22. Fourier analysis for cardiac disease (2005)

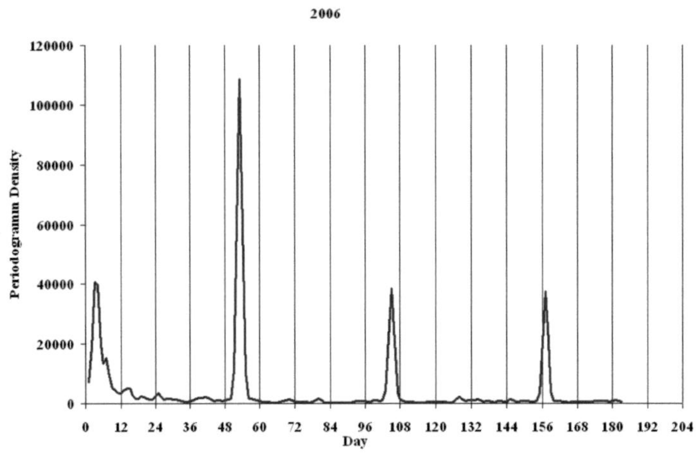

Fig. 23. Fourier analysis for cardiac disease (2006)

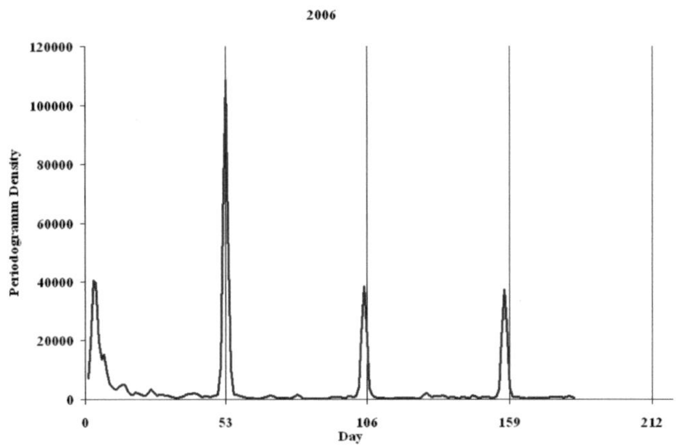

Fig. 24. Fourier analysis for respiratory disease (2005)

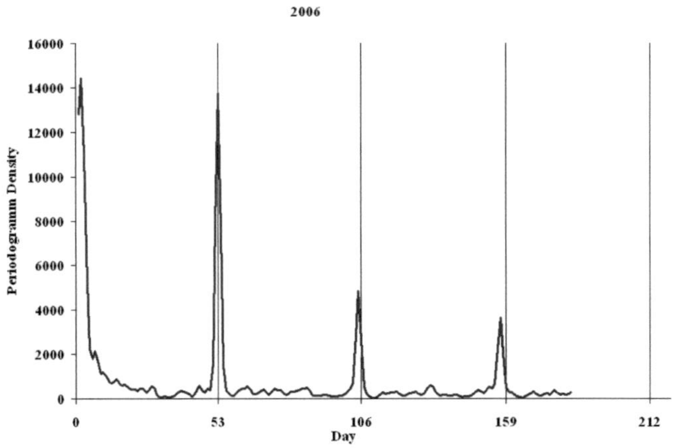

Fig. 25. Fourier analysis for respiratory disease (2006)

For 2005 and 2006 the spectral analysis carried out by periodogram, shows a peak at two days for respiratory deaths and cardiac death for 4 days (see Fig.26-29). Moreover, we observed that harmonic secondary for respiratory deaths is related to 68 days and for cardiac death is related to 53 days.

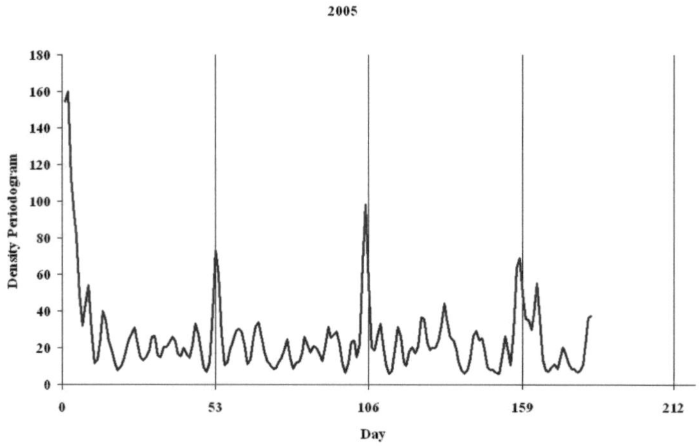

Fig. 26. Fourier analysis for cardiac death (2005)

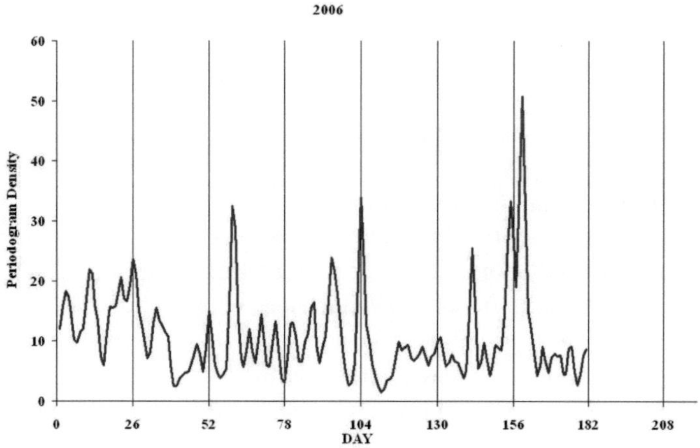

Fig. 27. Fourier analysis for cardiac death (2006)

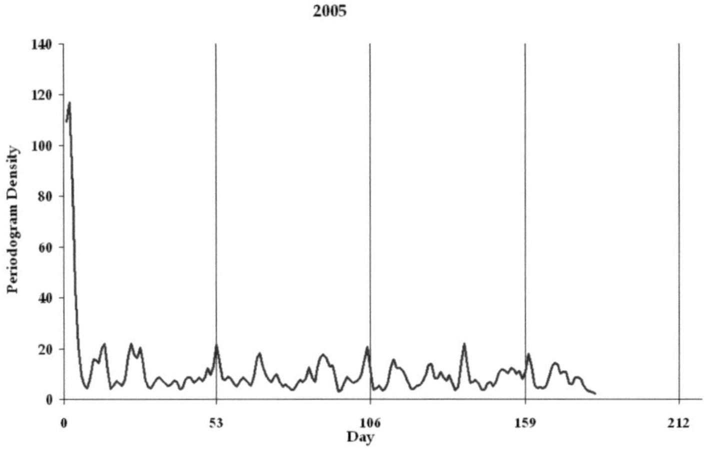

Fig. 28. Fourier analysis for respiratory death (2005)

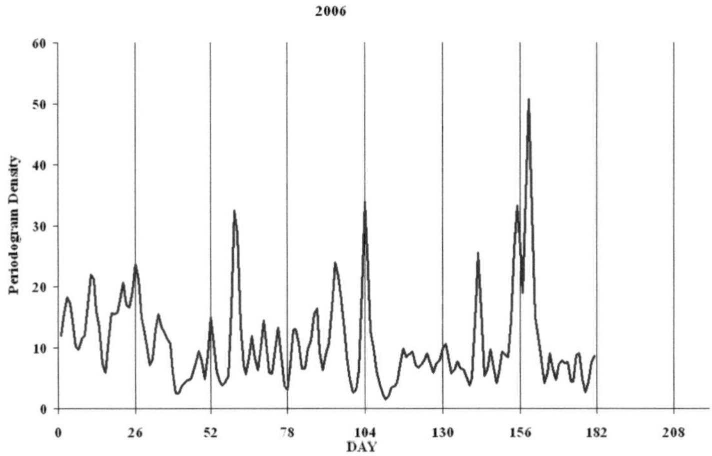

Fig. 29. Fourier analysis for respiratory death (2006)

4.3 Environmental and epidemiological analisys

The effects of PM10 and ozone linked to short-term exposure on cardio-respiratory diseases have been documented by the joint study of time series that examines changes of health outcomes related to changes in concentration levels of pollutants. To this end, the distributions daily of O3 and PM10 and hospital admissions were examined in terms of morbidity and mortality. Thus, it was possible to verify the existence of dynamic relationships between time series of pollutants and the time series of hospitalizations for cardiopulmonary disease.

In terms of morbidity, it was observed a possible causal link between the respiratory and cardiovascular diseases.

For ozone, the results show a meaningful increase in daily hospital admissions for cardio-respiratory system due to high concentration levels of this pollutant.

In terms of mortality for respiratory disease, it was observed that at high of concentration levels of PM10 increase the number of deaths. The relationship, however, is less evident than for cardiovascular disease, as there is found a lower proportion of deaths. Results for ozone show significant increases in deaths related to exposure to high levels of concentration.

4.3.1 NN results

Besides carrying out the analysis of trends of pollutant concentration levels and hospital admissions, we proceeded with the description of the main results obtained with the neural network model. The daily PM10 and O3 data and the aggregated data for cardio-respiratory disease (ICD9CM 390-519) that relate to hospital were taken into consideration.

From our results, we can observe that the neural network is able to reproduce a good approximation the causal link between the concentration levels of PM10 and of O3 and admissions [World Health Organisation, 2006].

Epidemiological data are used to investigate the relationship between PM10 and O3 and morbidity and mortality, suggests that most of the differences in mortality can be attributed to a worsening of pre-existing conditions rather than the oneset, due to air pollution, of new diseases.

As suggested by above considerations, the performances of the NN or the ability to reproduce the target variables (in our case the hospitalisation for cardiovascular and respiratory diseases) are strictly linked to the variables and patterns selections. As usually, we use 65% of random patterns during the training and the remaining 35% as test, never seen by NN during the learning phase.

Our aim is that we attempt to reproduce the average five days in advance of hospitalisation for the two considered pathologies given as input data the following variables (see Table 9):

NN Input Variables		
Julian Day	Sin (Jd)	Cos (JD)
Week Day	Sen (Week)	Cos (Week)
Pollutants	PM10	
	NO2	
	CO	SK (CO)
	O3	Sk (O3)
Meteorological	T	HR

Table 9. NN input variable

As evident, we collect the input data: general information (Julian day and week Day), air quality data (pollutants) and meteorological data.

During the search of the optimal architecture of neural net, we tested different input variables and we found that data related to general information are essential to reproduce the hospitalisation in best way. This sensitivity analysis will be not shown. In this chapter only we showed only the best architecture.

In order to facilitate the comparison of NN modelling, we show results related to the cardio-respiratory hospitalisations separately.

4.3.2 Results of simulations related to cardiac hospitalisation

As hidden neurons the best choice is 10 neurons for the MLP architecture. In the figure 30, we provided the results of NN's forecasting for all data (training and test sets) for the Rome area during the calendar years 2005-2006.

As evident, the NN predicted well the hospitalisations during all the days of period. The determination coefficient is very high (R^2=0.93) and we underestimate the extremes values of admissions both in term of the lower than upper limits. It is to note, that NN is able to forecast also the fall of the cardiac hospitalisation due to the Christmas holydays and this can be simulated mainly by the information related to Julian day and the week.

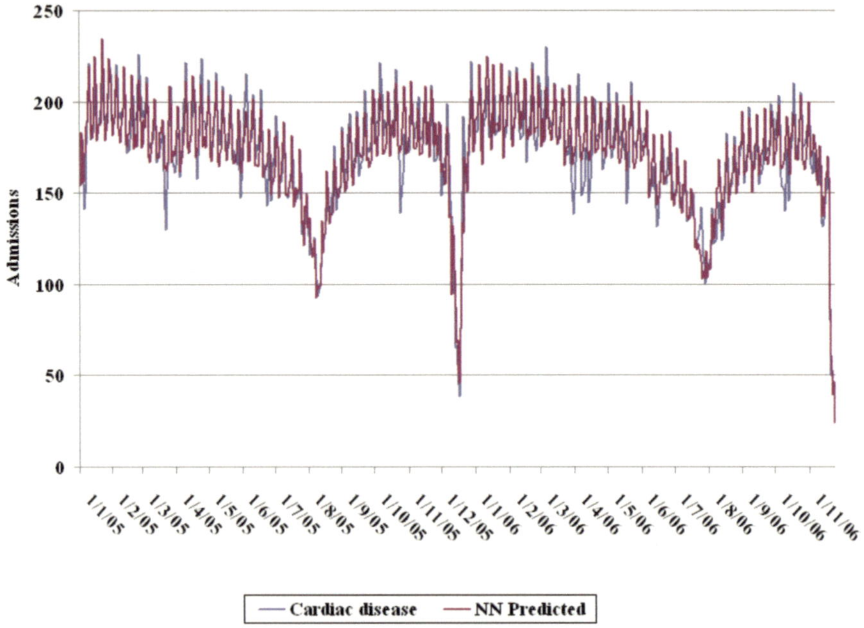

Fig. 30. Cardiac admissions for Rome (2005-2006)

When we compared the forecasting for cardiac diseases, it was more convenience to admit a band of error within to accept the results. We decided to take as reference levels the 10% of real value as confidence range for the acceptability of NN forecasting. Doing so, we find following results described in Table 10:

Cardiac hospitalisation by NN	
Percent of wrong simulation	**9.5**
Percent of right simulation	90.5

Table 10. NN performances for the forecasting within 10% of real data

In the short period, the NN is able to reproduce hospitalisation for cardiac disease for the 90.5% of the total hospitalisation. It is to underline that these excellent results meant that NN is able to understand the "global answer of the Rome city" respect to seasonal effects and the observed pollutants' levels.

4.3.3 Results of simulations related to respiratory hospitalisation

For this data, the number of the hidden neurons selected is related to 8.

The results for simulations of the respiratory hospitalisations are showed in fig 31. The determination coefficient is a little worse respect to previous simulation (R^2=0.92), even if levels are very significant.

If we account of compare the confidence limits of 10%, we find that the NN predicts only 82.1% of the respiratory admissions. Also for the confidence limits, the performances of NN for the respiratory are slightly lower respect to that of cardiac hospitalisation. By the Fig.31, it seems that NN makes some difficulty to simulate the minima during the winter season.

These results can suggest that, for the simulation of the respiratory admissions by NN, further analysis could be used (for example, it is be necessary to select the right patterns during the training phase in such a way to consider the real answer of the city of Rome to the pollution episodes).

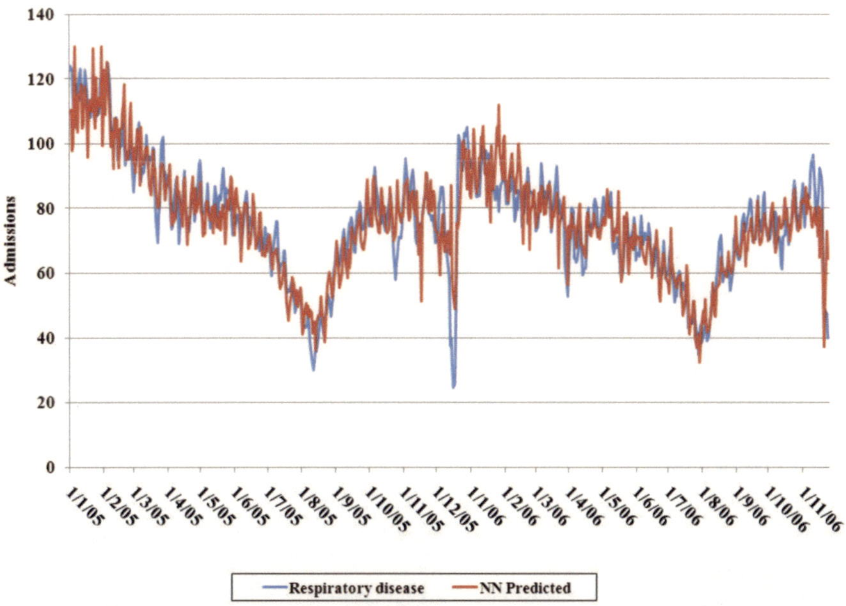

Fig. 31. Respiratory admissions for Rome (2005-2006)

Respiratory hospitalisation by NN	
Percent of wrong simulation	17.9
Percent of right simulation	82.1

Table 11. NN performances for the forecasting within 10% of real data

4.3.4 Autoregressive results

At the end, we compared the conventional autoregressive model with neural networks to forecast cardio-respiratory diseases under different meteorological and pollution variable.

Table 12 shows the resulting model coefficients for both cardio-respiratory admissions. All the variables introduced in the model are associated to a coefficient that is statistically significant.

Cardiac Admissions		Respiratory Admissions	
Coefficient	**Variable**	**Coefficient**	**Variable**
0.2324	Sin(Jd)	0.3627	Sin(Jd)
-0.1589	Cos(JD)	0.2128	Cos(JD)
0.1694	Sin (Week)	0.0629	Sin (Week)
0.2997	Cos (Week)	0.2567	Cos (Week)
-0.1402	PM10	-0.0717	PM10
0.2613	CO	0.385	CO
-0.0953	SK(CO)	-0.1299	SK(CO)
0.0055	NO2	-0.143	NO2
-0.0272	O3	0.099	O3
-0.0518	Sk(O3)	0.0137	Sk(O3)
-0.1176	T	-0.2198	T
0.0378	HR	-0.0565	HR
0.0485	constant	0.0203	constant

Table 12. Autoregressive model coefficients

Autoregressive model performances are evaluated using appropriate scalar measures and skill scores [Wilks, 1995], namely: explained variance in% (R^2), correlation coefficient (R), mean absolute error (MAE), root mean square error (RMSE) , relative absolute error and root relative squared error (see Table13).

Training phase		
	Cardiac Admissions	Respiratory Admissions
R^2	0,44	0,78
Correlation coefficient	0.67	0.88
Mean absolute error	0.25	0.27
Root mean squared error	0.43	0.32
Relative absolute error	62.32 %	53.28%
Root relative squared error	74.60 %	46.79 %
Total Number of patterns	451	451
Test phase		
	Cardiac Admissions	Respiratory Admissions
R^2	0,31	0,765
Correlation coefficient	0.557	0.875
Mean absolute error	0.271	0.261
Root mean squared error	0.449	0.317
Relative absolute error	73.14 %	54.13%
Root relative squared error	83.34%	48.43%
Total Number of patterns	242	242

Table 13. Validation of the autoregressive model related to cardio-respiratory admissions

The autoregressive models perform less satisfactory than NN models perform, especially for cardiac admissions, with an R^2 of 31% and 76% for respiratory admission.
As note in Fig.32, the results achieved with all the developed models show that in general, autoregressive model underestimate cardiac hospitalisation.
In general for cardio-respiratory admissions this model explains more of the observed variance in term of seasonal difference and less in term of transition seasons.

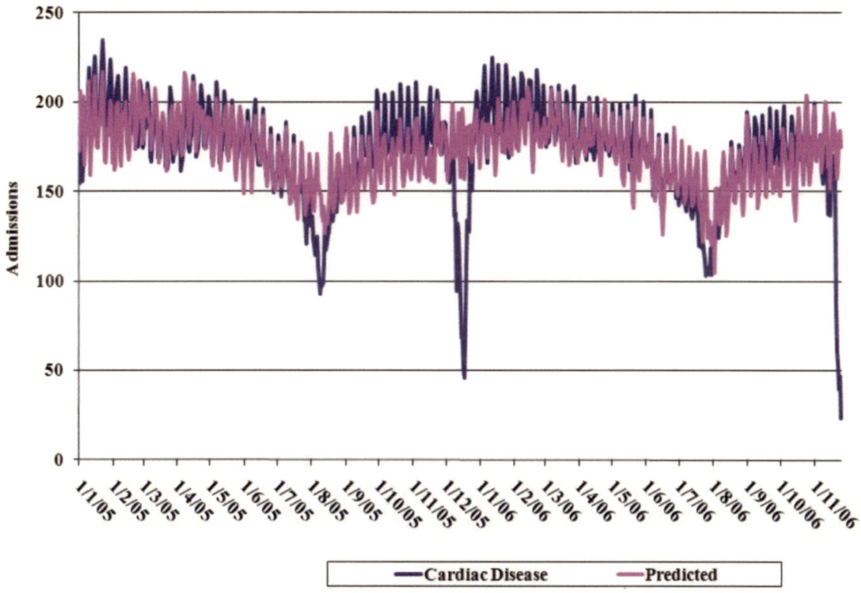

Fig. 32. Cardiac admissions for Rome (2005-2006)

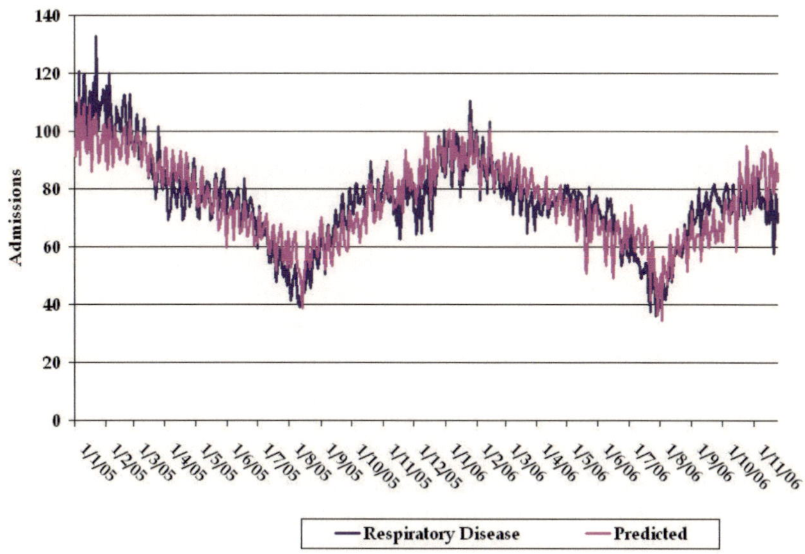

Fig. 33. Respiratory admissions for Rome (2005-2006)

5. Conclusion

In Rome and in general all the Italian cities, high concentration levels of air pollution, are one of the key risk factors of public health. Our data show that in Rome the concentration of PM10 and ozone have exceeded the danger levels suggested by the European Guidelines (DIR2008/50/CE).

One more interesting aim of for the health and environmental question are the connections between the air quality data and the relative effects on the human health, i.e. the hospitalisation. In general, while is well know that air quality impacts on the health, the quantification of this the effect is hard to simulate. This happen because the relation between the main variables (such as meteorological and pollutants ones) and health effects cannot be determined directly by deterministic models or by simplified statistical models. In fact, we can suppose that this relation could be non linear type and that the role of the important variables is hidden by the complexity of the phenomena.

In this context, we use one of the most advanced non linear models, such as the Neural Network, to attempt to model the relations between the environment and meteorological data and health effects on the populations. To this regards, we investigate the cardio-respiratory hospitalisations for total population of the Rome city, during the 2005 and 2006.

To that regards, we found that the conventional statistical descriptors, such as the daily average of pollutants, often cannot be link to the exposure levels, if they are taken standalone. By the pre-processing analysis, we demonstrated that the skewness coefficients for the pollutants can be given a more accurate connection with the real human exposure.

In our work, we applied an intelligent models constituted by a Neural network model (using the Mulilayer Perceptron architecture) to connect the environmental data with the hospitalisations for the two considered diseases.

The results obtained by NN model are very encouraging and suggest a way to modelling this complex relation. In fact, we obtained a very meaningful correlations (higher than 0.90) for both simulations. While the cardiac pathology is better reproduced by NN, the respiratory ones have needed more analysis in deep. However, both simulations exhibit that, to optimize the training phase, the choice of the input variables and the choice of patterns are the main factors to be considered for successful of intelligent methodology.

In our study, it is evident that the performances obtained is link to the right choice of input factors and that the NN performance is good only if some heavy pre-processing evaluation are given on input data.

These first results showed the importance of the environmental-epidemiological problem and the major areas in order to forecast with some accuracy the short-term effects on human health of the environmental component.

By using neural networks, it was possible to determine numerically the association statistically meaningful between the cases of death or hospitalization and pollutants (PM10 and/or O3).

The results coming from this work have used neural networks to investigate short-term the relationship between air pollution, mortality and hospital admissions, identifying and evaluating the sources of pollution in order to define and adopt effective mitigation measures for air quality improvement of Rome and the promotion of strategies for the prevention and treatment of cardio-respiratory diseases.

As last consideration, we underline that the results obtained seem encouraging to simulate the effects of air quality on the health through NN model, but at the same time indicate that further study are necessary in future as to extend the NN's prediction to more years and to consider also the spatial distribution of pollutant in relation with the local hospitalisation.

6. References

Abdul-Wahab, S.A., Al-Alawi, S.M. (2002). Assessment and prediction of tropospheric ozone concentration levels using artificial neural networks. *Environmental Modelling & Software* 17, 219-228

Abdi, H. (1994). Les re´seaux de neurones. Presse Universitaire de Grenoble

Battaglia F. (2007). Metodi di Previsione Statistica. Springer Verlag

Bishop, C.M. (1995). Neural Networks for Pattern Recognition. Clarendon Press, Oxford

Brunekreef, B. and Holgate, S. T. (2002). Air pollution and health, Lancet 360, 1233–1242

BuHamra, S., Smaoui, N., Gabr, M. (2003). The Box-Jenkins analysis and neural networks: prediction and time series modelling. *Applied Mathematical Modelling* 27 (10), 805-815

DM25/11/1994 - Decreto Ministeriale del 25/11/1994. Aggiornamento delle norme tecniche in materia di limiti di concentrazione e di livelli di attenzione e di allarme per gli inquinamenti atmosferici nelle aree urbane e disposizioni per la misura di alcuni inquinanti di cui al decreto ministeriale 15 aprile 1994.

European Environment Agency (1998). Europe's environment: the second assessment.23

Fausett, L. (1994). Fundamentals of Neural Networks. In: *Architectures, Algorithms and Applications*. Prentice Hall, Englewood Cliffs, NJ 07632

Gardner, M.W., Dorling, S.R. (2000). Statistical surface ozone models: an improved methodology to account for non-linear behaviour. *Atmospheric Environment* 34, 21-34

Gardner, M.W., Dorling, S.R. (1999). Neural network modelling and prediction of hourly NOx and NO2 concentrations in urban air in London. *Atmospheric Environment* 33, 709-719

Gariazzo C., Silibello C., Finardi S., Radice P., Piersanti A., Calori G., Cecinato A., Perrino C., Nussio F., Cagnoli M., Pelliccioni A., Gobbie G. P.and Di Filippo P. (2007). A gas/aerosol air pollutants study over the urban area of Rome using a comprehensive chemical transport model. *Atmospheric Environment* Volume 41, Issue 34, November 2007, 7286-7303

Giorgi, F. and Meleux, F.(2007). Modelling the regional effects of climate change on air quality, Comp. Rend. Geosci., 339, 721–733

Jol, A. and Kielland, G. (Eds.): Air Pollution in Europe 1997, European Environment Agency, Copenhagen, Denmark, 1997

MacQueen J. B. (1967). Some Methods for classification and Analysis of Multivariate Observations, *Proceedings of 5-th Berkeley Symposium on Mathematical Statistics and Probability*. Berkeley, University of California Press, 1:281-297

Murray A. Mittleman M.D.(2007). Air Pollution, Exercise, and Cardiovascular Risk. *The New England Journal of Medicine*,2007

Ripley, B.D. (1996). Pattern Recognition and Neural Networks. Cambridge University Press

Rojas R. (1996). Neural Networks: a systematic introduction, Springer-Verlag, Berlin Heidelberg

Seinfeld, J. H. and Pandis, S. N.(1998). Atmospheric chemistry and physics from air pollution to climate change, New York, John Wiley & Sons, Inc, 1113 pp.

StatSoft, Inc. (2006). STATISTICA (data analysis software system), version 6.0. www.statsoft.com

Wilks, D. S. (1995). Statistical Methods in the Atmospheric Sciences, Academic Press, San Diego, CA, USA, 476 pp.

World Health Organisation (2006). Air quality guidelines for particulate matter, ozone, nitrogen dioxide and sulphur dioxide, Global Update 2005. Geneva, 2006

World Health Organisation (2004). Environmental Epidemiology A Textbook on Study Methods and Public Health Applications. June 2004

World Health Organisation (2003). Health aspects of air pollution with particulate matter, ozone and nitrogen dioxide. Report on a WHO Working Group. Bonn, Germany, 13-15 January 2003

World Health Organisation (2001). Quantification of the health effects of exposure to air pollution. Report of a WHO working group. Bilthoven, Netherlands, 20-22 November 2000. Copenhagen, 2001

4

Air Pollution and Outpatient Treatment and Hospital Admissions for Respiratory Diseases in Children in Southeast Region of Brazil

Hermano Albuquerque De Castro[1], Sandra De Souza Hacon[2], Karen Dos Santos Gonçalves[3] and Washington Leite Junger[4]
[1]Oswaldo Cruz Foundation Sergio Arouca, National School of Public Health Ministry of Health,
[2,3]National School of Public Health Sergio Arouca - ENSP, Oswaldo Cruz Foundation - FIOCRUZ
[4]Institute of Social Medicine, State University of Rio de Janeiro
Brazil

1. Introduction

The harmful effects of air pollution on human health have been observed in both overall mortality[1-9] and mortality from specific causes such as cardiovascular disease[10-16] or respiratory diseases[13,17-19]. Effects on morbidity have also been observed and include increases in respiratory symptoms in children, decreases in lung function[21-23], increase respiratory diseases[24,25], or simply an increase in school absenteeism[26,27]. More recently, several studies have used the number of hospitalizations as an indicator of the effects of pollution on health[28-34].
Considering the amount of research that have been produced in many countries, various issues, however, deserve further elucidation, for example, which pollutants would be more associated with the effects investigated or which individuals more susceptible to these hazardous exposures. A recent study that uses data from several cities showed that daily exposure to volatile pollutants appears to be associated with respiratory hospital admissions than exposure to particulate matter with a diameter of up to 10 microns (PM_{10})[35].
The effects of air pollutants seem to relate differently between men and women. Kotesovec and colleagues (2000)[36], observed a significant increase in daily mortality associated with increased levels of Total Solid Particulate (TSP) and SO_2 in men until 65 and not among women of similar age, while that for the population over 65 years the mortality significantly increased only among women. Zanobetti and Schwartz (2000)[37] showed that the effect of PM_{10} on mortality could be modified by gender, the curve of deaths among women 1/3 higher than that of men.
In relation to cancer, and more specifically to lung cancer, several studies have shown differences in the occurrence of this disease between urban and rural areas[38]. It is assumed that this difference can be attributed to different carcinogens in environmental pollutants, but the difficulty of confirming this hypothesis is due to the presence of other risk factors that also are implicated in the etiology of disease, including active and passive smoking and occupational exposures.

Dean (1966)[39] showed that the highest rates observed in urban areas remained even after controlling for age and the start of smoking. Several studies have compared the coefficients of lung cancer between areas with different pollution levels showed a slight increase in those most polluted.[38]

In Brazil, some studies showed the effects of air pollution on health, Pena and Dulchiade (1991)[40] comparing annual averages of particulate matter at the rates of infant mortality from pneumonia in several areas of the city of Rio de Janeiro and found a statistically significant association. In Sao Paulo, Saldiva and colleagues conducted two important studies [41.42] using time series, and have shown associations between mortality from respiratory diseases and levels of nitrogen oxides (NO_X) and mortality in the elderly and levels of particulate matter. More recently, the same group showed evidence of an association between intrauterine mortality and air pollution[43].

Regarding morbidity, Sobral (1989)[44], using a cross-sectional study compared the proportions of children with respiratory symptoms in two areas of Greater Sao Paulo with different levels of pollution and found a positive correlation. Cubatão differences were observed in lung function of children living in areas with varying levels of pollution [45]. Rumel and colleagues (1993)[46] studied the occurrence of visits to emergency services for acute myocardial infarction and found an association with levels of carbon monoxide (CO) and ambient temperature. In an experimental study, Reymão and colleagues (1997)[47] suggest that air pollution may facilitate the formation of certain types of lung cancer in rats.

However, the ecological character of some these studies, the lack of specificity regarding the age groups most susceptible and the various health effects, the short period of investigation (usually one year), which hampers control of temporal trends and the short careful control of meteorological variables, among other issues, prevented a better assessment of the effects of air pollution on health in the Brazilian context. Moreover, none of previous studies investigated the effects of pollution on hospital admissions, or tried to define the most vulnerable population subgroups.

Encouraged by these results, a series study covering a longer period of time (three years) was conducted with data from the city of Sao Paulo[48.49]. In these studies, special attention was given to the control of meteorological variables, and an investigation of different causes of death as well as in different age groups was made. Also, was first investigated the effect of pollution on morbidity of children through the examination of hospital admissions. An enhancement of 3.4% in the number of deaths from all causes (excluding violent deaths) and cardiovascular causes, compared to an increase in pollution levels from 10th to 90th percentile. For respiratory causes of the increase was 6%. Furthermore, it was observed that the effects of pollution on mortality alone were more prominent from age 65, having no effect on mortality for children or young adults. Moreover, hospital admissions for respiratory diseases in children under 5 years age group only investigated with regard to hospitalization, also showed an association with increases in daily levels of pollutants.

The aim of this study was to assess the association between exposure to daily records on air pollution concentrations emitted from the industrial and car emissions and the daily numbers of children outpatient and hospital admissions due to respiratory diseases under 6 years in public hospitals and the Universal Healthcare System in the urban area of Vitoria from 2001 to 2003, in individuals of the age groups considered most susceptible to air pollution in the city of Vitoria in Espirito Santo.

2. Methodology

2.1 Area and period of the study

Vitoria is located at latitude South 20°19'9" and longitude West 40°20'50" and borders on the cities of Serra to the North, Vila Velha to the South, Cariacica to the West, and the Atlantic Ocean to the East. It is an extension of continental land consisting of a mountainous island with the same name and several mangrove and salt marsh areas[50], resulting from the retreat of ocean levels.

There were 293,305 inhabitants in an area of 93km^2, corresponding to 3,154 inhabitants per square kilometer, with the highest population density in the State of Espirito Santo and some 50% of the State's entire industrial activity[51]

Vitoria has the second highest annual per capita income of all the Brazilian State capitals, with R$1,588.00, and a human development index (HDI) of 0.856.[52]

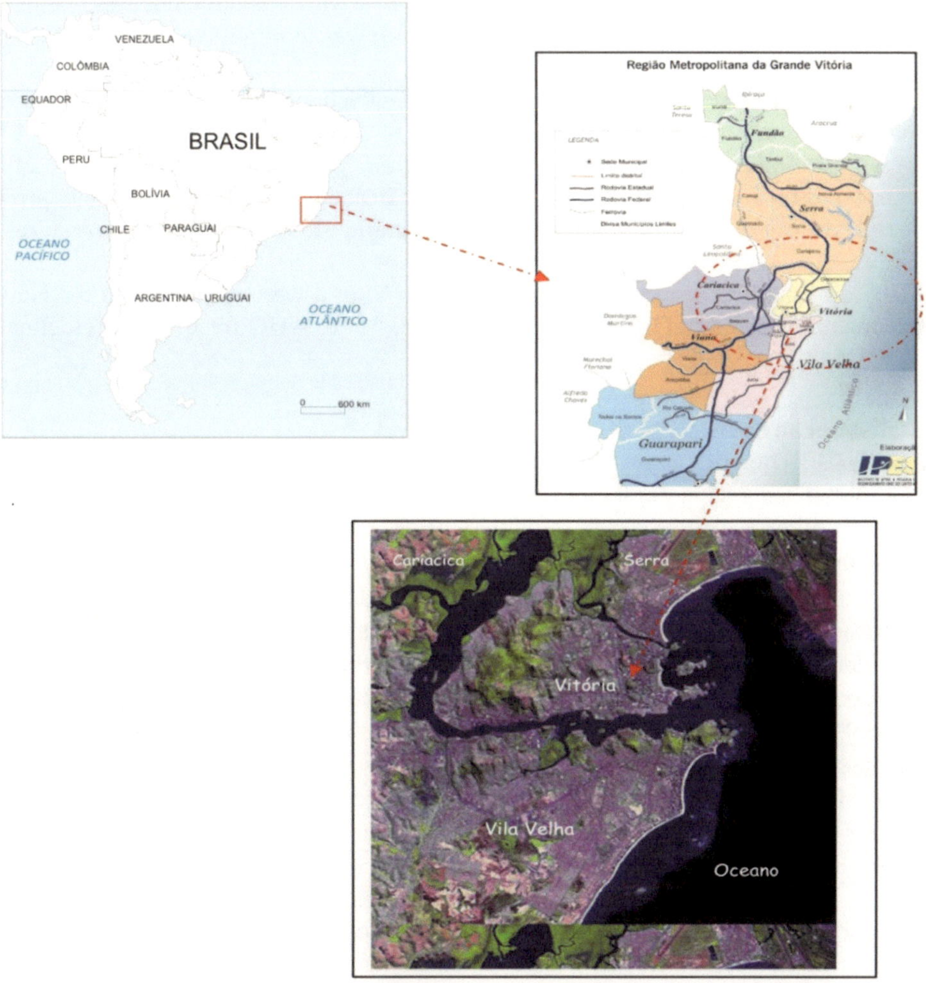

Source: Brazilian Institute of Geography and Statistics - IBGE. 2005

Fig. 1. Location of study area. City of Vitoria, Espirito Santo State, Brazil.

The daily records from the air quality monitoring program were provided by the State Environmental Secretariat (SEAMA) and State Environmental Institute (IEMA), and outpatient records on respiratory diseases were furnished by the Municipal Health Secretariat. Daily records on respiratory diseases were obtained from the Unified Productivity Bulletin (UPB), a registry used by 27 primary health units in the municipality of Vitoria, which is the only municipality that uses this kind of outpatient registry. Both data sets referred to January 1, 2001, to December 31, 2003. The UPB was established in the early 1990s with the aim of providing information related to population morbidity at outpatient services. This type of registry presents individual data on treatment in the primary health system. The information available contained date of consultation, patient's name, sex, date of birth, age, place of residence, and main diagnosis. The study analyzed respiratory diseases in general (J00-J99), pneumonia (J12-J18), and asthma (J45) for children under 6 years of age, based on the International Classification of Diseases, 10th Revision (ICD-10).
Despite the low frequency of missing observations in environmental databases, we used an imputation procedure. The purpose of the imputation was to minimize the loss of statistical precision of estimates of effects.
The air quality program is managed by the IEMA, which is responsible for five automatic monitoring stations that provided daily records of CO (8-hour averages), SO_2 (24-hour averages); particulate matter with an aerodynamic profile ≤ 10μg (PM10 - 24-hour averages); and O_3 and NO_2 (one-hour means), for Greater Vitoria. The IEMA also provides daily records on minimum, average, and maximum daily temperatures and relative humidity.
The daily air pollutant concentrations measured in Vitoria were compared to the National Environmental Council (CONAMA) standard 1990 [9] and WHO air quality guidelines for PM_{10}, SO_2, NO_2, and O^3 from 2005 [10].

2.2 Statistical analysis

Data analysis techniques were used usual time series analysis. For each outcome a model was estimated using semi-parametric class of generalized additive models (GAM)[53]. These models that allow both linear and nonlinear structures are introduced in the model. The implementation of the application GAM S-Plus was used. Each outcome was modeled initially took as its basic assumption that the distribution of counts of health events (visits, procedures or hospital admissions) follow a Poisson distribution.
The problem of over dispersion, a phenomenon in which the observed variance is larger than expected for the Poisson distribution, was treated using the quasi-likelihood estimation[54]. In analyzing the series of procedures nebulizer, the residual autocorrelation after adjustment for potential confounding factors available were modeled using Poisson regression for auto correlated data[55]. Robust regression was used to deal with too high or too low for the series of outcome[53].
The analysis strategy was to deal with seasonality and trend series using *splines* of the index of time, ie, the number of days elapsed since the series began. These smooth functions are flexible and are estimated from the data. We included indicator variables to control the effects of schedule - weekdays and holidays, which may modify the association between the pollutant and the response variable (outcome). It was also included in the model the effect of interactions of day of the weekend with an indicator variable for each quarter. This approach was employed because the heterogeneity of the occurrence of health events on

weekends in different seasons. Once it expects an increase in the number of hospitalizations due to influenza epidemics, the daily number of visits for *influenza* was introduced in a linear model.

The meteorological confounding factors were controlled through functions *splines* of temperature and humidity. Also introduced is a variable number of daily visits for all causes except respiratory and external causes, in order to control the residual variability in outcome due to series of problems that prevented the population's access to health services not covered by other variables[56].

Finally, add to the model of the baseline or *core model* terms corresponding to the studied pollutants (PM_{10}, SO_2, NO_2, CO and O_3) in a linear fashion. To construct the *core model*, after inclusion of each covariate were performed analysis of model fit via the periodogram or spectral analysis (to verify the presence of seasonal effects of medium and long term remaining), the autocorrelation function and partial autocorrelation function of the residual, testing normality of residuals (qq-plot) and eventually the Akaike information criterion (parsimony of the model) to decide between two or more models with similar diagnostic pictures.

3. Results

The biological manifestations of the effects of pollution on health appear to exhibit behavior that shows a lag in relation to the individual's exposure to pollutants. That is, events that occur on a given day may be associated with pollution levels that day and / or previous days. Thus, the daily values were tested for pollutants, lags of up to seven days and the average of two to seven days before the event as an indicator of cumulative exposure.

The results presented here represent the variations percentage in emergency procedures, mist or hospitalizations related to variations of 10 $\mu g/m^3$ in the levels of pollutants (except CO for which we calculated the percentage change in respect of 10 $\mu g/m^3$). The respective relative risks using the same convention are also presented. The adopted significance level of 5% in all analysis.

3.1 Descriptive analysis

3.1.1 Health events

Unified Productivity Bulletin-UPB

Table 1 presents the mean, standard deviation and percentiles for all outcomes analyzed. It is observed that the average child attended. There were no missing data for outcomes, but the first two days were excluded because there is no environmental data available. The number of valid observation was 1093.

	mean	SD	min	p5	p10	p25	p50	p75	p90	p95	max
DAR6	126.15	72.09	5.00	39.00	47.00	71.00	119.00	167.00	203.80	224.40	582.00
ASMA6	18.75	11.33	0.00	5.00	7.00	12.00	17.00	23.00	31.00	36.00	96.00
NEB6	80.67	46.54	0.00	20.00	25.20	43.00	74.00	111.00	146.00	166.40	237.00

Table 1. Descriptive statistics of health data BUP

The Figure 2 in Figure 3 show the temporal trends of the daily number of emergency visits for asthma (ASMA6) and respiratory diseases (DAR6) in children, respectively.

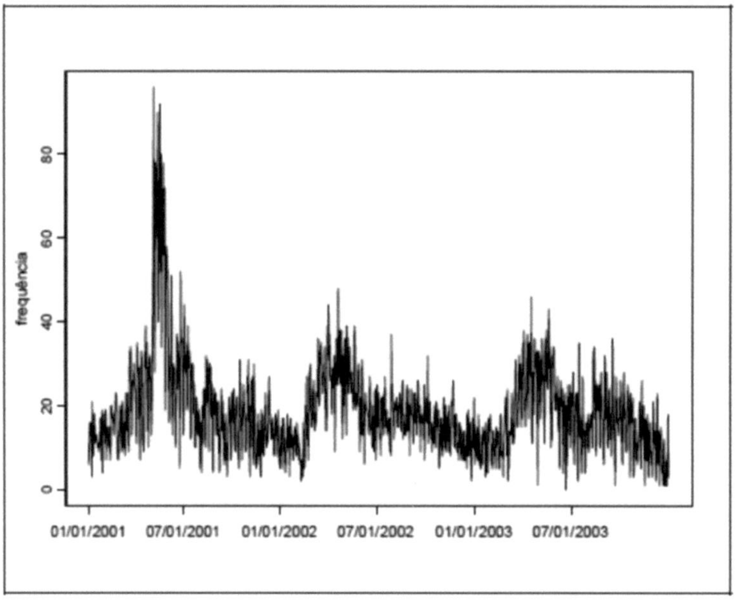

Fig. 2. Counts of daily visits for asthma in children under 6 years

The Figure 3 show the temporal evolution of the daily number of procedures performed in children nebulizer (NEB6).

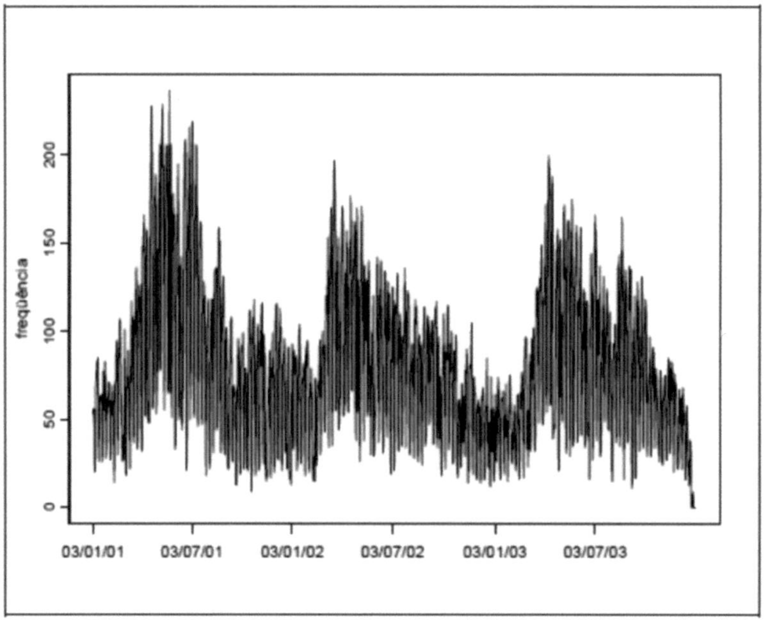

Fig. 3. Counts of daily procedures nebulization in children under 6 years

AIH

Table 2 shows the mean, standard deviation and percentiles for the number of daily hospital admissions for respiratory diseases in children (AIHDAR6), in the city of Victoria. The number of valid observations is 1093.

	mean	SD	min	p5	p10	p25	p50	p75	p90	p95	max
AIHDAR6	2.59	1.83	0.00	0.00	0.00	1.00	2.00	4.00	5.00	6.00	10.00

Table 2. Descriptive statistics of health data AIH

The Figure 4 show the temporal trends of the number of daily hospital admissions for respiratory diseases in children (AIHDAR6).

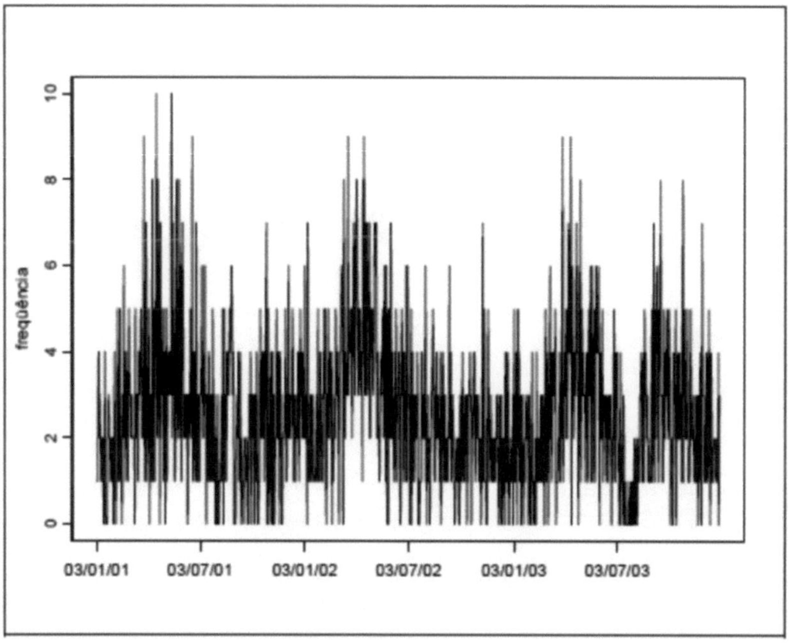

Fig. 4. Counts of daily admissions for respiratory diseases in children under 6 years

Meteorology

Table 3 shows the mean, standard deviation and percentiles for the meteorological variables: minimum temperature, average and maximum (degrees Celsius) and relative humidity (%). The number of valid observations is 1093.

	mean	SD	min	p5	p10	p25	p50	p75	p90	p95	max
Maximum temperature	28.47	3.12	19.65	23.15	24.35	26.05	28.70	30.85	32.55	33.25	35.60
Average temperature	24.17	2.35	17.91	20.41	21.07	22.19	24.28	26.15	27.28	27.66	28.84
Minimum temperature	20.88	2.31	15.00	16.80	17.70	19.00	21.10	22.85	23.70	24.05	25.75
Relative Humidity	77.36	6.01	57.98	68.58	70.26	72.98	77.00	81.45	85.87	88.33	95.63

Table 3. Descriptive statistics of meteorological data

The Figure 5 show the temporal trends of the average daily mean temperature and relative humidity. Each indicator is constructed by averaging the monitors in the city of Victoria.

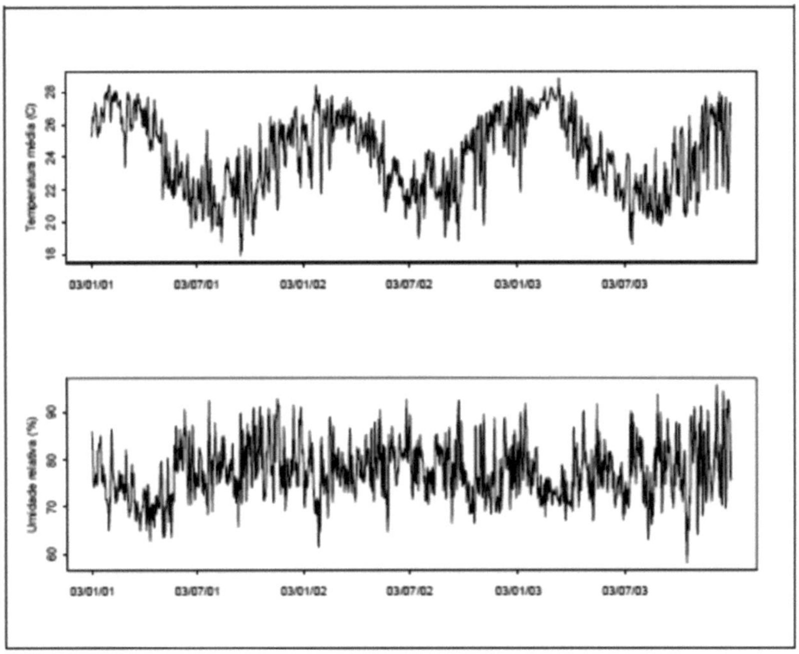

Fig. 5. Mean temperature and daily mean relative humidity for the period 2001- 2003

Pollutants

Table 4 shows the mean, standard deviation and percentiles of the concentrations of PM_{10}, SO_2, NO_2, CO and O_3, in g/m^3. Following imputation, the number of observations used in the analysis was 1093.

	mean	SD	min	p5	p10	p25	p50	p75	p90	p95	max
PM	27.09	6.97	6.50	16.54	18.98	22.65	26.44	30.81	35.31	39.40	60.65
SO2	15.02	6.04	4.10	7.23	8.43	10.50	14.10	18.40	22.91	26.16	47.46
NO2	21.50	7.51	6.54	10.72	12.63	15.96	20.71	26.30	31.84	34.79	53.16
CO	1024.41	381.10	357.63	546.50	620.50	756.00	944.25	1223.75	1496.61	1710.63	3157.00
O3	38.89	13.58	10.25	21.35	23.53	28.50	37.00	46.75	57.25	64.23	97.50

Table 4. Descriptive statistics of the pollution data in the City of Vitoria.

The Figure 6, Figure 7, Figure 8, Figure 9 and Figure 10 show the temporal trends of daily concentrations of PM_{10}, SO_2, NO_2, CO and O_3, respectively. The average concentrations of these pollutants in the city of Victoria was not violated in any day primary or secondary standards for air pollution established by Brazilian CONAMA Resolution 003/90[55].

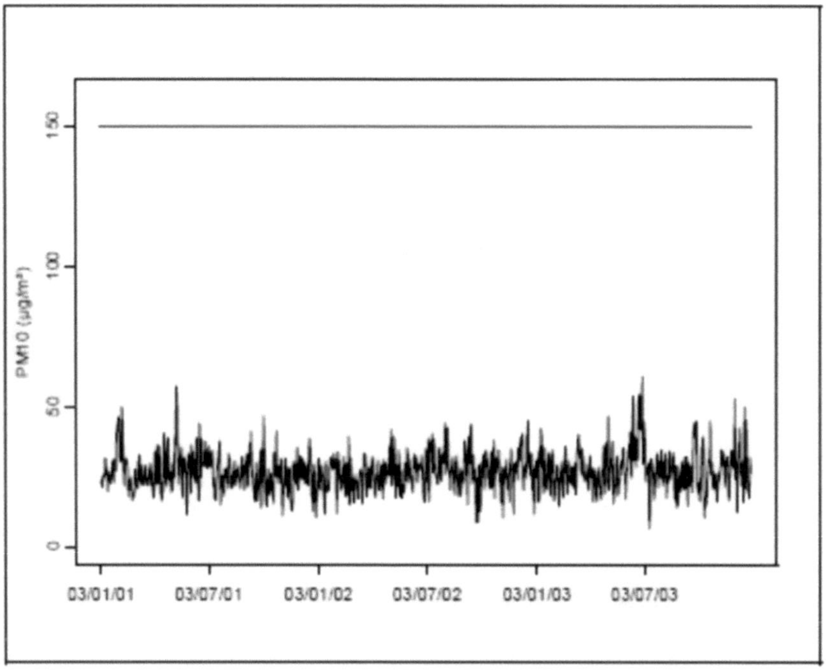

Fig. 6. Daily average concentrations of PM10 in the city of Victoria

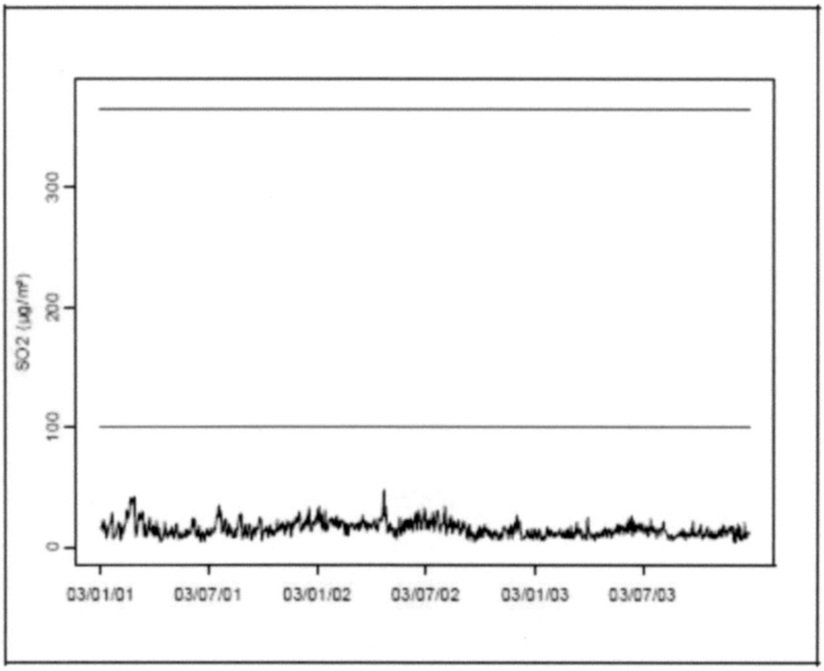

Fig. 7. Daily average concentrations of SO_2 in the city of Victoria

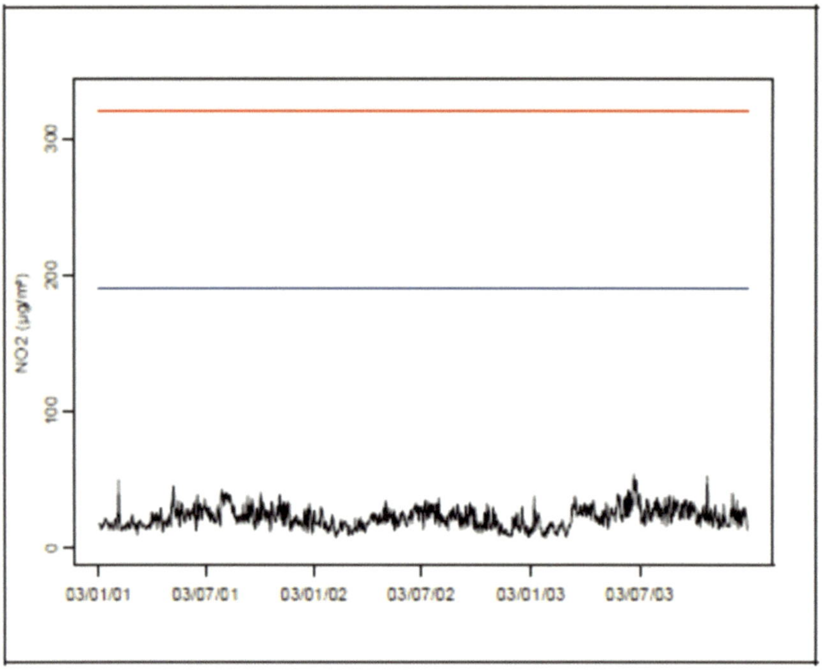

Fig. 8. Daily average concentrations of NO_2 in the city of Victoria

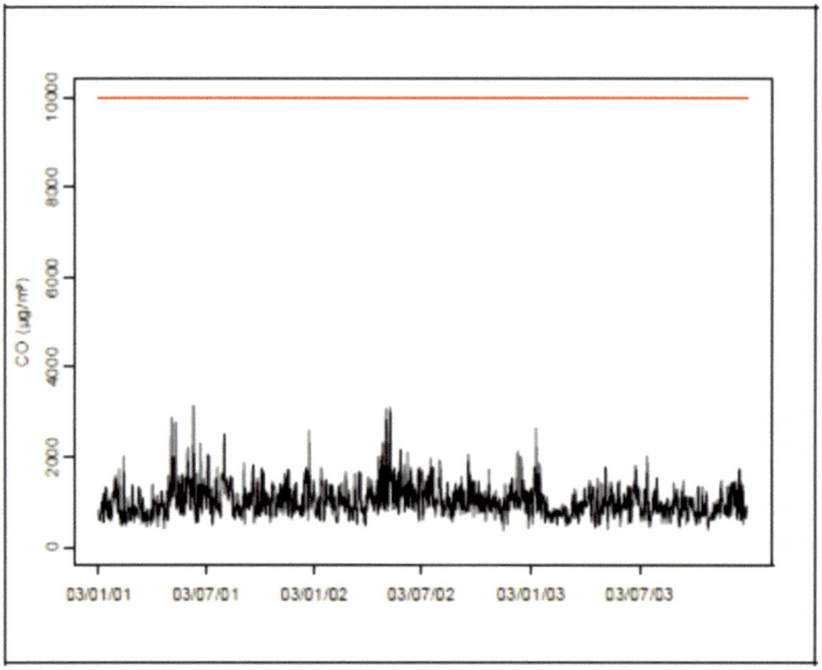

Fig. 9. Daily average concentrations of CO

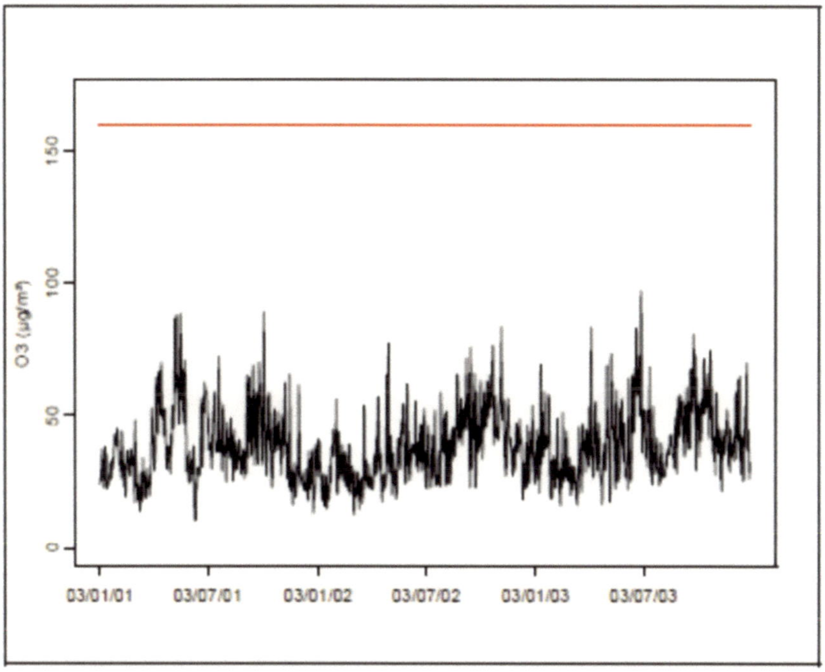

Fig. 10. Daily average concentrations of O_3

3.2 Effects of pollutants

3.2.1 Respiratory diseases

In Table 5 are shown the percentage changes and relative risks with confidence intervals of 95% for the outcome of respiratory diseases in children. We estimated a 2.1% increase in average daily number of outpatients increased to 10 µg / m³ PM_{10} exposure in a cumulative average of 7 days. NO_2 was estimated for a 2.6% increase in the number of attendances outpatients referring to an increase of 10 µg/m³. For O_3 was estimated to increase 1.4% for the exposure with a lag of 3 days and from 1.14% to 1.21% cumulative average exposure for 4-6 days.

Exposição a PM10	%RR	IC (95%)	RR	IC (95%)	p-valor
current day	0.48	-0.821; 1.792	1.00	0.992; 1.018	0.473
lag of 1 day	0.44	-0.839; 1.740	1.00	0.992; 1.017	0.501
lag of 2 days	0.46	-0.859; 1.800	1.00	0.991; 1.018	0.495
lag of 3 days	0.17	-1.106; 1.471	1.00	0.989; 1.015	0.791
average of 2 days	0.66	-0.834; 2.174	1.01	0.992; 1.022	0.389
average of 3 days	0.85	-0.809; 2.544	1.01	0.992; 1.025	0.317
average of 4 days	0.85	-0.926; 2.650	1.01	0.991; 1.027	0.352
average of 5 days	1.22	-0.651; 3.121	1.01	0.993; 1.031	0.203
average of 6 days	1.77	-0.185; 3.769	1.02	0.998; 1.038	0.076
average of 7 days	2.09	0.050; 4.172	1.02	1.001; 1.042	0.045

Exposição a SO2	%RR	IC (95%)	RR	IC (95%)	p-valor
current day	-0.98	-2.429; 0.483	0.99	0.976; 1.005	0.188
lag of 1 day	-0.15	-1.593; 1.313	1.00	0.984; 1.013	0.840
lag of 2 days	-0.08	-1.541; 1.398	1.00	0.985; 1.014	0.912
lag of 3 days	-1.08	-2.568; 0.430	0.99	0.974; 1.004	0.160
average of 2 days	-0.73	-2.298; 0.859	0.99	0.977; 1.009	0.365
average of 3 days	-0.63	-2.295; 1.053	0.99	0.977; 1.011	0.459
average of 4 days	-1.07	-2.813; 0.711	0.99	0.972; 1.007	0.238
average of 5 days	-0.95	-2.765; 0.906	0.99	0.972; 1.009	0.314
average of 6 days	-0.72	-2.602; 1.191	0.99	0.974; 1.012	0.456
average of 7 days	-0.98	-2.900; 0.978	0.99	0.971; 1.010	0.324
Exposição a NO2	%RR	IC (95%)	RR	IC (95%)	p-valor
current day	0.78	-0.528; 2.097	1.01	0.995; 1.021	0.245
lag of 1 day	-0.16	-1.503; 1.207	1.00	0.985; 1.012	0.820
lag of 2 days	0.54	-0.924; 2.023	1.01	0.991; 1.020	0.473
lag of 3 days	0.72	-0.726; 2.185	1.01	0.993; 1.022	0.331
average of 2 days	0.44	-1.031; 1.936	1.00	0.990; 1.019	0.559
average of 3 days	0.67	-0.977; 2.347	1.01	0.990; 1.023	0.427
average of 4 days	0.99	-0.794; 2.807	1.01	0.992; 1.028	0.279
average of 5 days	1.44	-0.439; 3.352	1.01	0.996; 1.034	0.134
average of 6 days	1.92	-0.020; 3.900	1.02	1.000; 1.039	0.053
average of 7 days	2.64	0.645; 4.680	1.03	1.006; 1.047	0.009
Exposição a CO	%RR	IC (95%)	RR	IC (95%)	p-valor
current day	0.00	-0.025; 0.023	1.00	0.975; 1.023	0.935
lag of 1 day	0.01	-0.019; 0.030	1.01	0.981; 1.030	0.669
lag of 2 days	-0.03	-0.049; - 0.004	0.97	0.952; 0.996	0.020
lag of 3 days	-0.02	-0.042; 0.005	0.98	0.959; 1.005	0.119
average of 2 days	0.00	-0.027; 0.033	1.00	0.974; 1.034	0.829
average of 3 days	-0.02	-0.054; 0.014	0.98	0.947; 1.014	0.243
average of 4 days	-0.03	-0.072; 0.003	0.97	0.930; 1.003	0.071
average of 5 days	-0.05	-0.090; - 0.010	0.95	0.914; 0.990	0.015
average of 6 days	-0.06	-0.098; - 0.014	0.95	0.906; 0.986	0.009
average of 7 days	-0.04	-0.085; 0.003	0.96	0.919; 1.003	0.070
Exposição O3	%RR	IC (95%)	RR	IC (95%)	p-valor
current day	0.22	-0.500; 0.953	1.00	0.995; 1.010	0.546
lag of 1 day	0.22	-0.485; 0.926	1.00	0.995; 1.009	0.544
lag of 2 days	0.31	-0.398; 1.032	1.00	0.996; 1.010	0.388
lag of 3 days	1.44	0.740; 2.150	1.01	1.007; 1.022	0.000
average of 2 days	0.32	-0.497; 1.146	1.00	0.995; 1.011	0.442
average of 3 days	0.47	-0.420; 1.363	1.00	0.996; 1.014	0.303
average of 4 days	1.21	0.270; 2.151	1.01	1.003; 1.022	0.012
average of 5 days	1.18	0.212; 2.150	1.01	1.002; 1.022	0.017
average of 6 days	1.14	0.161; 2.128	1.01	1.002; 1.021	0.023
average of 7 days	0.94	-0.052; 1.937	1.01	0.999; 1.019	0.064

Table 5. Percentage change and relative risks for care per DAR6

Asthma

In Table 6, the estimated effects for the outcome of asthma in children. Estimated to increase from 3.9% to 6.1% in the average daily number of outpatients increased to 10 µg / m³ PM10 in an average cumulative exposure ranging from 4 to 7 days. NO2 was estimated for a 2.9% increase in the number of outpatient visits related to an increase of 10 µg / m³ exposure lagged 3 days and 3.7% to 5.8% for the cumulative exposure of 3 to 7 days. The effect of CO is less than 0.1%, very small although statistically significant. For O3 was estimated to increase 1.8% for the exhibition on the same day and from 2% to 3.5% cumulative average exposure for 2-7 days.

Exposição a PM10	%RR	IC (95%)	RR	IC (95%)	p-valor
current day	0.57	-2.027; 3.235	1.01	0.980; 1.032	0.670
lag of 1 day	2.51	-0.078; 5.158	1.03	0.999; 1.052	0.058
lag of 2 days	2.06	-0.486; 4.673	1.02	0.995; 1.047	0.114
lag of 3 days	2.10	-0.462; 4.720	1.02	0.995; 1.047	0.109
average of 2 days	2.22	-0.786; 5.325	1.02	0.992; 1.053	0.149
average of 3 days	3.10	-0.195; 6.511	1.03	0.998; 1.065	0.066
average of 4 days	3.89	0.346; 7.550	1.04	1.003; 1.076	0.031
average of 5 days	4.98	1.213; 8.884	1.05	1.012; 1.089	0.009
average of 6 days	6.10	2.139; 10.219	1.06	1.021; 1.102	0.002
average of 7 days	5.92	1.797; 10.206	1.06	1.018; 1.102	0.005
Exposição a SO2	%RR	IC (95%)	RR	IC (95%)	p-valor
current day	-2.33	-5.123; 0.551	0.98	0.949; 1.006	0.112
lag of 1 day	-1.55	-4.373; 1.365	0.98	0.956; 1.014	0.295
lag of 2 days	-3.33	-6.129; - 0.442	0.97	0.939; 0.996	0.024
lag of 3 days	-5.02	-7.824; - 2.122	0.95	0.922; 0.979	0.001
average of 2 days	-2.47	-5.492; 0.653	0.98	0.945; 1.007	0.120
average of 3 days	-3.66	-6.842; - 0.379	0.96	0.932; 0.996	0.029
average of 4 days	-5.32	-8.603; - 1.927	0.95	0.914; 0.981	0.002
average of 5 days	-6.13	-9.512; - 2.632	0.94	0.905; 0.974	0.001
average of 6 days	-6.37	-9.828; - 2.777	0.94	0.902; 0.972	0.001
average of 7 days	-7.28	-10.794; - 3.625	0.93	0.892; 0.964	0.000
Exposição a NO2	%RR	IC (95%)	RR	IC (95%)	p-valor
current day	1.94	-0.947; 4.915	1.02	0.991; 1.049	0.190
lag of 1 day	2.64	-0.330; 5.694	1.03	0.997; 1.057	0.082
lag of 2 days	1.71	-1.102; 4.599	1.02	0.989; 1.046	0.236
lag of 3 days	2.90	0.143; 5.739	1.03	1.001; 1.057	0.039
average of 2 days	3.27	-0.069; 6.711	1.03	0.999; 1.067	0.055
average of 3 days	3.71	0.118; 7.428	1.04	1.001; 1.074	0.043
average of 4 days	4.86	1.067; 8.788	1.05	1.011; 1.088	0.012
average of 5 days	4.82	0.928; 8.871	1.05	1.009; 1.089	0.015
average of 6 days	5.07	1.079; 9.217	1.05	1.011; 1.092	0.012
average of 7 days	5.78	1.689; 10.031	1.06	1.017; 1.100	0.005

Exposição a CO	%RR	IC (95%)	RR	IC (95%)	p-valor
current day	0.03	-0.020; 0.074	1.03	0.981; 1.076	0.256
lag of 1 day	0.06	0.018; 0.111	1.07	1.018; 1.117	0.007
lag of 2 days	-0.01	-0.058; 0.028	0.99	0.943; 1.029	0.502
lag of 3 days	0.01	-0.035; 0.052	1.01	0.966; 1.054	0.691
average of 2 days	0.08	0.020; 0.137	1.08	1.020; 1.147	0.009
average of 3 days	0.06	-0.010; 0.121	1.06	0.990; 1.129	0.097
average of 4 days	0.06	-0.011; 0.133	1.06	0.989; 1.143	0.099
average of 5 days	0.05	-0.026; 0.129	1.05	0.974; 1.138	0.196
average of 6 days	0.02	-0.060; 0.104	1.02	0.941; 1.110	0.602
average of 7 days	0.07	-0.018; 0.155	1.07	0.982; 1.167	0.120
Exposição O3	%RR	IC (95%)	RR	IC (95%)	p-valor
current day	1.76	0.331; 3.205	1.02	1.003; 1.032	0.016
lag of 1 day	1.07	-0.321; 2.479	1.01	0.997; 1.025	0.132
lag of 2 days	1.02	-0.324; 2.384	1.01	0.997; 1.024	0.138
lag of 3 days	2.56	1.222; 3.912	1.03	1.012; 1.039	0.000
average of 2 days	2.00	0.389; 3.643	1.02	1.004; 1.036	0.015
average of 3 days	2.20	0.491; 3.944	1.02	1.005; 1.039	0.012
average of 4 days	3.21	1.426; 5.034	1.03	1.014; 1.050	0.000
average of 5 days	3.45	1.610; 5.321	1.03	1.016; 1.053	0.000
average of 6 days	3.34	1.470; 5.244	1.03	1.015; 1.052	0.000
average of 7 days	3.20	1.305; 5.130	1.03	1.013; 1.051	0.001

Table 6. Percentage change and relative risks for care per ASMA6

Table 7 Estimated effects for the outcome nebulization in children. We estimated an increase of 2% and 2.3% for the exhibition on the same day and with a lag of 3 days respectively, and 3.1% to 3.6% for the cumulative exposure from 4 to 7 days in the average number daily for an increase of 10 μg/m³ PM_{10}. For NO_2 was estimated to increase from 2.9% to the cumulative exposure of 7 days. For O_3 was estimated to increase from 1.8% to the exposure with a lag of 2 days and 1.4% cumulative average exposure for 4 days.

Exposição a PM10	%RR	IC (95%)	RR	IC (95%)	p-valor
current day	1.98	0.043; 3.957	1.02	1.000; 1.040	0.045
lag of 1 day	0.21	-1.713; 2.173	1.00	0.983; 1.022	0.831
lag of 2 days	1.46	-0.435; 3.401	1.01	0.996; 1.034	0.132
lag of 3 days	2.31	0.426; 4.236	1.02	1.004; 1.042	0.016
average of 2 days	1.50	-0.750; 3.792	1.01	0.993; 1.038	0.194
average of 3 days	2.11	-0.342; 4.625	1.02	0.997; 1.046	0.093
average of 4 days	3.14	0.515; 5.826	1.03	1.005; 1.058	0.019
average of 5 days	3.59	0.823; 6.430	1.04	1.008; 1.064	0.011
average of 6 days	3.63	0.742; 6.607	1.04	1.007; 1.066	0.014
average of 7 days	3.36	0.354; 6.452	1.03	1.004; 1.065	0.028

Exposição a SO2	RR	IC (95%)	RR	IC (95%)	p-valor
current day	-0.57	-2.673; 1.585	0.99	0.973; 1.016	0.603
lag of 1 day	-0.92	-3.000; 1.203	0.99	0.970; 1.012	0.393
lag of 2 days	-0.60	-2.691; 1.530	0.99	0.973; 1.015	0.577
lag of 3 days	-0.35	-2.487; 1.831	1.00	0.975; 1.018	0.750
average of 2 days	-0.96	-3.226; 1.349	0.99	0.968; 1.013	0.411
average of 3 days	-1.09	-3.478; 1.348	0.99	0.965; 1.013	0.377
average of 4 days	-1.11	-3.608; 1.445	0.99	0.964; 1.014	0.390
average of 5 days	-1.38	-3.956; 1.269	0.99	0.960; 1.013	0.305
average of 6 days	-2.07	-4.717; 0.641	0.98	0.953; 1.006	0.133
average of 7 days	-2.77	-5.462; - 0.011	0.97	0.945; 1.000	0.049
Exposição a NO2	%RR	IC (95%)	RR	IC (95%)	p-valor
current day	0.82	-1.258; 2.932	1.01	0.987; 1.029	0.444
lag of 1 day	1.59	-0.549; 3.772	1.02	0.995; 1.038	0.147
lag of 2 days	1.71	-0.342; 3.808	1.02	0.997; 1.038	0.103
lag of 3 days	1.63	-0.370; 3.663	1.02	0.996; 1.037	0.111
average of 2 days	1.62	-0.751; 4.042	1.02	0.992; 1.040	0.183
average of 3 days	2.38	-0.177; 4.996	1.02	0.998; 1.050	0.069
average of 4 days	2.93	0.247; 5.684	1.03	1.002; 1.057	0.032
average of 5 days	2.60	-0.155; 5.427	1.03	0.998; 1.054	0.065
average of 6 days	2.57	-0.262; 5.476	1.03	0.997; 1.055	0.076
average of 7 days	2.36	-0.529; 5.340	1.02	0.995; 1.053	0.111
Exposição a CO	%RR	IC (95%)	RR	IC (95%)	p-valor
current day	0.00	-0.030; 0.040	1.00	0.971; 1.040	0.781
lag of 1 day	0.00	-0.036; 0.036	1.00	0.964; 1.037	0.990
lag of 2 days	0.02	-0.018; 0.050	1.02	0.982; 1.051	0.356
lag of 3 days	-0.03	-0.063; 0.003	0.97	0.939; 1.003	0.079
average of 2 days	0.00	-0.040; 0.048	1.00	0.961; 1.049	0.860
average of 3 days	0.02	-0.034; 0.066	1.02	0.966; 1.069	0.529
average of 4 days	-0.01	-0.061; 0.049	0.99	0.941; 1.051	0.837
average of 5 days	0.00	-0.057; 0.062	1.00	0.945; 1.064	0.937
average of 6 days	-0.01	-0.069; 0.056	0.99	0.934; 1.058	0.844
average of 7 days	-0.02	-0.082; 0.046	0.98	0.921; 1.047	0.584
Exposição O3	%RR	IC (95%)	RR	IC (95%)	p-valor
current day	0.38	-0.670; 1.432	1.00	0.993; 1.014	0.483
lag of 1 day	-0.44	-1.502; 0.642	1.00	0.985; 1.006	0.427
lag of 2 days	1.82	0.803; 2.842	1.02	1.008; 1.028	0.000
lag of 3 days	0.99	-0.003; 1.990	1.01	1.000; 1.020	0.051
average of 2 days	-0.05	-1.252; 1.174	1.00	0.987; 1.012	0.940
average of 3 days	1.05	-0.234; 2.358	1.01	0.998; 1.024	0.110
average of 4 days	1.40	0.071; 2.755	1.01	1.001; 1.028	0.039
average of 5 days	1.06	-0.299; 2.434	1.01	0.997; 1.024	0.127
average of 6 days	0.92	-0.451; 2.307	1.01	0.995; 1.023	0.190
average of 7 days	0.87	-0.515; 2.281	1.01	0.995; 1.023	0.219

Table 7. Percentage change and risks relating to procedures NEB6

Hospitalizations

Table 8 Estimated effects presented for the outcome of hospital admissions of children. Statistically significant effect was found only for O_3. Estimated to increase by 3.2% and 4% for exposure lagged by 1 and 3 days, respectively, and 4.3% to 7.9% average cumulative exposure for 2-7 days, referring to an increase of 10 µg/m³ of O_3. Despite the impact of high frequency of occurrence of this outcome in the population is low.

Exposição a PM10	%RR	IC (95%)	RR	IC (95%)	p-valor
current day	1.06	-4.675; 7.133	1.01	0.953; 1.071	0.724
lag of 1 day	3.14	-2.755; 9.390	1.03	0.972; 1.094	0.303
lag of 2 days	1.00	-4.845; 7.208	1.01	0.952; 1.072	0.743
lag of 3 days	1.32	-4.410; 7.388	1.01	0.956; 1.074	0.659
average of 2 days	3.00	-3.793; 10.263	1.03	0.962; 1.103	0.396
average of 3 days	3.13	-4.398; 11.259	1.03	0.956; 1.113	0.425
average of 4 days	3.44	-4.569; 12.121	1.03	0.954; 1.121	0.411
average of 5 days	3.90	-4.539; 13.076	1.04	0.955; 1.131	0.377
average of 6 days	5.46	-3.481; 15.219	1.05	0.965; 1.152	0.240
average of 7 days	6.00	-3.351; 16.262	1.06	0.966; 1.163	0.216
Exposição a SO2	%RR	IC (95%)	RR	IC (95%)	p-valor
current day	2.09	-4.161; 8.739	1.02	0.958; 1.087	0.522
lag of 1 day	1.33	-4.870; 7.928	1.01	0.951; 1.079	0.682
lag of 2 days	3.27	-3.026; 9.975	1.03	0.970; 1.100	0.316
lag of 3 days	-2.76	-8.797; 3.667	0.97	0.912; 1.037	0.391
average of 2 days	2.16	-4.583; 9.384	1.02	0.954; 1.094	0.540
average of 3 days	3.37	-3.795; 11.069	1.03	0.962; 1.111	0.366
average of 4 days	1.69	-5.663; 9.609	1.02	0.943; 1.096	0.662
average of 5 days	1.31	-6.257; 9.498	1.01	0.937; 1.095	0.742
average of 6 days	-0.32	-8.006; 8.000	1.00	0.920; 1.080	0.937
average of 7 days	-0.96	-8.780; 7.536	0.99	0.912; 1.075	0.819
Exposição a NO2	%RR	IC (95%)	RR	IC (95%)	p-valor
current day	0.26	-5.870; 6.780	1.00	0.941; 1.068	0.937
lag of 1 day	5.53	-0.834; 12.299	1.06	0.992; 1.123	0.090
lag of 2 days	0.45	-5.609; 6.888	1.00	0.944; 1.069	0.889
lag of 3 days	2.28	-3.649; 8.584	1.02	0.964; 1.086	0.459
average of 2 days	3.86	-3.184; 11.408	1.04	0.968; 1.114	0.291
average of 3 days	3.39	-4.088; 11.454	1.03	0.959; 1.115	0.384
average of 4 days	4.09	-3.740; 12.563	1.04	0.963; 1.126	0.315
average of 5 days	2.87	-5.068; 11.474	1.03	0.949; 1.115	0.490
average of 6 days	3.28	-4.869; 12.118	1.03	0.951; 1.121	0.442
average of 7 days	3.22	-5.076; 12.247	1.03	0.949; 1.122	0.458

Exposição a CO	%RR	IC (95%)	RR	IC (95%)	p-valor
current day	-0.06	-0.159; 0.044	0.94	0.853; 1.045	0.270
lag of 1 day	-0.02	-0.126; 0.076	0.98	0.882; 1.079	0.630
lag of 2 days	-0.02	-0.125; 0.083	0.98	0.883; 1.086	0.692
lag of 3 days	-0.09	-0.195; 0.013	0.91	0.823; 1.013	0.086
average of 2 days	-0.07	-0.189; 0.058	0.94	0.828; 1.060	0.300
average of 3 days	-0.08	-0.217; 0.066	0.93	0.804; 1.068	0.295
average of 4 days	-0.14	-0.298; 0.017	0.87	0.742; 1.017	0.081
average of 5 days	-0.19	-0.360; - 0.020	0.83	0.697; 0.981	0.029
average of 6 days	-0.20	-0.379; - 0.020	0.82	0.684; 0.980	0.030
average of 7 days	-0.17	-0.352; 0.020	0.85	0.703; 1.021	0.081
Exposição O3	**%RR**	**IC (95%)**	**RR**	**IC (95%)**	**p-valor**
current day	3.02	-0.010; 6.145	1.03	1.000; 1.061	0.051
lag of 1 day	3.22	0.159; 6.379	1.03	1.002; 1.064	0.039
lag of 2 days	2.99	-0.076; 6.154	1.03	0.999; 1.062	0.056
lag of 3 days	4.04	1.053; 7.124	1.04	1.011; 1.071	0.008
average of 2 days	4.35	0.864; 7.963	1.04	1.009; 1.080	0.014
average of 3 days	5.30	1.510; 9.233	1.05	1.015; 1.092	0.006
average of 4 days	6.55	2.580; 10.667	1.07	1.026; 1.107	0.001
average of 5 days	7.34	3.257; 11.594	1.07	1.033; 1.116	0.000
average of 6 days	7.94	3.783; 12.261	1.08	1.038; 1.123	0.000
average of 7 days	7.91	3.699; 12.294	1.08	1.037; 1.123	0.000

Table 8. Percentage change and relative risks for hospitalizations DAR6

4. Conclusion

Descriptive analysis of indicators of air pollution in the city of Victoria shows that, on average, these indicators did not exceed the primary standard or secondary air quality proposed by the World Health Organization (WHO) and by CONAMA 003/90[55]. However, even when the pollution levels are considered acceptable, it was possible to detect adverse health effects of some pollution indicators studied. These deleterious effects are observed on increasing the average daily number of outpatient procedures, hospitalizations in the mist and more susceptible populations, children residents in the city of Victoria.

The results of this study indicate the existence of statistical association between daily concentrations of air pollutants and daily average number of outpatient procedures, hospitalizations and mist in populations of children residents in the city of Victoria. This finding implies that some of these illnesses tracks stocks in the region may have been caused by air pollution. The pollutants whose effects were statistically significant were the PM_{10}, O_3 and NO_2.

The frequency of occurrence of hospital admissions in the population of the city of victory is very low, as shown in Table 2, and therefore, effects of great magnitude had low impact on the population.

The damage to the respiratory system due to exposure to air pollutants is the result of combined effects of all pollutants present in complex mix of air pollution. The results associated with PM_{10} and O_3 are consistent with the pathophysiology of these two pollutants. Both in an early act as primary irritant of the respiratory tract and may cause increased bronchial reactivity and symptoms of bronchospasm. Local inflammatory signs emerge that usually prevail over those of bronchospasm[61]. The combination of possible respiratory effects at two different times may explain a greater number of medical visits on the same day and some days after the increase in the levels of pollutants.

In studies whose outcome variable is the pediatric emergency medical care, considering lags of one or more days between exposure and demand for health services, several factors must be considered. One is the motivation of parents or guardians to seek pediatric clinics that depends, among other reasons, concern about the health of the child[57], the knowledge of the meanings and possible worsening of respiratory signs and symptoms and also the possibility to attend a health facility.

The clinical effects of environmental pollutants on the respiratory system vary according to factors related to the pollutants and exposed individuals. Children less sensitive when exposed to low environmental concentrations have mild symptoms and few clinical implications and do not require medical attention. It is reasonable to assume that the estimated effect is smaller than one would estimate that if these children had sought a health service. With low levels of air pollution observed was not expected a high number of severe cases, but a large number of milder cases.

The results of this study are consistent with those of studies conducted in other cities in the world using similar methodology. However, the health information system used, the Unified Productivity Bulletin (BUP) available in the city of Victoria, have not been fully validated. It is therefore necessary to consider that bias resulting from lack of validity of information may be operating in the study population. It is therefore reasonable to consider that the accuracy of this study is subject to a validation study of BUP.

5. Acknowledgments

This study received financial support from the Strategic Development Program at the Sergio Arouca National School of Public Health, Oswaldo Cruz Foundation (ENSP/FIOCRUZ), in partnership with the Vitória Municipal Health Secretaria. The State Environmental Secretariat (SEAMA) and State Environmental Institute (IEMA) provided the air quality database, with technical support from Nilson Castiglioni Júnior and José Gustavo da Costa. The authors wish to acknowledge the logistic field support provided by the State Health Secretariat through Maria de Fátima Bertollo Dettoni and Diana de Oliveira Frauches. The authors also acknowledge the collaboration and technical support from the Health Surveillance Secretariat of the Brazilian Ministry of Health.

6. References

[1] Dockery DW, Schwartz J, Spengler JD. Air pollution and daily mortality: associations with particulates and acid aerosols. Environ Res 1992; 59(2):362-373.

[2] Dockery DW, Pope CA, III, Xu X, Spengler JD, Ware JH, Fay ME et al. An association between air pollution and mortality in six U.S. cities. N Engl J Med 1993; 329(24):1753-1759.

[3] Pope CA, Thun MJ, Namboodiri MM, Dockery DW, Evans JS, Speizer FE et al. Particulate Air-Pollution As A Predictor of Mortality in A Prospective-Study of Us Adults. Am J Respir Crit Care Med 1995; 151(3):669-674.
[4] Sartor F, Snacken R, Demuth C, Walckiers D. Temperature, ambient ozone levels, and mortality during summer 1994, in Belgium. Environ Res 1995; 70(2):105-113.
[5] Schwartz J. Particulate air pollution and daily mortality in Detroit. Environ Res 1991; 56(2):204-213.
[6] Schwartz J, Dockery DW. Increased mortality in Philadelphia associated with daily air pollution concentrations. Am Rev Respir Dis 1992; 145(3):600-604.
[7] Schwartz J. Air pollution and daily mortality in Birmingham, Alabama. Am J Epidemiol 1993; 137(10):1136-1147.
[8] Spix C, Wichmann HE. Daily mortality and air pollutants: findings from Koln, Germany. J Epidemiol Community Health 1996; 50 Suppl 1:s52-s58.
[9] Touloumi G, Samoli E, Katsouyanni K. Daily mortality and "winter type" air pollution in Athens, Greece--a time series analysis within the APHEA project. J Epidemiol Community Health 1996; 50 Suppl 1:s47-s51.
[10] Ballester F, Corella D, Perez-Hoyos S, Hervas A. Air pollution and mortality in Valencia, Spain: a study using the APHEA methodology. J Epidemiol Community Health 1996; 50(5):527-533.
[11] Borja-Aburto VH, Loomis DP, Bangdiwala SI, Shy CM, Rascon-Pacheco RA. Ozone, suspended particulates, and daily mortality in Mexico City. Am J Epidemiol 1997; 145(3):258-268.
[12] Dockery DW, Pope CA. Acute Respiratory Effects of Particulate Air-Pollution. Annual Review of Public Health 1994; 15:107-132.
[13] Pope CA, Schwartz J, Ransom MR. Daily Mortality and Pm(10) Pollution in Utah Valley. Archives of Environmental Health 1992; 47(3):211-217.
[14] Schwartz J, Dockery DW. Particulate air pollution and daily mortality in Steubenville, Ohio. Am J Epidemiol 1992; 135(1):12-19.
[15] Schwartz J. Total suspended particulate matter and daily mortality in Cincinnati, Ohio. Environ Health Perspect 1994; 102(2):186-189.
[16] Sunyer J, Castellsague J, Saez M, Tobias A, Anto JM. Air pollution and mortality in Barcelona. J Epidemiol Community Health 1996; 50 Suppl 1:s76-s80.
[17] Fairley D. The relationship of daily mortality to suspended particulates in Santa Clara County, 1980-1986. Environ Health Perspect 1990; 89:159-168.
[18] Schwartz J. What are people dying of on high air pollution days? Environ Res 1994; 64(1):26-35.
[19] Anderson HR, Ponce dL, Bland JM, Bower JS, Strachan DP. Air pollution and daily mortality in London: 1987-92. BMJ 1996; 312(7032):665-669.
[20] Braun-Fahrlander C, Ackermann-Liebrich U, Schwartz J, Gnehm HP, Rutishauser M, Wanner HU. Air pollution and respiratory symptoms in preschool children. Am Rev Respir Dis 1992; 145(1):42-47.
[21] Pope CA, Dockery DW. Acute Health-Effects of PM10 Pollution on Symptomatic and Asymptomatic Children. American Review of Respiratory Disease 1992; 145(5):1123-1128.

[22] Roemer W, Hoek G, Brunekreef B. Effect of ambient winter air pollution on respiratory health of children with chronic respiratory symptoms. Am Rev Respir Dis 1993; 147(1):118-124.
[23] Hoek G, Brunekreef B. Acute effects of a winter air pollution episode on pulmonary function and respiratory symptoms of children. Arch Environ Health 1993; 48(5):328-335.
[24] Dockery DW, Speizer FE, Stram DO, Ware JH, Spengler JD, Ferris BG, Jr. Effects of inhalable particles on respiratory health of children. Am Rev Respir Dis 1989; 139(3):587-594.
[25] Jaakkola JJ, Paunio M, Virtanen M, Heinonen OP. Low-level air pollution and upper respiratory infections in children. Am J Public Health 1991; 81(8):1060-1063.
[26] Ransom MR, Pope CA. Elementary-School Absences and Pm(10) Pollution in Utah Valley. Environmental Research 1992; 58(2):204-219.
[27] Romieu I, Lugo MC, Velasco SR, Sanchez S, Meneses F, Hernandez M. Air pollution and school absenteeism among children in Mexico City. Am J Epidemiol 1992; 136(12):1524-1531.
[28] Bates DV, Sizto R. Relationship between air pollutant levels and hospital admissions in Southern Ontario. Can J Public Health 1983; 74(2):117-122.
[29] Burnett RT, Dales R, Krewski D, Vincent R, Dann T, Brook JR. Associations between ambient particulate sulfate and admissions to Ontario hospitals for cardiac and respiratory diseases. Am J Epidemiol 1995; 142(1):15-22.
[30] Burnett RT, Dales RE, Raizenne ME, Krewski D, Summers PW, Roberts GR et al. Effects of low ambient levels of ozone and sulfates on the frequency of respiratory admissions to Ontario hospitals. Environ Res 1994; 65(2):172-194.
[31] Ponce dL, Anderson HR, Bland JM, Strachan DP, Bower J. Effects of air pollution on daily hospital admissions for respiratory disease in London between 1987-88 and 1991-92. J Epidemiol Community Health 1996; 50 Suppl 1:s63-s70.
[32] Pope CA. Respiratory-Disease Associated with Community Air-Pollution and A Steel Mill, Utah Valley. American Journal of Public Health 1989; 79(5):623-628.
[33] Pope CA, Dockery DW, Spengler JD, Raizenne ME. Respiratory Health and PM10 Pollution - A Daily Time-Series Analysis. American Review of Respiratory Disease 1991; 144(3):668-674.
[34] Schwartz J. Air pollution and hospital admissions for respiratory disease. Epidemiology 1996; 7(1):20-28.
[35] Hagen JA, Nafstad P, Skrondal A, Bjorkly S, Magnus P. Associations between outdoor air pollutants and hospitalization for respiratory diseases. Epidemiology 2000; 11(2):136-140.
[36] Kotesovec F, Skorkovsky J, Brynda J, Peters A, Heinrich J. Daily mortality and air pollution in northern Bohemia: different effects for men and women. Cent Eur J Public Health 2000; 8(2):120-127.
[37] Zanobetti A, Schwartz J. Race, gender, and social status as modifiers of the effects of PM_{10} on mortality. J Occup Environ Med 2000; 42(5):469-474.
[38] Cohen AJ, Pope CA, Speizer FE. Ambient air pollution as a risk factor for lung cancer. Salud Publica de Mexico 1997; 39(4):346-355.

[39] Dean G. Lung cancer and bronchitis in Northern Ireland, 1960-2. Br Med J 1966; 5502:1506-1514.

[40] Penna MLF, Dulchiade M. Air pollution and infant mortality from pneumonia in the Rio de Janeiro metropolitan area. Bulletin of PAHO 1991; 25(1):47-54.

[41] Saldiva PH, Lichtenfels AJ, Paiva PS, Barone IA, Martins MA, Massad E et al. Association between air pollution and mortality due to respiratory diseases in children in Sao Paulo, Brazil: a preliminary report. Environ Res 1994; 65(2):218-225.

[42] Saldiva PHN, Pope CA, Schwartz J, Dockery DW, Lichtenfels AJ, Salge JM et al. Air-Pollution and Mortality in Elderly People - A Time-Series Study in Sao-Paulo, Brazil. Archives of Environmental Health 1995; 50(2):159-163.

[43] Pereira LA, Loomis D, Conceicao GM, Braga AL, Arcas RM, Kishi HS et al. Association between air pollution and intrauterine mortality in Sao Paulo, Brazil. Environ Health Perspect 1998; 106(6):325-329.

[44] Sobral HR. Air pollution and respiratory diseases in children in Sao Paulo, Brazil. Soc Sci Med 1989; 29(8):959-964.

[45] Spektor DM, Hofmeister VA, Artaxo P, Brague JA, Echelar F, Nogueira DP et al. Effects of heavy industrial pollution on respiratory function in the children of Cubatao, Brazil: a preliminary report. Environ Health Perspect 1991; 94:51-54.

[46] Rumel D, Riedel LF, Latorre MR, Duncan BB. [Myocardial infarct and cerebral vascular disorders associated with high temperature and carbon monoxide in a metropolitan area of southeastern Brazil]. Rev Saude Publica 1993; 27(1):15-22.

[47] Reymao MS, Cury PM, Lichtenfels AJ, Lemos M, Battlehner CN, Conceicao GM et al. Urban air pollution enhances the formation of urethane-induced lung tumors in mice. Environ Res 1997; 74(2):150-158.

[48] Gouveia N, Fletcher T. Time series analysis of air pollution and mortality: effects by cause, age and socioeconomic status. J Epidemiol Community Health 2000; 54(10):750-755.

[49] Gouveia N, Fletcher T. Respiratory diseases in children and outdoor air pollution in Sao Paulo, Brazil: a time series analysis. Occup Environ Med 2000; 57(7):477-483.

[50] Available at: http://www.ipes.es.gov.br/

[51] Available at: http://www.vitoria.es.gov.br/negocios/investe.htm/

[52] Available at: http://www.vitoria.es.gov.br/

[53] Hastie T, Tibshirani R. Generalized Additive Models. London: Chapman and Hall, 1990.

[54] McCullagh P, Nelder J.A. Generalized Linear Models. 2 ed. London: Chapman and Hall, 1989.

[55] Zeger LS. A regression model for time series of counts. Biometrika 1988; 75(4):621-629.

[56] Martins LC, Latorre MR, Cardoso MR, Goncalves FL, Saldiva PH, Braga AL. [Air pollution and emergency room visits due to pneumonia and influenza in Sao Paulo, Brazil]. Rev Saude Publica 2002; 36(1):88-94.

[57] Hernandez-Cadena L, Tellez-Rojo MM, Sanin-Aguirre LH, Lacasana-Navarro M, Campos A, Romieu I. [Relationship between emergency consultations for respiratory diseases and air pollution in Juarez City, Chihuahua]. Salud Publica Mex 2000; 42(4):288-297.

[58] Ostro BD, Eskeland GS, Sanchez JM, Feyzioglu T. Air pollution and health effects: A study of medical visits among children in Santiago, Chile. Environ Health Perspect 1999; 107(1):69-73.

5

Tobacco Smoke Induced Cough: Mechanisms Driving Acute and Chronic Cough Pathology

Megan S Grace, Mark A Birrell, Eric Dubuis and Maria G Belvisi
Respiratory Pharmacology Group, NHLI, Imperial College London
United Kingdom

1. Introduction

Cough is an important protective mechanism that clears foreign material from the airway and aids in immune defence. However, chronic excessive cough of various aetiologies is a common presentation to specialist respiratory clinics, and is reported as a troublesome symptom by a significant proportion of the population (Ford et al., 2006). In extreme situations chronic cough can persist for several years, and is not only socially embarrassing, but can be painful and debilitating. Chronic cough is often associated with an underlying respiratory disease, several of which can be caused or exacerbated by exposure to tobacco smoke or environmental pollution, for example chronic obstructive pulmonary disease (COPD), emphysema, bronchitis, lung cancer and asthma. In addition, chronic cough can be of unknown cause (idiopathic) (Morice et al., 2007). Recently, the label chronic 'cough hypersensitivity syndrome' (CCHS) was proposed as a means of focussing the cough community and general practitioners on the symptomology of cough and understanding of the mechanisms behind cough sensation, with the ultimate goal of developing effective anti-tussive treatments (Millqvist et al., 1998; Chung, 2011).

At present, little is known about the mechanisms that drive the cough reflex, and even less about how these mechanisms are altered to lead to chronic cough. Numerous environmental irritants are known to induce coughing such as air pollution, tobacco smoke, smoke from burning vegetation, and vehicle exhaust. This chapter focuses on tobacco smoke (TS), which is one of the most common inhaled irritants (both as an active smoker, and as a secondary environmental pollutant), and is known to contain thousands of noxious chemicals (U.S. Department of Health and Human Services, 2010). Exposure to acute TS readily evokes coughing in both animals and human non-smokers (Andre et al., 2009; Lee et al., 1993; Lee et al., 2007), and prolonged exposure to TS can lead to an altered sensitivity to a range of tussive stimuli (Karlsson et al., 1991; Doherty et al., 2000; Bergren, 2001; Dicpinigaitis, 2003; Lewis et al., 2007). It is believed that if the mechanisms behind acute or chronic cough associated with TS exposure can be revealed it would lead to the development of truly effective cough therapies. The aim of this chapter is to discuss the current understanding of how exposure to TS can cause/alter the cough response and we will consider some of the most promising new therapeutic targets for the treatment of cough.

2. Cough: An overview

2.1 Background

Under normal conditions, cough is an important protective mechanism that clears foreign material from the airways and aids in immune defence (Fontana et al., 1999). Despite this, even an acute cough can be unpleasant and painful for the sufferer. It is therefore not surprising that cough is the most frequent reason for which patients consult with their family doctor or a general or respiratory physician (McCormick et al., 1995); and that antitussives are among the most widely used over-the-counter self medication therapies. In contrast to acute cough, chronic cough of various aetiologies often has no functional consequence, and can lead to a dramatic decrease in quality of life (Irwin et al., 1998; Morice et al., 2007). Chronic cough is defined as a cough which persists for longer than 8 weeks (Harding, 2006), and is often associated with underlying inflammatory airways diseases. Excessive coughing has also been observed as a side-effect of certain medical treatments, for example angiotensin-converting enzyme inhibitors which are used in the prevention of cardiovascular disorders (Fuller & Choudry, 1987; Irwin et al., 1998). However, there is not always an obvious associated underlying condition, and so chronic cough can also be thought of as idiopathic in nature (Morice et al., 2007). Currently, there are no safe and effective medications to suppress cough (Karlsson & Fuller, 1999; Schroeder & Fahey, 2002; Belvisi & Geppetti, 2004; Reynolds et al., 2004; Nasra & Belvisi, 2009).

2.2 The cough reflex

The physiology of the cough reflex has been well described. Briefly, rapid inspiration is followed by an expiratory effort against a closed glottis, and rapid generation of intrapulmonary pressure. Explosive expiration results from sudden opening of the glottis, causing a high linear velocity of gas flow which sweeps irritant material up towards the pharynx (Widdicombe, 2002). In order to initiate cough, the nervous system first needs to detect an irritant stimulus and relay this message to the brain. The "cough centre" of the central nervous system (CNS) is believed to be in close proximity to the nucleus tractus solitarius (NTS), where the afferent nerves which mediate cough are known to synapse with second-order neurons (Figure 1). It is also thought that this putative cough centre is likely to be linked to the respiratory centre of the brain, because a profound change in breathing pattern is an integral part of the cough reflex (Karlsson & Fuller, 1999). It is this afferent arm that initiates and controls the cough reflex which is likely to be altered in disease, and as such is the focus of research investigating cough hypersensitivity.

2.3 Sensory nerves and the cough reflex

Cough is initiated by a wide variety of chemicals, or mechanical stimuli, which act by stimulating specialised peripheral sensory neurons that terminate in the airways (Figure 1). Chemical irritants bind to receptors, which open ion channels on the terminals of the airway sensory nerves, leading to cation influx and membrane depolarisation. If membrane depolarisation is of sufficient magnitude, the peripheral nervous system will send signals to the CNS in the form of action potentials. Action potentials are carried by subsets of sensory nerve fibres via the vagus nerves and sensory ganglia (nodose and jugular), where the cell bodies are located, to the medulla where they terminate in the NTS. Second order neurons then relay the message to a respiratory pattern generator within the CNS, which interprets the afferent information, resulting in activation of motor neurons and ultimately initiation of coughing. Moreover, mediators can interact with the nerve terminals or ion channels in the airways to inhibit or promote depolarisation, alter the response to activating stimuli, or lead to changes in gene expression modifying the function of the sensory fibre itself (Taylor-Clark & Undem, 2006).

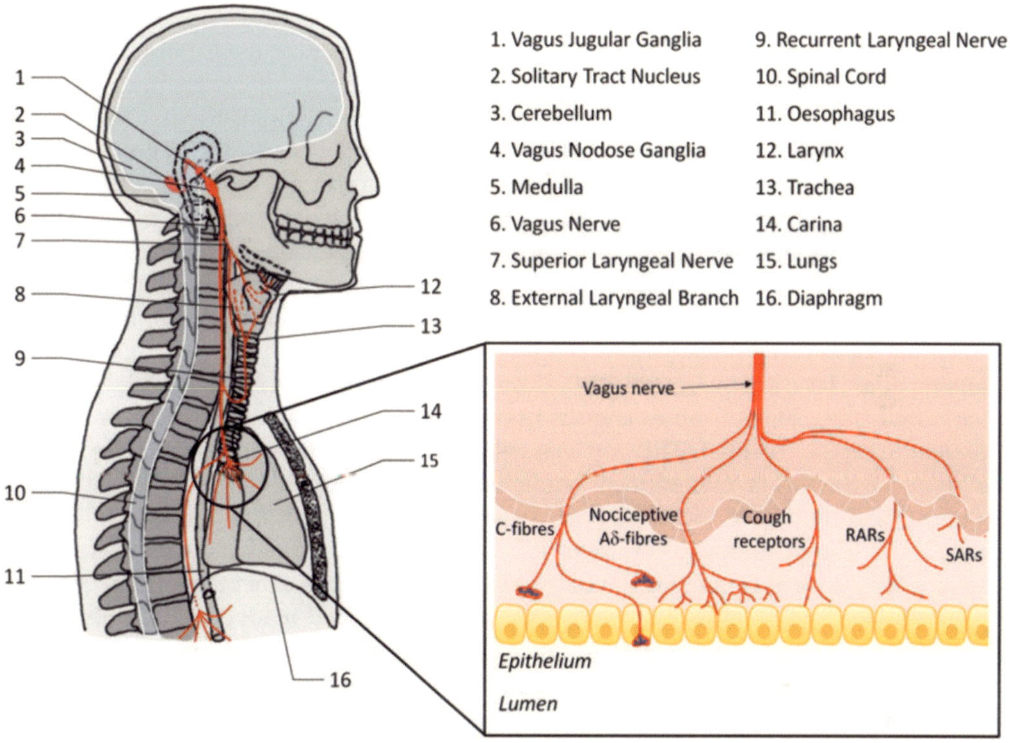

Fig. 1. Airway sensory nerves and cough.
Cell bodies for airway nerve fibres originate in two ganglia, the jugular and nodose, which are located under the ear bone within the head. Airway sensory nerves are mainly carried via the vagus nerve, where they terminate both in and under the airway epithelium (illustrated in the enlarged panel). These fibres consist of the C-fibres, Aδ-nociceptors, polymodal Aδ-fibres ('cough receptors), rapidly adapting receptors (RARs), and slowly adapting receptors (SARs), which sense both chemical and mechanical stimuli. Of these fibres, the chemosensitive C-fibres and mechanosensitive polymodal Aδ-fibres are thought to mediate cough. Once stimulated, information is carried along the vagus nerve via the nodose and jugular sensory ganglia to the solitary tract nucleus (NTS), located in the medulla. In the NTS the sensory fibres synapse to second-order neurons which relay the message to a respiratory pattern generator, activating efferent motor neurons, and leading to cough. The C-fibres also contain neuropeptides, which are released upon nerve activation in some species and lead to neurogenic inflammation (Nasra & Belvisi, 2009).

Airway afferent nerves express a large number of different receptors and ion channels that modulate nerve activity. Cell bodies for the vagus nerves originate in the nodose and jugular ganglia, which are located in the head (Figure 1). In addition to the airways, vagus nerves innervate several organs in the body, including the oesophagus, heart and gastrointestinal tract (Berthoud & Neuhuber, 2000). Airway vagal sensory fibres branch in to the superior and recurrent laryngeal nerves, which carry the fibres to the bronchi and trachea (Belvisi, 2003). These fibres consist of the rapidly-adapting receptors, slowly-adapting receptors, C-fibres, Aδ nociceptors, and 'cough receptors'. Characteristics of each of the different fibre types have been described elsewhere (Undem *et al.*, 2002; Reynolds *et al.*, 2004; Lee & Undem, 2008). In this section we will briefly cover the C-fibres and 'cough receptors' that are thought to be directly associated with cough. C-fibres are predominantly chemosensitive sensory nerves, with high-threshold mechanosensitivty. C-fibres that innervate the airways originate in both the nodose and jugular vagal ganglia, and are found predominantly within the airway epithelium. These nerves are activated by a wide range of stimuli, including food extracts (capsaicin, wasabi, ginger, allicin, mustard oil), environmental irritants (vehicle exhaust, air pollution, tobacco smoke, burning vegetation), endogenous inflammatory mediators (prostaglandin E_2, bradykinin), and acid (Mohammed *et al.*, 1993; Caterina *et al.*, 1997; Bautista *et al.*, 2006; Kaufman *et al.*, 1980). Exposure to aerosols of these compounds causes cough in conscious guinea-pigs, dogs and humans (Canning et al 2006; Kaufman et al 1980; Costello et al 1985; Laude et al 1993; Lalloo *et al.*, 1995; Birrell *et al.*, 2009). C-fibres contain neuropeptides, and have been found to express Transient Receptor Potential (TRP) ion channels, which are thought to play a central role in the cough reflex. This makes them attractive pharmacological targets for antitussive treatment, and they have therefore been a main focus of research in the cough field. In contrast, the 'cough receptors' are extrapulmonary, low threshold mechanosensors that originate in the nodose ganglia. These nerves do not express neuropeptides, and are insensitive to classical C-fibre stimulants such as capsaicin and bradykinin (Canning *et al.*, 2004; Mazzone, 2004). However, they are extremely sensitive to low pH and dynamic punctate mechanical stimulation, and adapt only when the mechanical stimulus becomes static. It has been proposed that different types of cough and therefore multiple cough pathways may exist. These pathways theoretically contribute distinctly to defensive productive cough which aids in protecting the airways, and dry non-productive urge-to-cough sensations associated with disease states. It could therefore be possible to inhibit the non-productive cough pathway while preserving defensive cough (Canning, 2011).

2.4 Cough in inflammatory airways disease

The central and peripheral nervous systems are capable of adapting to their environment. External influences such as disease, injury and inflammation are able to induce changes in expression of various genes involved in the production of neuropeptides, neurotransmitters, and ion channels (Taylor-Clark & Undem, 2006). However, we do not yet understand this neuroplasticity with respect to mechanisms of cough linked with airway inflammation and other cough-associated pathologies (Lee & Undem 2008). It is possible that exposure to tussigenic agents could lead to long or short-term changes in the peripheral sensory nerves or CNS, or for example at the NTS where airway sensory nerves synapse (Bautista *et al.*, 2006).

Studies in subgroups of patients have suggested that the cough reflex associated with viral infections, gastro-oesophageal reflux, COPD and 'cough-variant' asthma becomes hypersensitive to challenge with tussive agents when compared to normal controls (Doherty *et al.*, 2000; Pecova *et al.*, 2008). This suggests that there may be a common mechanism behind the augmented cough reflex in these diseases. Indeed, some of these airways diseases (eg. asthma and COPD) are associated with enhanced release of inflammatory mediators (e.g. prostaglandin E_2 and bradykinin), and a lowering of physiological pH within the lungs. Interestingly, the threshold for sensory nerve stimulation and cough is reduced in the presence of inflammatory mediators, and inhalation of these mediators and low pH can induce coughing in both humans and animals. It could therefore be postulated that enhanced release of endogenous pro-tussive mediators could be at least partially involved in cough hypersensitivity seen in inflammatory diseases (Choudry et al 1989; Fox et al, 1996; Ho et al, 2000; Hunt *et al.*, 2000; Kostikas *et al.*, 2002).

2.5 Section summary

Cough is an interesting and quickly-developing field of research. This section provided a brief introduction to cough, and of the afferent nerves that control the cough reflex. Great advances have been made in our understanding of the cough reflex in the last decade, however, there are still many questions left to answer. We still know little about what receptors on the airway sensory nerve endings are involved in provoking cough, and how these mechanisms are altered to cause hypersensitivity and chronic cough. The rest of this chapter will deal with tobacco smoke as a stimulus for coughing, the current theories on the mechanisms of action behind smoke-induced cough, and research addressing how smoke exposure leads to excessive cough associated with disease states.

3. Acute effects of tobacco smoke on the cough reflex

Various environmental irritants are known to induce coughing such as air pollution, tobacco smoke (TS), smoke from burning vegetation, and vehicle exhaust. These irritants contain many of the same chemical constituents, which can be used to study the mechanisms driving acute cough. These studies are important, as we first need to understand how cough occurs in the healthy state before we can determine how these mechanisms change to cause chronic or excessive coughing associated with disease.

3.1 Models of acute TS-induced cough

TS is one of the most common inhaled irritants, and reliably evokes airway irritation and coughing in both animals and human non-smokers (Lee et al., 1993, 2007; Andre et al., 2009). However, it remains uncertain which constituents in tobacco and other types of smoke are primarily responsible for evoking these irritant effects. Using several different methods, activation of airway sensory nerves and, in some cases, the cough reflex has been investigated in dog, cat, guinea-pig and mouse animal models, amongst others, which have provided some valuable insights in to the mechanisms driving the acute cough response. However, species differences have been observed for a multitude of physiological processes. As such, the results observed in these animal models may not all be applicable to human cough. This highlights the importance of replicating these studies in both *in vitro* studies using human tissue (where possible) and clinical trials, as the mechanisms driving acute and/or chronic cough may be different.

3.2 Mechanisms of action of TS in acute cough

3.2.1 Nicotinic receptors

Nicotine is a major constituent of TS, and nicotinic receptors are known to be present on a variety of cells in the airways, including neurons (Gu et al., 2008). As such, the nicotinic acetylcholine (nACh) receptors were hypothesised to be responsible for acute cough induced by smoke inhalation. Lee and colleagues originally studied this hypothesis in both awake and anesthetised dogs. Using single fibre analysis, the authors observed that a single puff of TS generated from high nicotine, but not low nicotine cigarettes triggered action potential generation in bronchopulmonary C-fibres and RARs. Moreover, the competitive selective nACh receptor antagonist hexamethonium inhibited sensory nerve stimulation in response to TS, but had no effect on other tussive stimuli, indicating a role for nicotine in the smoke-induced irritant response in dogs (Lee et al., 1983, 1985, 1986, 1989; Kou & Lee, 1990, 1991). The ability of nicotine to stimulate airway sensory nerves was corroborated in rat isolated vagal ganglia neurons by assessing calcium influx. Calcium is an important signal transduction molecule in neurons, and plays a pivotal role in the regulation of membrane excitability. Airway neurons were selectively tagged with a specialised fluorescent tracer, allowing them to be differentiated from vagal neurons that innervate other organs. Calcium entry in to airway neuronal cells was successfully stimulated by nicotine, a response which was all-but abolished with hexamethonium pre-treatment (Xu et al., 2007). In the same study, the authors also confirmed a stimulatory effect of nicotine on C-fibres and RARs (Xu et al., 2007).

However, as discussed in section 3.1, there are species differences associated with many physiological functions, and as such effects observed in animal models do not always reflect the mechanisms involved in human responses. Thus, Lee and colleagues went on to investigate the role of nACh receptors in TS-induced airway irritation in humans in a set of three studies (Lee et al., 1993). The first trial assessed the irritant effects of inhaling a single bolus of smoke generated from high or low nicotine cigarettes, or 'gas phase' control in healthy young non-smokers. Participants were blinded as to what stimulus they were receiving, and when the smoke bolus was to be delivered. Airway irritation was subjectively measured, with participants asked to push a button in response to the level of airway irritation they perceived. Smoke from high nicotine cigarettes triggered intense airway irritation in the lower neck and upper chest. In contrast, low nicotine cigarettes caused little to no irritation in comparison to gas phase. High nicotine cigarettes also triggered reflex coughing in the majority of participants. Whereas, coughing was absent with inhalation of both low nicotine and gas phase irritants. This corroborated their findings in the dog model (Lee et al., 1983, 1985, 1986, 1989; Kou & Lee, 1990, 1991). The second study assessed the role of nicotine in TS-associated airway irritation and cough. Pre-medication with the general nACh receptor inhibitor hexamethonium was reported to significantly attenuate airway irritation compared to placebo control. The number of coughs was also reduced with hexamethonium pre-treatment in comparison to placebo. Finally, the third study investigated whether aerosolised nicotine alone could induce airway irritant responses. Indeed, nicotine evoked intense and sustained irritation and vigorous coughing in comparison to placebo, which induced no irritation and few coughs. Lee and colleagues have summarised their research in two reviews (Lee et al., 2007, 2010).

From these studies, it was concluded that TS causes airway irritation and cough via activation of sensory nerve endings in the airways, and that nicotine is likely to be the primary causative agent for this nociceptive response. In addition, the irritant responses to TS stimulation were proposed to be mediated by vagal bronchopulmonary C-fibres and RARs (Lee et al., 1993). However, inhibition of the nACh receptors did not completely abolish coughing induced by TS inhalation. Furthermore, TS contains a multitude of potentially tussive noxious constituents in addition to nicotine; and not all smoke contains nicotine but can still induce coughing, for example wood smoke. Tussive stimuli also act via diverse mechanisms, as different irritants target various membrane receptors expressed on airway sensory nerve endings. It is therefore likely that other noxious substances and one or more other receptors are involved in the TS-induced acute cough response. Indeed, it has recently been discovered that nicotine also activates the Transient Receptor Potential (TRP) class of ion channels, and that TS-induced cough can be inhibited by TRP-selective antagonists (Talavera et al., 2009; Andre et al., 2009).

3.2.2 Transient Receptor Potential (TRP) receptors

The TRP ion channels have been linked to various roles in sensory perception, including detection of noxious stimuli (Caterina et al., 1997; Nilius, 2007). A number of TRP receptor subtypes have been found to be expressed on sensory neurons, specifically Vanilloid (TRPV)1, TRPV2, TRPV3, TRPV4, Melastatin (TRPM)8, and Ankyrin (TRPA)1 (Caspani & Heppenstall, 2009). The TRPV1 ion channel has a well-established role in cough, and two known TRPV1 ligands (capsaicin and citric acid) are routinely used to assess the cough reflex in animal and clinical studies. More recently, the TRPA1 ion channel was also identified as a pro-tussive receptor in both humans and an animal model; an effect which was blocked by TRPA1-selective antagonists (Birrell et al., 2009; Andre et al., 2009). This is a significant finding, as TRPA1 is activated by a multitude of both environmental irritants and endogenous mediators. In fact, many constituents contained in tobacco smoke, wood smoke and air pollution are now known to activate TRPA1 ion channels, and thus it has become a key candidate for mediating the tussive effects associated with these pollutants.

Acrolein and crotonaldehyde are abundant in TS (Facchinetti et al., 2007; Andre et al., 2009), and have been shown to selectively activate TRPA1 (Bautista et al., 2006; Andre et al., 2008). In a set of studies demonstrating the role of TRPA1 in cough, Andre and colleagues established that both acrolein and crotonaldehyde induce robust coughing in guinea pigs, and that this effect could be inhibited by the selective TRPA1 antagonist HC-030031 (Andre et al., 2009). Because these irritants are common constituents in TS, the authors hypothesised that they might contribute to the cough associated with smoke inhalation. Indeed, TS exposure for 10 minutes caused vigorous bouts of coughing in conscious guinea pigs, which was inhibited approximately 50% by the cation blocker (ruthenium red) as well as a selective TRPA1 antagonist (HC-030031). Interestingly, the TRPV1-selective antagonist capsazepine was also reported to have a small inhibitory effect on TS-induced coughing, though not to the extent of TRPA1 inhibition (Andre et al., 2009).

A role for TRPA1 in TS-induced cough has been further substantiated by the finding that nicotine is also capable of activating this receptor (Talavera et al., 2009). Application of nicotine was observed to activate both mouse- and human-TRPA1 heterologously expressed in CHO cells via a direct gating mechanism. In addition, TRPA1-mediated nicotine responses were identified in mouse trigeminal neurons, a response that was blunted in genetically modified mice with the TRPA1 gene distrupted (*Trpa1*$^{-/-}$), and virtually abolished in *Trpa1*$^{-/-}$ neurons in the presence of the nACh inhibitor hexamethonium. Moreover, using an *in vitro* isolated vagus nerve preparation, we investigated the ability of nicotine to induce membrane depolarisation, which is a measure of sensory nerve activation. The magnitude of depolarisation elicited by nicotine was observed to be significantly smaller in *Trpa1*$^{-/-}$ mice in comparison to vagus nerves from wild-type mice ($p < 0.05$; data not shown), indicating a role for TRPA1 in nicotine stimulation of sensory nerves. Moreover, pre-treatment with either a nAChR or TRPA1 antagonist inhibited nicotine responses in wild-type mice; and pre-treatment with a nAChR antagonist virtually abolished nicotine responses in *Trpa1*$^{-/-}$ mouse vagus (Figure 2). Overall, these studies provide strong evidence for a role for both the TRPA1 and nACh ion channels in the response to nicotine. Thus, it is possible that part of the inhibition of acute TS-induced cough observed by Andre and colleagues (2009) could be caused by a reduction in the effects of nicotine with TRPA1 antagonism.

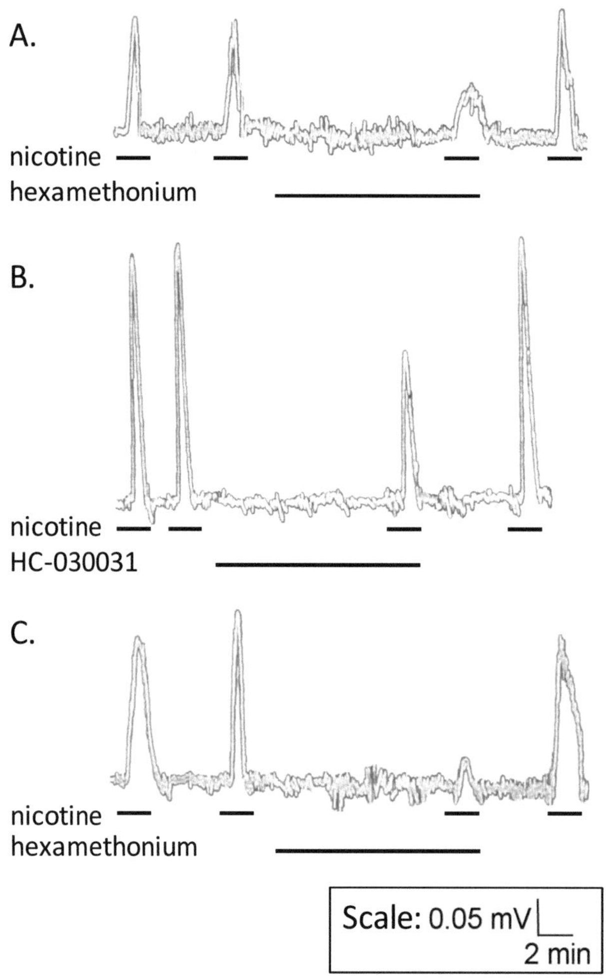

Fig. 2. Representative traces showing isolated vagus nerve responses to nicotine stimulation. Vagus nerve trunks from wild type (C57Bl/6j) or *Trpa1*$^{-/-}$ mice were exposed to stimulations of nicotine with or without the presence of antagonist. Two 2-minute stimulations to nicotine alone were performed to establish reproducibility of the nicotine response. The nerve was then incubated for 10 minutes with an nAChR antagonist (hexamethonium) or TRPA1 antagonist (HC-030031) and a third stimulation with nicotine in the presence of antagonist. The nerve was washed, and a final stimulation with nicotine performed to ensure nerve viability. *A. and B.* Magnitude of nerve depolarisation (a measure of sensory nerve activation) in wild-type vagal tissue was inhibited by either nAChR or TRPA1 antagonism. *C.* Depolarisation was virtually abolished with nAChR antagonism in *Trpa1*$^{-/-}$ vagal tissue.

Finally, it is important to note that, because TRPA1 and TRPV1 are co-expressed on sensory neurons, there is a possibility these TRP channels act in concert to elicit functional responses to noxious stimuli. Indeed, it has been suggested that TRPA1 channels could be activated by an overflow of calcium in the locale of other activated channels, without ever being modified by a reactive ligand. Furthermore, TRPA1 channels may act to amplify other calcium-mobilising pathways, including activation of TRPV1 (Zurborg et al., 2007; Cavanaugh et al., 2008). There is evidence for this type of coupling with bradykinin signalling in trigeminal neurons (Bautista et al., 2006). However, whether this sort of cooperation exists in generating cough has yet to be determined.

3.3 Section summary

The above studies suggest a significant role for both the TRPA1 and nACh receptors in acute tussive responses to TS inhalation. However, reduction in TS-induced cough with selective TRPA1 and nACh inhibitors is only partial, and there are thousands of constituents contained in TS, suggesting that there are likely to be multiple mechanisms and yet more receptors mediating the tussive effects of TS. For example, the TRPV1 ion channel has a well-established role in cough. It is highly possible that tobacco smoke also contains irritants, or induces the production of endogenous metabolites that directly or indirectly activate TRPV1. Furthermore, smoke inhalation reduces airways pH and increases temperature, both of which are known to activate the TRPV1 receptor. Indeed, there is some suggestion in the literature that TRPV1-selective antagonists may attenuate the acute tussive response to tobacco smoke, though the inhibitory effect was small (Andre et al., 2009).

4. Cough and disease

Chronic cough is reported as a troublesome symptom by 7% of the population (Ford et al., 2006). In extreme situations, cough can persist for several years, and is not only socially embarrassing, but can be painful and debilitating. Chronic cough is often associated with an underlying respiratory disease, several of which are associated with the inhalation of tobacco smoke and other air pollutants, for example asthma, COPD and lung cancer (WHO 2008a; WHO 2011). But the mechanisms by which smoking or air pollution causes exaggerated cough remains unknown (Morice et al., 2004; Smith & Woodcock, 2006).

4.1 Models of tobacco smoke and disease

A number of attempts have been made to simulate smoke-induced respiratory disease in animal models in order to study the mechanisms by which TS leads to cough hypersensitivity. The guinea-pig, as the only small animal that exhibits a functional cough reflex, is by far the cheapest and easiest animal in which to investigate cough in chronic models, and as such most disease research has been conducted using these animals. Both sub-chronic and chronic models of TS exposure using guinea-pigs have successfully induced an enhanced cough reflex when animals were subsequently exposed to tussive mediators (Karlsson et al., 1991; Bergren, 2001; Lewis et al., 2007).

4.1.1 Sub-chronic models of tobacco smoke exposure

Sub-chronic models of up to two weeks TS exposure have produced hypersensitivity to tussive stimuli in guinea-pigs. Compared to air-exposed controls, guinea-pigs exposed to two weeks of TS for one hour per day exhibited a 3.7-fold and 2.5-fold increase in coughing in response to aerosolised citric acid and capsaicin stimulation, respectively (Karlsson et al., 1991). Enhanced responses to citric acid and capsaicin stimuli abated over the following three weeks, suggesting that cough hyperresponsiveness in this model is a very plastic phenomenon. Because prostaglandin E_2 has been previously shown to potentiate capsaicin-induced coughing in human volunteers (Choudry et al., 1989), the authors investigated whether prostaglandins could be involved in the augmented response to tussive stimuli seen after TS exposure. The general cyclo-oxygenase inhibitor indomethacin was injected 1 hour prior to stimulation with citric acid. Though a slight decrease in the number of coughs was observed with indomethacin pre-treatment compared to vehicle pre-treatment in TS-exposed animals, the effect was not significant, and was mirrored in air-exposed controls (Karlsson et al., 1991). It should, however, be noted that this was an acute exposure to indomethacin following 2 weeks of TS exposure, which would only prevent release of prostaglandins during the acute tussive stimulation. This experiment may engender more meaningful results if indomethacin was given throughout the two-week TS exposure, which would prevent chronic enhanced release of prostaglandins in the airways. Long-term effects of prostaglandins in the airways may be more likely to be involved in the hypertussive response than an acute release during irritant exposure.

A more recent study has corroborated the above findings, and established a brief time-course for the effects of TS on enhanced cough responses, which revealed remarkable differences in the enhancement observed with citric acid or capsaicin stimulation (Lewis et al., 2007). Specifically, enhanced cough to citric acid stimulation developed after exposure to TS for only 1 day; hypersensitivity peaked after 2 days of TS exposure and remained elevated for 10 days. In contrast, enhanced cough to capsaicin stimulation was not observed until guinea-pigs had been exposed to TS for 4 days, but thereafter cough sensitivity also remained elevated for 10 days.

Our group has also substantiated the findings of these previous studies, having developed a model whereby guinea-pigs are exposed to TS twice daily for 8 consecutive days. In this model we observed hypersensitivity to tussive stimuli in the smoke-treated animals in comparison to air-exposed controls. An increase in isolated sensory nerve responses to stimulation with capsaicin and citric acid was observed in the smoke-treated animals. This result was paralleled *in vivo* by an increase in cough sensitivity to capsaicin aerosol in smoked animals compared to air-exposed controls (Figure 3).

4.1.2 Chronic models of tobacco smoke exposure

Excessive cough is often one of the first presenting symptoms of COPD. Sub-chronic models of respiratory disease are therefore useful, as they can assess the mechanisms of enhanced cough at the beginning stages of disease. However, chronic models are also needed, because several physiological changes occur as the disease progresses. It is these structural changes which may lead to the chronic, irreversible hypertussive effects. For example, more advanced stages of COPD are associated not only with inflammation in the airway mucosa and parenchyma, but destruction of lung parenchyma and fibrosis. It is with these types of structural changes that we may begin to observe long-term enhancement of the cough reflex, rather than the reversible changes observed in, for example, Karlsson and colleagues (1991) sub-chronic model.

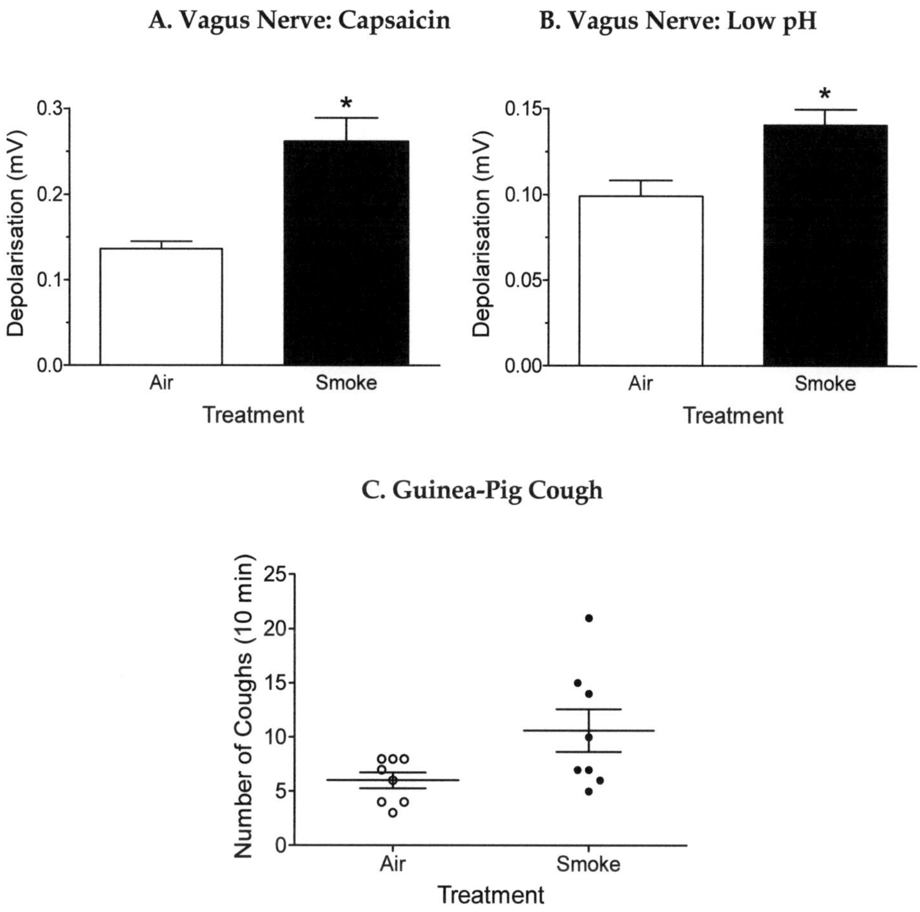

Fig. 3. Investigating *in vitro* sensory nerve and *in vivo* cough responses to tussive stimili following sub-chronic tobacco smoke exposure.
Guinea-pigs were exposed twice daily for 8 days to either air (white bars and open circles) or tobacco smoke (black bars and filled circles). Twenty four hours after the final exposure either the animals were culled and vagus nerves removed; or conscious animals were exposed to tussive stimuli. Magnitude of vagus nerve depolarisation (a measure of sensory nerve activation) to (a) 1μM capsaicin, or (b) low pH 5 was compared between air and smoke-exposed animals (n = 12). (c) animals were exposed to 30μM aerosolised capsaicin for 5 minutes (coughs counted during this period and for a further 5 minutes; n = 8). * indicates statistical significance compared to air-exposed controls ($p < 0.05$, Mann-Whitney unpaired t-test).

There is a wealth of literature examining the effects of chronic TS on inflammation; however, to our knowledge only one study has directly assessed the effects of long-term smoke exposure on the cough reflex (Bergren, 2001). Guinea-pigs were exposed to either compressed air or TS for 30 minutes per day for a total of 90 days. In the TS group, spontaneous coughing was observed both during TS exposure and at other non-exposure times, with increasing regularity as the study progressed. After 90 days, animals exposed to TS exhibited a significantly greater number of coughs to either capsaicin or bradykinin challenge than air-exposed controls. Moreover, hypersensitivity to capsaicin was further enhanced with ovalbumin sensitisation, which is an animal model of allergic asthma. This result holds implications for co-morbidity of patients suffering from more than one airway pathology.

4.2 Mechanisms of action

Thus far, the mechanisms driving chronic cough have been elusive. Models of excessive cough such as those reviewed above are useful for determining these mechanisms, and add to our understanding of the disease process. There is some evidence to suggest that an increase in receptor expression may be involved in the development of cough hypersensitivity, as evidenced by an increase in TRPV1 expression in the lungs of chronic coughers compared to healthy controls (Groneberg et al., 2004). As-yet there are no documented studies investigating changes in the expression of TRPA1 or other receptors associated with cough. Alternately, it has been proposed that the lung environment during inflammatory airways disease may be sensitising the peripheral nerves, making them more likely to respond when exposed to a low level of irritant that would not normally reach cough threshold. For example, patients with inflammatory airways disease exhibit a decrease in lung pH, and high levels of endogenous inflammatory mediators within the airways (Profita et al., 2003; Montuschi et al., 2003; Hunt *et al.*, 2000; Kostikas *et al.*, 2002). Two inflammatory mediators, prostaglandin E_2 and bradykinin, have not only been shown to sensitise airway nerves to other tussive stimuli, but can in fact induce coughing themselves (Costello et al 1985; Maher et al 2009; Choudry et al 1989; Katsumata et al 1991; Fox et al., 1996). Therefore, if the endogenous concentration of these irritants reaches high enough levels, coughing could be directly induced without any environmental challenge.

A qualitative change in the vagal afferent innervation of guinea-pig airways has also been documented in disease models. C-fibres are known to express neuropeptides on their nerve endings, which are released in response to nerve stimulation, where they can contribute to peripheral neurogenic inflammation. Activation of nociceptors can also cause central sensitisation via release of neuropeptides from their central terminals, where they enhance synaptic neurotransmission. Under normal circumstances, these neuropeptides are synthesised nearly exclusively in C-fibres, and are not expressed on other sub-sets of sensory afferents. However, in models of respiratory virus and allergic inflammation, Undem and colleagues have demonstrated that Aδ-nociceptive neurons transiently produced neuropeptides, an effect that appeared to reverse with resolution of virus infection (Carr et al., 2002; Myers et al., 2002). This is a particularly important finding, as it suggests that sensory neuropeptide release from afferent nerve endings and central terminals may not require chemical stimulation, but could be provoked following activation of low-threshold mechanosensors.

4.3 Section summary

The studies discussed in this section have established the importance of the TRPV1 ion channel in development of excessive cough in disease states. What has not yet been investigated is the role that other ion channels may play. No-doubt future studies will assess hypersensitivity to TRPA1-selective irritants, now that TRPA1 has been identified as a promising target for cough. But it is also important to determine the function that other tussive compounds play in this pathology. In particular, endogenous inflammatory mediators such as prostaglandin E_2 and bradykinin are known to be released in greater amounts in inflammatory airway disease. These mediators are not only able to sensitise airway afferents to stimulation by other tussive ligands, but can induce coughing themselves with acute exposure. In addition, the discovery by Lewis and colleagues (2007) that hypersensitivity to citric acid stimulation develops well before capsaicin could be important, and warrants further investigation. This could be to do with the fact that capsaicin acts solely on the TRPV1 ion channel, whereas the tussive response to citric acid is only partially mediated via TRPV1. Therefore the other ion channel(s) involved in the citric acid response (such as the acid sensing ion channels, or ASICs) could be upregulated or otherwise affected by TS more quickly than TRPV1.

There is also the debate on whether hypersensitivity involves central or peripheral sensitisation of the cough reflex. That is, does hypersensitivity develop because there is an enhanced reactivity of the peripheral nerves to a stimulus; or is the stimulus amplified within the CNS, producing a response to otherwise non-noxious stimuli? Ultimately, it is the interplay between all of these factors that is likely to lead to excessive coughing associated with inflammatory airway diseases.

5. Therapeutic targets

Currently available anti-tussive therapies are largely offered over-the-counter (OTC) as self medication programmes, and are among the most widely used OTC drugs. However, OTC remedies show little efficacy in alleviating cough (Schroeder & Fahey, 2002); and opiates, the gold standard in cough treatment, are associated with moderate to severe side-effects (Karlsson & Fuller, 1999; Belvisi & Geppetti, 2004; Reynolds et al., 2004). In fact, it has been recognised that cough and cold remedies can cause adverse events in children under 11 years of age (American Academy of Paediatrics, 1997; Gunn et al., 2001; Centres for Disease Control, 2007; Vassilev et al., 2009). In early 2008, this lead the U.S. Food and Drug administration to release an advisory notice recommending that OTC cough and cold medicines should not be used to treat children under 2 years of age, due to potentially life-threatening side-effects (U.S. FDA, 2008). The development of efficacious cough therapies with fewer, less severe side-effects is therefore urgently required.

The site of action of anti-tussive agents can be broadly classified as those that act peripherally, and those that act centrally. It is currently not known whether the enhanced cough seen in disease states is due to peripheral or central sensitisation, and as such targeted therapeutics specific to the enhanced response are difficult to identify. However, targeting either compartment would theoretically lead to attenuation in cough due to a general suppression of the reflex. This has lead to concerns that targeting the tussive reflex in diseases could inhibit both excessive cough, and the functional cough associated with health benefits. Therefore, the ideal anti-tussive therapy would suppress only the enhanced cough associated with disease, while leaving the protective part of the reflex functional. Centrally-acting suppressants are generally associated with neurological side-effects such as sedation, nausea and physical dependence, which limits their effective use. In contrast, peripherally acting anti-tussives exert their effects by targeting peripheral sensory nerve afferents, and could potentially provide a better approach than centrally acting therapies. In this section we have discussed only a select few of the peripherally-acting anti-tussive therapies that are either currently being pursued as potential therapies, or show promise in pre-clinical research and human trials. This is not an exhaustive list but covers some of the key targets currently being investigated.

5.1 TRPV1 inhibitors

Research over the last decade has revealed TRPV1 as a promising target in the field of cough. It has already been established that chronic coughers show higher expression of TRPV1 in the lung in comparison to 'healthy' individuals (Groneberg et al., 2004); and TRPV1 antagonists are efficacious in preventing cough in guinea pigs induced by capsaicin and citric acid aerosol (Lalloo et al., 1995; Trevisani et al., 2004). However, TRPV1 is now known to be tonically active in thermoregulatory pathways, and as such one of the main issues with currently available TRPV1 antagonists is that they cause hyperthermia (Gavva et al., 2008; Lehto et al., 2008). This is a potential confounding factor in the clinical development of TRPV1 therapeutics. Research is currently under way to produce TRPV1 inhibitors that do not affect body temperature, with limited success thus far (Lehto et al., 2008). It is also of concern that TRPV1 appears to be widely expressed throughout the body, and thus may lead to other unexpected side effect issues. Despite these reservations, several TRPV1 inhibitors are currently under development both as antitussives and analgesics (Gunthorpe & Chizh, 2009).

5.2 TRPA1 inhibitors

The recent discovery of TRPA1 as a pro-tussive receptor and its role in TS-induced cough is a significant finding (Birrell et al., 2009; Andre et al., 2009). This opens up a whole new field of research for potential anti-tussive remedies that could help to alleviate cough, not only associated with the common cold and seasonal flu, but more importantly for those who suffer from excessive coughing associated with chronic inflammatory diseases. Specifically, activation of the TRPA1 receptor could be significant in several pathological situations given that it is known to be stimulated by a multitude of environmental irritants (including constituents of air pollution and burning vegetation), as well as endogenous products of oxidation which can be generated in the airways by inhalation of pollutants or during inflammation (Bessac et al., 2008; Andre et al., 2008; Taylor-Clark et al., 2008). This could be of particular importance in highly polluted areas such as large cities, or in occupations where workers are chronically exposed to environmental irritants.

TRPA1 is largely expressed by a subset of TRPV1-expressing neurons, and both are activated by tussive agents, so it could be possible that these two channels act in concert to elicit functional responses. The theory that TRPA1 and TRPV1 may co-operate comes from evidence that TRPA1 can be activated by an overflow of Ca^{2+} in the locale of other activated channels, such as TRPV1, without ever being modified by a reactive ligand. Moreover, TRPA1 could amplify other Ca^{2+} mobilising pathways (Zurborg et al., 2007; Cavanaugh et al., 2008). Both TRPA1 and TRPV1 inhibition can totally or partially block responses to a range of tussive agents (Maher et al., 2010). However, it has yet to be determined whether cooperation exists between these two channels in initiating the cough reflex. Information to date would suggest TRPA1 expression is more restricted which may make for a more optimal safety profile than TRPV1 inhibition, although this remains to be seen with the increased testing of TRPA1 antagonists in both pre clinical and clinical studies. Unfortunately, the tools available to probe this target are limited (Viana & Ferrer-Montiel,

2009), and it is therefore difficult to predict whether single TRPA1 or TRPV1 therapies or a combined drug would be more effective in treating heightened sensory nerve responsive disease states (Belvisi et al., 2011).

5.3 nACh receptor inhibitors

Neuronal nACh receptors are pentameric ligand-gated ion channels which are formed by assembly of five transmembrane segments. To date there are 17 known members of the nACh family expressed in humans, which assemble in numerous combinations to form functional ion channels with widely varying agonist and antagonist gating properties (Gu et al., 2008). In addition, nACh receptors are widely expressed throughout the body, including both the central and peripheral nervous systems. This limits development of nACh-based therapies without a more in-depth understanding of what receptor subtypes are involved in cough, and subsequent development of selective antagonists with which to inhibit these responses. Though selective ligands targeting specific subunits of nACh receptors are being developed as therapeutic agents for neurodegenerative diseases, the authors do not know of any current interest in developing such compounds as therapies for cough (Lee et al., 2007; Gu et al., 2008).

5.4 β_2-adrenoceptor antagonists

Bronchodilators are a cornerstone of symptomatic treatment for COPD and asthma (Barnes, 2010a, 2010b). One of the most effective bronchodilators currently available are the β_2-adrenoceptor agonists, which are widely used to alleviate the bronchoconstriction associated with respiratory diseases. In some clinical trials, treatment with β_2-agonists has also been shown to possess anti-tussive properties in both healthy volunteers (Lowry et al., 1987) and chronic cough pathologies associated with allergic (Ellul-Micallef, 1983) or obstructive conditions (Campbell et al., 2005; Chong et al., 2005; Mulrennan et al., 2004; Pounsford et al., 1985). However, an anti-tussive effect of β_2-agonists in clinical trials has not been universally observed (Chang et al., 1998; Smith et al., 1991). The lack of definitive data demonstrating an anti-tussive activity of β_2-agonists in these studies may be due to the research protocols used, including the use of subjective symptom scoring; that few of these studies have been performed under double-blind, randomised and placebo-controlled conditions; and that cough is rarely a primary end-point of the research.

Recently, the ability of β_2-agonists to inhibit the cough reflex was assessed in a pre-clinical model (Freund-Michel et al., 2010). The β_2-agonist terbutaline was shown to attenuate guinea-pig cough responses to both capsaicin and citric acid *in vivo*. In addition, both terbutaline and fenoterol blocked sensory nerve activation in response to a number of tussive agonists in the guinea-pig isolated vagal nerve preparation; and fenoterol inhibited depolarisations of human isolated vagus nerve induced by capsaicin. The ability of these compounds to directly inhibit sensory nerve responses provides evidence against the existing dogma that the anti-tussive effects of β_2-agonists are secondary to bronchodilation. Furthermore, the authors proposed a mechanism-of-action, whereby β_2-agonists stimulate adenylyl cyclase, leading to cyclic AMP accumulation, activation of protein kinase G, and opening of large conductance calcium-activated potassium (BK_{Ca}) channels, thereby inhibiting sensory nerve depolarisation. Both short- and long-acting β_2-agonists are already used in the clinic as bronchodilators for asthma and COPD; and have a proven acceptable safety profile in man. Furthermore, their mechanism of action appears to be via the opening of BK_{Ca} channels, which provides non-selective inhibition of the cough reflex and thus would be effective against a range of tussive mediators. However, more studies need to be done to corroborate the findings of Freund-Michel and colleagues (2010), coupled with appropriate well-controlled and blinded clinical investigation with the use of objective cough monitoring.

5.5 Methylxanthines

Methylxanthines are another class of bronchodilator that are commonly used to alleviate the symptoms of COPD and asthma (Barnes, 2010a, 2010b). As with β_2-agonists, methylxanthines have been proposed to inhibit the cough reflex. Clinical studies have suggested that theophylline acts as an anti-tussive in a range of conditions. In children and adults with poorly controlled asthma (Bose et al., 1987; Fairfax et al., 1990), theophylline significantly improved scores for cough and wheeze compared to placebo. Theophylline is also recommended for the treatment of cough in COPD (ACCP guidelines 2006) and has been shown to be effective for treating ACE-inhibitor related cough (Cazzola et al., 1993). Hypersensitivity of the cough reflex is a feature of all these conditions and whilst specific effects on the underlying disorders cannot be excluded, a general inhibitory effect on cough reflex sensitivity would seem more plausible. Indeed, in subjects with ACE-inhibitor cough, theophylline was shown to reduce cough reflex hypersensitivity in addition to ameliorating symptoms. Furthermore, theophylline has been shown in clinical trials to be an effective treatment for pain (mechanical nociception, renal colic, non-cardiac chest pain, post lumbar puncture headache) which may indicate an effect on nociceptive processes (Rao et al., 2007; Pechlivanova & Georgiev, 2005). Our preliminary data (described below) demonstrates that theophylline directly inhibits sensory nerve activation and the cough reflex (Dubuis et al., 2011). More recently, Usmani and colleagues (2005) investigated the anti-tussive effects of another methylxanthine theobromine in a comprehensive set of studies. Using an *in vivo* conscious model of cough in guinea-pigs, the authors established that theobromine dose-dependently inhibited citric acid-induced cough in a similar fashion to the established systemic opiate codeine. This result was replicated in normal volunteers in a study where theobromine significantly attenuated capsaicin-induced cough. In comparison, codeine did not significantly affect capsaicin-induced cough in human participants. Finally, it was demonstrated that the effects of theobromine were being mediated peripherally by direct inhibition of sensory nerves, using an *in vitro* isolated vagus preparation. However, it should be noted that the participants in this clinical trial were all healthy individuals with no indication of respiratory disease. Therefore, these studies need to be replicated using participants exhibiting excessive cough, to see if the beneficial effects of theobromine are maintained in disease states. Furthermore, the mechanism by which theobromine attenuates cough is unclear, thus further pre-clinical trials are also required. Finally, it is not clear whether theobromine will exhibit a preferable anti-tussive profile compared to theophylline which is already approved for use in respiratory disease.

5.6 Section summary

There is currently a number of promising peripherally-acting anti-tussive targets being investigated. Of those that target specific ion channels, TRPA1 and TRPV1 antagonists are two of the most exciting. These inhibitors provide the potential for selectively suppressing ion channels that are directly involved in the cough reflex. However, there have been some issues in the development of these compounds, due to inherent side effects, e.g. hyperthermia associated with TRPV1 compounds; or the apparent difficulty in developing efficacious selective antagonists in the case of TRPA1. Alternatively, compounds such as β-agonists or methylxanthines are thought to suppress cough by generally inhibiting sensory nerve activation to tussive stimuli. The mechanisms by which these antitussives exert their effects are not fully understood, but they provide potential therapeutic remedies that could reach the market in a much quicker timescale, due to the fact that they are already widely prescribed bronchodilator agents.

6. Conclusions

Despite a decreasing trend for smoking in some developed countries over the last decade, smoking worldwide is still on the increase, particularly in developing nations (Office for National Statistics, 2010; WHO, 2010). Moreover, indoor and outdoor air pollution is a major environmental health problem in both developed and developing countries alike (WHO, 2008b). In contrast to most other diseases, the global burden of chronic respiratory diseases is also on the increase (WHO, 2005; WHO, 2008a; WHO 2011). In combination, these trends represent a major concern for respiratory health worldwide. Prolonged, excessive coughing is a symptom associated with a large number of respiratory diseases, and is thus likely to be an increasing issue over the next several years. The findings discussed in this chapter represent a breakthrough in the field of cough, and could hold major implications for understanding the pathogenesis of chronic cough. Though further investigations are required, we are now beginning to establish likely mechanisms that lead to acute cough to smoke exposure, and excessive cough associated with smoking- and pollution-related chronic diseases. It is probable that the ideal therapy for chronic cough will involve multiple targets, but the TRP family of ion channels in particular should be considered highly promising for the development of future novel anti-tussive treatments.

7. References

American Academy of Paediatrics (1997). Committee on Drugs Use of codeine- and dextromethorphan-containing cough remedies in children. *Paediatrics*, 99, pp. 918-920

American College of Chest Physicians (2006). Diagnosis and management of cough executive summary: ACCP evidence-based clinical practice guidelines. *Chest*, 129, pp. 1S-23S

Andre, E., Campi, B., Materazzi, S., Trevisani, M., Amadesi, S., Massi, D., Creminon, C., Vaksman, N., Nassini, R., Civelli, M., Baraldi, PG., Poole, D., Bunnett, N., Geppetti, P., & Patacchini, R. (2008). Cigarette smoke- induced neurogenic inflammation is mediated by alpha,beta-unsaturated aldehydes and the TRPA1 receptor in rodents. *Journal of Clinical Investigation*, 118, pp. 2574–2582

Andrè, E., Gatti, R., Trevisani, M., Preti, D., Baraldi, P., Patacchini, R., & Geppetti, P. (2009). Transient receptor potential ankyrin receptor 1 is a novel target for pro-tussive agents. *British Journal of Pharmacology*, 158, pp. 1621-1628

Barnes PJ (2010a). New therapies for asthma: is there any progress? *Trends Pharmacol. Sci.*, 31(7): 335-343.

Barnes PJ (2010b). New therapies for chronic obstructive pulmonary disease. *Med. Princ. Pract.*, 19(5): 330-338

Bautista, D., Jordt, S., Nikai, T., Tsuruda, P., Read, A., Poblete, J., Yamoah, E., Basbaum, A., & Julius, D. (2006). TRPA1 mediates the inflammatory actions of environmental irritants and proalgesic agents. *Cell*, 124, pp. 1269-1282

Belvisi, M. (2003). Airway sensory innervations as a target for novel therapies: an outdated concept? *Current Opinion in Pharmacology*, 3, pp. 239-243

Belvisi, M., & Geppetti, P. (2004). Cough 7: Current and future drugs for the treatment of chronic cough. Thorax, 59, pp. 438-40

Belvisi, M., Dubuis, E., & Birrell, M. (2011). TRPA1 channels: insights into cough and airway inflammatory disease. Chest, in press.

Bergren, D. (2001). Chronic tobacco smoke exposure increases cough to capsaicin in awake guinea pigs. *Respiratory Physiology*, 126, pp. 127-140

Berthoud, H., & Neuhuber, W. (2000). Functional and chemical anatomy of the afferent vagal system. *Autonomic Neuroscience*, 85, pp. 1-17

Bessac, B., Sivula, M., von Hehn, C., Escalera, J., Cohn, L., & Jordt, S. (2008). TRPA1 is a major oxidant sensor in murine airway sensory neurons. *Journal of Clinical Investigation*, 118, pp. 1899-1910

Birrell, M., Belvisi, M., Grace, M., Sadofsky, L., Faruqi, S., Hele, D., Maher, S., Freund-Michel, V., & Morice, A. (2009). TRPA1 agonists evoke coughing in guinea pig and human volunteers. *American Journal of Respiratory and Critical Care Medicine*, 180, pp. 1042-1047

Bose, B., Cater, J., & Clark, R. (1987). A once daily theophylline preparation in prevention of nocturnal symptoms in childhood asthma. *European Journal of Pediatrics*, 146, pp. 524-527

Campbell, M., Eliraz, A., Johansson, G., Tornlng, G., Nihlen, U., Bengtsson, T., & Rabe, K. (2005). Formoterol for maintenance and as-needed treatment of chronic obstructive pulmonary disease. *Respiratory Medicine*, 99, pp. 1511–1520

Canning, B., Mazzone, S., Meeker, S., Mor,i N., Reynolds, S., & Undem, B. (2004). Identification of the tracheal and laryngeal afferent neurones mediating cough in anaesthetised guinea-pigs. *Journal of Physiology*, 557, pp. 543-558

Canning, B., Mori, N., & Mazzone, S. (2006). Vagal afferent nerves regulating the cough reflex. *Respiratory Physiology & Neurobiology*, 152, pp. 223-242

Canning, B. (2011). Functional implications of the multiple afferent pathways regulating cough. *Pulmonary Pharmacology & Therapeutics*, doi: 10.1016/j.pupt.2011.01.008

Carr, M., Hunter, D., Jacoby, D., & Undem, B. (2002). Expression of tachykinins in nociceptive vagal afferent neurons during respiratory viral infection in guinea pigs. *American Journal of Respiratory and Critical Care Medicine*, 165, pp. 1071-1075

Caspani, O., & Heppenstall, P. (2009). TRPA1 and cold transduction: An unresolved issue? *Journal of General Physiology*, 133, pp. 245-249

Caterina, M., Schumacher, M., Tominaga, M., Rosen, T., Levine, J., & Julius, D. (1997). The capsaicin receptor: a heat-activated ion channel in the pain pathway. *Nature*, 389, pp. 816-824

Cavanaugh, E., Simkin, D., & Kim, D. (2008). Activation of transient receptor potential A1 channels by mustard oil, tetrahydrocannabinol and Ca^{2+} reveals different functional channel states. *Neuroscience*, 154, pp. 1467-1476

Cazzola, M., Matera M., Liccardi, G., De Prisco, F., D-Amato, G., & Rossi, F. (1993). Theophylline in the inhibition of angiotensin-converting enzyme inhibitor-induced cough. *Respiration*, 60, pp. 212-215

Centres for Disease Control and Prevention (2007). Infant deaths associated with cough and cold medications - two states, 2005. *Morbidity and Mortality Weekly Report*, 56, pp. 1-4

Chang, A., Phelan, P., Carlin, J., Sawyer, S., & Robertson, C. (1998). A randomised, placebo controlled trial of inhaled salbutamol and beclomethasone for recurrent cough. *Archives of Disease in Childhood*, 79, pp. 6–11

Chong, C., Chen, C., Ma, H., Wu, Y., & Wang, T. (2005). Comparison of lidocaine and bronchodilator inhalation treatments for cough suppression in patients with chronic obstructive pulmonary disease. *Emergency Medicine Journal*, 22, pp. 429–432

Choudry, N., Fuller, R., & Pride, N. (1989). Sensitivity of the human cough reflex: effect of inflammatory mediators prostaglandin E2, bradykinin, and histamine. The *American Reveview of Respiratory Disease*, 140, 137-141

Chung, K. (2011). Chronic 'cough hypersensitivity syndrome': A more precise label for chronic cough. *Pulmonary Pharmacology & Therapeutics*, doi: 10.1016/j.pupt.2011.01.012

Costello, J., Dunlop, L., & Gardiner, P. (1985). Characteristics of prostaglandin induced cough in man. *British Journal of Clinical Pharmacology*, 20, pp. 355-359

Dicpinigaitis, P. (2003). Cough reflex sensitivity in cigarette smokers. *Chest*, 123, pp. 685–688

Doherty, M., Mister, R., Pearson, M., & Calverley P. (2000). Capsaicin responsiveness and cough in asthma and chronic obstructive pulmonary disease. *Thorax*, 55, pp. 643–649

Dubuis, E., Birrell, M., Wortley, M., Grace, M., Maher, S., & Belvisi, M. (2011). Theophylline and theobromine block excitation of sensory nerves and prevent cough. *American Journal of Respiratory and Critical Care Medicine*, submitted abstract

Ellul-Micallef, R. (1983). Effect of terbutaline sulphate in chronic "allergic" cough. *British Medical Journal*, 287, pp. 940–943

Fairfax, A., Clarke, R., Chatterjee, S., Connolly, C., Higenbottam, T., Holgate, S., Hughes, J., Johnson, C., Johnston, R., MacIntyre, D., *et al.* (1990). Controlled-release theophylline in the treatment of nocturnal asthma. *Journal of International Medical Research*, 18, pp. 273-281

Fontana, A., Pantaleo, T., Lavorini, R., Mutolo, D., Polli, G., & Pistolesi, M. (1999). Coughing in laryngectomized patients. *American Journal of Respiratory and Critical Care Medicine*, 160, pp. 1578-1584

Ford, A., Forman, D., Moayyedi, P., & Morice, A. (2006). Cough in the community: a cross sectional survey and the relationship to gastrointestinal symptoms. *Thorax*, 61, pp. 975-979

Fox, A., Lalloo, U., Belvisi, M., Bernareggi, M., Chung, K., & Barnes, P. (1996). Bradykinin-evoked sensitisation of airway sensory nerves: a mechanism for ACE-inhibitor cough. *Nature Medicine*, 2, pp. 814-817

Freund-Michel, V., Birrell, M., Giembycz, M., Hele, D., Haj-Yahia, S., Belvisi, M. (2010). B_2-agonists block tussive responses in guinea pigs *via* an atypical cAMP-dependent pathway. *European Respiratory Journal*, 35, pp. 647-654

Fuller, R., & Choudry, N. (1987). Increased cough reflex associated with angiotensin converting enzyme inhibitor cough. *British Medical Journal*, 295, pp. 1025-1026

Gavva, N., Treanor, J., Garami, A., Fang, L., Suapaneni, S., Akrami, A., Alvarez, F., Bak, A., Darling, M., Gore, A., Jang, G., Kesslak, J., Ni, L., Norman, M., Palluconi, G., Rose, M., Salfi, M., Tan, E., Romanovsky, A., Banfield, C., & Davar, G. (2008). Pharmacological blockade of the vanilloid receptor TRPV1 elicits marked hyperthermia in humans. *Pain*, 136, pp. 202-210

Groneberg, D., Niimi, A., Dinh, Q., Cosio, B., Hew, M., Fischer, A., & Chung, K. (2004). Increased expression of Transient Receptor Potential Vanilloid-1 in airway nerves of chronic cough. *American Journal of Respiratory and Critical Care Medicine*, 170, pp. 1276-1280

Gunn, V., Taha, S., Liebelt, E., & Serwint, J. (2001). Toxicity of over-the-counter cough and cold medications. *Pediatrics*, 108, pp. E52

Gunthorpe, M., & Chizh, B. (2009). Clinical development of TRPV1 antagonists: targeting a pivotal point in the pain pathway. *Drug Discovery Today*, 14, pp. 56-67

Gu, Q., Ni, D., & Lee, L. (2008) Expression of neuronal nicotinic acetylcholine receptors in rat vagal pulmonary sensory neurons. *Respiratory Physiology & Neurobiology*, 161, pp. 87–91

Harding, S. (2006). Gastroesophageal reflux and chronic cough. *GI Motility Online*, doi:10.1038/gimo77

Ho, C., Gu, Q., Hong, J, & Lee, L. (2000). Prostaglandin E(2) enhances chemical and mechanical sensitivities of pulmonary C fibers in the rat. *American Journal of Respiratory and Critical Care Medicine*, 162, pp. 528–533

Hunt, J., Fang, K., Malik, R., Snyder, A., Malhotra, N., Platts-Mills, T., & Gaston, B. (2000). Endogenous airway acidification. *American Journal of Respiratory and Critical Care Medicine*, 161, pp. 694-699

Irwin, R., Boulet, L., Cloutier, M., Gold, P., Ing, A., O'Byrne, P., Prakash, U., Pratter, M., & Rubin, B. (1998). Managing cough as a defense mechanism and as a symptom: A consensus panel report of the American College of Chest Physicians. *Chest*, 114, pp. 133S-181S

Karlsson, J., Zackrisson, C. & Lundberg, J. (1991). Hyperresponsiveness to tussive stimuli in cigarette smoke-exposed guinea-pigs: a role for capsaicin-sensitive, calcitonin gene-related peptide-containing nerves. *Acta Physiologica Scandinavica*, 141, pp. 445-454

Karlsson, J., & Fuller, R. (1999). Pharmacological regulation of the cough reflex - from experimental models to antitussive effects in man. Pulmonary Pharmacology & Therapeutics, 12, pp. 215-228

Katsumata, U., Sekizawa, K., Ujiie, Y., Sasaki, H., & Takishima, T. (1991). Bradykinin-induced cough reflex markedly increases in patients with cough associated with captopril and enalapril. *The Tohoku Journal of Experimental Medicine*, 164, pp. 103-109

Kaufman, M., Coleridge, H., Coleridge, J., & Baker, D. (1980). Bradykinin stimulates afferent vagal C-fibers in intrapulmonary airways of dogs. *Journal of Applied Physiology: Respiratory, Environmental and Exercise Physiology*, 48, pp. 511-517

Kostikas, K., Papatheodorou, G., Ganas, K., Psathakis, K., Panagou, P., & Loukides, S. (2002). pH in expired breath condensate of patients with inflammatory airways diseases. *American Journal of Respiratory and Critical Care Medicine*, 165, pp. 1364-1370

Kou, Y., and Lee, L. (1990). Stimulation of rapidly adapting receptors in the canine lungs by a single breath of cigarette smoke. *Journal of Applied Physiology*, 68, pp. 1203-1210

Kou, Y., & Lee, L. (1991) Mechanisms of cigarette smoke-induced stimulation of rapidly adapting receptors in canine lungs. *Respiratory Physiology*, 83, pp. 61–75

Lalloo, U., Fox, A., Belvisi, M., Chung, F., & Barnes, P. (1995). Capsazepine inhibits cough induced by capsaicin and citric acid but not by hypertonic saline in guinea pigs. *Journal of Applied Physiology*, 79, pp. 1082-1087

Laude, E., Higgins, K., & Morice, A. (1993). A comparative study of the effects of citric acid, capsaicin and resiniferatoxin on the cough challenge in guinea-pig and man. *Pulmonary Pharmacology*, 6, pp. 171-175

Lee, L., Morton, R., Hord, A., & Frazier, D. (1983). Reflex control of breathing following inhalation of cigarette smoke in conscious dogs. *Journal of Applied Physiology*, 54, pp. 562-570

Lee, L., Morton, R., & Frazier D. (1985). Influence of nicotine in cigarette smoke on acute ventilatory responses in awake dogs. *Journal of Applied Physiology*, 59, pp. 229-236

Lee, L., & Morton, R. (1986). Hexamethonium aerosol prevents cigarette smoke induced pulmonary reflexes in dogs. *Respiratory Physiology*, 66, pp. 303-314

Lee, L., Kou, Y., Frazier, D., Beck, E., Pisarri, T., Coleridge, H., & Coleridge, J. (1989). Stimulation of vagal pulmonary C-fibers by a single breath of cigarette smoke in dogs. *Journal of Applied Physiology*, 66, 2032-2038

Lee, L., Gerhardstein, D., Wang, A., & Burki, N. (1993). Nicotine is responsible for airway irritation evoked by cigarette smoke inhalation in men. *Journal of Applied Physiology*, 75, pp. 1955–1961

Lee, L., Burki, N., Gerhardstein, D., Gu, Q., Kou, Y., & Xu, J. (2007) Airway irritation and cough evoked by inhaled cigarette smoke: role of neuronal nicotinic acetylcholine receptors. *Pulmonary Pharmacology & Therapeutics*, 20, pp. 355–364

Lee, M., & Undem, B. (2008). Basic mechanisms of cough: Current understanding and remaining questions. *Lung*, 186, pp. S10-S16

Lee, L., Gu, Q., & Lin, Y. (2010). Effect of smoking on cough reflex sensitivity: Basic and preclinical studies. *Lung*, 188, pp. S23-S27

Lehto, S., Tamir, R., Deng, H., Klionsky, L., Kuang, R., Le, A., Lee, D., Louis, J., Magal, E., Manning, B., Rubino, J., Surapaneni, S., Tamayo, N., Wang, T., Wang, J., Wang, J., Wang, W., Youngblood, B., Zhang, M., Zhu, D., Norman, M., & Gavva, N. (2008). Antihyperalgesic effects of (R,E)-N-(2-Hydroxy-2,3-dihydro-1H-inden-4-yl)-3-(2-(piperidin-1-yl)-4-(trifluoromethyl)phenyl)-acrylamide (AMG8562), a novel Transient Receptor Potential Vanilloid Type 1 modulator that does not cause hyperthermia in rats. *The Journal of Pharmacology and Experimental Therapeutics*, 326, 218-229

Lewis, C., Ambrose, C., Banner, K., Battram, C., Butler, K., Giddings, J., Mok, J., Nasra, J., Winny, C., & Poll, C. (2007). Animal models of cough: Literature review and presentation of a novel cigarette smoke-enhanced cough model in the guinea pig. *Pulmonary Pharmacology & Therapeutics*, 20, pp. 325-333

Lowry, R., Higenbottam, T., Johnson, T., & Godden, D. (1987). Inhibition of artificially induced cough in man by bronchodilators. *British Journal of Clinical Pharmacology*, 24, pp. 503–510

Maher, S., Birrell, M., & Belvisi, M. (2009). Prostaglandin E_2 mediates cough via the EP_3 receptor: implications for future disease therapy. *American Journal of Respiratory and Critical Care Medicine*, 180, pp. 923-928

Maher, S., Grace, M., Birrell, M. & Belvisi, M. (2010). Prostaglandin E2-induced sensory nerve activation is mediated by TRPA1 and TRPV1. *American Journal of Respiratory and Critical Care Medicine*, **181, pp.** A5541

Mazzone, S. (2004). Sensory regulation of the cough reflex. *Pulmonary Pharmacology & Therapeutics*, 17, pp. 361-368

McCormick, A., Fleming, D., & Charlton, J. (1995). Office of population censuses and surveys. In: Morbidity statistics from general practice, fourth national study 1991-1992. Series MB5 no 3. London: HMSO

Millqvist, E., Bende, M., & Lowhagen, O. (1998). Sensory hyperreactivity - a possible mechanism underlying cough and asthma-like symptoms. *Allergy*, 53, pp. 1208-1212

Mohammed, S., Higenbottam, T., & Adcock, J. (1993). Effects of aerosol-applied capsaicin, histamine and prostaglandin E2 on airway sensory receptors of anaesthetized cats. *Journal of Physiology*, 469, pp. 51-66

Montuschi, P., Kharitonov, S., Ciabattoni, G., & Barnes, P. (2003). Exhaled leukotrienes and prostaglandins in COPD. *Thorax*, 58, pp. 585-588

Morice, A. & committee members. (2004). The diagnosis and management of chronic cough. *European Respiratory Journal*, 24, pp. 481-492

Morice, A., Fontana, G., Belvisi, M., Birring, S., Chung, K., Dicpinigaitis, P., Kastelik, J., McGarvey, L., Smith, J., Tatar, M., & Widdicombe, J. (2007). ERS guidelines on the assessment of cough. *European Respiratory Journal*, 29, pp. 1256-1276

Mulrennan, S., Wright, C., Thompson, R., Goustas, P., & Morice, A. (2004). Effect of salbutamol on smoking related cough. *Pulmonary Pharmacology & Therapeutics* 17, pp. 127-131

Myers, A., Kajekar, R., & Undem, B. (2002). Allergic inflammation-induced neuropeptide production in rapidly adapting afferent nerves in guinea pig airways. *American Journal of Physiology: Lung, Cellular and Molecular Physiology*, 282, pp. L775-L781

Nasra, J., & Belvisi, M. (2009). Modulation of sensory nerve function and the cough reflex: Understanding disease pathogenesis. *Pharmacology & Therapeutics*, 124, pp. 354-375

Nilius, B. (2007). TRP channels in disease. *Biochimica et Biophysica Acta*, 1772, pp. 805–812

Office for National Statistics (2010). Social Trends No. 40: 2010 edition

Pechlivanova, D., & Georgiev, V. (2005). Effects of single and long-term theophylline treatment on the threshold of mechanical nociception: contribution of adenosine A1 and alpha2-adrenoceptors. *Methods and Findings in Experimental and Clinical Pharmacology*, 27, pp. 659-664

Pecova, R., Zucha, J., Pec, M., Neuschlova, M., Hanzel, P., & Tatar, M. (2008). Cough reflex sensitivity testing in seasonal allergic rhinitis patients and healthy volunteers. *Journal of Physiology*, 59, pp. 557-564

Pounsford, J., Birch, M., & Saunders, K. (1985). Effect of bronchodilators on the cough response to inhaled citric acid in normal and asthmatic subjects. *Thorax*, 40, pp. 662–667

Profita, M., Sala, A., Bonanno, A., Riccobono, L., Siena, L., Melis, M., Di Giorgi, R., Mirabella, F., Gjomarkaj, M., Bonsignore, G., & Vignola, A. (2003). Increased prostaglandin E2 concentrations and cyclooxygenase-2 expression in asthmatic subjects with sputum eosinophilia. *Journal of Allergy and Clinical Immunology*, 112, pp.709-716

Rao, S., Mudipalli, R., Remes-Troche, J., Utech, C., & Zimmerman, B. (2007). Theophylline improves esophageal chest pain - a randomized, placebo-controlled study. *American Journal of Gastroenterology*, 102, pp. 930-938

Reynolds, S., Mackenzie, A., Spina, D., & Page, C. (2004). The pharmacology of cough. Trends in Pharmacological Sciences, 25, pp. 569-76

Schroeder, K., & Fahey, T. (2002). Systematic review of randomised controlled trials of over the counter cough medicines for acute cough in adults. British Medical Journal, 324, pp. 329-331

Smith, C., Adamson, D., Choudry, N., & Fuller, R. (1991). The effect of altering airway tone on the sensitivity of the cough reflex in normal volunteers. *European Respiratory Journal*, 4, pp. 1078–1079

Smith, J. & Woodcock, A. (2006). Cough and its importance in COPD. *International Journal of Chronic Obstructive Pulmonary Disease*, 1, pp. 305-314

Talavera, K., Gees, M., Karashima, Y., Meseguer, V., Vanoirbeek, J., Damann, N., Everaerts, W., Benoit, M., Janssens, A., Vennekens, R., Viana, F., Nemery, B., Nilius, B., & Voets, T. (2009). Nicotine activates the chemosensory cation channel TRPA1. *Nature Neuroscience*, 12, pp. 1293-1300

Taylor-Clark, T., & Undem, B. (2006). Transduction mechanisms in airway sensory nerves. *Journal of Applied Physiology*, 101, pp. 950-959

Taylor-Clark, T., McAlexander, M., Nassenstein, C., Sheardown, S., Wilson, S., Thornton, J., Carr, M., & Undem, B. (2008). Relative contributions of TRPA1 and TRPV1 ion channels in the activation of vagal bronchopulmonary C-fibres by the endogenous autacoid 4-oxononenal. *Journal of Physiology*, 586, pp. 3447-3459

Trevisani, M., Milan, A., Gatti, R., Zanasi, A., Harrison, S., Fontana, G., Morice, A., Geppetti, P. (2004). Antitussive activity of iodo-resiniferatoxin in guinea pigs. *Thorax*, 59, pp. 769-772

Undem, B., Carr, M., & Kollarik, M. (2002). Physiology and plasticity of putative cough fibres in the guinea pig. *Pulmonary Pharmacology & Therapeutics*, 15, 193-198

U.S. Department of Health and Human Services (2010). How Tobacco Smoke Causes Disease: The Biology and Behavioural Basis for Smoking-Attributable Disease: A Report of the Surgeon General. In: *U.S. Department of Health and Human Services, Centres for Disease Control and Prevention, National Center for Chronic Disease Prevention and Health Promotion, Office on Smoking and Health.* Atlanta, GA.

U.S. Food and Drug Administration (2008). Public Health Advisory: FDA recommends that over-the-counter cough and cold products not be used for infants and children under 2 years of age. Accessed 7 Sept 2009, available from: http://www.fda.gov/Drugs/DrugSafety/PublicHealthAdvisories/ucm051137.html

Usmani, O., Belvisi, M., Patel, H., Crispino, N., Birrell, M., Korbonits, M., & Barnes, P. (2005). Theobromine inhibits sensory nerve activation and cough. *FASEB Journal*, 19, pp. 231-233

Vassilev, Z., Chu, A., Ruck, B., Adams, E., & Marcus, S. (2009). Adverse reactions to over-the-counter cough and cold products among children: the cases managed out of hospitals. *Journal of Clinical Pharmacy and Therapeutics*, 34, pp. 313-318

Viana, F., & Ferrer-Montiel, A. (2009). TRPA1 modulators in preclinical development. *Expert Opinion*, 19, pp. 1788-1799

Widdicombe, J. (2002). Neuroregulation of cough: implications for drug therapy. *Current Opinion in Pharmacology*, 2, pp. 256-263

World Health Organisation (2005). Prevention and control of chronic respiratory diseases at country level: Towards a Global Alliance against Chronic Respiratory Diseases (GARD). In: *WHO Meeting on Prevention and Control of Chronic Respiratory Diseases*, Geneva Switzerland, 17-19

World Health Organisation (2008a). Fact Sheet No. 307: Asthma, http://www.who.int/mediacentre/factsheets/fs307/en/index.html

World Health Organisation (2008b). Fact Sheet No. 313: Air quality and health, http://www.who.int/mediacentre/factsheets/fs313/en/index.html

World Health Organisation (2010). Fact Sheet No. 339: Tobacco http://www.who.int/mediacentre/factsheets/fs339/en/index.html

World Health Organisation (2011). Fact Sheet No. 315: Chronic obstructive pulmonary disease (COPD) http://www.who.int/mediacentre/factsheets/fs315/en/index.html

Xu, J., Yang, W., Zhang, G., Gu, Q., & Lee, L. (2007) Calcium transient evoked by nicotine in isolated rat vagal pulmonary sensory neurons. *American Journal of Physiology: Lung, Cellular and Moleular Physiology*, 292, pp. L54–L61

Zurborg, S., Yurgionas, B., Jira, J., Caspani, O., & Heppenstall, P. (2007). Direct activation of the ion channel TRPA1 by Ca^{2+}. *Nature Neuroscience*, 10, pp. 277-279

6

Air Pollution, Reactive Oxygen Species (ROS), and Autonomic Nervous System Interactions Modulate Cardiac Oxidative Stress and Electrophysiological Changes

Elisa Ghelfi
Harvard School of Public Health,
Department of Environmental Health, MIPS Program, Boston,
USA

1. Introduction

1.1 Air pollution: A global overview

In the last decades we witnessed unprecedented rapid deterioration in the environment as a consequence of intense anthropogenic activity. Air pollution, and more precisely particulate matter (PM) is both an alarming environmental problem and a public health concern that affects many regions of the world. Ambient air pollution has been associated with increased respiratory mucosal symptoms, exacerbation of asthma, chronic obstructive pulmonary disease (COPD) as well as cardiovascular diseases and mortality [World Health Organization (WHO) working group et al., 2003]. This association is based on observational epidemiological studies of disease occurrence in the human populations and in *in-vitro* and *in-vivo* studies of animals and humans [Health Effect Institute [HEI] et al., 2002].

Some groups in the population are more susceptible to air pollution induced health risks. Children are particularly at risk for deleterious respiratory outcomes due to the immaturity of their respiratory organ systems. They spend significantly more time outdoors than adults, especially during the summer months when smog and ozone levels are highest. Elderly, diabetics, people affected by underlying heart or lung disease, lower socioeconomic population living in proximity to sources of pollution [Mohai et al., 2009], are among the groups that experience increased risk for both pulmonary and cardiovascular system diseases.

Sources of pollutants differ in different regions and are influenced by many factors. Air pollution levels are higher in the vicinity of specific sources such as roads, chemical plants, oil refineries, manufacturing facilities, and other industrial facilities. Meteorological factors determine the distribution of pollutants, since they can travel far from the original source, influenced by the wind, along with the topography of the regions and phenomena of temperature inversion, a meteorological condition that traps pollutants at ground level instead of circulating them away, and it is often responsible for episodes of sudden noxious toxin and particle concentrations in small areas. The increase of the world population and the consequent increase in the production and consumption of resources in particular of fossil fuels, influence the concentration and the quality of the emissions. Urbanization imposes also a significant pressure, by 2025 coastal populations alone are expected to reach six billion while the year 2007 has been the first in human history when more than half of all world population live in cities [United Nation Environment Program (UNEP) 2007].

1.2 Anthropogenic emission in rural areas, industrial environments, and developing countries

Anthropogenic emissions of pollutants in the atmosphere are not only a concern for the industrialized world but also for developing countries and rural areas around the globe, with differences in the sources and in the chemicals dispersed in the environment.
A 2005 World Health Organization (WHO) Global update assessed the burden of diseases due to atmospheric pollution and reported that more than 2 million premature deaths each year can be attributed to air pollution. More than half of this disease burden is borne by the population of developing countries [World Health Organization (WHO) 2005].
In industrialized countries, air pollution is largely due to fossil fuel combustion for transportation, industrial activity and electricity production, while in developing countries (excluding the large metropolitan areas) the air pollution mostly consists of uncontrolled burning of biomass for cooking, heating, farming and deforesting [Armaroli & Balzani 2011].
Rural areas have lower outdoor air pollutants since less vehicular traffic and industrial smoke are present. Nevertheless individual exposures are often huge as a consequence of indoor solid fuel combustion like wood, crop residues, and dung which are extensively used for heating and cooking. The percentage of people using solid fuels varies widely among countries and regions ranging from respectively 77%, 74%, and 74% in sub-Saharan Africa, South-East Asia, and the Western Pacific Region, while in the majority of industrialized countries, the use of solid fuel falls below 5% [Perez-Padilla et al., 2010]. Women are particularly exposed to indoor air pollution, since in rural areas of developing countries they have larger amounts of time for indoor cooking and attending home heating. [Perez-Padilla et al., 2010].
In Europe and North America the introduction of air quality policy, limiting the emissions of the main air pollutants from road transport and large industrial combustion, has significantly improved the air quality and reduced air pollution-induced health effects. However a report from WHO indicated that air pollution contributed annually in Europe to 100,000 premature deaths and the loss of 725,000 working days [Eurostat, 2009].
Data arising from constant monitoring of outdoor pollutants are increasing from many other regions of the world, since the knowledge that air pollutants are dangerous for health is gaining global awareness. The type of pollution and the mix of the gases released in the atmosphere differ among countries. As an example, data from Tokyo showed that sulfur dioxide, one of the main pollutants in urban areas, had and annual average concentration below 10 $\mu g/m^3$, for the years 2000-2005 which corresponds to concentrations recorded in the least polluted cities in Europe such as Copenhagen and Barcelona. On the other hand the annual average ambient nitrogen dioxide concentration in Tokyo was 60 $\mu g/m^3$, a value higher than those in the most polluted cities in Europe such as Paris and Athens [Katanoda et al., 2011].

1.3 Initial reports of health risk associated with air pollution

One of the first recorded episodes that gave undeniable evidence of the potential for atmospheric pollution to cause deaths and diseases was registered in December 1930 in the

Meuse valley in Belgium [Bell & Davis 2001], [Nemery et al., 2001]. The area of Liège on the River Meuse, was once one of the most heavily industrialized areas of continental Europe with steel mills, coke ovens, foundries, smelters, fertilizer and explosives plants established since the industrial revolution. The weather was characterized by temperature inversion conditions, with a very feeble wind that blew from the city of Liège into the narrow valley. The temperature inversion at about 70–80 m above ground, just above the tallest chimneys in the valley, prevented the fumes from rising, trapping the emitted gases and impurities to accumulate in the corridor formed by the valley between Liège and Huy. More than 60 people died which was more than 10 times the normal mortality rate. The average age of the victims was about 62 years and ranged from 20 to 89 years.

The report released by the committee of experts appointed to investigate the disaster, noted that also several hundreds of people were affected severely, with respiratory problems such as "asthma like" symptoms, wheezing, laryngeal irritation, chest pain and coughing. The report postulates that fine soot particles, onto which irritant gases had been adsorbed, had a major role in the noxiousness of the fog. Sulfur compounds proved the most abundant compounds emitted in the valley. Investigators estimated that more than 60,000 kg of sulfur dioxide was produced per day, with a resultant sulfur dioxide (SO_2) concentration of up to 100 mg/m^3 after 4 days of fog. This SO_2 concentration exceeds the current WHO standard for toxicity (20μg/m^3 for daily mean concentration) and could account for the victims' symptoms. Additional components of the thick fog of air pollutants included sulfuric acid mist, and fluoride gases together with carbon soot.

In the United States a similar episode occurred in the town of Donora located in the Monongahela River Valley in Pennsylvania. In late October Donora was submerged in noxious smog. As in the Meuse valley disaster, an intense, meteorological temperature inversion settled on the valley trapping the pollutants. The smog was a deadly mixture of emissions from the steel plants and coal furnaces located in the valley and in the town, consisting of carbon soot, sulfur dioxide, carbon monoxide and metal dust and particulate. The smog was so thick that it was reported that the residents had to keep lights on all day. In the five days between October 26 and 31, twenty people died, some 400 required hospitalization and more than 7,000 in a town of 14,000 residents were sickened before rain dispersed the killing smog on October 30 and 31, 1948 [Helfand et al., 2001].

The investigations following the Donora Smog Disaster once more showed the association between air pollution and increased mortality. The data from the investigations were essential to determine the first federal clean-air act, enacted in 1955 by the Congress, to address the national environmental problem of air pollution and to provide funds to the Public Health Service to conduct research into the causes and the control of air pollution in the United States.

In Europe the deadliest episode that raised the awareness about the threat posed by air pollution, occurred in London in December 1952. The London fog of 1952 is widely regarded as a catalyst for the study of air pollution epidemiology. Again, a temperature inversion settled over windless London and trapped the carbon soot from coal burning, residential heating and cooking, industrial smoke and vehicle exhaust. About 4,000 people died prematurely in a single week followed by another 8,000 deaths during the next few months. The smog-related deaths were primarily attributed to pneumonia, bronchitis, tuberculosis, and heart failure. Many with pre-existing conditions, including asthma, died of respiratory distress. Many others died of cardiac distress and asphyxiation. Non-fatal health effects from the smog included

short-term chest pains, lung inflammation and diminished breathing ability, damaged respiratory cells, permanent lung damage, and increased incidence of asthma attacks [De Angelo, 2009]. In a report of the disaster The Ministry of Health noted that morbidity and mortality remained elevated in the greater London region until March 1953.
The acute air pollution episodes which occurred in the Meuse valley, in Donora and in 1952 London are extreme examples that are unlikely to occur in cities and in countries where the air quality is under constant control. However the risk for acute and chronic exposure to deadly concentration of air pollutants is higher in rapidly economically growing regions or areas where massive urbanization occurs and monitoring for pollution and health is not systematically conducted.
What was observed in those episodes was the first evidence that air pollution and particle pollution, are serious threats to the health of the population, especially for the elderly children and individuals with pre-existing cardiovascular and respiratory conditions. Carbon soot, sulfur dioxide and fine particulate pollution were the major culprits for the adverse health effects occurring in the population in the Meuse valley, Donora and London disasters. Studies in the following decades have identified in air particle pollution one of the major risk for health.
The extent of the effects of air pollution depends on the actual exposure. In a landmark study "The Harvard Six Cities Study", Dockery and colleagues indicated for the first time a strong positive correlation between levels of air pollution and cardiovascular mortality. In this longitudinal cohort mortality study, the morbidity and mortality of the population of six US cities was associated with long-term exposure to fine particulate air pollution including sulfate. The results showed that deaths from lung cancer, pulmonary disease, and heart disease were 26 percent higher in the city with the highest level of pollutants. Rather than indicating sulfur dioxide as the culprit emission, The Harvard Six Cities Study directed the attention to particulate matter. This is another important contribution of the study that identified in particulate matter what is now universally recognized as a dangerous form of air pollution.

2. Sources of air pollution

Air pollution comprises of a very complex mixture of thousands of chemicals and chemicals interactions.
At least six main air pollutants have been identified by the WHO, by the European European Environmental Agency (EEA) and the US EPA agencies, as noxious for human health, these are: lead, carbon monoxide (CO), sulfur dioxide (SO_2), nitrogen dioxide (NO_2), ozone (O_3) and particulate matter (PM). All of these but lead are major components of automotive pollution, and have been included in the guidelines for maximum concentration in urban areas, by the World Health Organization (WHO) and many national environmental agencies around the world.

2.1 Main components of urban air pollution

2.1.1 Lead

In the past, motor vehicles were the biggest source of lead. But since leaded gasoline has been phased out, lead emissions have decreased by about 98 percent. Today, metal processing is the biggest source of atmospheric lead. The highest air concentrations are found in the vicinity of ferrous and nonferrous smelters and battery manufacturers [Clean

Air Trust, 1999]. Lead can harm the kidneys, liver, nervous system and other organs. It may cause neurological impairments such as seizures, mental retardation and behavioral disorders. Even at low doses, lead is associated with damage to the nervous systems of fetuses and young children, resulting in lowered IQ and learning problems. Recent studies also show that lead may be a factor in high blood pressure and subsequent heart disease [Clean Air Trust, 1999].

2.1.2 Carbon monoxide (CO)

Carbon monoxide is a gas emitted directly from vehicles as a result of incomplete combustion of fuel. When it is inhaled in very high doses, CO replaces oxygen in the bloodstream by binding with hemoglobin, thus interfering with normal transport of oxygen to the heart and the brain and to the whole body. Exposure to high CO levels is lethal. Low levels found in ambient settings do not affect healthy individuals and indeed have been shown to have anti-inflammatory effects. Although CO has been shown to hasten the onset of angina (chest pain) in people with coronary artery disease and the incidence of cardiac effects. It is unclear whether this is an effect of CO or traffic related pollutants for which CO is a marker. Some epidemiologic studies have found positive correlation between CO level and morbidity, mortality and adverse pregnancy outcome [HEI, 2004]. *In vivo* experiments showed that urban carbon monoxide air pollution exacerbates rat heart ischemia reperfusion injury. Interestingly, recent observations of CO delivered at very low concentration in a controlled way showed positive beneficial effects in animal models in the modulation of inflammation [Motterlini & Otterbein, 2010]. In another study using a rat model of myocardial infarction and exposure to CO at 35 PPM the current EPA standard, Wellenius and colleagues showed that CO at that concentration reduced arrhythmias observed in the first 24 hrs after the infarction. [Wellenius et al., 2004]

2.1.3 Sulfur oxides (SOx)

Sulfur oxides SOx, comprising sulfur oxide (SO), sulfur dioxide (SO_2), and sulfur trioxide (SO_3), are gaseous by-products of the combustion of fossil fuels that contain sulfur. Clinical studies have shown that exposure to SO_2 at level as low as 0.7 mg/m^3, (0.25 part-per-million (ppm), elicits increased broncho-constriction in people with asthma [Gong H. Jr. et al., 1995]. Acute decline in pulmonary function has also been observed in association with air pollution episodes in which levels of SO_2 were briefly but considerably elevated [Bascom, 1996]. Sulfur dioxide is also associated with increased daily mortality and hospital admissions from respiratory and cardiovascular disease, even at low levels. In an analysis of a large US cohort study long term exposure to SO_2 has been associated with reduced pulmonary function and mortality from cardiovascular disease. Reduction in ambient SO_2 concentrations owing to regulatory action has recently been associated with decreased mortality and improved respiratory health in children in Hong Kong [HEI, 2004].

2.1.4 Nitrogen oxides (NOx)

Nitrogen oxides consisting of nitrogen oxide (NO) and nitrogen dioxide (NO_2) are by-products of fossil fuel combustion in transportation, industrial applications, and waste incineration. Like SO_2 urban cause of outdoor NO_2, are mobile source emissions from both on-road vehicles such as cars, trucks, buses and off-road equipment, consisting mainly of ships, airplanes, locomotives, agricultural and construction machinery. Unlike SO_2, NO_2 is relatively insoluble and is thus more likely to reach the lower airways. Moreover NO_2 is an oxidant. In clinical experiments it elicits inflammatory responses at levels of 1mg/m^3 (0.9 ppm), and increases responsiveness to ozone and allergens [Bascom, 1996]. In epidemiological studies NO_2 has been associated with increased respiratory morbidity such as asthma exacerbation and reduced lung function and rate of lung growth in children. Short-term increase of NO_2, like SO_2, is associated with increased daily mortality and hospital admission for respiratory and cardiovascular diseases [Zemp et al., 1999; HEI, 2004].

2.1.5 Ozone (O_3)

Ozone and photochemical oxidants are typical pollutants in photochemical smog. Ground level ozone can be formed by sunlight-induced oxidation of precursor pollutants such as NOx and carbon hydroxides in the atmosphere. Ozone is a strong oxidant and an unstable molecule. Important ozone precursors and reactive intermediates are compounds of the organic hydroxyl group, hydroxyl radical (OH), hydroperoxyl radical ($HO_2^{\bullet}$) and singlet oxygen. Volatile organic compounds (VOCs) are a variety of readily evaporable toxic compounds from both anthropogenic sources like unburned fossil fuel, fuel combustion processes and biogenic emission from vegetation. VOCs are responsible for triggering chemical reactions in the atmosphere that contribute to ozone formation. The interaction of these compounds with NOx forms additional ozone in the presence of heat and sunlight, conditions typical of the summer season when ozone tends to accumulate over urban areas.

Studies have shown that ozone has a negative impact on human health, being associated with an increase in pulmonary diseases, reduced pulmonary functions, exacerbation of asthma and increase in hospital admission. Collectively these studies have revealed a small association between daily mortality and ozone level, which is independent of the effect of particulate matter.

There are additional concerns about increased ozone exposure and respiratory morbidity in children. Asthma, the most common chronic childhood disease, has significant public health impacts and is characterized by chronic lung inflammation, reversible airflow obstruction, and immune sensitization to allergens. According to time series evidence, exposure to concentration of ozone below 80 ppb may produce short-term lung function deficits and increased risk of respiratory illnesses including asthma episodes severe enough to require medical attention. Early childhood chronic ozone exposure may produce reduced lung function growth, especially in those parameters reflecting small airway flow rates [Wigle et al., 2007].

2.1.6 Particulate matter (PM)

Particulate matter is a complex mixture of organic and inorganic solid particles and liquid droplets deriving from many different sources and materials. Ambient air particles vary greatly in size and chemical composition depending upon their formation process, the seasonal changes, and the characteristics of the region. PM can be characterized by origin as geogenic, from soil and geological material, as opposed to anthropogenic, when originated by human activities. PM can be discriminated by type of airborne transformation in primary or secondary particles, or can be characterized by physicochemical properties such as solubility, aerodynamic diameter or particle size. In some geographical regions, a single industrial source of PM may dominate, but more commonly the PM is a mixture of local and transported particulate as well as primary and secondary particles. Because of the variability and complexity of sources and weather patterns, the resultant particulate mixture in any given area has significant daily variability in PM quality.

Primary particles originate directly from a defined source, for example from incomplete combustion of fuels in vehicle exhausts or from the combustion of organic substances. Additional sources are road dust, industrial smoke emissions, smokestacks, forest fires, windblown soil, volcanic dust and sea spray, to mention a few.

Secondary particles are known to make up most of the fine airborne particle pollution mass. These particles are formed in complex reactions in the atmosphere by chemicals such as sulfur dioxides and nitrogen oxides. Organic carbon (OC) and elemental carbon (EC, also called black carbon or soot), form the major fraction of secondary particulate matter. OC and EC are abundant in many source emissions from combustion of organic material. Carbon accounts for 10 to 40% of PM mass on a global scale but this fraction exceeds 50% in many urban atmospheres due to energy-related fossil-fuel and bio-fuel combustion, while in rural areas large-scale wildfires consume millions of acres of forest generating smoke that mostly consists of carbonaceous material [Mauderly & Chow, 2008].

Organic aerosols include also non PM components like volatile organic compounds (VOCs) such as propane and benzene and semi-volatile organic compounds (SVOCs), in equilibrium in the atmosphere between gas and particulate phases, such as polycyclic aromatic hydrocarbons (PAHs), well known carcinogens. VOCs and SVOCs form a dynamic continuum in the atmosphere with particulate and they can be adsorbed on the surface or inside PM [Mauderly & Chow, 2008].

The term PM_{10} refers to all airborne particulate matter less than 10 microns in aerodynamic diameter. The coarse particle fraction has an aerodynamic diameter between 10 μm and 2.5 μm. Fine particles ($PM_{2.5}$) comprise those particles with diameters less than 2.5 μm, while ultrafine particles (UFP or $PM_{0.1}$) are particles with an aerodynamic diameter less than 0.1 μm. In urban areas PM_{10} originates from crushing or grinding operations and dust stirred up by vehicles traveling on roads, with the organic carbon fraction in the form of biological components such as detritus, fungi, pollen, and spores. PM_{10} , once inhaled deposit in the upper part of the respiratory tract such as the nose, trachea, and bronchi. As particles in this fraction land on these mucous and cilia covered surfaces, they may be propelled upwards by the movement of cilia in the upper airways with the mucus and particles moved into the pharynx where it may be swallowed or expectorated. PM_{10} may not cause as extensive cardiovascular effects as $PM_{2.5}$, but has been strongly associated with hospital admissions for respiratory symptoms [Brunekreef & Forsberg, 2005] and there is growing evidence for effects of coarse PM on cardiovascular mortality and morbidity especially in arid regions where coarse PM concentration are relatively high [Gold et al., 1999].

Fine particles, $PM_{2.5}$, consist of a complex mixture of many different constituents, and are often formed from agglomerates of nanosized particles. Foremost among these are secondary particles, formed by secondary sulfate nitrate, and ammonium. Most sulfates derive from the oxidation of sulfur dioxide that is produced by natural sources and by anthropogenic combustion of fossil fuels. Sulfur dioxide when reacting with hydrogen peroxide, ozone, or oxygen results in particulate sulfuric acid. Sulfuric acid can be neutralized by ambient ammonia to ammonium sulfate and bisulfate that contribute to the $PM_{2.5}$ associated acidity. Nitrate associated with $PM_{2.5}$ results largely from the oxidation of nitrogen dioxide derived primarily from combustion processes of fossil fuels. Nitrogen dioxide is converted into vapor-phase nitric acid by reaction with hydroxyl radicals under daylight conditions, while at night it is oxidized to nitric acid by a sequence of reactions initiated by ozone that produces nitrate. Ammonium nitrate produced by reaction of atmospheric ammonia with nitric acid also contributes to the acidity of the particles [Schlesinger, 2007b].

Fine particles also have an organic component of primary and secondary carbonaceous aerosols as well as an inorganic fraction that consists of crustal material derived from soil dust, rocks, or particles produced by mechanical generation from agriculture, mining, construction and road traffic. Aluminum and silicon are the two major crustal derived elements found in $PM_{2.5}$ and, together with calcium, can become aerosolized from various combustion processes, while potassium is a signature for biomass burning such as wood burning and cooking [Schlesinger, 2007b]. Transition metals are an important but relatively small fraction of $PM_{2.5}$. The major metal constituents include Cr, Co, Ni, Mn, Zn, V, Cu, and mainly Fe [Gurgueira et al., 2002].

Ultrafine particles (UFPs or $PM_{0.1}$), with an aerodynamic diameter smaller than 0.1μm, constitute about 10% of fine particulate mass but represent over 85-90% of the total $PM_{2.5}$ particle number. UFP particles are constituted mainly by organic carbon and elemental carbon. The larger UFP numbers in the atmosphere, despite a smaller mass, raise concerns since their exposures have increased dramatically with the increased sources of their emission such as internal combustion engines, power plants, incinerators and many other thermo-degradation practices [Terzano et al., 2010].

How deep a given particle can penetrate into the airways depends largely on its aerodynamic diameter. The alveolar region is of particular interest, as in this region the lungs are most permeable in order to facilitate gas exchange between the blood and the inhaled air. Fine and ultrafine particles dominate the deposited particles in the alveoli both in term of number and mass. They have high deposition efficiencies of 30–60% (between 20 and 40 nm) and 20–30% (between 1 and 3 μm) of the inhaled particles respectively (ICRP 1994 model for particle deposition). In the deeper region of the lungs a major fraction of the deposited particles is engulfed by macrophages, specialized defense cells, which recognize and internalize non-soluble particles which which are either retained or digested and solubilized. Retained fine or ultrafine particles may pass into the lymphatics of the lung, or be taken within specialized macrophages to the lymphatics , and accumulated in the lymphatic nodes of the lung. A remaining small fraction of UFP is retained long term in the epithelium and interstitial spaces [Schmid et al., 2009].

Hypotheses have been proposed suggesting that UFP have the ability to translocate to the blood stream and target other organs in the body [Godleski, 2006]. One of the most important features for particulate toxicity is the surface reactivity that depends on the chemical composition, deposition site, size, shape, and surface area of the particles. The ratio between the surface area and the mass of the particle is an important determinant for the toxicity because chemical reactions and leaking of constituents occurs from the surface. In addition the percentage of surface molecules increases when the particles' diameter decreases, making the fine and ultrafine particles more hazardous.

The following sections will focus mainly on the effects of particulate matter on human health with particular attention on the cardiovascular system. A vast body of literature has shown correlations between fine particulate matter and a wide range of PM-related human health effects in the general population, including the aggravation of heart diseases, cardiovascular morbidity and mortality. Recent studies have suggested that it is not simply the particulate mass that is responsible for the adverse health effects, but its chemical composition is also an important determinant. Elemental carbon, organic carbonaceous fraction and transition metals are the most frequently cited suspects for the detrimental effects of PM, in particular through their ability to generate free radicals. Moreover, sulfur dioxide and derived sulfates have been associated with health outcomes in the consensus assessments of the WHO [WHO, 2003]. However the causal role of sulfur compounds has been criticized on the basis of their low toxic potency [Schlesinger & Cassee, 2003; Happo et al., 2010]. Thus, it is PM that has become regarded as possible leading mechanisms of disease exacerbation in patients with cardiovascular disorders.

3. Reactive oxygen species, oxidative stress and airborne environmental pollutants

Free radicals and oxidative stress have been implicated in inflammatory response after exposure to particulate matter [Donaldson et al., 2005]. Several studies carried out in cell culture, in animal models as well as in humans have established that once inhaled and deposited in to the lungs, fine and ultrafine particles can trigger pro-inflammatory responses [Gonzalez-Flecha, 2004].

Both organic materials and transition metals present in PM are able to generate free radicals. Electron paramagnetic measurements indicate that $PM_{2.5}$ contains persistent radicals in the concentration range of $1,3x10^{16}$ and $1,5x10^{17}$ radical/gram ($1,0x10^{17}$ = 0,16 mM). This radical concentration is comparable to that found in cigarette smoke particulate matter, which is also in the range of 10^{16} to 10^{17} [Squadrito et al., 2001]. Free radicals are reactive molecules with an unpaired electron. In a stable configuration electrons (e^-) orbit around atoms in pairs with opposite spin. When only one electron is present in the outer orbital the atom has an unstable configuration, and tends to be reactive, attracting one electron from other molecules in order to reorganize itself in a stable configuration.

In biological settings free radicals are potentially very dangerous since they can react indiscriminately with neighboring molecules in order to acquire one electron. This process of electron stealing leads to oxidation and often inactivation of target molecules and cellular damage. In biological systems Reactive Oxygen Species (ROS) or free radicals from oxygen are reactive molecules generated as intermediates in reduction–oxidation (redox) reactions, in which one chemical species is oxidized, and its electrons are passed to another chemical species, which is thereby reduced, leading from molecular oxygen to (O_2) to water (H_2O). Here is the sequence of reactions (1). The donation of a single electron (reduction) to molecular oxygen, results in the formation of a superoxide ($^{\bullet}O_2^-$). Superoxide radical undergoes spontaneously or enzymatically, by the action of superoxide dismutase (SOD) to dismutation, a chemical reaction between two identical molecules to produce two different products, to generate hydrogen peroxide (H_2O_2) and oxygen. The reduction of hydrogen peroxide by a third electron results in the formation of the highly reactive hydroxyl radical ($^{\bullet}OH$). Finally the donation of a fourth electron yields water.

$$O_2 \xrightarrow{e^-} {}^{\bullet}O_2^- \xrightarrow{e^-} H_2O_2 \xrightarrow{e^-} {}^{\bullet}OH \xrightarrow{e^-} H_2O \qquad (1)$$

An additional form of ROS is singlet oxygen, a very short lived and reactive form of molecular oxygen in which the outer electrons are raised to a higher energy state can be formed by a variety of mechanism including the Haber-Weiss reaction (2) occurring in biological systems.

$$H_2O_2 + {}^{\bullet}O_2^- \longrightarrow O_2 + {}^{\bullet}OH + OH^- \tag{2}$$

Another reaction that occurs in biological systems leading to production of highly oxidizing species and formation of $^{\bullet}OH$ radicals is the Fenton reaction (3). Some transition metals including iron can catalyze Fenton reactions.

$$Fe^{2+} + H_2O_2 \longrightarrow Fe^{3+} + {}^{\bullet}OH + OH^- \tag{3}$$

$$Fe^{3+} + H_2O_2 \longrightarrow Fe^{2+} + {}^{\bullet}OOH + H^+$$

3.1 Cellular sources of ROS and antioxidant defenses

ROS are formed physiologically in biological systems. It is widely accepted that low level of ROS are involved in important physiological functions such as signal transductions to promote cell proliferation and survival. Excessive amounts of ROS, referred to as oxidative stress, contribute to depletion of antioxidants, cause aberrant cell death and have been implicated in a variety of pathological events such as arteriosclerosis, ischemia-reperfusion injury, cardiovascular diseases, inflammation and neurodegenerative diseases [Chen & Nadziejko, 2005].

The mitochondrion is the major cellular source of ROS. In the mitochondria $^{\bullet}O_2^-$ can be generated enzymatically during oxidative phosphorylation in the electron transfer chain, as a byproduct of normal cellular aerobic metabolism, with the rate of respiration responsible for the rate of generation of ROS [Mccarthy et al., 1976]. The mitochondrial enzyme superoxide dismutase (mSOD) rapidly scavenges $^{\bullet}O_2^-$ accelerating the removal of this radical by dismutation to generate H_2O_2, a less reactive molecule.

Mitochondria are involved also in the generation of nitric oxide ($^{\bullet}NO$) via the nitric oxide synthase (NOS) reaction. Superoxide anion and $^{\bullet}NO$ react to form another harmful oxidant, peroxinitrite ($ONOO^-$) which is also a potential source for more powerful and aggressive hydroxyl radical ($^{\bullet}OH$).

Several non-mitochondrial sources of ROS exist in the cell. The endoplasmic reticulum is a source of ROS, where resident cytocrome P-450 oxidizes unsaturated fatty acids and xenobiotics such as pollutants, drugs and toxins to generate $^{\bullet}O_2^-$ and H_2O_2.

Peroxisomes are cytoplasmic membrane-enclosed organelles that contain at least 50 different enzymes involved in a variety of biochemical pathways in different types of cells and oxidation reactions leading to the production of hydrogen peroxide, like the peroxisomal oxidation of fatty acids [Gilca et al., 2007]. The peroxisome also contains catalase, an ubiquitous antioxidant which decomposes H_2O_2 and prevents accumulation of this toxic molecule by either converting it to water or by using it to oxidize other organic compounds.

Membrane associated oxidases such as NADPH oxidases generate ROS by reacting with the intracellular NADPH, to reduce molecular oxygen superoxide anion ($^{\bullet}O_2^-$) [Cash et al., 2007]. This reaction is typical of activated phagosomes in neutrophils and macrophages during the respiratory burst, in response to xenobiotics such as particles of pollution, inflammatory agents or infectious conditions. Upon activation, neutrophils initiate an oxidative burst by consuming molecular oxygen resulting in the formation ROS as a defense mechanism to achieve localized microbicidal function.

As a consequence of the activation of neutrophils and oxidative burst, myeloperoxidase (MPO), a hemeprotein present in the azurophil granules in neutrophils, is released either into the lysosomes of the phagocytic cell or into the extracellular space. MPO catalyzes the formation of hypochlorous acid (HOCl) from H_2O_2 and chloride ions, a further strong oxidizing and chlorinating species. MPO activation may lead to irreversible protein and lipid modification, increasing levels of oxidized low density lipoprotein, through free radical formation. Elevated MPO is considered as a risk factor for cardiovascular diseases [Al-Hweish et al., 2010].

Cells have a defense mechanism against oxidative stress that is constituted by the endogenous antioxidants. Antioxidants are molecules that protect biological targets against oxidative damage. They play a role in preventing damage by suppressing the formation of ROS or by scavenging them, rapidly before they attack biologically essential molecules. Finally they play a role in the repair of the damage, clearing the waste and reconstructing the lost functions [Niki, 2010].

Among the enzymatic antioxidants is Cu/Zn SOD, a cytoplasmic metalloenzyme that catalyzes the dismutation of superoxide anions to molecular oxygen and hydrogen peroxide and thus is a critical component of the oxidative stress defense mechanism. Mn/SOD is a mitochondrial isoenzyme with the same function but with potentially different sensitivity to soluble metals. In addition, there is a third SOD isoform located on the extracellular surface, EC-SOD. Glutathione peroxidase, an enzyme that catalyzes the reduction of hydroperoxides including hydrogen peroxide using glutathione as reducing substrate and glutathione reductase, a flavoprotein containing redox active disulfide bonds that catalyzes NADPH-dependent reduction of oxidized glutathione and therefore is essential for maintaining levels of reduced glutathione in the cell [Hatzis et al., 2006]. Glutathione (GSH) and the oxidized form gluthatione disulfide (GSSG) are major antioxidants. GSH as the most abundant free thiol in eukaryotic cells maintains an optimal intracellular redox environment. Reduced GSH is the biologically active form that is oxidized to GSSG during oxidative stress [Circu & Aw, 2008]. Thioredoxin and thioredoxin reductase together form an additional redox regulatory system. Thioredoxin and thioredoxin reductase can catalyze the regeneration of many antioxidant molecules including ubiquinone (Q10), lipoic acid and ascorbic acid and, as such, constitute an important antioxidant defense against ROS [Santos et al., 2011]. Catalase is an enzyme comprised in the enzymatic antioxidant protection of the cell, able to metabolize hydrogen peroxide to water and oxygen. The non-enzymatic hydrophilic antioxidant agents include ascorbate, urate, bilirubin, and melatonin. Lipophilic non enzymatic antioxidant radical scavengers include tocopherols (such as α-tocopherol), carotenoids, (such as β-carotene), ubiquinol, and flavonoids.

3.2 Ambient sources of ROS oxidative stress

The human lung with a surface area of 40-120 m^2 is exposed to between 10,000 and 20,000 liters of ambient air each day [Salvi & Holgate, 1999],and ambient air contains a wide range of pollutants. Many of individual pollutants are free radicals or have the ability to promote free radical reactions that can trigger redox cycling.

Several pathways have been considered for inhaled particles to produce ROS and cause oxidative stress. Particles deposited into the lungs can introduce oxidizing species such as transition metals, ozone or organic compounds [Prahalad et al., 1999]. Highly oxidizing species like PAHs can be adsorbed on the particles surface. These species can be transformed *in vivo* into quinones through the action of cytochrome P450, epoxide hydrolase and oxidoreductase enzymatic pathways. Finally particles can activate inflammatory cells such as phagocytic cells and leukocytes, inducing oxidative burst with the generation of oxidative stress and inflammation [Mudway et al., 2005]. Indeed, it is well known that phagocytosis of even inert particles by lung macrophages will produce a burst of ROS which increases with increasing phagocytic events and is further increased by opsonization of the ingested material [Kobzik et al., 1990].

Several studies suggested the role of metals in the oxidative capacity of PM. Transition metals present in the particles, mostly in the oxidized form as oxides and sulfates, catalyze Fenton-type reactions. Transition metals have been shown in several studies to increase ROS formation in cell free systems, in cell suspension and in animal models [Gonzalez-Flecha 2004]. Wilson and colleagues [Wilson et al., 2002], showed that intratracheal administration of iron iron-bearing with ultra-fine particles amplifies the cell recruitment in the broncho-alveolar lavage fluid (BALF), while Saldiva and colleagues [Saldiva et al., 2002], recognized a significant dose-dependent association between PM metal component especially vanadium, with neutrophils and lymphocytes present in BALF. An *in-vivo* study showed that the inhalation of concentrated respirable size urban particulate matter containing, among other elements Mn, Fe, Cu, and Zn, produced a significant increase of oxidative stress in the lung and in the heart of experimental animals [Gurgueira et al., 2002].

Among organic compounds found on the surface of particles are quinones, a class of cyclic organic compounds. Quinoid redox cycling has been previously implicated in the toxicity of combustion products such as cigarette smoke, and $PM_{2.5}$ has been shown to contain large quantities of semiquinone radicals able to induce redox cycling. During redox cycling the semiquinone intermediate reduces molecular oxygen to the superoxide radical and ultimately yields the hydroxyl radical [Squadrito et al., 2001]. Quinones or hydrogen peroxide applied directly to lung macrophages or macrophage cell-lines in vitro induce production of pro-inflammatory cytokines by these cells.

4. Effects of PM and air pollutants on the cardiovascualr system

"There's so much pollution in the air now, that if it weren't for our lungs, there'd be no place to put it all." (Orben R.). The effects of outdoor air pollution on the pulmonary and cardiovascular systems have been analyzed in both short-term and long term studies using data from population in many regions of the world. In all cases an association has been found for pathologies arising in the pulmonary and in the cardiovascular systems with the severity of concentration of air pollutants and in particular with the exposure to PM.

4.1 Short-term exposure to air pollutants effects on the cardiovascular system

Short-term studies establish association between daily health related events, for example cardiovascular mortality or hospitalization, and daily changes in the levels of ambient air pollutants. Typically associations are evaluated for exposures ranging from the day of the health events to a few weeks prior to the health related event.

Time series studies estimated that an increase of $10\mu g/m^3$ in mean $PM_{2.5}$ concentration during the preceding day contributes on average to the premature death of about 1 susceptible person per day in a region of 5 million people (based on annual US death rates in 2005). Short-term increase in $PM_{2.5}$ levels lead to the early mortality of tens of thousands of individuals per year in the United States alone [Pope et al., 2006].

Traffic emissions are the major cause for exceedingly high pollutant levels in urban areas. Several studies have found positive association between elevated PM traffic exposures over a period as brief as a few days or even a few hours and elevated risk for myocardial infarction [Peters et al., 2001], [D'Ippoliti et al., 2003], [Zanobetti & Schwartz, 2005]. Acute increases of risk for ischemic heart disease events have been observed consistently even as rapidly as 1 to 2 hours after exposure to elevated PM in case crossover analysis [Symons et al., 2006]. Daily hospitalizations for heart failure have also been associated with short-term changes in $PM_{2.5}$ exposure, in a large daily time-series analysis of and cardiovascular and respiratory hospitalization by use a US Medicare file database [Symons et al., 2006].

Among the groups more susceptible to air pollution are the elderly, and people with preexisting pulmonary and cardiovascular diseases. Peters and colleagues observed an association between exposures to traffic while traveling in cars, buses, and trolley cars and while riding on a bicycle or motorcycle and the increased risk of a myocardial infarction within one hour afterward in a susceptible population [Peters et al., 2004].

The younger, healthier population is not immune to the risks associated with short-term exposures to air pollutants. Some studies have addressed risk for adverse health effect of outdoor air pollution exposure in athletes or subjects exercising in urban areas and cyclist commuters, who often are close to busy traffic. They are often acutely exposed to exhaust from combustion engines during exercising or commuting and this may therefore represent an important fraction of their daily exposure to outdoor particulate pollution. The total number of particles deposited in the lungs increases in proportion to minute ventilation and the deposition fraction nearly doubles from rest to intense exercise [Rundell et al., 2006; Daigle et al., 2003].

In New York City runners, after 30 min of exercise near busy roadways, an acute rise in blood carboxyhaemoglobin from 1.7% to 5.1% occurred, a concentration similar to those found in regular cigarette smokers [Nicholson, 1983]. In a study of marathon runners the levels of PM_{10} were significantly associated with decreased performance for women but not for men. For every 10 ug/m3 increase in PM_{10} women marathon performance can be expected to decrease 1,4%. Men's and women's performances were not associated with any other pollutants. Only PM_{10} was found to correlate with performance.

Barath and colleagues showed that short-term exposure of human subjects to diesel exhaust impairs vasomotor functions of both endothelium dependent and independent vasodilators and endogenous endothelial fibrinolytic function parameters. Inthat study young healthy volunteers exercising on bicycle ergometers were exposed to diesel exhaust derived from engine condition mimicking vehicles functioning in urban environment, with acceleration retardation and variation in engine load as well as periods of constant speed and idling [Barath et al., 2010]. Conversely a similar study found no changes in micro-vascular vasodilation, blood coagulation parameters or markers of systemic inflammation related to particle exposure in healthy volunteers exercising on an ergometer bicycle and breathing air from one of Copenhagen's busiest roads [Brauner et al., 2008].

A study explored the possibility of reducing the cardiovascular effects of short-term air pollution exposure to urban pollution by wearing a simple facemask. Cardiovascular parameters were measured in a group of young subjects, who walked a predefined city center route in Beijing, wearing a facemask. This simple precaution led to a reduction in systolic blood pressure during exercise and increase heart rate variability. Translated into a susceptible population this finding suggests that wearing a simple facemask has the potential to reduce the incidence of acute cardiovascular events [Langrish & Mills 2009].

4.2 Long-term exposure to air pollutants: evidence for effects on the cardiovascular system

Long-term effects of air pollution are evaluated by monitoring large cohorts of participants over several years. These studies relate progression of disease, hospitalization and long term mortality to average concentration of air pollutants.

The first large prospective cohort study that demonstrated an adverse health impact of long-term air pollution exposure was the Harvard Six Cities study [Dockery et al., 1993]. This study established that chronic exposure to air pollutants is independently related to cardiovascular mortality. Of the 1,401 validated deaths, 646 were due to cardiovascular causes. The American Cancer Society (ACS), Cancer Prevention II study population, the largest study of the long-term health effects of air pollution, included about 500,000 adults resident across the US. Long term exposure to multiple air pollutants was investigated against mortality statistics for a 16 year period [Pope et al., 1995].

The ACS follow-up study increased the degree of control for confounding variables, such as diet and gaseous co-pollutants [Pope et al., 2002]. The primary results showed that each $10 \mu g/m^3$ increase in annual $PM_{2.5}$ mean concentration was associated with increases in all-cause, and cardiopulmonary mortality of 4% and 6% respectively. The relationship between $PM_{2.5}$ and adverse health effects was linear and without an apparent lower "safe" threshold. Mortality was most strongly associated with $PM_{2.5}$, sulfate particles, and SO_2. There also appeared to be an association between cardiopulmonary mortality and summertime O_3, when based on mean summer O_3 levels from 1982 to 1998.

Several studies following the lead of these two predecessors, investigated the incidence of specific cardiovascular diseases linked to long term exposure to outdoor pollution. A re-analysis of the ACS study suggested that long term exposure to elevated $PM_{2.5}$ may promote both ischemic and non ischemic cardiovascular events. Ischemic cardiac events occurring when the heart muscle receives insufficient blood, accounted for the largest absolute risk for mortality per $10 ug/m^3$ elevation in $PM_{2.5}$. Slightly lower was the relative risk for deaths due to arrhythmias, heart failure or cardiac arrest.

Survival analysis of US Medicare data from 196,000 survivors of acute myocardial infarction showed that the risk of a post-myocardial death or hospital admission for congestive heart failure was increased with higher exposure to PM_{10} [Zanobetti & Schwartz, 2007]. Data from the Worcester (USA) Heart Attack study also found that long-term exposure to traffic-related air pollution was associated with significantly increased risk of acute myocardial infarction [Tonne et al., 2007].

A number of epidemiological studies using prospective cohort designs suggest a relationship between long-term exposure to sulfate and total cardiopulmonary mortality. Very often however total $PM_{2.5}$ was also associated with these same health endpoints making unclear as to whether effects could be attributed specifically to sulfate [Schlesinger, 2007a].

In the last 40 years the implementation of strict standards for pollutants such as PM, ozone, nitrogen oxides and sulfur oxides by the governments and the environmental agencies of developed countries contributed to reduce their concentration in the cities. A dangerous level of air pollutants in the vast megalopolis is a challenge that developing countries are facing. The first cohort studies have been recently published examining the association of outdoor air pollution with mortality in China [Cao et al., 2011]. In the study, 70,947 middle-aged men and women in the China National Hypertension Survey and its follow-up study were enrolled; mortality for cardiovascular diseases was associated with total suspended particle concentration, nitrogen dioxide and sulfur dioxide. From 1991 to 2000, a significant association was found between air pollution levels and mortality from cardiopulmonary diseases and from lung cancer. Each 10 $\mu g/m^3$ elevation of total PM, SO_2 and nitric oxides was associated with a 0,9%, 3,2% and 2,3% increased risk of cardiovascular mortality respectively.

Some studies investigated air pollution-induced cardiovascular risk in healthy young adults in their late 20s. A Dutch long term study on exposure to outdoor air pollution that addressed this issue, investigated carotid artery thickening and aortic pulse wave velocity, in a population based prospective cohort study. The aim of the study was to examine early life determinants of cardiovascular risk. Carotid artery intima–media thickness, which is a measure of atherosclerosis, together with pulse wave velocity are intermediate endpoints of cardiovascular diseases and reflect functional and structural arterial characteristics. Accelerating atherosclerosis is one of the consequences of long term exposure to outdoor air pollutants. In the study the estimated individual exposure to traffic related pollution comprising nitrogen dioxide, black carbon, $PM_{2.5}$ and sulfur dioxide showed a positive association with carotid artery intima-media thickness. Furthermore exposure to nitrogen dioxide was associated with a 4,9% increase in pulse wave velocity per 20 mg/m^3 increase in background concentration of sulfur dioxide [Lenters et al., 2010], showing that even low levels of air pollution may cause early vascular damage. Furthermore recent study on young healthy volunteers showed that diesel exhaust impairs vasomotor responses to both endothelium dependent and independent vasodilators [Mills et al., 2005]. On the other hand data exist, showing that in young healthy volunteers, exposure to air pollution particles at outdoor concentrations is not associated with detectable lipid or protein oxidation, altered homeostasis, or micro-vascular activity, all of which may predict cardiovascular events.

Finally the American Heart Association in its Scientific Statement 2010, elaborated by a large number of experts in the field, focusing on major air pollution studies and aiming to provide an updated evaluation linking PM exposure to cardiovascular disease concluded that, considering the available epidemiological studies that reported the associations between PM exposures with specific cardiovascular outcomes such as morbidity, mortality and hospitalization, the existing level of overall evidence is strong for an effect of PM on ischemic heart disease moderate for heart failure and ischemic stroke and modest or mixed for peripheral vascular and cardiac arrhythmia/arrest [Brook et al., 2010].

5. Mechanisms linking air pollution to cardiovascular morbidity and mortality

A number of interrelated pathways have been proposed to explain the epidemiological phenomenon of air pollution related cardiovascular mortality and morbidity. The biological mechanisms underlying cardiovascular alterations induced by both short-term and long-term exposure to airborne pollutants are not entirely clear, neither are fully elucidated the contribution to disease of different air pollution components, nor the mechanisms by which exposures to particulate matter, the component of air pollution most intensively investigated, triggers cardiovascular events.

Air pollutants may directly affect cardiac tissue via the generation of pulmonary and systemic inflammation or by direct translocation of oxidant components of the particles into the systemic circulation.

Extensive literature shows that inhalation of particulate matter may eventually lead to endothelial cell dysfunction and the release of blood and systemic factors increasing platelet aggregability, that increased vascular oxidative stress, accelerate the progression of atherosclerosis and the development of acute coronary syndromes. Decreases of cardiac blood flow and increases in coronary vascular resistance with inhalation of concentrated ambient particles have been shown in a canine model of coronary ischemia [Bartoli et al., 2009].

In addition, an accumulating body of data suggests that particulate matter triggers pulmonary nerve reflexes, which can activate and unbalance the autonomic nervous system, resulting in alterations of heart rate variability and induction of arrhythmias, leading to cardiomyopathy.

5.1 Pulmonary and systemic oxidative stress and inflammation: potential for cardiovascular system harm by air pollution

Inflammation is a common feature in most diseases that have been associated with PM exposures and several studies indicate that PM could cause both lung and systemic inflammation [Scapellato & Lotti, 2007]. While inhaled coarse particles are mostly removed by ciliary clearance, fine and ultrafine particles have the ability to reach the lower airways, be deposited in the alveolar space and trigger local inflammation. Alveolar macrophages exposed in vitro to PM have been shown to undergo intracellular oxidation, become apoptotic, have impaired phagocytosis, depressed respiratory burst responses and release pro-inflammatory cytokines [Tao et al., 2003].

Experimental animals exposed to titanium dioxide fine and ultrafine particles, which are able to generate free radicals, have shown that more ultra-fine particles are retained in the interstitial tissue of the lung, developing a marked airspace inflammatory response [Ferin et al., 1992].

The lungs can be both a target and a source of systemic inflammation and oxidative stress that can induce and worsen pre-existing chronic inflammatory conditions [Gomez-Mejiba et al., 2009]. In a model of short-term exposure to urban concentrated air particles (CAPs) experimental animals showed two-fold increase in the steady state concentration of oxidants in the lungs and heart. The increase in oxidative stress was associated with CAPs' content of iron, manganese, copper, and zinc in the lung and with iron, aluminum, silicon and titanium in the heart. CAPs exposure was associated with significant lung and heart edema and increased serum lactate dehydrogenase indicating mild damage to both tissues [Gurgueira et al., 2002]. Inflammation produced in the lung has a number of effects in organs, such as the cardiovascular system and the nervous system. The mechanism by which inhaled ambient particles are sensed and how these effects are systemically transduced remain elusive.

Ozone, a major component of air pollution, has a considerable impact on public health. Besides the well-described respiratory tract inflammation and dysfunctions, there is accumulating evidence indicating that ozone exposure affects brain functions. In a recent published study it is showed that, similarly to with lung inflammation, ozone exposure caused a sustained time- and dose-dependent neuronal activation in the hypothalamus, amigdala and dorso-lateral regions of the nucleus tractus solitarius overlapping terminal lung afferents running in vagus nerves. [Gackiere et al., 2011].

In a study where spontaneously hypertensive rats underwent a single-inhalation exposure to residual oil fly ash (ROFA) which are particles rich in transition metals, cardiovascular toxicity was induced in a concentration-dependent manner. Exposure to the highest concentration of PM impaired heart functions, reduced heart rate, and increased arrhythmias. These changes were accompanied by increased pulmonary inflammation, increased lung resistance, and increased vagal tone, [Farraj et al., 2011].

Among postulated mechanisms aiming to explain links among oxidative stress, inflammation and the effects on the cardiovascular system is the hypothesis that fine and ultrafine particles containing metals and organic components with oxidant potential, translocate from the alveoli to the blood and lymphatic circulation and then deposited in many compartments of the organism including the liver, the kidneys, the heart and the brain where they exert the inflammatory potential.

Diesel exhaust, the major source of fine and ultrafine emission particulate in urban environments, has been shown to generate high concentrations of superoxide anion in solution as measured by electron paramagnetic resonance. The result highlights the innate potential of these particles to generate oxygen-centered free radicals and importantly, shows that combustion derived nanoparticles do not necessarily require recruitment of inflammatory cells from the lung to cause oxidative stress and damages [Miller et al., 2009], and that particles can induce directly oxidative stress if translocated to other body regions, although the mechanism by which ultra-fine particles can penetrate through pulmonary tissue and enter capillaries remains to be shown. In addition to translocation through blood circulation, particles once phagocytized by macrophages and dendritic cells may be transported and accumulated in lymph nodes in the lung or to those closely associated with the lungs [Peters et al., 2006].

Accumulation of macrophages containing ultrafine carbonaceous particles has been shown in the bronchoalveolar lavage of children with no respiratory symptoms, with the percentage of cells containing particles ranging between 1% and 16% [Bunn et al., 2001]. In addition, PM can impair macrophages phagocytic activity. Alveolar macrophages exposed to aggregates of ultrafine carbon particles showed less ability to kill bacteria as compared to macrophages loaded with washed diesel exhaust particles. Conversely, lipid peroxidation of lung surfactants was significantly increased either with washed diesel-loaded macrophages or with carbon-loaded macrophages with a predominance of diesel particle-induced lipid peroxidation, probably caused by 10 to 100 fold higher concentration of transition metal, in washed diesel than in carbon particles [Lundborg et al., 2007].

A recently published study evaluated the inflammatory response systemically and in the lung, for a panel of elderly volunteers upon exposure to PM. The study considered the effect of the organic fraction of fine particles, comprising primary organics from combustion sources, and secondary organics from photochemically oxidized volatile organic compounds. The differences in lung versus systemic inflammatory responses to primary and secondary organic particle components, particle size fractions, and the potential to induce reactive oxygen species were evaluated. Exhaled nitric oxide (NO), which is an airway inflammation marker and plasma interleukin-6 (IL-6) which is a systemic inflammation marker were measured. Secondary particles, organic markers, fine particles and O_3 were positively associated with exhaled NO. Primary particles, organic markers, ultrafine particles, CO, and NO_x were positively associated with IL-6. Reactive oxygen species were associated with both outcomes [Delfino et al., 2010].

5.2 Vascular changes and alterations in blood-borne factors induced by air pollutants affect the cardiovascular system

In addition to promoting exacerbations of lung disease and inflammation, air pollution and especially PM have been associated with damage of the vasculature and exacerbation of cardiovascular diseases. Recent controlled exposures have demonstrated that air pollution inhalation causes vascular endothelial dysfunction [Langrish et al., 2009], arterial vasoconstriction, increased blood pressure [Brook et al., 2011], myocardial ischemia [Nuvolone et al., 2011] and attenuates micro vascular endothelium-dependent dilation [Nurkiewicz et al., 2004; Hildebrandt et al., 2009]. Ambient air pollution is also associated with increased concentration of blood markers of inflammation and coagulation such as fibrinogen, in patients with chronic pulmonary disease [Hildebrandt et al., 2009]. Fibrinogen is an acute phase reactant and coagulation factor synthesized by hepatocytes and released in large amounts into the circulation in response to inflammatory factors. Increased in concentrations of fibrinogen are considered a risk factor for arterial occlusive disorders such as myocardial infarction.

One investigation in particular, examined the relationship of outdoor pollution and *in vivo* width of the human microvasculature. In a large population-based cohort study of adults without pre-existing cardiovascular disease, independent association was found between long-term and short-term concentrations of fine particulate air pollution and vessel diameters of the retinal microvasculature, as measured using a standardized photographic methods. Increased air pollution concentrations were associated with retinal arteriolar narrowing, an outcome that has been connected with increased risk of myocardial infarction, stroke, hypertension and cardiovascular mortality independent of other risk factors [Adar et al., 2010].

A study was undertaken to investigate possible links between air pollution and changes in blood indices in elderly people. Exposure to fine particles from two UK cities demonstrated associations between air pollution and hematological indices such as hemoglobin content, and concentration of red blood cells, including mean cell volume, mean cell hemoglobin, and mean cell hemoglobin concentration. The changes in hemoglobin adjusted for albumin suggests that inhalation of fine particles may cause the decrease of red cells in the circulation and that an action of such particles either on lung endothelial cells or on erythrocytes themselves may be responsible for changing red cell adhesiveness [Seaton et al., 1999].

Particle pollution has been shown in several investigations to affect the progression of atherosclerosis. Atherosclerosis can remain asymptomatic for years and is widespread in populations consuming high fat diets. In atherosclerosis fatty material such as cholesterol collects along the walls of arteries, eventually stiffening and blocking the arteries. A chronic inflammation in the wall of arteries is a typical characteristic of atherosclerosis. Fragments of plaque can break off and move through the affected artery to smaller blood vessels, blocking them and causing tissue damage or death mostly due to heart attack and stroke.

Animal studies has first established a causal association between exposure to PM and atherosclerosis. The effects of inhaled fine particles on aortic atherosclerosis have been assessed in a mouse model of hypercholesterolemia. Long-term exposures of the ApoE mice to concentrated ambient air particles, showed a 57% increase in the percentage of atherosclerotic plaque area in the aortic root, as compared to the control animals [Chen & Nadziejko, 2005; Araujo & Nel, 2009].

In a recent study ApoE mice receiving tracheal instillation of diesel exhausts particles showed for the first time that pulmonary exposure to the PM within diesel exhaust enhances atherogenesis. Plaque area was significantly increased in diesel exhaust-exposed mice as compared with controls. Interestingly there was no evidence of systemic inflammation, increased circulating blood lipids or endothelial dysfunction in the diesel exhaust-exposed animals [Miller et al., 2009]. Studies on human populations have evidenced the association between PM exposures and the progression of atherosclerosis. Hoffmann and colleagues investigated the associations of long-term residential exposure to traffic and fine particulate matter with the degree of coronary atherosclerosis in a population-based cohort in Germany. The study demonstrated that residential exposure to highly trafficked roads is associated with coronary atherosclerosis measured as coronary artery calcification, with a positive association between fine particulate and the progression of the disease. A reduction in the distance between the residence and a major road by half was associated with a 7.0% higher coronary artery calcification [Hoffmann et al., 2007].

A cross-sectional study conducted among young participants aged 10-18 years, randomly selected from different urban areas of Isfahan city, the second largest and air-polluted city in Iran, showed a higher correlation between fine particulate matter and platelet tissue factor expression, a coagulation factor associated with atherosclerotic cardiovascular disease. This finding is consistent with various experimental studies that showed exposure to PM increases platelet tissue factor expression in atherosclerotic lesions [Poursafa et al., 2011].

Despite accumulating data indicating that particulate matter exposure contributes to the progression of atherosclerosis in animal models and in humans, the strength of associations between PM and atherosclerosis in humans is still being debated, and the strength and relative importance of the mechanisms in contributing to cardiovascular morbidity and mortality is still to be ascertained.

5.3 Disturbances of the autonomic nervous system: Impacts on the cardiopulmonary system

The interplay between nerves and vasculature is very complex and not yet completely clarified. Developmental studies in mice show that smooth muscle cells surrounding main vessels, release diffusible factors that direct growth of sympathetic nerves along arteries. In general, nerves and vasculature course along each other forming a neurovascular bundle, with blood vessels being not only routes for sympathetic axon guidance but also themselves, final sympathetic neuron targets [Larrivee et al., 2009].

Sympathetic and parasympathetic nervous system activity have complex effects on vascular tone.

Whereas increased parasympathetic activity normally leads to coronary vasodilation, in the presence of coronary artery disease, parasympathetic stimulation may lead to net coronary constriction [Pope et al., 2004]. Additionally, the stimulation of nervous C-fiber endings in the lungs may result in an axon local reflex with release of neuropeptides, which in turn may act on the mucosal vasculature, to promote vasodilatation and micro-vascular leakage. Neuropeptides may further interact with sensory neurons, propagating neurogenic inflammation within the airways.

Neurogenic inflammation has a potential importance in airway diseases; for instance neurogenic inflammation triggers a vicious cycle of neuro-immune interactions that amplify airway inflammation and airway hyperresponsiveness in allergic asthma [Pisi et al., 2009a].

In response to inspired air conditions, the sensory nerves in the lungs recruit appropriate reflexes, which induce different vascular processes, such as vasodilatation, vasoconstriction, plasma extravasation and exudation [Pisi et al., 2009b]. Observations have been reported on the significant narrowing of the pulmonary vasculature in rats exposed to urban fine particulate aerosol, with the effect being more prominent in the intra-acinar arterioles [Rivero et al., 2005]. Thus suggesting that exposure to environmental particles may modify the balance between vasoconstriction and vasodilation at pulmonary level.

The sympathetic and parasympathetic nerve controls vital functions such as heart rate (HR), heart rate variability (HRV), and heart rate recoveries, parameters linking autonomic changes with mortality and morbidity. Many studies reported to date, have shown associations between air pollution levels and changes in heart rate variability, propensity to ischemia and arrhythmias, in elderly subjects or in patient with apparent cardiovascular diseases [Godleski, 2006].

HR is normally determined by spontaneous and periodic depolarizations of the sinoatrial node, the frequency of which is modulated by the sympathetic and parasympathetic divisions of the autonomic nervous system. HRV is controlled by the cardiac autonomic nervous system, and refers to the beat-to-beat difference or R-R interval change in the intrinsic rhythm of the heart.

Assessment of HRV provides a measure of the degree of balance between sympathetic and parasympathetic (vagus nerve) activity. Decreased HRV has been considered to reflect a diminished vagal and increased sympathetic modulation of the sinus node. Sympatho-exitation has been shown to exert pro-arrhythmic effects and has been implicated in the development of heart failure, myocardial infarction and hypertension. Aberrant sympatho-activity and reduced vagal modulation of sinus node lead to an autonomic imbalance favoring cardiac electrical instability, which is predictive of negative cardiac outcomes. Additional findings has been shown that decreased HRV can be influenced by a greater complexity in the relationship between neural input and sinus node responsiveness as well as the possible interference with non neural mechanisms [Lombardi, 2002].

HRV can be assessed by time or frequency domain indices. Time domain measures the amount of time in milliseconds in the beat to beat intervals of the heart; frequency domain provides information about the frequency distribution of the components of HRV. HRV is often express as low frequency, high frequency ratio (LF/HF) [Feldman et al., 2010]. HRV parameters offer a non invasive method to estimate autonomic control mechanisms and to identify patients with an increased cardiac mortality.

Gathering data show a correlation between exposure to particulate matter and triggering of autonomic nervous system reflexes, eventually altering the cardiac frequency and function. It has been shown in the Framingham Heart Study that in elderly subjects decreased heart rate variability is associated with substantially increased occurence of major cardiac events. Studies on animals exposed to particle pollution support the hypothesis of the autonomic nervous system imbalance as a consequence of particles inhalation. Dogs exposed to concentrated air particles (CAPs) revealed LF and HF powers during HRV that were significantly higher for CAPs exposure as compared to sham exposure. The cardiac and respiratory changes recorded in the study, suggest an effect mediated via both the sympathetic nervous system and the vagus nerve [Godleski et al., 2000]. In animals exposed ROFA particles, associations have been reported between these fine particles and ventricular arrhythmia with changes of the autonomic regulation of the heart including a decrease in parasympathetic modulation [Wellenius et al., 2002].

Similar evidence has been reported from an epidemiological study, in patients with a history of serious arrhythmias, carrying an Implanted Cardioverter Defibrillator (ICD). ICD device monitors electrocardiographic (ECG) abnormalities that may occur in the heart rhythm. On detection of ventricular arrhythmia or rapid atrial fibrillation the defibrillator initiates pacing, an electrical shock therapy, in order to restore a normal cardiac rhythm. The device provides objective and accurate records of the occurrence and timing of arrhythmic events, and it found correspondence between increased risk of cardiac arrhythmias and elevated concentration of air pollutants. The association was stronger to nitrogen dioxide, carbon monoxide, black carbon, and fine particle mass, suggesting autonomic dysregulation as presumed pathways to these clinical endpoints [Peters et al., 2000].

Clinical exposure studies in young healthy individual have shown variable effects. The influence of air pollution on ECG parameters in young healthy individuals has been investigated in controlled human exposures to elemental carbon ultrafine particles, using set parameters that describe the autonomic regulation of the heart. As expected, young healthy individuals did not show dramatic changes in the ECG parameters. Interestingly, exposure to $10\mu m/m^3$ ultrafine particles was associated with changes in parameters indicating an increase in parasympathetic tone, either with exposures at rest as well as during exercising, furthermore the heart repolarization parameter, was influenced even if not significantly, by air pollution exposure [Zareba et al., 2009]. Conversely adverse effects on ventricular repolarization were assessed in a community-based study of adult healthy individuals. The adverse effects were associated with $PM_{2.5}$ particle upon 3 to 4 hours of outdoor activity as recorded with a PM and ECG portable Holter recorder [Liao et al., 2010].

Finally, several studies showed that short-term exposure to concentrated $PM_{2.5}$ raises diastolic blood pressure and trigger vasoconstriction in healthy adults [Brook et al., 2002; Urch et al., 2005]. A study provided additional insight into the acute cardiovascular effects of air pollution exposure and the autonomic nervous system control. In the study PM2.5 and not ozone was responsible for a diastolic blood pressure and only transiently during the actual period of inhalation. The result implicates autonomic nervous system imbalance, as the most pro-hypertensive response. The magnitude of diastolic BP elevation during exposures was most strongly associated with decreases in HRV markers of parasympathetic autonomic nervous system withdrawal [Brook, 2008]. This hypothesis is supported by the fact that human airways are lined with receptors and nerve endings that, after stimulation by inhaled particulate matter, may be capable of altering reflexes in the autonomic nervous system pathways, leading to a blunting of cardiovascular parasympathetic tone and relative favoring of sympathetic activity [Widdicombe & Lee, 2001]. A further study with dogs exposed to particle pollution, has contributed to the evidence that diastolic BP, acutely increases during short term concentrated ambient particles inhalation. Also show in these studies was that homeostatic mechanisms such as baroreceptor reflex sensitivity was activated during the inhalation exposure in order to acutely lower the blood pressure response to pollutants, thus limiting the height of the blood pressure response. Alpha-adrenergic receptor antagonist mitigated this response. [Bartoli et al., 2009] suggesting activation of the sympathetic branch of the autonomic nervous system.

6. Evidence for the autonomic nervous system and ROS participation in the alteration of cardiovascular system

Air pollution especially the particulate fraction, has been shown to trigger or exacerbate pathological cardiovascular conditions in short-term and long term exposure studies. Free radicals play a role in the cardio-toxicity induced by air pollution since particulate matter is rich in organic and inorganic molecules able to trigger free radical reactions. Among the hypothesized pathways for the onset and the exacerbation of cardiovascular pathologies are the stimulation of the nerve fibers and the imbalance of the autonomic nervous system. Studies presented in this section show that concentrated air pollutants are able to trigger an oxidative response in the heart of experimental animals and to stimulate both the limbs of the autonomic nervous system. Furthermore PM induced oxidative stress lead to heart damages and alteration of cardiac parameters controlled by the autonomic nervous system.

6.1 Role of ROS in the autonomic nervous system related cardiac changes upon exposure to air pollution

Ambient particles may elicit cardiovascular effects in part, through the stimulation of nervous fibers of the autonomic system. Support for this hypothesis has come from a number of studies showing that short-term exposure to particles is associated with changes in the autonomic functions as assessed by heart rate (HR) and heart rate variability (HRV) [Delfino et al., 2005] in a wide population range, from healthy adults [Wu et al., 2010] to older people and in patients with current or underlying cardiovascular diseases [Riojas-Rodriguez et al., 2006; Park et al., 2005; Schwartz et al., 2005]. HRV is the variability between the R-to-R waveform intervals, allowing a quantitative non-invasive measure of the cardiac autonomic nervous system control. Reduced heart rate variability has been linked to increased risk of myocardial infarction and it has been considered a predictor of increased risk of mortality in patients with heart failure [Tsuji et al., 1996].

The PM concentration and composition in the urban environment varies hourly during the day. Experimental models using animals exposed to outdoor airborne pollutants are a valuable representation to appreciate the activity of the cardiac autonomic nervous system, in a realistic representation of the urban population exposure.

Airborne particles can be collected by means of virtual impactor technology, which selects, concentrate and deliver outdoors particle pollution to the experimental setting. In the virtual impactor the airborne particles are separated by size, and redirected into two main airstreams, according to cut off characteristics. The fine particles follow that streamlines of the major air flow, while the coarse particles pass into the forward minor flow. In this way only the particle size of interest is kept and delivered for inhalation. Once selected, the fine particles are concentrated and maintained in suspension without physical or chemical alteration so that the quality of the complex mixtures of pollutants present in the urban environment is preserved. Concentrated ambient particles (CAPs) delivered to experimental animals have been shown to produce ROS and induce oxidative stress [Gurgueira et al., 2002]. The decay of excited oxygen molecules and carbonyl groups, generated during the lipid peroxidation induced by ROS, can be measured as light emission that can be detected as chemiluminescence (CL). CL constitutes a quantitative measure of the oxidative stress generated in whole intact organ, in real time, and in a non-invasive manner, after CAPs inhalation.

Gurgueira and colleagues [Gurgueira et al., 2002] showed that the CL in the heart and lung of rats increases two-fold, when the animals undergo to short-term CAPs exposure. Interestingly upon inhalation of pollutants, the oxidative stress in lungs increased immediately, while a significant level of oxidative stress in the heart was developed only after one-hour lag time, suggesting pulmonary to cardiac signaling, via either nervous or systemic mediators. In addition these changes were associated with oxidants dependent lung and heart edema, and with significant increase in serum levels of lactate dehydrogenase and creatine phosphokinase activities, measures of tissue damage, detected in both heart and lung. Interestingly, the level of activity of several antioxidants enzymes such as SOD and catalase, was up regulated in both organs. The increased oxidative stress in heart and lung and the increased concentration of antioxidants shows that CAPs induces ROS activity, and that in turn, ROS trigger an adaptation/protection mechanism in those organs, increasing the concentration of antioxidants.

The exciting data showing the time delay, between the rise of oxidative stress in rat's lung versus rat's heart, implies that a mechanism of pulmonary to cardiac system signaling through the autonomic nervous system or through systemic metabolites is in action; in this mechanism ROS, may play a determinant role. The signaling to the heart may be triggered in the lungs. The bronchial airways autonomic neural control includes both sympathetic and parasympathetic innervations. In response to inspired air conditions, the sensory nerves can recruit appropriate reflexes, causing afferent transmission, and release of neurotransmitters from peripheral endings, probably via local axon reflexes with antidromic conduction down afferent nerve collaterals [Pisi et al., 2009a]. Sensory nerves can also recruit appropriate reflexes which can induce different vascular processes such as vasodilatation, increase in vascular permeability and bronchoconstriction [Saria et al., 1988].

When rats undergo short-term exposures to CAPs, the CL measured from the whole heart is significantly higher than in the rats exposed to filtered air, and it shows signs of tissues edema indicating heart tissue damage. If the animals are pretreated with N-acetyl-cisteine (NAC), an antioxidant precursor of glutathione, both the increase in heart CL and the development of edema in the cardiac tissue are abrogated, confirming that PM is able to generate oxidative stress in the heart, and that pretreatment with antioxidants exert a protection against PM inhalation. The damages detected in the heart of rats after CAPs exposures, suggest the possibility of alterations in cardiac function. Experimental animals in which a controlled and steady suspension of standard Urban Ambient Particles (UAP) rich in S, Fe, Br, and Pb, was instilled intratracheally, showed significant changes in the autonomic control of the heart. Although UAP instillation did not change the HR, it significantly altered the HRV, with increases in both the high frequency (HF) and the low frequency (LF) components of HRV, which signify the parasympathetic and sympathetic limbs of the autonomic nervous system respectively. In this model the pre-treatment of the rats with the adrenergic receptor antagonist atenolol and with the muscarinic receptor antagonist glycopirrolate, prevents UAP-induced increase CL in the heart, suggesting that cardiac oxidants are mediated through the two limbs of the autonomic nervous system [Rhoden et al., 2005].

The result is confirmed in experimental setting in which rats are short-term exposed to CAPs. Indeed in CAPs model as for the UAP model, both atenolol and glycopirrolate pre-treatment, effectively prevents the increase of heart CL. The analysis of HRV and the HF and LF components in the rats exposed to CAPs, shows increases in both sympathetic and parasympathetic stimulation, with a predominance of the parasympathetic limb. In addition both sympathetic and parasympathetic antagonists prevented PM-induced oxidative stress in the heart. Taken together these outcomes suggest that deposition of PM in the lung is rapidly sensed, resulting in an imbalance in cardiac autonomic activity. The prevention of oxidant accumulation exerted by the pretreatment with NAC indicates that this pathway uses ROS as intermediates [Rhoden et al., 2005]. Interestingly, a recent paper by Rimmer and colleagues [Dyavanapalli et al., 2010], showed that ROS and especially singlet oxygen and hydroxyl radicals, block the ganglionic transmission in rats' intra-cardiac ganglion neurons, with consequences for the parasympathetic regulation of the cardiac functions, the parasympathetic unbalance, and a predominance of sympathetic pro-arrhythmic activity. In this model the administration of catalase, prevented the blockage of the transmission in intra-cardiac ganglion by ROS. These results further indicate that ROS plays a determinant role in the autonomic control of the heart.

6.2 CAPs upregulate parasympathetic cardiac tone through stimulation of lung's afferent nervous fibers

Inhaled toxicants trigger cardiopulmonary reflexes aimed to reduce the amount of inspired pollutants transported into the blood stream. Pulmonary chemoreflexes including apnea, bradycardia and hypotension were first reported by Brodie in the 1900 [Brodie 1900]. Extensive evidence indicates that bronchopulmonary C-fiber afferents are responsible for these responses and that these afferents are extremely sensitive to chemical irritants. Approximately 75% of the afferent fibers in the vagal branches innervating the respiratory tract are nonmyelinated C-fibers. A variety of inhaled toxicants such as ozone, sulfur dioxide, ammonia, tobacco, wood smoke diesel exhaust, PM, acrolein, volatile anesthetics, and capsaicin, have been shown to stimulate bronchopulmonary C-fiber afferents.

A proposed hypothesis suggests that PM deposition in the lung triggers neural reflexes mediated by vagus nervous unmyelinated C-fibers. In this approach PM could modulate the sympathetic/parasympathetic tone in the heart increasing the oxidative stress and leading to functional cardiac alterations. The Transient Receptor Potential Vanilloid Receptor 1 (TRPV1) is pervasive on parasympathetic fibers in the lung and in particular on C-fibers. The TRPV1 receptor plays a role in initiating inflammatory processes and integrating painful stimuli and it is known to be broadly expressed in all "port of entry" tissues such as the skin, the gut, the conjuntiva, and the airways [Veronesi & Oortgiesen, 2006]. TRPV1 is activated by various ligand-like agents and a plethora of seemingly unrelated stimuli such as chemical irritants, inflammatory mediators, and tissue damaging stimuli and by nonselective stimuli such as high temperature (>43°C), acidic pH (<5.3), intracellular redox states, and electrostatic charge.

The activation of TRPV1 receptors on sensory fibers, such as C-fibers and some non-neuronal cells like respiratory epithelia, produces calcium and sodium influx and the corresponding release of tachykinin neuropeptide, such as substance P and inflammatory cytokines, initiating and modulating neurogenic inflammation. Studies on human respiratory epithelial cells show that PM-induced inflammatory cytokine release is initiated by activation of TRPV1 receptors. Reflexes generated by nocireceptors such as TRPV1 affect cardiovascular function by increasing sympathetic and decreasing parasympathetic activity [Klabunde, 2005].

Capsazepine (CPZ) is a selective pharmacological antagonist of TRPV1. The administration of CPZ in rats before short-term exposure to CAPs, blocks the TRPV1 receptor in the lungs and effectively prevents CAPs induced increase of oxidative stress in the heart. In animals not pretreated with CPZ, CAPs exposure induces increase of CL together with changes in cardiac functions measured as HR and ECG waveform morphology. The triggering of TRPV1-mediated autonomic reflexes in the lungs during CAPs exposure induces changes in the cardiac rhythm, stimulated cardiac current abnormalities and led to changes in conduction velocity and ventricular repolarization. In particular the functional cardiac electrophysiologic changes elicited by the reflex activation consisted in increased P-wave duration, a marker of intra-atrial conduction time, which is influenced by changes in the autonomic tone, and increase of QT interval, a measure of ventricular depolarization and repolarization. On the other hand the QRS interval that reflect, the rapid depolarization of the right and left ventricles and T_{pe} duration, a marker of transmural dispersion and repolarization, were decreased upon exposure to CAPs.

Notably all of these changes were abrogated by the pretreatment with the TRPV1 antagonist CPZ. Therefore this suggests a central role for TRPV1 receptor in eliciting the observed responses while the complete abrogation, of the CAPs induced increase in cardiac oxidative stress, by the pretreatment with CPZ provides evidences in support of the primary role of pulmonary irritant receptors in mediating the response of autonomic nervous system PM mediated oxidative stress.

The depolarization repolarization equilibrium producing the ECG waveform is influenced by ions channels [Zareba & Cygankiewicz, 2008]. The inhibition of sodium and calcium channels by pharmacological intervention has been shown to shorten the QT interval and increases the risk of ventricular fibrillation. Given the results from animal CAPs exposures, it is tempting to speculate that the mechanism by which CAPs leads to shortening of the QT interval, involves increased vagal tone to the heart and inhibition of sodium, calcium or potassium channels. This hypothesis is supported by the changes in vagal tone and by the prevention of these changes by CPZ. Interestingly recent data from Whyte and colleagues show that ROS alter the depolarization-activated calcium and potassium conductance, which underlie neuronal excitability of intra-cardiac neurons in the intra-cardiac ganglion plexus [Whyte et al., 2009]. This notion is particularly interesting since it has been reported that some interventions terminating or evoking arrhythmias may produce their effects also via modification of intra-cardiac neural activity [Kukanova & Mravec, 2006].

6.3 Role of ROS pressor stimuli in the autonomic nervous system cardiac: Changes upon exposure to air pollution.

Cohort and panel studies have found that exposure to PM is associated not only with changes in HR and decreased heart rate variability, but also with changes in vascular parameters, and increased arterial blood pressure [Nurkiewicz et al., 2004; Brook et al., 2002]. One study in particular [Bartoli et al., 2009] showed that short-term exposure to CAPs increased heart rate, systolic blood pressure, diastolic blood pressure and mean arterial pressure in experimental animals. These changes were accompanied by increase in baroceptor reflex sensitivity after CAPs exposure while blockade by alpha adrenergic inhibitor completely abrogated those changes.

The autonomic nervous system is the most rapidly responding regulator of blood pressure. It receives continuous information from the baroreceptors, which are pressure sensitive nerve endings, situated in the carotid sinus and the aortic arch. A decrease in blood pressure causes activation of the sympathetic nervous system resulting in increased contractility of the heart (beta receptors) and vasoconstriction of both the arterial and venous side of the circulation (alpha receptors). Other factors contributing to blood pressure control are: the exchange of fluid that occurs across the capillary membrane between the blood and the interstitial fluids, hormonal responses, and the kidneys through the renin-angiotensin pathway.

Angiotensin-II (ang-II), the final active messenger of the renin–angiotensin system, has multiple biological actions including vasoconstriction, stimulation of myocytes, and facilitation of norepinephrine release from sympathetic neurons.

Furthermore ang-II interacts with the sympathetic nervous system both peripherally and centrally to increase vascular tone. Animal studies show that ang-II has effects on both limbs of the autonomic nervous system, simultaneously facilitating sympathetic activity and inhibiting vagal activity on the heart. Interestingly ang-II increases the production of superoxide anion via stimulation of NAD(P)H oxidase, and the resulting oxidative stress has been postulated as an important mediator of ang-II signaling, in the central nervous system. A study on rats has shown that ang-II activates sympathetic outflow by stimulation of superoxide anion in the paraventricular nucleus [Patel et al., 2011]. Thus ang-II is a possible important link between the pulmonary and cardiovascular effects of PM mediated by the autonomic nervous system.

Short exposures of rats to CAPs have been shown to significantly increase the blood levels of ang-II. Pretreatment of the animals with angiotensin converting enzyme (ACE) inhibitor, significantly reduced the circulating concentration of ang-II, while the blockade of the ang-II receptor AT-1, further increased the ang-II blood level as compared to the CAPs only group. Plasma creatinine levels in the experimental animals were within the physiological range, showing that no significante change in the renal system has occurred.

Increased levels of circulating ang-II were accompanied by increased production of ROS in the heart of rats exposed to CAPs, leading to altered ventricular repolarization as an effect of possible changes in ion currents . On the other hand, heart CL assessment after CAPs exposures in rats treated with ACE and AT1 inhibitors showed a significantly decreased level of oxidants, suggesting a direct role of ang-II in the rise of the cardiac oxidative stress.

The evaluation of ECGs in CAPs exposed animals for changes in the waveforms showed a lengthening of the QRS, QT, T_{pe} and RT_p intervals and a decrease in T_{pe} and increase in P_{dur} and RT_p intervals, while blockade of angiotensin synthesis with ACE inhibitor reversed the effect of CAPs exposure. Consistently following the blockade of AT1 receptor, CAPs exposure was not associated with statistically significant changes with T_{pe} , P_{dur} or RT_p conduction velocity and ventricular depolarization intervals.

This model of CAPs short- term exposure has shown a significant increase of ROS in the cardiac tissue as measured as CL. The increase in ROS, possibly mediated by receptor AT1 /NAD(P)H oxidase activation, could lead to electrophysiological changes, in the duration of cardiac waveform and possibly arrhythmia, by mechanisms similar to those initiated by activation of pulmonary reflexes.

Interestingly, exposure to fine PM may potentiate hypertension generating ROS through a NAD(P)H oxidase and eNOS dependent mechanism, with important implications for PM mediated cardiovascular effects, suggesting that PM my induce cardiac damage by modulating sensitivity to pressor stimuli [Sun et al., 2008].

7. Conclusion

Air pollution and in particular particulate matter, has been recognized as a risk for human health. PM inhalation has been positively associated with the onset and exacerbation of cardiovascular pathologies. The risk for cardiovascular outcomes has been found to rise among susceptible population such as individuals with preexisting pulmonary and cardiovascular conditions and the elderly. The mechanism(s) by which PM elicit cardiovascular diseases are not fully elucidated but scientific evidences showed that PM-induced free radicals are responsible for triggering systemic inflammation, impairing vascular parameters and influenceing the cardiac autonomic nervous system. In our researches we measured *in vivo* free radicals formation in rats exposed to concentrated ambient particles (CAPs). We showed that CAPs increased free radical induced oxidative stress in lung and heart and that antioxidants prevented it. CAPs inhalation increased both sympathetic and parasympathetic stimulation, with a predominance of the parasympathetic limb while pretreatment with antagonists of both limbs restored the autonomic cardiac control and prevented PM-induced oxidative stress in the heart. Taken together these outcomes suggest that deposition of PM in the lung is immediately sensed, resulting in an imbalance in cardiac autonomic activity. The prevention of oxidants accumulation exerted by the pretreatment with NAC indicates that this pathway uses free radicals as intermediates. Furthermore CAPs inhalation through the stimulation of TRPV1 receptors in the lungs induced changes in the cardiac rhythm, stimulated cardiac current abnormalities and led to changes in conduction velocity and ventricular repolarization. Finally we showed that CAPs exposure significantly increased the blood levels of angiotensin-II accompanied by increased production of ROS in the heart of rats. Treatment with ACE and AT-1 receptor inhibitors prevented CAPs effects in experimental animals. Further researches are needed to elucidate which component(s) of PM trigger the pathological cardiac effects and the increased oxidative stress, which are the consequences of angiotensin-II rise on the vascular tone, blood pressure and cardiac rhythm and how PM, through pulmonary reflexes, influence the autonomic nervous system.

8. Acknowledgements

This work would not have been possible without the assistance of Mr. Emil Millet to which the author is obliged for the essential contribution to the critical revision of the manuscript, the insightful considerations on the scientific material, and for the editing of the text. Special thanks go to Dr. Beatriz Gonzalez-Flecha for her guidance in the researches described in the last section of this chapter, and her essential contribution to the critical review of the manuscript. The author would like to express her gratitude to Prof. John Godleski and Dr. Guillaume Lenormand for the critical reading of the manuscript and the insightful suggestions. Any errors of fact or interpretation are entirely my own.

9. References

Adar, S. D., Klein, R., Klein, B. E., Szpiro, A. A., Cotch, M. F., Wong, T. Y., O'Neill, M. S., Shrager, S., Barr, R. G., Siscovick, D. S.Kaufman, J. D. (2010). Air pollution and the microvasculature: A cross-sectional assessment of *in vivo* retinal images in the population-based multi-ethnic study of atherosclerosis (MESA). *PLoS Medicine,* Vol.7, No. 11, pp. 1549-1676, 1549-1277

Al-Hweish, A., Sultan, S. S., Mogazi, K., & Elsammak, M. Y. (2010). Plasma myeloperoxidase, NT-proBNP, and troponin-I in patients on CAPD compared with those on regular hemodialysis. *Hemodialysis International.International Symposium on Home Hemodialysis,* Vol.14, No. 3, pp. 308-315, 1542-4758; 1492-7535

Araujo, J. A., & Nel, A. E. (2009). Particulate matter and atherosclerosis: Role of particle size, composition and oxidative stress. *Particle and Fibre Toxicology,* Vol.6, pp. 24, 1743-8977; 1743-8977

Armaroli, N., & Balzani, V. (2011). The legacy of fossil fuels. *Chemistry, an Asian Journal,* Vol.6, No. 3, pp. 768-784, 1861-471X; 1861-471X

Barath, S., Mills, N. L., Lundback, M., Tornqvist, H., Lucking, A. J., Langrish, J. P., Soderberg, S., Boman, C., Westerholm, R., Londahl, J.Blomberg, A. (2010). Impaired vascular function after exposure to diesel exhaust generated at urban transient running conditions. *Particle and Fibre Toxicology,* Vol.7, pp. 19, 1743-8977

Bartoli, C. R., Wellenius, G. A., Diaz, E. A., Lawrence, J., Coull, B. A., Akiyama, I., Lee, L. M., Okabe, K., Verrier, R. L., & Godleski, J. J. (2009). Mechanisms of inhaled fine particulate air pollution-induced arterial blood pressure changes. *Environmental Health Perspectives,* Vol.117, No. 3, pp. 361-366, 1552-9924; 0091-6765

Bascom, R. (1996). Environmental factors and respiratory hypersensitivity: The americas. *Toxicology Letters,* Vol.86, No. 2-3, pp. 115-130, 0378-4274; 0378-4274

Bell, M. L., & Davis, D. L. (2001). Reassessment of the lethal london fog of 1952: Novel indicators of acute and chronic consequences of acute exposure to air pollution. *Environmental Health Perspectives,* Vol.109 Suppl 3, pp. 389-394, 0091-6765

Brauner, E. V., Moller, P., Barregard, L., Dragsted, L. O., Glasius, M., Wahlin, P., Vinzents, P., Raaschou-Nielsen, O., & Loft, S. (2008). Exposure to ambient concentrations of particulate air pollution does not influence vascular function or inflammatory pathways in young healthy individuals. *Particle and Fibre Toxicology,* Vol.5, pp. 13, 1743-8977

Brodie, T. G. (1900). On reflex cardiac inhibition. *The Journal of Physiology,* Vol.26, No. 1-2, pp. 92-106, 0022-3751; 0022-3751

Brook, R. D. (2008). Cardiovascular effects of air pollution. *Clinical Science (London, England : 1979),* Vol.115, No. 6, pp. 175-187, 1470-8736; 0143-5221

Brook, R. D., Brook, J. R., Urch, B., Vincent, R., Rajagopalan, S., & Silverman, F. (2002). Inhalation of fine particulate air pollution and ozone causes acute arterial vasoconstriction in healthy adults. *Circulation,* Vol.105, No. 13, pp. 1534-1536, 1524-4539; 0009-7322

Brook, R. D., Rajagopalan, S., Pope, C. A.,3rd, Brook, J. R., Bhatnagar, A., Diez-Roux, A. V., Holguin, F., Hong, Y., Luepker, R. V., Mittleman, M. A.American Heart Association Council on Epidemiology and Prevention, Council on the Kidney in Cardiovascular Disease, and Council on Nutrition, Physical Activity and Metabolism. (2010). Particulate matter air pollution and cardiovascular disease: An update to the scientific statement from the american heart association. *Circulation,* Vol.121, No. 21, pp. 2331-2378, 1524-4539; 0009-7322

Brook, R.D., Bard, R.L., Burnett, R.T., Shin H.H., Vette A, Croghan C., Phillips M, Rodes, C., Thornburg, J., & Williams R. (2011). Differences in blood pressure and vascular responses associated with ambient fine particulate matter exposures measured at the personal versus community level. Occup Environ Med. Vol. 68, No.3, pp. 224-30

Brunekreef, B., & Forsberg, B. (2005). Epidemiological evidence of effects of coarse airborne particles on health. *The European Respiratory Journal : Official Journal of the European Society for Clinical Respiratory Physiology,* Vol.26, No. 2, pp. 309-318, 0903-1936; 0903-1936

Bunn, H. J., Dinsdale, D., Smith, T., & Grigg, J. (2001). Ultrafine particles in alveolar macrophages from normal children. *Thorax,* Vol.56, No. 12, pp. 932-934, 0040-6376; 0040-6376

Cao, J., Yang, C., Li, J., Chen, R., Chen, B., Gu, D., & Kan, H. (2011). Association between long-term exposure to outdoor air pollution and mortality in china: A cohort study. *Journal of Hazardous Materials,* Vol.186, No. 2-3, pp. 1594-1600, 1873-3336; 0304-3894

Cash, T. P., Pan, Y., & Simon, M. C. (2007). Reactive oxygen species and cellular oxygen sensing. *Free Radical Biology & Medicine,* Vol.43, No. 9, pp. 1219-1225, 0891-5849; 0891-5849

Chen, L. C., & Nadziejko, C. (2005). Effects of subchronic exposures to concentrated ambient particles (CAPs) in mice. V. CAPs exacerbate aortic plaque development in hyperlipidemic mice. *Inhalation Toxicology,* Vol.17, No. 4-5, pp. 217-224, 0895-8378; 0895-8378

Circu, M. L., & Aw, T. Y. (2008). Glutathione and apoptosis. *Free Radical Research,* Vol.42, No. 8, pp. 689-706, 1029-2470; 1029-2470

Clean Air Trust, (1999). Lead, In: *Clean Air Trust,* (2011), Available from: <http://www.cleanairtrust.org/lead.html>

Daigle, C. C., Chalupa, D. C., Gibb, F. R., Morrow, P. E., Oberdorster, G., Utell, M. J., & Frampton, M. W. (2003). Ultrafine particle deposition in humans during rest and exercise. *Inhalation Toxicology,* Vol.15, No. 6, pp. 539-552, 0895-8378; 0895-8378

De Angelo L. (2009). The London smog disaster, In: *The English magazine,* Available from: < http://english-magazine.org/index.php/sci-tech/913-science-article.html >.

Delfino, R. J., Sioutas, C., & Malik, S. (2005). Potential role of ultrafine particles in associations between airborne particle mass and cardiovascular health. *Environmental Health Perspectives,* Vol.113, No. 8, pp. 934-946, 0091-6765; 0091-6765

Delfino, R. J., Staimer, N., Tjoa, T., Arhami, M., Polidori, A., Gillen, D. L., George, S. C., Shafer, M. M., Schauer, J. J., & Sioutas, C. (2010). Associations of primary and secondary organic aerosols with airway and systemic inflammation in an elderly panel cohort. *Epidemiology (Cambridge, Mass.),* Vol.21, No. 6, pp. 892-902, 1531-5487; 1044-3983

D'Ippoliti, D., Forastiere, F., Ancona, C., Agabiti, N., Fusco, D., Michelozzi, P., & Perucci, C. A. (2003). Air pollution and myocardial infarction in rome: A case-crossover analysis. *Epidemiology (Cambridge, Mass.),* Vol.14, No. 5, pp. 528-535, 1044-3983; 1044-3983

Dockery, D. W., Pope, C. A.,3rd, Xu, X., Spengler, J. D., Ware, J. H., Fay, M. E., Ferris, B. G.,Jr, & Speizer, F. E. (1993). An association between air pollution and mortality in six U.S. cities. *The New England Journal of Medicine,* Vol.329, No. 24, pp. 1753-1759, 0028-4793 <http://hollis.harvard.edu/?q=issn%3A0028-4793>; 0028-4793 <http://hollis.harvard.edu/?q=issn%3A0028-4793>

Donaldson, K., Tran, L., Jimenez, L. A., Duffin, R., Newby, D. E., Mills, N., MacNee, W., & Stone, V. (2005). Combustion-derived nanoparticles: A review of their toxicology following inhalation exposure. *Particle and Fibre Toxicology,* Vol.2, pp. 10, 1743-8977; 1743-8977

Dyavanapalli, J., Rimmer, K., & Harper, A. A. (2010). Reactive oxygen species alters the electrophysiological properties and raises [Ca2+]i in intracardiac ganglion neurons. *American Journal of Physiology.Regulatory, Integrative and Comparative Physiology,* Vol.299, No. 1, pp. R42-54, 1522-1490; 0363-6119

Eurostat, (2011). Air pollution statistics, In: *European Commission,* (2009), Available from: <http://eep.eurostat.ec.europa.eu/statistics_explained/ >

Farraj, A. K., Hazari, M. S., Haykal-Coates, N., Lamb, C., Winsett, D. W., Ge, Y., Ledbetter, A. D., Carll, A. P., Bruno, M., Ghio, A.Costa, D. L. (2011). ST depression, arrhythmia, vagal dominance, and reduced cardiac micro-RNA in particulate-exposed rats. *American Journal of Respiratory Cell and Molecular Biology,* Vol.44, No. 2, pp. 185-196, 1535-4989; 1044-1549

Feldman, D., Elton, T. S., Menachemi, D. M., & Wexler, R. K. (2010). Heart rate control with adrenergic blockade: Clinical outcomes in cardiovascular medicine. *Vascular Health and Risk Management,* Vol.6, pp. 387-397, 1178-2048; 1176-6344

Ferin, J., Oberdorster, G., & Penney, D. P. (1992). Pulmonary retention of ultrafine and fine particles in rats. *American Journal of Respiratory Cell and Molecular Biology,* Vol.6, No. 5, pp. 535-542, 1044-1549; 1044-1549

Gackiere, F., Saliba, L., Baude, A., Bosler, O., & Strube, C. (2011). Ozone inhalation activates stress-responsive regions of the central nervous system. *Journal of Neurochemistry,* 1471-4159; 0022-3042

Gilca, M., Stoian, I., Atanasiu, V., & Virgolici, B. (2007). The oxidative hypothesis of senescence. *Journal of Postgraduate Medicine,* Vol.53, No. 3, pp. 207-213, 0022-3859; 0022-3859

Godleski, J. J. (2006). Responses of the heart to ambient particle inhalation. *Clinics in Occupational and Environmental Medicine,* Vol.5, No. 4, pp. 849-864, 1526-0046; 1526-0046

Godleski, J. J., Verrier, R. L., Koutrakis, P., Catalano, P., Coull, B., Reinisch, U., Lovett, E. G., Lawrence, J., Murthy, G. G., Wolfson, J. M.Killingsworth, C. (2000). Mechanisms of morbidity and mortality from exposure to ambient air particles. *Research Report (Health Effects Institute),* Vol.(91), No. 91, pp. 5-88; discussion 89-103, 1041-5505; 1041-5505

Gong H Jr. Lachenbrunch PA, Harber P. Linn WS. （1995）Comparative short-term health responses to sulfur dioxide exposure and other common stresses in a panel of asthmatics. Toxicol Ind Health Vol.11, No.5, pp.467-487.

Gold, D. R., Damokosh, A. I., Pope, C. A.,3rd, Dockery, D. W., McDonnell, W. F., Serrano, P., Retama, A., & Castillejos, M. (1999). Particulate and ozone pollutant effects on the respiratory function of children in southwest mexico city. *Epidemiology (Cambridge, Mass.),* Vol.10, No. 1, pp. 8-16, 1044-3983; 1044-3983

Gomez-Mejiba, S. E., Zhai, Z., Akram, H., Pye, Q. N., Hensley, K., Kurien, B. T., Scofield, R. H., & Ramirez, D. C. (2009). Inhalation of environmental stressors & chronic inflammation: Autoimmunity and neurodegeneration. *Mutation Research,* Vol.674, No. 1-2, pp. 62-72, 0027-5107; 0027-5107

Gonzalez-Flecha, B. (2004). Oxidant mechanisms in response to ambient air particles. *Molecular Aspects of Medicine,* Vol.25, No. 1-2, pp. 169-182, 0098-2997; 0098-2997

Gurgueira, S. A., Lawrence, J., Coull, B., Murthy, G. G., & Gonzalez-Flecha, B. (2002). Rapid increases in the steady-state concentration of reactive oxygen species in the lungs and heart after particulate air pollution inhalation. *Environmental Health Perspectives,* Vol.110, No. 8, pp. 749-755, 0091-6765; 0091-6765

Happo, M. S., Salonen, R. O., Halinen, A. I., Jalava, P. I., Pennanen, A. S., Dormans, J. A., Gerlofs-Nijland, M. E., Cassee, F. R., Kosma, V. M., Sillanpaa, M.Hirvonen, M. R. (2010). Inflammation and tissue damage in mouse lung by single and repeated dosing of urban air coarse and fine particles collected from six european cities. *Inhalation Toxicology,* Vol.22, No. 5, pp. 402-416, 1091-7691; 0895-8378

Hatzis, C., Godleski, J. J., Gonzalez-Flecha, B., Wolfson, J. M., & Koutrakis, P. (2006). Ambient particulate matter exhibits direct inhibitory effects on oxidative stress enzymes. *Environmental Science & Technology,* Vol.40, No. 8, pp. 2805-2811, 0013-936X; 0013-936X

Health Effect Institute (HEI). (2002). *Understanding the health effects of the particulate matter mix: Progress and next steps: HEI perspective.*

HEI, International Scientific Oversight Committee. (2004). *Health effects of outdoor air pollution in developing countries of asia: A literature review.*

Helfand, W. H., Lazarus, J., & Theerman, P. (2001). Donora, pennsylvania: An environmental disaster of the 20th century. *American Journal of Public Health,* Vol.91, No. 4, pp. 553, 0090-0036

Hildebrandt, K., Ruckerl, R., Koenig, W., Schneider, A., Pitz, M., Heinrich, J., Marder, V., Frampton, M., Oberdorster, G., Wichmann, H. E.Peters, A. (2009). Short-term effects of air pollution: A panel study of blood markers in patients with chronic pulmonary disease. *Particle and Fibre Toxicology,* Vol.6, pp. 25, 1743-8977; 1743-8977

Hoffmann, B., Moebus, S., Mohlenkamp, S., Stang, A., Lehmann, N., Dragano, N., Schmermund, A., Memmesheimer, M., Mann, K., Erbel, R.Heinz Nixdorf Recall Study Investigative Group. (2007). Residential exposure to traffic is associated with coronary atherosclerosis. *Circulation,* Vol.116, No. 5, pp. 489-496, 1524-4539; 0009-7322

Katanoda, K., Sobue, T., Satoh, H., Tajima, K., Suzuki, T., Nakatsuka, H., Takezaki, T., Nakayama, T., Nitta, H., Tanabe, K.Tominaga, S. (2011). An association between long-term exposure to ambient air pollution and mortality from lung cancer and respiratory diseases in japan. *Journal of Epidemiology / Japan Epidemiological Association,* Vol.21, No. 2, pp. 132-143, 1349-9092; 0917-5040

Klabunde, R. (2005). Neurohumoral control of the heart and circulation, *In: Cardiovascular physiology concepts.* pp. 128-129, Lippincott Williams & Wilkins,

Kobzik L, Godleski JJ, Brain JD. (1990) Selective down-regulation of alveolar macrophages oxidative response to opsonin-independent phagocytosis. J Immunol. Jun 1;144(11):pp., 4312-9.

Kukanova, B., & Mravec, B. (2006). Complex intracardiac nervous system. *Bratislavske Lekarske Listy,* Vol.107, No. 3, pp. 45-51, 0006-9248; 0006-9248

Langrish, J. P., Lundback, M., Mills, N. L., Johnston, N. R., Webb, D. J., Sandstrom, T., Blomberg, A., & Newby, D. E. (2009). Contribution of endothelin 1 to the vascular effects of diesel exhaust inhalation in humans. *Hypertension,* Vol.54, No. 4, pp. 910-915, 1524-4563; 0194-911X

Langrish, J. P., Mills, N. L., Chan, J. K., Leseman, D. L., Aitken, R. J., Fokkens, P. H., Cassee, F. R., Li, J., Donaldson, K., Newby, D. E.Jiang, L. (2009). Beneficial cardiovascular effects of reducing exposure to particulate air pollution with a simple facemask. *Particle and Fibre Toxicology,* Vol.6, pp. 8, 1743-8977; 1743-8977

Larrivee, B., Freitas, C., Suchting, S., Brunet, I., & Eichmann, A. (2009). Guidance of vascular development: Lessons from the nervous system. *Circulation Research,* Vol.104, No. 4, pp. 428-441, 1524-4571; 0009-7330

Lenters, V., Uiterwaal, C. S., Beelen, R., Bots, M. L., Fischer, P., Brunekreef, B., & Hoek, G. (2010). Long-term exposure to air pollution and vascular damage in young adults. *Epidemiology (Cambridge, Mass.),* Vol.21, No. 4, pp. 512-520, 1531-5487; 1044-3983

Liao, D., Shaffer, M. L., Rodriguez-Colon, S., He, F., Li, X., Wolbrette, D. L., Yanosky, J., & Cascio, W. E. (2010). Acute adverse effects of fine particulate air pollution on ventricular repolarization. *Environmental Health Perspectives,* Vol.118, No. 7, pp. 1010-1015, 1552-9924; 0091-6765

Lombardi, F. (2002). Clinical implications of present physiological understanding of HRV components. *Cardiac Electrophysiology Review,* Vol. 6, pp. 245-249

Lundborg, M., Bouhafs, R., Gerde P., Ewing, P., Camner, P., Dahlén S.E., Jarstrand **C**. (2007). Aggregates of ultrafine particles modulate lipid peroxidation and bacterial killing by alveolar macrophages. *Environmental research.* Vol. 104, No. 2, pp. 250-257

Mauderly, J. L., & Chow, J. C. (2008). Health effects of organic aerosols. *Inhalation Toxicology,* Vol.20, No. 3, pp. 257-288, 1091-7691; 0895-8378

Mccarthy, J. L., Green, W., & Sohal, R. S. (1976). Crowding stress and adrenal mitochondrial 11 beta-hydroxylation in vitro. *Proceedings of the Society for Experimental Biology and Medicine.Society for Experimental Biology and Medicine (New York, N.Y.),* Vol.153, No. 3, pp. 528-531, 0037-9727; 0037-9727

Miller, M. R., Borthwick, S. J., Shaw, C. A., McLean, S. G., McClure, D., Mills, N. L., Duffin, R., Donaldson, K., Megson, I. L., Hadoke, P. W.Newby, D. E. (2009). Direct impairment of vascular function by diesel exhaust particulate through reduced bioavailability of endothelium-derived nitric oxide induced by superoxide free radicals. *Environmental Health Perspectives,* Vol.117, No. 4, pp. 611-616, 1552-9924; 0091-6765

Mills, N. L., Tornqvist, H., Robinson, S. D., Gonzalez, M., Darnley, K., MacNee, W., Boon, N. A., Donaldson, K., Blomberg, A., Sandstrom, T.Newby, D. E. (2005). Diesel exhaust inhalation causes vascular dysfunction and impaired endogenous fibrinolysis. *Circulation,* Vol.112, No. 25, pp. 3930-3936, 1524-4539; 0009-7322

Mohai, P., Lantz, P. M., Morenoff, J., House, J. S., & Mero, R. P. (2009). Racial and socioeconomic disparities in residential proximity to polluting industrial facilities: Evidence from the americans' changing lives study. *American Journal of Public Health,* Vol.99 Suppl 3, pp. S649-56, 1541-0048; 0090-0036

Motterlini, R., & Otterbein, L. E. (2010). The therapeutic potential of carbon monoxide. *Nature Reviews.Drug Discovery,* Vol.9, No. 9, pp. 728-743, 1474-1784; 1474-1776

Mudway, I. S., Duggan, S. T., Venkataraman, C., Habib, G., Kelly, F. J., & Grigg, J. (2005). Combustion of dried animal dung as biofuel results in the generation of highly redox active fine particulates. *Particle and Fibre Toxicology,* Vol.2, pp. 6, 1743-8977; 1743-8977

Nemery, B., Hoet, P. H., & Nemmar, A. (2001). The meuse valley fog of 1930: An air pollution disaster. *Lancet,* Vol.357, No. 9257, pp. 704-708, 0140-6736 <http://hollis.harvard.edu/?q=issn%3A0140-6736>; 0140-6736 <http://hollis.harvard.edu/?q=issn%3A0140-6736>

Nicholson JP, C. D. (1983). Carboxyhemoglobin levels in new york city runners *Physician Sportsmed,* Vol.11, pp. 135-138,

Niki, E. (2010). Assessment of antioxidant capacity in vitro and *in vivo. Free Radical Biology & Medicine,* Vol.49, No. 4, pp. 503-515, 1873-4596; 0891-5849

Nuvolone, D., Balz,i D., Chini, M., Scala, D., Giovannini, F., Barchielli, A. (2011). Short-Term Association Between Ambient Air Pollution and Risk of Hospitalization for Acute Myocardial Infarction: Results of the Cardiovascular Risk and Air Pollution in Tuscany (RISCAT) Study. Am J Epidemiol. Vol.174,v No.1, pp. 63-71

Nurkiewicz, T. R., Porter, D. W., Barger, M., Castranova, V., & Boegehold, M. A. (2004). Particulate matter exposure impairs systemic microvascular endothelium-dependent dilation. *Environmental Health Perspectives,* Vol.112, No. 13, pp. 1299-1306, 0091-6765; 0091-6765

Park, S. K., O'Neill, M. S., Vokonas, P. S., Sparrow, D., & Schwartz, J. (2005). Effects of air pollution on heart rate variability: The VA normative aging study. *Environmental Health Perspectives,* Vol.113, No. 3, pp. 304-309, 0091-6765; 0091-6765

Patel, K. P., Mayhan, W. G., Bidasee, K. R., & Zheng, H. (2011). Enhanced angiotensin II-mediated central sympathoexcitation in streptozotocin-induced diabetes: Role of superoxide anion. *American Journal of Physiology.Regulatory, Integrative and Comparative Physiology,* Vol.300, No. 2, pp. R311-20, 1522-1490; 0363-6119

Perez-Padilla, R., Schilmann, A., & Riojas-Rodriguez, H. (2010). Respiratory health effects of indoor air pollution. *The International Journal of Tuberculosis and Lung Disease : The Official Journal of the International Union Against Tuberculosis and Lung Disease,* Vol.14, No. 9, pp. 1079-1086, 1815-7920; 1027-3719

Peters, A., Dockery, D. W., Muller, J. E., & Mittleman, M. A. (2001). Increased particulate air pollution and the triggering of myocardial infarction. *Circulation,* Vol.103, No. 23, pp. 2810-2815, 1524-4539; 0009-7322

Peters, A., Liu, E., Verrier, R. L., Schwartz, J., Gold, D. R., Mittleman, M., Baliff, J., Oh, J. A., Allen, G., Monahan, K.Dockery, D. W. (2000). Air pollution and incidence of cardiac arrhythmia. *Epidemiology (Cambridge, Mass.),* Vol.11, No. 1, pp. 11-17, 1044-3983; 1044-3983

Peters, A., Veronesi, B., Calderon-Garciduenas, L., Gehr, P., Chen, L. C., Geiser, M., Reed, W., Rothen-Rutishauser, B., Schurch, S., & Schulz, H. (2006). Translocation and potential neurological effects of fine and ultrafine particles a critical update. *Particle and Fibre Toxicology,* Vol.3, pp. 13, 1743-8977; 1743-8977

Peters, A., von Klot, S., Heier, M., Trentinaglia, I., Hormann, A., Wichmann, H. E., Lowel, H., & Cooperative Health Research in the Region of Augsburg Study Group. (2004). Exposure to traffic and the onset of myocardial infarction. *The New England Journal of Medicine,* Vol.351, No. 17, pp. 1721-1730, 1533-4406; 0028-4793

Pisi, G., Olivieri, D., & Chetta, A. (2009a). The airway neurogenic inflammation: Clinical and pharmacological implications. *Inflammation & Allergy Drug Targets,* Vol.8, No. 3, pp. 176-181, 1871-5281

Pisi, G., Olivieri, D., & Chetta, A. (2009b). The airway neurogenic inflammation: Clinical and pharmacological implications. *Inflammation & Allergy Drug Targets,* Vol.8, No. 3, pp. 176-181, 1871-5281

Pope, C. A.,3rd, Burnett, R. T., Thun, M. J., Calle, E. E., Krewski, D., Ito, K., & Thurston, G. D. (2002). Lung cancer, cardiopulmonary mortality, and long-term exposure to fine particulate air pollution. *JAMA : The Journal of the American Medical Association,* Vol.287, No. 9, pp. 1132-1141, 0098-7484; 0098-7484

Pope, C. A.,3rd, Burnett, R. T., Thurston, G. D., Thun, M. J., Calle, E. E., Krewski, D., & Godleski, J. J. (2004). Cardiovascular mortality and long-term exposure to particulate air pollution: Epidemiological evidence of general pathophysiological pathways of disease. *Circulation,* Vol.109, No. 1, pp. 71-77, 1524-4539; 0009-7322

Pope, C. A.,3rd, Muhlestein, J. B., May, H. T., Renlund, D. G., Anderson, J. L., & Horne, B. D. (2006). Ischemic heart disease events triggered by short-term exposure to fine particulate air pollution. *Circulation,* Vol.114, No. 23, pp. 2443-2448, 1524-4539; 0009-7322

Pope, C. A.,3rd, Thun, M. J., Namboodiri, M. M., Dockery, D. W., Evans, J. S., Speizer, F. E., & Heath, C. W.,Jr. (1995). Particulate air pollution as a predictor of mortality in a prospective study of U.S. adults. *American Journal of Respiratory and Critical Care Medicine,* Vol.151, No. 3 Pt 1, pp. 669-674, 1073-449X

Poursafa, P., Kelishadi, R., Lahijanzadeh, A., Modaresi, M., Javanmard, S. H., Assari, R., Amin, M. M., Moattar, F., Amini, A., & Sadeghian, B. (2011). The relationship of air pollution and surrogate markers of endothelial dysfunction in a population-based sample of children. *BMC Public Health,* Vol.11, pp. 115, 1471-2458; 1471-2458

Prahalad, A. K., Soukup, J. M., Inmon, J., Willis, R., Ghio, A. J., Becker, S., & Gallagher, J. E. (1999). Ambient air particles: Effects on cellular oxidant radical generation in relation to particulate elemental chemistry. *Toxicology and Applied Pharmacology,* Vol.158, No. 2, pp. 81-91, 0041-008X; 0041-008X

Rhoden, C. R., Wellenius, G. A., Ghelfi, E., Lawrence, J., & Gonzalez-Flecha, B. (2005). PM-induced cardiac oxidative stress and dysfunction are mediated by autonomic stimulation. *Biochimica Et Biophysica Acta,* Vol.1725, No. 3, pp. 305-313, 0006-3002; 0006-3002

Riojas-Rodriguez, H., Escamilla-Cejudo, J. A., Gonzalez-Hermosillo, J. A., Tellez-Rojo, M. M., Vallejo, M., Santos-Burgoa, C., & Rojas-Bracho, L. (2006). Personal PM2.5 and CO exposures and heart rate variability in subjects with known ischemic heart disease in mexico city. *Journal of Exposure Science & Environmental Epidemiology,* Vol.16, No. 2, pp. 131-137, 1559-0631; 1559-0631

Rivero, D. H., Soares, S. R., Lorenzi-Filho, G., Saiki, M., Godleski, J. J., Antonangelo, L., Dolhnikoff, M., & Saldiva, P. H. (2005). Acute cardiopulmonary alterations induced by fine particulate matter of Sao Paulo, Brazil. *Toxicological Sciences : An Official Journal of the Society of Toxicology,* Vol.85, No. 2, pp. 898-905, 1096-6080; 1096-0929

Rundell, K. W., Caviston, R., Hollenbach, A. M., & Murphy, K. (2006). Vehicular air pollution, playgrounds, and youth athletic fields. *Inhalation Toxicology,* Vol.18, No. 8, pp. 541-547, 1091-7691; 0895-8378

Saldiva, P. H., Clarke, R. W., Coull, B. A., Stearns, R. C., Lawrence, J., Murthy, G. G., Diaz, E., Koutrakis, P., Suh, H., Tsuda, A.Godleski, J. J. (2002). Lung inflammation induced by concentrated ambient air particles is related to particle composition. *American Journal of Respiratory and Critical Care Medicine,* Vol.165, No. 12, pp. 1610-1617, 1073-449X; 1073-449X

Salvi, S., & Holgate, S. T. (1999). Mechanisms of particulate matter toxicity. *Clinical and Experimental Allergy : Journal of the British Society for Allergy and Clinical Immunology,* Vol.29, No. 9, pp. 1187-1194, 0954-7894; 0954-7894

Santos, C. X., Anilkumar, N., Zhang, M., Brewer, A. C., & Shah, A. M. (2011). Redox signaling in cardiac myocytes. *Free Radical Biology & Medicine,* Vol.50, No. 7, pp. 777-793, 1873-4596; 0891-5849

Saria, A., Martling, C. R., Yan, Z., Theodorsson-Norheim, E., Gamse, R., & Lundberg, J. M. (1988). Release of multiple tachykinins from capsaicin-sensitive sensory nerves in the lung by bradykinin, histamine, dimethylphenyl piperazinium, and vagal nerve stimulation. *The American Review of Respiratory Disease,* Vol.137, No. 6, pp. 1330-1335, 0003-0805; 0003-0805

Scapellato, M. L., & Lotti, M. (2007). Short-term effects of particulate matter: An inflammatory mechanism? *Critical Reviews in Toxicology,* Vol.37, No. 6, pp. 461-487, 1040-8444; 1040-8444

Schlesinger, R. B. (2007a). The health impact of common inorganic components of fine particulate matter (PM2.5) in ambient air: A critical review. *Inhalation Toxicology,* Vol.19, No. 10, pp. 811-832, 1091-7691; 0895-8378

Schlesinger, R. B. (2007b). The health impact of common inorganic components of fine particulate matter (PM2.5) in ambient air: A critical review. *Inhalation Toxicology,* Vol.19, No. 10, pp. 811-832, 1091-7691; 0895-8378

Schlesinger, R. B., & Cassee, F. (2003). Atmospheric secondary inorganic particulate matter: The toxicological perspective as a basis for health effects risk assessment. *Inhalation Toxicology,* Vol.15, No. 3, pp. 197-235, 0895-8378; 0895-8378

Schmid, O., Moller, W., Semmler-Behnke, M., Ferron, G. A., Karg, E., Lipka, J., Schulz, H., Kreyling, W. G., & Stoeger, T. (2009). Dosimetry and toxicology of inhaled ultrafine particles. *Biomarkers : Biochemical Indicators of Exposure, Response, and Susceptibility to Chemicals,* Vol.14 Suppl 1, pp. 67-73, 1366-5804; 1354-750X

Schwartz, J., Litonjua, A., Suh, H., Verrier, M., Zanobetti, A., Syring, M., Nearing, B., Verrier, R., Stone, P., MacCallum, G.Gold, D. R. (2005). Traffic related pollution and heart rate variability in a panel of elderly subjects. *Thorax,* Vol.60, No. 6, pp. 455-461, 0040-6376; 0040-6376

Seaton, A., Soutar, A., Crawford, V., Elton, R., McNerlan, S., Cherrie, J., Watt, M., Agius, R., & Stout, R. (1999). Particulate air pollution and the blood. *Thorax,* Vol.54, No. 11, pp. 1027-1032, 0040-6376; 0040-6376

Squadrito, G. L., Cueto, R., Dellinger, B., & Pryor, W. A. (2001). Quinoid redox cycling as a mechanism for sustained free radical generation by inhaled airborne particulate matter. *Free Radical Biology & Medicine,* Vol.31, No. 9, pp. 1132-1138, 0891-5849; 0891-5849

Sun, Q., Yue, P., Ying, Z., Cardounel, A. J., Brook, R. D., Devlin, R., Hwang, J. S., Zweier, J. L., Chen, L. C., & Rajagopalan, S. (2008). Air pollution exposure potentiates hypertension through reactive oxygen species-mediated activation of Rho/ROCK. *Arteriosclerosis, Thrombosis, and Vascular Biology,* Vol.28, No. 10, pp. 1760-1766, 1524-4636; 1079-5642

Symons, J. M., Wang, L., Guallar, E., Howell, E., Dominici, F., Schwab, M., Ange, B. A., Samet, J., Ondov, J., Harrison, D.Geyh, A. (2006). A case-crossover study of fine particulate matter air pollution and onset of congestive heart failure symptom exacerbation leading to hospitalization. *American Journal of Epidemiology,* Vol.164, No. 5, pp. 421-433, 0002-9262; 0002-9262

Tao, F., Gonzalez-Flecha, B., & Kobzik, L. (2003). Reactive oxygen species in pulmonary inflammation by ambient particulates. *Free Radical Biology & Medicine,* Vol.35, No. 4, pp. 327-340, 0891-5849; 0891-5849

Terzano, C., Di Stefano, F., Conti, V., Graziani, E., & Petroianni, A. (2010). Air pollution ultrafine particles: Toxicity beyond the lung. *European Review for Medical and Pharmacological Sciences,* Vol.14, No. 10, pp. 809-821, 1128-3602; 1128-3602

Tonne, C., Melly, S., Mittleman, M., Coull, B., Goldberg, R., & Schwartz, J. (2007). A case-control analysis of exposure to traffic and acute myocardial infarction. *Environmental Health Perspectives,* Vol.115, No. 1, pp. 53-57, 0091-6765; 0091-6765

Tsuji, H., Larson, M. G., Venditti, F. J.,Jr, Manders, E. S., Evans, J. C., Feldman, C. L., & Levy, D. (1996). Impact of reduced heart rate variability on risk for cardiac events. the framingham heart study. *Circulation,* Vol.94, No. 11, pp. 2850-2855, 0009-7322; 0009-7322

United Nation Environment Program (UNEP). (2007). Geo4 global environment outlook: Environment for development, Available from: <www.unep.org/geo/geo4/ >

Urch, B., Silverman, F., Corey, P., Brook, J. R., Lukic, K. Z., Rajagopalan, S., & Brook, R. D. (2005). Acute blood pressure responses in healthy adults during controlled air pollution exposures. *Environmental Health Perspectives,* Vol.113, No. 8, pp. 1052-1055, 0091-6765; 0091-6765

Veronesi, B., & Oortgiesen, M. (2006). The TRPV1 receptor: Target of toxicants and therapeutics. *Toxicological Sciences : An Official Journal of the Society of Toxicology,* Vol.89, No. 1, pp. 1-3, 1096-6080; 1096-0929

Wellenius, G. A., Saldiva, P. H., Batalha, J. R., Krishna Murthy, G. G., Coull, B. A., Verrier, R. L., & Godleski, J. J. (2002). Electrocardiographic changes during exposure to residual oil fly ash (ROFA) particles in a rat model of myocardial infarction. *Toxicological Sciences : An Official Journal of the Society of Toxicology,* Vol.66, No. 2, pp. 327-335, 1096-6080; 1096-0929

Whyte, K. A., Hogg, R. C., Dyavanapalli, J., Harper, A. A., & Adams, D. J. (2009). Reactive oxygen species modulate neuronal excitability in rat intrinsic cardiac ganglia. *Autonomic Neuroscience : Basic & Clinical,* Vol.150, No. 1-2, pp. 45-52, 1872-7484; 1566-0702

Widdicombe, J., & Lee, L. Y. (2001). Airway reflexes, autonomic function, and cardiovascular responses. *Environmental Health Perspectives,* Vol.109 Suppl 4, pp. 579-584, 0091-6765; 0091-6765

Wigle, D. T., Arbuckle, T. E., Walker, M., Wade, M. G., Liu, S., & Krewski, D. (2007). Environmental hazards: Evidence for effects on child health. *Journal of Toxicology and Environmental Health.Part B, Critical Reviews,* Vol.10, No. 1-2, pp. 3-39, 1521-6950; 1093-7404

Wilson, M. R., Lightbody, J. H., Donaldson, K., Sales, J., & Stone, V. (2002). Interactions between ultrafine particles and transition metals *in vivo* and in vitro. *Toxicology and Applied Pharmacology,* Vol.184, No. 3, pp. 172-179, 0041-008X; 0041-008X

World Health Organization (WHO). (2005). *WHO Air quality guidelines for particular matter, ozone, nitrogen dioxide, sulfur dioxide,* Global Update 2005, Available in: <http://whqlibdoc.who.int/hq/2006/WHO_SDE_PHE_OEH_06.02_eng.pdf>

World Health Organization (WHO) Working Group. (2003). *Aspects of air pollution with particulate matter ozone and nitrogen dioxide,* Available from: <http://www.euro.who.int/__data/assets/pdf_file/0005/112199/E79097.pdf>

Wu, S., Deng, F., Niu, J., Huang, Q., Liu, Y., & Guo, X. (2010). Association of heart rate variability in taxi drivers with marked changes in particulate air pollution in beijing in 2008. *Environmental Health Perspectives,* Vol.118, No. 1, pp. 87-91, 1552-9924; 0091-6765

Zanobetti, A., & Schwartz, J. (2005). The effect of particulate air pollution on emergency admissions for myocardial infarction: A multicity case-crossover analysis. *Environmental Health Perspectives,* Vol.113, No. 8, pp. 978-982, 0091-6765; 0091-6765

Zanobetti, A., & Schwartz, J. (2007). Particulate air pollution, progression, and survival after myocardial infarction. *Environmental Health Perspectives,* Vol.115, No. 5, pp. 769-775, 0091-6765; 0091-6765

Zareba, W., Couderc, J. P., Oberdorster, G., Chalupa, D., Cox, C., Huang, L. S., Peters, A., Utell, M. J., & Frampton, M. W. (2009). ECG parameters and exposure to carbon ultrafine particles in young healthy subjects. *Inhalation Toxicology,* Vol.21, No. 3, pp. 223-233, 1091-7691; 0895-8378

Zareba, W., & Cygankiewicz, I. (2008). Long QT syndrome and short QT syndrome. *Progress in Cardiovascular Diseases,* Vol.51, No. 3, pp. 264-278, 1532-8643

Zemp, E., Elsasser, S., Schindler, C., Kunzli, N., Perruchoud, A. P., Domenighetti, G., Medici, T., Ackermann-Liebrich, U., Leuenberger, P., Monn, C.Zellweger, J. P. (1999). Long-term ambient air pollution and respiratory symptoms in adults (SAPALDIA study). the SAPALDIA team. *American Journal of Respiratory and Critical Care Medicine,* Vol.159, No. 4 Pt 1, pp. 1257-1266, 1073-449X; 1073-449X

7

Acute Effects of Fine Particulate Air Pollution on Cardiac Electrophysiology

Duanping Liao[1], Michele L. Shaffer[1] and Haibo Zhou[2]
[1]*Department of Public Health Sciences, Penn State University College of Medicine, Hershey PA,*
[2]*Department of Biostatistics, School of Public Health, University of North Carolina at Chapel Hill, NC, USA*

1. Introduction

Numerous epidemiological studies have demonstrated a consistent link between particulate air pollution, especially fine particulate matter with aerodynamic diameter<2.5μm ($PM_{2.5}$), and increased cardiopulmonary morbidity and mortality (1-5). The mechanisms responsible for such an association have been the focus of recent environmental health studies. The most promising and frequently studied mechanism is PM related effects on cardiac autonomic modulation (6-10). In a study specifically designed to investigate the time course of PM on cardiac autonomic modulation, Cavallari et al. reported an early and a later phase response, with the early effects at 2 hours and delayed effects at 9-13 hours after exposure (11). Since cardiac autonomic modulation regulates important cardiac electrophysiological activities, other electrophysiological parameters have been proposed as important markers of electric activity disturbances associated with PM. These markers include ventricular repolarization, ischemic potential, arrhythmia, and other waveform changes. For instance, it was reported (12-14) that air pollution is associated with severe arrhythmia in patients with implantable cardioverter defibrillators (ICDs). Recently, it was reported that elevated GIS-estimated ambient $PM_{2.5}$ exposures one day prior to the ECG measurement were associated with increased odds of PVC in women enrolled in the Women's Health Initiative (WHI) clinical trials study (15). However, very little is known about PM effects on various cardiac electrophysiological parameters from a study specifically designed to examine the individual-level exposures to $PM_{2.5}$ and all ECG-based parameters.

We therefore designed the Air Pollution and Cardiac Risk and its Time Course (APACR) study to investigate the effects and time course of individual-level exposures to $PM_{2.5}$ on various cardiac electrophysiological parameters. The individual findings on each of the electrophysiological premasters have been reported elsewhere (7;16-19). This chapter summarizes those major findings and presents the overall findings indicating various time-courses from those publications.

2. Materials and methods

2.1 Population

The APACR study successfully examined 106 individuals, with a response rate of approximately 75%. The study was designed as a 24-hour continuous real-time monitoring of $PM_{2.5}$ exposures and cardiac electrophysiological parameters, with the blood samples drawn from the beginning and end of 24 hours to obtain measures of the blood markers (7;16). Briefly, all study participants were recruited from communities in central Pennsylvania, primarily from the Harrisburg metropolitan area. The inclusion criteria for the study included nonsmoking adults $\geq$ 45 years old who had not been diagnosed with severe cardiac problems (defined as diagnosed valvular heart disease, congenital heart disease, acute myocardial infarction or stroke within 6 months, or congestive heart failure). Approximately 75% of the individuals who were contacted and who met our inclusion criteria were enrolled in the APACR study. Our targeted sample size was 100 individuals, and we enrolled and examined 106 individuals for the APACR study. Individual-level $PM_{2.5}$ and Holter ECG monitoring were initiated between 0800 and 1000 hours on the first day, immediately after participants were administered a standardized questionnaire, underwent a brief physical examination, and a fasting blood draw by a trained and certified research nurse. The next morning, the participants returned to remove the monitors and had their second blood draw. The APACR study has maintained approval by the Penn State University College of Medicine institutional review board. All participants gave written informed consent prior to their participation in the study.

2.2 Personal PM2.5 exposures

The APACR study used a personal $PM_{2.5}$ DataRam (pDR, model 1200, Thermo Scientific, Boston, MA) for real-time 24-hour personal $PM_{2.5}$ exposure assessment. Details of the exposure assessment (7;16) and of the instrument's performance have been reported elsewhere (20-23). Real-time $PM_{2.5}$ concentrations were recorded at 1-minute intervals and averaged over 30-minute segments, beginning on the hour or half hour. Therefore, we calculated, on a 30-minute basis, the corresponding time-of-the-day specific average exposure to $PM_{2.5}$ for each participant as a time-dependent repeated measures over a 24-hour period. Thus, each participant contributed 48 exposure data points.

2.3 Electrophysiological variables

We used the high sampling rate (1000 Hz) 12-lead HScribe Holter System (Mortara Instrument, Inc.) for 24-hour Holter beat-to-beat ECG data collection. This high sampling rate Holter system is available for research use only. The high sampling rate significantly increases the resolution and enhances the accurate capture of fiducial point and various wave form measures. The ECG data were scanned to a designated computer for offline processing, using specialized software by an experienced investigator. One experienced investigator followed established protocols to identify machine scanned errors, to verify the Holter identified, and to identify and label additional electronic artifacts and arrhythmic beats in the ECG recording. The reader adjudicated files are saved and used for the calculation of the following five ECG variable categories: the heart rate variability (HRV), ectopy, ventricular repolarization, potential ischemia, and P-wave related measures. All variables were calculated on a 30-minute basis. Thus, they were treated as time-of-the-day specific repeated measures over a 24-hour period. Each participant contributed 48 dependent variable data points.

2.4 HRV variables

We used the above mentioned "reader adjudicated" beat-to-beat ECG for HRV analysis. From the "reader adjudicated" data, we eliminated artifacts and other arrhythmic beats, and only retained normal R to R intervals. We then performed time and frequency domain HRV analysis [Fast Fourier Transformation (FFT)] using the HRV Analysis System (Department of Physics, University of Kuopio, Finland). All calculations were based on current recommendations (24). Briefly, the adjacent RR interval data were interpolated using a piecewise cubic spline approach, with a 2 Hz sampling rate. The FFT was performed on the equidistantly interpolated RR time series. We used a second order polynomial model to remove the slow non-stationary trends of the HRV signal. The following HRV indices were calculated as measures of CAM: standard deviation of all RR intervals (SDNN, ms), square root of the mean of the sum of the squares of differences between adjacent RR intervals (RMSSD, ms), power in the high frequency range (0.15-0.40 Hz, HF), power in the low frequency range (0.04-0.15 Hz, LF), and the LF/HF ratio.

2.5 Arrhythmia frequency

We calculated the frequency of ventricular and supraventricular ectopy. No participant had other less frequent arrhythmic beats, such as atrial fibrillation/flutter and supraventricular and ventricular tachycardia in our study period.

2.6 Ventricular repolarization

We calculated QT Prolongation Index (QTI, %) as a primary measure of ventricular repolarization. The duration of ventricular repolarization is often estimated by Bazett's heart rate-corrected QT interval (QT_c) (25). Although QT_c and QTI (26) are strongly correlated ($r = 0.96$), QTI is less rate-sensitive (26;27) and has a higher repeatability than QT_c (28;29). We focused on QTI, but also reported other HR-corrected QT indices are also available for analysis.

2.7 P wave related measures

The following P-wave based atrial fibrillation/flutter (AF) predictors were calculated from the normal heart beats:

- P wave duration (ms), as the time between the first "onset" and last "offset" deflection from the isoelectro line.
- PR duration (ms), as the time between the first onset defection of the P and R wave, (the latter representing the onset of ventricular depolarization), with longer PR duration the higher risk of AF.
- P wave complexity (unitless), as the average ratio of the second to the first eigenvalue, the value of which reflects the relative complexity of atrial depolarization (30), with more complexity in the atrial depolarization indicating the higher risk of AF.

2.8 ST-height

The calculated ST-height included beat-to-beat ST-height from 10 leads (inferior leads II, III, and aVF; lateral leads I, V5, and V6; septal leads V1 and V2; and anterior leads V3 and V4), defined as the distance between the J point, and 60 ms after the J point. We then calculated on a 30-minute basis the average ST-height for each lead. Therefore, the ST-height measures are treated as repeated outcome measures, and each individual contributed 48 data points for each of the 10 leads.

2.9 Other individual-level covariables

A standardized questionnaire was used to collect the following individual-level information: (a) demographic variables, including age, race, sex, and highest education level; (b) medication uses, including anti-anginal medication, anti-hypertensive medication, and anti-diabetic medication; and (c) physician diagnosed chronic disease history, including CVD (including revascularization procedures and myocardial infarction), hypertension, and diabetes. The averages of the 2nd and 3rd measures of seated systolic and diastolic blood pressures on Day-1 were used to represent a participant's blood pressure levels. Day-1 fasting glucose was measured by the GCRC central laboratory. CVD was defined by anti-anginal medication use or a history of CVD. Hypertension was defined by anti-hypertensive medication use, physician diagnosed hypertension, systolic blood pressure ≥ 140 mmHg, or diastolic blood pressure ≥90mm Hg. Diabetes was defined by anti-diabetic medication use, physician diagnosed diabetes, or fasting glucose >126 mg/dl. Body mass index (BMI) was defined as the ratio of weight to height squared (BMI, kg/m^2).

2.10 Weather variables

We obtained real-time temperature and relative humidity using the HOBO H8 logger (Onset Computer Corporation, Bourne, MA), directly fixed on top of the container housing the $PM_{2.5}$ monitor. The real-time temperature and relative humidity were recorded at 1-minute intervals and averaged over 30-minute segments corresponding to the time segments during which $PM_{2.5}$ and ECG variables were measured. The weather variables were treated as repeated measures, and each individual contributed 48 data points for each.

3. Statistical analysis

In the APACR study, the individual-level, real-time $PM_{2.5}$ exposure and cardiac electrophysiology outcomes were measured over a 24 hour period. The $PM_{2.5}$ and outcome summaries were constructed every 30 minutes for all participants, producing 48 repeated measures. We extended the distributed lag model (31-33) for statistical analyses. Specifically, we constructed polynomial distributed lag models, which enable us to provide interpretation of the cumulative effects of the lags included in the model, as well as individual lag effects. In a lag distributed model, all lags to be analyzed are entered into a single model. The coefficients from the lags are the respective effects from the individual lags. The cumulative effect of all lags is the weighted average of individual effects. In contrast, the moving average model takes the average of intended lag exposures and relates the average with the outcome measured a given total lag units ago. Since $PM_{2.5}$ exposures and ECG outcome data were assessed in parallel over 48 lags (24 hours), we decided *a priori* to model no more than 10 lags, which allowed us to fit the distributed lag models using at least 80% of the data. For continuous outcomes (e.g., heart rate-corrected QT intervals) we used a linear mixed-effects models framework (34). For count (e.g., PVC count, total ectopy count) data we used negative binomial regression model (35) and generalized estimating equations (GEE) framework (36). Details of these models have been published (7;16-19). We systematically started from the largest number of lags (lag 0–10), and reduced the total number of individual lags by back-eliminating the longer lags (e.g., lag 10), one lag at a time until a significant cumulative effect from all the included lags ($p < 0.05$) was identified. We then used this model as our final model for a specific ECG outcome. All results are expressed per 10 µg/m^3 increase in $PM_{2.5}$. We used SAS version 9 (SAS Institute, Inc., Cary, NC) for all analyses. **Figure 1** graphically represents the individual lag and cumulative effects from a distributed lag model.

Figure 1. Panel A. Analytic Methods – Lag 0 Effect

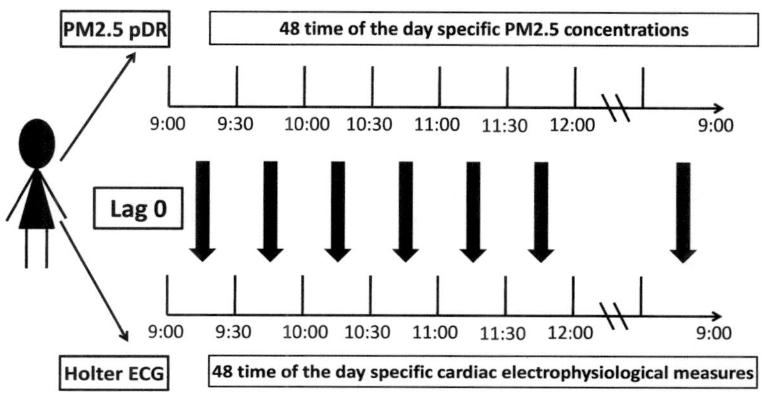

Figure 1. Panel B. Analytic Methods – Lag 1 Effect

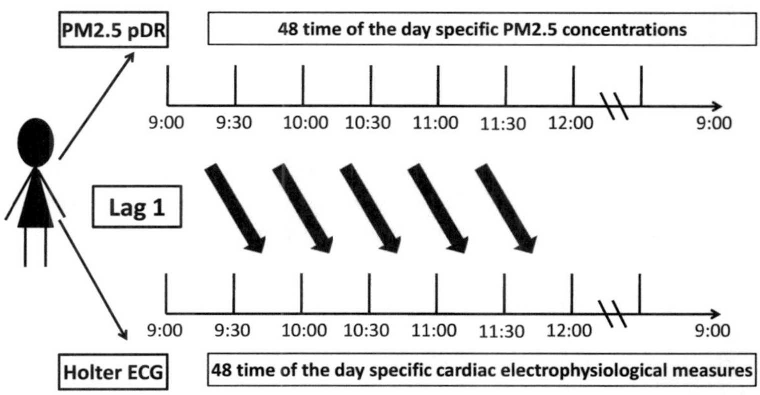

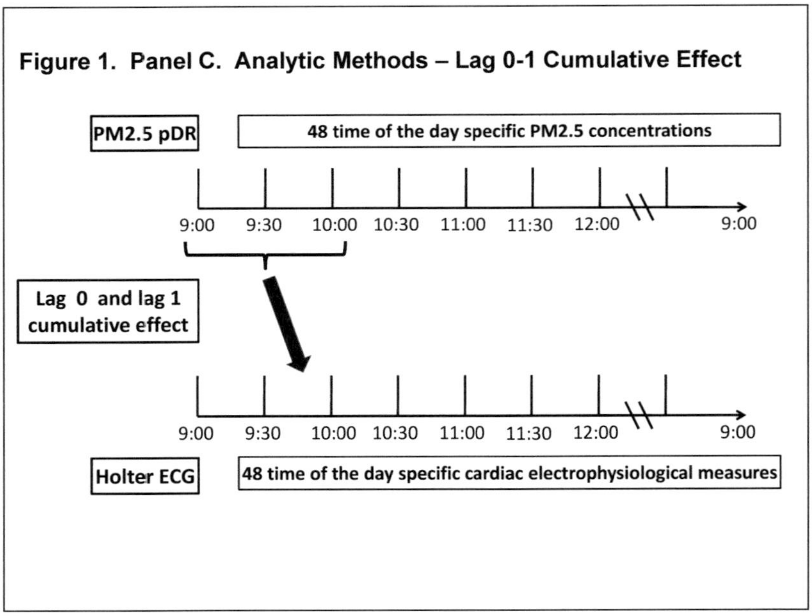

Fig. 1. Illustrations of PM2.5 effects from a distributed lag model

4. Results

Table 1 presents demographic and clinical characteristics in this community-based sample of 106 middle-aged healthy non-smokers. The mean age of the participants was 56 years, with 73% non-Hispanic white, 60% females, and 43% classified as having chronic disease (CVD, hypertension, or diabetes). The prevalence of CVD, hypertension, and diabetes was 7.6%, 35.2%, and 7.6%, respectively.

The average individual-level exposure to $PM_{2.5}$ (over all 30 minute segments) was 13.49 (SD=22) $\mu g/m^3$. The medians of the within-individual interquartile ranges (IQR) for the entire study sample on lag 0, lag 0-1, lag 0-2, lag 0-3, and lag 0-4 $PM_{2.5}$ concentration were 6.38 $\mu g/m^3$, 6.57 $\mu g/m^3$, 5.97 $\mu g/m^3$, 5.83 $\mu g/m^3$, and 6.06 $\mu g/m^3$, respectively, which indicates no substantial variation in the IQRs across the window of exposure, supporting our decision of reporting the relationship between $PM_{2.5}$ and ECG parameters per 10 $\mu g/m^3$ increase of $PM_{2.5}$ across all models.

According to the model selection strategy described above, the final models for each of the continuous ECG outcomes are summarized in **Table 2**, and the results from arrhythmia counts as outcome are presented in **Table 3**. All these models were adjusted for age, sex, race, temperature, relative humidity, diabetes, hypertension, and CVD. From the cumulative effects of $PM_{2.5}$ summarized in Tables 2 and 3, the time course patterns are clearly shown as ranging from 30 minutes to several hours of elevated $PM_{2.5}$ levels.

Characteristic	All subjects	Hypertension, Diabetes, or CVD		
		No	Yes	P value[c]
	N=106	N=60	N=45	
Age	56 (7.6)	56 (8.2)	57 (6.8)	0.32
Gender (% Male)	40	40	40	1.00
Race (% non-Hispanic White)	73	72	76	0.66
Glucose (mg/dL)	89 (25)	85 (10)	94 (36)	0.10
BMI (kg/m2)	28 (5.9)	26 (4.3)	30 (7.1)	<0.01
CVD (%)	7.6	0.00	18	<0.01
Hypertension (%)	35	0.00	85	<0.01
Diabetes (%)	7.6	0.00	18	<0.01
Systolic Blood Pressure (mm Hg)	122 (16)	117 (12)	128 (18)	<0.01
Diastolic Blood Pressure (mm Hg)	75 (9.2)	73 (8.3)	77 (9.8)	0.02
College or Higher (%)	79	73	87	0.10
Hypertensive Medicine Use (%)	19	0.00	44	<0.01
Diabetic Medicine Use (%)	6.7	0.00	16	<0.01
Arrhythmia Medicine Use (%)	1.9	0.00	4.4	0.18

a Results are presented as mean (standard deviation) for continuous variables and percentage for categorical variables

b he median of the within-individual interquartile ranges of PM2.5 concentration.

c p-value for comparing CVD and No CVD groups.

Table 1. Demographic and clinical characteristics of the study population[a]

ECG Parameter	Lags	ß (SE, p value)
HRV Log_HF (ms^2)	Lag 0	-0.003 (0.007)
	Lag 1	-0.006 (0.005)
	Lag 2	-0.007 (0.003) *
	Lag 3	-0.009 (0.004) **
	Lag 4	-0.009 (0.004) *
	Lag 5	-0.009 (0.004) *
	Lag 6	-0.008 (0.004) *
	Lag 7	-0.007 (0.003) *
	Lag 8	-0.005 (0.004)
	Lag 9	-0.002 (0.005)
	Lag 10	0.002 (0.008)
	Cumulative	-0.062 (0.022) **
SDNN (ms)	Lag 0	-0.07 (0.21)
	Lag 1	-0.09 (0.13)
	Lag 2	-0.12 (0.10)
	Lag 3	-0.13 (0.10)
	Lag 4	-0.15 (0.12)
	Lag 5	-0.16 (0.12)
	Lag 6	-0.17 (0.11)
	Lag 7	-0.18 (0.10)
	Lag 8	-0.18 (0.10)
	Lag 9	-0.18 (0.15)
	Lag 10	-0.17 (0.24)
	Cumulative	**-1.59 (0.54)** **

ECG Parameter	Lags	ß (SE, p value)
QTI (%)	Lag 0	0.07 (0.04) *
	Lag 1	0.04 (0.02) *
	Lag 2	0.02 (0.02)
	Lag 3	0.01 (0.03)
	Lag 4	0.01 (0.03)
	Lag 5	0.02 (0.02)
	Lag 6	0.05 (0.03) *
	Lag 7	0.08 (0.04) *
	Cumulative	**0.32 (0.13)** **
ST-height ST-II	Lag 0	0.04 (0.08)
	Lag 1	0.14 (0.06) **
	Lag 2	0.20 (0.07) **
	Lag 3	0.21 (0.09) **
	Lag 4	0.20 (0.16)
	Cumulative	**0.79 (0.23)** **
ST-III	Lag 0	0.02 (0.07)
	Lag 1	0.08 (0.05)
	Lag 2	0.13 (0.06) *
	Lag 3	0.15 (0.08) *
	Lag 4	0.14 (0.14)
	Cumulative	**0.52 (0.27)***
P complexity	Lag 0	0.0002 (0.0002)
	Lag 1	0.0004 (0.0002) **
	Lag 2	0.0005 (0.0002) **
	Lag 3	0.0004 (0.0004)
	Cumulative	0.0016 (0.0006) **

* : $p<0.05$ **: $p<0.01$

Table 2. Regression coefficient of continuous ECG variables associated with a 10μg/m^3 increment of $PM_{2.5}$.

Ectopy Variable	Lags	Rate Ratiob (95%CI)
PVC (count)	Lag 0 (same time)	1.08 (1.05, 1.10) **
	Lag 0-1 (30 min. prior)	1.03 (1.00, 1.05) *
PAC (count)	Lag 0 (same time)	0.94 (0.85, 1.04)
	Lag 0-1 (30 min. prior)	0.97 (0.89, 1.05)

a The rate ratios were calculating by exponentiating the regression coefficients from distributed lag negative binomial models. A rate ratio of 1.05 indicates a 5% increase in ectopy count/30 minutes in association with a 10 μg/m3 increase in PM2.5 concentration

b Adjusted for age, sex, race, chronic disease status, and the same lag period temperature and relative humidity.

*: P value<0.05 **: P value<0.01

Table 3. The cumulative rate ratiosa (95% CI) of ectopy counts associated with a 10 μg/m3 increment of PM2.5.

To elucidate whether $PM_{2.5}$ affects inflammatory response as a potential mechanism that explains the associations between $PM_{2.5}$ and ECG-based parameters, we examined the association between individual level 24-hour $PM_{2.5}$ concentration and blood inflammatory markers in the APACR study population. In these analyses, we treated $PM_{2.5}$ exposure as 24-hour average from the pDR measures. Two blood samples were collected from each participant, one immediately before and one immediately after the 24-hour study period. Concentrations of several inflammation markers were assessed and averaged. Linear regression models were used to assess the association between mean 24-hour $PM_{2.5}$ exposure and the mean inflammation markers. Age, race, gender, relative humidity, temperature, and participant's chronic disease status were adjusted for in the regression models. We did not observe significant associations between 24-hour mean $PM_{2.5}$ exposure and mean inflammation markers. The regression coefficients (SE) per 10 $\mu g/m^3$ increase in $PM_{2.5}$ were: -0.02 (0.02) g/dL for albumin, 81 (217) ng/mL for C-reactive protein (CRP), -0.56 (0.13) pg/mL for interleukin-1 α (IL-1 α), -0.28 (0.30) pg/mL for interleukin-1 β (IL-1 β), -19 (56) pg/mL for macrophage migration inhibitory factor (MIF), -1.66 (5.37) pg/mL for tumor necrosis factor-α (TNFα), 100 (73) pg/mL for tumor necrosis factor soluble receptor I (TNFsRI),and 0.02 (0.09) x 103/mm³ for white blood cell count, respectively (all p-values > 0.05).

Similarly, we also examined the association between individual level 24-hour $PM_{2.5}$ concentration and blood hemostatic factors--blood markers of coagulation and thrombosis potential in the APACR . We did not observe significant associations between 24-hour mean $PM_{2.5}$ exposure and mean hemostatic factor levels. The regression coefficients (SE) per 10 $\mu g/m^3$ increase in $PM_{2.5}$ were: -0.13 (0.78) % for antithrombin III, 1.95 (2.97) % for factor VIII, -2.79 (3.88) mg/dL for fibrinogen, 0.56 (0.54) IU/mL for plasminogen activator inhibitor, 0.06 (0.19) ng/mL for tissue plasminogen activator, and -0.13 (0.15) µg/mL for D-Dimer (all p-values > 0.05).

5. Discussion

The mechanisms responsible for the consistently reported association between fine particle exposure and cardiovascular disease mortality and morbidity are not fully understood. Previous studies have suggested several possible underlying mechanisms, including cardiac autonomic impairment as measured by lower HRV (Creason et al. 2001; Gold et al. 2000; He et al. 2010; Liao et al. 1999, 2004; Pope et al. 1999) and effects on ventricular repolarization (Campen et al. 2006; Ghelfi et al. 2008; Henneberger et al. 2005; Liao et al. 2010; Lux and Pope 2009; Samet et al. 2009; Yue et al. 2007), T-wave alternans (Zanobetti et al. 2009), myocardium ischemia (Zhang et al. 2009), and arrhythmias (Berger et al. 2006; Dockery et al. 2005; Eblet et al. 2005; Liao et al. 2009; Sarnat et al. 2006). We conducted this study to systematically examine all of these cardiac electrophysiological parameters in one study population under a single standardized personal $PM_{2.5}$ exposure. With both $PM_{2.5}$ exposure and ECG based parameters assessed in parallel for 24 hours, and subsequently divided as 30-minute based segment specific measures, we can apply distributed lag methods to identify the suggested time-course of associations, the lagged time of any significant associations between $PM_{2.5}$ and ECG parameters.

Since the associations we found on each of the five ECG-based parameter domains have been published (7;16-19), we selected to use 1-2 parameters from each domain to illustrate the overall pattern of the time-courses of elevated $PM_{2.5}$ on ECG parameters. The following patterns are clearly shown in Tables 2 and 3:

1. The effects on HRV as measures of cardiac autonomic modulation were limited to within approximately 5.5 hours of the $PM_{2.5}$ exposure;
2. The effects on heart rate corrected QT as measure of ventricular repolarization were limited to within approximately 4 hours of the $PM_{2.5}$ exposure;
3. The effects on ST-height as measures of ischemic potential were limited to within approximately 2.5 hours of the $PM_{2.5}$ exposure;
4. The effects on P-wave based parameters as measures of atrial fibrillation (Afib) vulnerability were limited to within approximately 2 hours of the $PM_{2.5}$ exposure; and
5. The effects on the frequency of ventricular ectopy were limited to within approximately 60 minutes.

To our knowledge, this is the first study designed to have sufficient temporal resolution of both exposure and ECG variables, e.g. on the 30-minute basis of exposure, outcome, and covariables. Such a study design enabled us to examine the acute effect of $PM_{2.5}$ exposure on various ECG-based parameters. Another major strength of this study is that $PM_{2.5}$ exposures, the ECG outcome data, and the covariables were measured at the individual level on a real-time basis over 24 hours. With these individual-level data, we can adjust for individual-level time-varying and non-time-varying confounding factors. Overall, our data provide evidence of acute effects of $PM_{2.5}$ exposure on cardiac electrophysiological profiles.

Mechanisms that would explain the associations between various ECG parameters and $PM_{2.5}$ exposure are unknown at this time. It is biologically plausible that exposures to $PM_{2.5}$ directly reduce parasympathetic modulation and increase sympathetic modulation, resulting in longer ventricular repolarization, elevated ST-height, increased Afib vulnerability, and a decreased threshold for arrhythmia. Since HRV is a reliable measure of cardiac autonomic modulation, and most published studies have suggested that PM exposure is associated with lower HRV indices, we repeated all of our analyses to include adjustment for HRV variables in the final models. In general, associations between $PM_{2.5}$ and various ECG-based parameters were attenuated but still remained statistically significant when we adjusted for HRV variables. These HRV-adjusted findings are consistent with an intermediate effect of PM exposure on autonomic modulation. However, adjustment for HRV parameters did not completely eliminate the associations between $PM_{2.5}$ and various ECG parameters suggesting that other mechanisms might also explain the associations. For the inflammatory responses to $PM_{2.5}$ pathway, our relatively low levels of 24-hour mean $PM_{2.5}$ exposure are not associated with blood inflammation markers. These null finding suggest that more studies on the chronic exposure and inflammatory responses are needed to elucidate the sub-acute and chronic effects of PM on systemic inflammation as a mechanistic link between PM and cardiac electrophysiology and cardiopulmonary disease. For the blood coagulation and thrombosis potential responses to $PM_{2.5}$ pathway, the 24-hour mean levels of $PM_{2.5}$ exposure were not associated with blood hemostatic factors. These null findings suggest that more studies on chronic PM exposure and hemostatic factors are needed to elucidate their role in the pathophysiologic effects of air pollution on deep vein thrombosis and cardiopulmonary disease. In a just published study by Zuurbier and co-workers [37], it was concluded that air pollution exposure during commuting was not consistently associated with acute changes in inflammation markers, blood cell counts or blood coagulation markers in individuals. It should be noted that individuals in this study were exposed to higher levels of traffic-related pollutants than the APACR study participants.

The APACR study has several limitations. First, our findings may not apply to smokers or persons with a recent acute cardiac event, as such persons were excluded from the study population. Second, the majority of participants reported that they stayed indoors most of the time during the 24-hour study period, except when they had to travel by automobile, and they had limited exposure to second hand cigarette smoke. Thus, participants had relatively low levels of exposure to $PM_{2.5}$ and we cannot determine whether exposures at higher levels would exhibit similar associations. Third, it is well known that sympathetic nervous activity increases during physical activity, which could be related to higher $PM_{2.5}$ exposure if it occurs outdoors. Thus, it is possible that the $PM_{2.5}$ and ECG-parameters associations in this study were confounded by physical activity. However, the vast majority of our participants reported staying indoors 97% of the 24 hour study period reduces the possibility that the consistent associations were mainly due to outdoor activity confounding. Fourth, the ECG data were not collected under a controlled, supine-position setting, and short-term variation due to other factors that may impact the ECG parameters cannot be fully accounted for in our analysis. However, it is not feasible to keep a healthy participant in a supine indoor position for 24 hours, and even if this were achieved, the results from such a study design would not be generalizable to a real-world situation.

6. Conclusions

The data from the APACR study enabled us to systematically examine the acute effects of $PM_{2.5}$ exposures on various clinically relevant cardiac electrophysiological disturbances. In general, higher $PM_{2.5}$ is adversely associated with all five major ECG parameters we analyzed, with the adverse effects occurring acutely (within 2-5 hours of elevated $PM_{2.5}$) or ultra acutely (within 0.5 hr of elevated $PM_{2.5}$). These adverse effects on ECG parameters may trigger the onset of acute cardiac events and cumulatively over time, may result in increased risk of cardiac disease. Thus, it is possible that $PM_{2.5}$ exposure is associated with cardiovascular and cerebral vascular disease by first affecting the cardiac electrophysiology.

7. References

[1] Brook RD, Franklin B, Cascio W, Hong Y, Howard G, Lipsett M, Luepker R, Mittleman M, Samet J, Smith SCJ, Tager I. Air pollution and cardiovascular disease: a statement for healthcare professionals from the Expert Panel on Population and Prevention Science of the American Heart Association. Circulation. 2004;109(21):2655-71.

[2] Mann JK, Tager IB, Lurmann F, Segal M, Quesenberry CPJ, Lugg MM, Shan J, Van Den Eeden SK. Air pollution and hospital admissions for ischemic heart disease in persons with congestive heart failure or arrhythmia. Environ Health Perspect. 2002;110(12):1247-52.

[3] Pope CA 3rd , Burnett RT, Thun MJ, Calle EE, Krewski D, Ito K, Thurston GD. Lung cancer, cardiopulmonary mortality, and long-term exposure to fine particulate air pollution. JAMA. 2002;287(9):1132-41.

[4] Samet JM, Rappold A, Graff D, Cascio WE, Berntsen JH, Huang YT, Herbst M, Bassett M, Montilla T, Hazucha MJ, Bromberg PA, Devlin RB. Concentrated ambient ultrafine particle exposure induces cardiac changes in young healthy volunteers. Am J Respir Crit Care Med. 2009;179(11):1034-42.

[5] Schwartz J. Air pollution and hospital admissions for heart disease in eight U.S. counties. Epidemiology. 1999;10(1):17-22.

[6] Gold DR, Litonjua A, Schwartz J, Lovett E, Larson A, Nearing B, Allen G, Verrier M, Cherry R, Verrier R. Ambient pollution and heart rate variability. Circulation. 2000;101(11):1267-73.

[7] He F, Shaffer ML, Li X, Rodriguez-Colon S, Wolbrette DL, Williams R, Cascio WE, Liao D. Individual-level $PM_{2.5}$ exposure and the time course of impaired heart rate variability: the APACR Study. J Expo Sci Environ Epidemiol. 2011;21(1):65-73.

[8] Liao D, Creason J, Shy C, Williams R, Watts R, Zweidinger R. Daily variation of particulate air pollution and poor cardiac autonomic control in the elderly. Environ Health Perspect. 1999;107(7):521-5.

[9] Luttmann-Gibson H, Suh HH, Coull BA, Dockery DW, Sarnat SE, Schwartz J, Stone PH, Gold DR. Short-term effects of air pollution on heart rate variability in senior adults in Steubenville, Ohio. J Occup Environ Med. 2006;48(8):780-8.

[10] Magari SR, Hauser R, Schwartz J, Williams PL, Smith TJ, Christiani DC. Association of heart rate variability with occupational and environmental exposure to particulate air pollution. Circulation. 2001;104(9):986-91.

[11] Cavallari JM, Fang SC, Eisen EA, Schwartz J, Hauser R, Herrick RF, Christiani DC. Time course of heart rate variability decline following particulate matter exposures in an occupational cohort. Inhal Toxicol. 2008;20(4):415-22.

[12] Dockery DW, Luttmann-Gibson H, Rich DQ, Link MS, Mittleman MA, Gold DR, Koutrakis P, Schwartz JD, Verrier RL. Association of air pollution with increased incidence of ventricular tachyarrhythmias recorded by implanted cardioverter defibrillators. Environ Health Perspect. 2005;113(6):670-4.

[13] Peters A, Liu E, Verrier RL, Schwartz J, Gold DR, Mittleman M, Baliff J, Oh JA, Allen G, Monahan K, Dockery DW. Air pollution and incidence of cardiac arrhythmia. Epidemiology. 2000;11(1):11-7.

[14] Vedal S, Rich K, Brauer M, White R, Petkau J. Air pollution and cardiac arrhythmias in patients with implantable cardioverter defibrillators. Inhal Toxicol. 2004;16(6-7):353-62.

[15] Liao D, Whitsel EA, Duan Y, Lin H, Quibrera PM, Smith R, Peuquet DJ, Prineas RJ, Zhang Z, Anderson G. Ambient particulate air pollution and ectopy--the environmental epidemiology of arrhythmogenesis in Women's Health Initiative Study, 1999-2004. J Toxicol Environ Health A. 2009;72(1):30-8.

[16] Liao D, Shaffer ML, Rodriguez-Colon S, He F, Li X, Wolbrette DL, Yanosky J, Cascio WE. Acute adverse effects of fine particulate air pollution on ventricular repolarization. Environ Health Perspect. 2010;118(7):1010-5.

[17] He F, Shaffer ML, Rodriguez-Colon S, Bixler EO, Vgontzas AN, Williams RW, Wu R, Cascio WE, Liao D. Acute effects of fine particulate air pollution on ST segment height: a longitudinal study. Environ Health. 2010;9:68.

[18] 18. Liao D, Shaffer ML, He F, Rodriguez-Colon S, Wu R, Whitset EA, Bixler EO, Cascio WE. Fine Particulate Air Pollution is Associated with Higher Vulnerability to Atrial Fibrillation- the APACR Study J Toxicol Environ Health A. 2011;74:1-13.

[19] He F, Shaffer M, Rodriguez-Colon S, Yanosky J, Bixler E, Cascio W, Liao D. Acute Effects of Fine Particulate Air Pollution on Cardiac Arrhythmia-The APACR Study.. Environ Health Perspect. In press 2011.

[20] Rea AW, Zufall MJ, Williams RW, Sheldon L, Howard-Reed C. The influence of human activity patterns on personal PM exposure: a comparative analysis of filter-based and continuous particle measurements. J Air Waste Manag Assoc. 2001;51(9):1271-9.

[21] Howard-Reed C, Rea AW, Zufall MJ, Burke JM, Williams RW, Suggs JC, Sheldon LS, Walsh D, Kwok R. Use of a continuous nephelometer to measure personal exposure to particles during the U.S. Environmental Protection Agency Baltimore and Fresno Panel studies. J Air Waste Manag Assoc. 2000;50(7):1125-32.

[22] Wallace L, Williams R, Rea A, Corghan C. Continuous weeklong measurements of personal exposures and indoor concentrations of fine particles for 37 health-impaired North Carolina residents for up to four seasons Atmos Environ. 2006;40(3):399-414.

[23] Williams R, Rea A, Vette A, Croghan C, Whitaker D, Stevens C, McDow S, Fortmann R, Sheldon L, Wilson H, Thornburg J, Phillips M, Lawless P, Rodes C, Daughtrey H. The design and field implementation of the Detroit Exposure and Aerosol Research Study. J Expo Sci Environ Epidemiol. 2009;19(7):643-59.

[24] Task Force of the European Society of Cardiology and the North American Society of Pacing and Electrophysiology. Heart rate variability: standards of measurement, physiological interpretation and clinical use. Circulation. 1996;93(5):1043-65.

[25] Bazett H. An analysis of the time-relations of electrocardiogram. Heart. 1920;7:353-70.

[26] Rautaharju PM, Warren JW, Calhoun HP. Estimation of QT prolongation. A persistent, avoidable error in computer electrocardiography. J Electrocardiol. 1990;23 Suppl:111-7.

[27] Rautaharju PM, Zhou SH, Wong S, Prineas R, Berenson GS. Functional characteristics of QT prediction formulas. The concepts of QTmax and QT rate sensitivity. Comput Biomed Res. 1993;26(2):188-204.

[28] Vaidean G, Schroeder E, Whitsel E, Prineas R, Chambless L, Perhac S. Computer measurement of spatial T axis deviation is a reliable measurement in healthy subjects. The ARIC study. [abstract]. Circulation .2002 ;106:744.

[29] Moss AJ, Zareba W, Benhorin J, Couderc JP, Kennedy H, Locati-Heilbron E, Maison-Blanche P. ISHNE guidelines for electrocardiographic evaluation of drug-related QT prolongation and other alterations in ventricular repolarization: task force summary. A report of the Task Force of the International Society for Holter and Noninvasive Electrocardiology (ISHNE), Committee on Ventricular Repolarization. Ann Noninvasive Electrocardiol. 2001;6(4):333-41.

[30] 30. Priori SG, Mortara DW, Napolitano C, Diehl L, Paganini V, Cantu F, Cantu G, Schwartz PJ. Evaluation of the spatial aspects of T-wave complexity in the long-QT syndrome. Circulation. 1997;96(9):3006-12.

[31] Almon S. The distributed lag between capital appropriations and expenditures. Econometrica. 1965;33:178-96.

[32] Pope CA3, Schwartz J. Time series for the analysis of pulmonary health data. Am J Respir Crit Care Med. 1996;154(6 Pt 2):S229-33.

[33] Schwartz J. The distributed lag between air pollution and daily deaths. Epidemiology. 2000;11(3):320-6.

[34] Laird NM, Ware JH. Random-effects models for longitudinal data. Biometrics. 1982;38(4):963-74.

[35] Hilbe JM. Negative Binomial Regression. Cambridge, UK. Cambridge University Press; 2007.

[36] Hardin J, Hilbe J. Generalized Estimating Equations. London:Chapman and Hall; 2003.

[37] Moniek Zuurbier, Gerard Hoek, Marieke Oldenwening, Kees Meliefste, Esmeralda Krop, Peter van den Hazel, and Bert Brunekreef: In-Traffic Air Pollution Exposure and CC16, Blood Coagulation, and Inflammation Markers in Healthy Adults. EHP. 2011. Online Ahead of Print: doi: 10.1289/ehp.1003151 from http://dx.doi.org/

8

Carbon Monoxide Urban Air Pollution: Cardiac Effects

G. Meyer , S. Tanguy, P. Obert and C. Reboul
Laboratory of Cardiovascular Pharm-ecology,
Faculty of Sciences, Avignon University,
France

1. Introduction

Heart disease is a leading cause of death world-wide. The development of heart pathological phenotype results from a complex interplay between genetic and environmental factors. Among environmental factors, recently the deleterious health effects of urban air pollution were pointed out in epidemiological studies (Bhatnagar, 2006, Brook et al., 2004) and a particular attention is then paid to micro and nano-particles air pollution. However, some gazes, such as SO_2, NO_x, O_3, CO_x, could also be reported to have potential deleterious cardiovascular health effects. Particularly, carbon monoxide (CO) resulting from the partial oxidation of carbon-containing compound is reported in epidemiological studies as one of the main pollutants responsible for the development of cardiovascular diseases (Bell et al., 2009, Stieb et al., 2009). Indeed, at low concentration, as may be found in urban environment, CO has been correlated with hospital admissions, mortality and morbidity related to cardiovascular dysfunctions (Bell et al., 2009, Burnett et al., 1997).
Today, the cardiac effects of CO poisoning, corresponding to acute exposure to very high concentrations of CO (1000 - 10000 ppm), were largely studied and are known as the consequence of tissue hypoxemia resulting from the high affinity of CO for blood haemoglobin. However, at low concentrations, as classically found in urban environment, such a hypoxemia could not be considered as a trigger of CO-induced cardiac incoherencies. Then, although some epidemiological evidences that CO air pollution could play a key role in the deleterious effects of prolonged exposure to urban air pollution, today, whether this gaze could be considered as a main risk factor in the development of cardiac diseases, is less understood. Therefore, the aim of this review was to explore, based on experimental literature, the potential link between exposure to such an environmental pollutant and occurrence of cardiac disturbances.

2. CO in urban environment

The purpose of this review is not to discuss on the level of CO measured in urban area. However, in order to focus our review on concentrations corresponding to those measured in urban environment, we first have to consider the range of urban CO concentration observed in environmental studies.

In urban area the most common sources of CO are cigarette smoke and vehicle exhaust (Cunnington and Hormbrey, 2002). In the US, daily mean ambient levels of CO range from 0.5 to 2 ppm (Samet et al., 2000). Exhaled CO levels range from 0 to 21 ppm in non smokers, and from 2 to 50 ppm in smokers (Jones and Lam, 2006). The highest levels of CO exposure were found in car park/garages (12 ppm), private car/taxi (11 ppm) and bar/pub/nights club (8 ppm) (Chau et al., 2002). Then, in urban environments CO concentration usually varies from 2 to 40 ppm, but during heavy traffic or when peoples are exposed to second-hand cigarette smoke it may be as high as 170 ppm (Bevan, 1991, Stern et al., 1988, Wright et al., 1975). Although CO levels are relatively low in urban environment, data from the APHEA-2 project (Air Pollution and Health: A European Approach) studying the relation between air pollution and total cardiovascular mortality in 19 European cities, reported a significant association of CO with cardiovascular mortality (Samoli et al., 2007).

3. Regular exposure to low CO level and phenotypical remodelling of the heart

3.1 Acute low level CO exposure

The acute effects of such low levels of CO on the myocardium are today few studied and results are contradictory and conflicting. Thom et al., (Thom et al., 1999, Thom et al., 2000) discussed that carboxyhemoglobin (HbCO) values associated with levels of CO found in urban area are so low that tissue hypoxemic stress is doubtful and compensatory physiological mechanisms certainly are sufficient to maintain tissue oxygenation. These authors reported yet, on cultured endothelial cells, that acute exposure to low concentrations of CO cause a nitric oxide (NO)-dependent oxidative stress, since CO deleterious effects were inhibited by the addition of N^{ω}nitro-L-arginine methyl ester to inhibit NO synthesis (Thom et al., 2000). In this study, the reaction of NO with superoxide anion to form the highly cytotoxic peroxynitrite is mentioned as a main trigger of lethal CO effects. Indeed, it is today well established that acute CO exposure was associated with higher reactive oxygen species production (Piantadosi, 2002). Indeed, CO molecules form relatively tight complexes with heme proteins (instead of O_2) responsible for mitochondrial and non-mitochondrial reactive oxygen species production (Piantadosi, 2008). Regarding its mitochondrial effects, it was shown that CO binds to cytochrome-c-oxidase altering mitochondrial electron transport chain and then, especially in metabolically active tissues like heart, induced reactive oxygen species production (D'Amico et al., 2006, Zuckerbraun et al., 2007). CO-dependent reactive oxygen species production could also occur via non-mitochondrial sources, notably NADPH oxidase and nitric oxide synthase (NOS) (Piantadosi, 2008); however this is not yet clearly established in the scientific literature.

During CO exposure, the interaction between reactive oxygen species and NO, mentioned above, could also contribute to alter the regulation of coronary blood flow and then the regulation of myocardial perfusion. Indeed, it is today well known that NO play a major role in the coronary vasomotor response of the myocardium. Therefore, we can note that a myocardial dysfunction and a potential cardiac hypoxia in heart of rats inhaling CO for 90 min at 250 ppm was previously reported (Favory et al., 2006). In this model, myocardial hypoxia was explained by coronary endothelium dependent abnormalities. Such a coronary-dependent impairment of myocardial perfusion could then contribute to exacerbate tissue hypoxia.

3.2 Prolonged low level CO exposure

CO molecule, promoting reactive oxygen species dependent signalling molecules, could have biological significance in the adaptation of cells to hypoxia. However, whether recurrent exposure to low levels of CO could participate to the deleterious effects of urban CO exposure is not today well understood. Recently, Bye et al. (Bye et al., 2008) reported, in a model of rats exposed to CO levels experienced by heavy smokers (18 months, 5 days a week at 200 ppm), a pathological remodelling of the heart, characterized by impaired Ca^{2+} handling and increased growth factor signalling. This pathological hypertrophy of the heart was associated in-vivo with reduced aerobic capacity. In model simulating CO exposure at level found in cigarette smoke (200 ppm for 14 consecutive days), the use of LU135252, a selective inhibitor of type A endothelin (ET-1) receptors (ET_A), in drinking water, markedly prevents right ventricular hypertrophy but not left ventricular, suggesting then a role of ET-1 in the right ventricle and/or in the pulmonary circulation during CO exposure (Loennechen et al., 2002). In another model, closer to urban area pollution, Andre et al. (Andre et al., 2010) reported that 4 weeks of CO exposure at low levels (30-100 ppm 12 hours/day) in healthy rats, promotes heart arrhythmias, even in absence of CO in the environment. This propensity was exacerbated during a β-adrenergic stress. This phenomenon is explained in this work by a pathological cardiomyocytes remodelling. Indeed, in this model of rats, following 4 weeks of CO exposure at low level, both contraction and relaxation of single cardiomyocytes were altered. Several changes explained this alteration of cells function, including decreased Ca^{2+} transient amplitude, decreased Ca^{2+} sensitivity of myofilaments and increased diastolic intracellular Ca^{2+} subsequent to reduced SERCA-2a expression and increased Ryanodine receptor (RyR) phosphorylation (on the PKA-dependent site Ser^{2809}). Authors evoked β-adrenergic stress as a potential trigger of this phenotypical cardiac myocytes remodelling. Indeed, at the cardiomyocytes level, β-adrenergic stimulation activates PKA, which phosphorylates both Ca^{2+} handling proteins involved in excitation-contraction-coupling and myofilaments regulatory proteins. This hypothesis is endorsed by the lower β-adrenergic response in animals exposed to CO pollution. Because reactive oxygen species could also activate PKA in the heart (Marx et al., 2000) and CO is well known to activate reactive oxygen species production, the authors also hypothesized that oxidative stress could be a main trigger of this specific remodelling. This is supported by the impairment of heart enzymatic antioxidant status in CO exposed rat hearts and increased activity of thioredoxin reductase confirming then, in this model, that CO, even at very low levels, was responsible for heart oxidative stress. Finally, prolonged CO exposure (50 ppm during 3 weeks) in rats with pathological right ventricular hypertrophia was reported to induce RV tissue necrosis (Gautier et al., 2007). The authors reported then, that CO-induced alteration of the right ventricular perfusion could play a key role in this phenomenon.

4. Prolonged low level CO exposure and ischemic pathology of the heart

Myocardial infarction due to ischemia reperfusion remains today a major cause of morbidity and mortality in western nations. Those myocardial ischemia-reperfusion injuries result in cardiac dysfunction, arrhythmias, as well as irreversible myocytes damages (Murphy and Steenbergen, 2008). Sensitivity of the myocardium to ischemia-reperfusion-induced cellular injuries is recognized today to be the result of a complex interplay between genetic, pathological and environmental factors.

4.1 Acute CO exposure and Ischemic pathology of the heart

Regarding ischemic pathologies of the heart the effect of CO is today still controversial. Indeed, CO is classically used to pre-condition the heart and then reduce its vulnerability against ischemia-reperfusion (Clark et al., 2003, Fujimoto et al., 2004, Stein et al., 2005). Indeed, since the study of Clark et al. (Clark et al., 2003) has reported the cardioprotective effects of a water soluble CO releasing molecule, named CORM-3, many studies tested whether CORM-3 or acute CO exposure could reduce the severity of myocardial ischemia-reperfusion injuries. Today, CORM-3 is known as reducing the severity of ventricular fibrillation (Bak et al., 2003) and the size of infracted area (Clark et al., 2003) without altered HbCO concentration (Guo et al., 2004). In the same way, exogenous CO in perfusion buffer of isolated heart (0.01 or 0.001%) was reported to improve myocardial post-ischemic recovery (Bak et al., 2005). Finally, acute inhaled CO exposures (from few hours to 24 hours) at high levels (from 500 to 1000 ppm) were reported to be able to precondition the heart against such a coronary artery occlusion (Fujimoto et al., 2004). P38 mitogen activated protein kinase (p38MAPK) and akt-eNOS-GMPc pathway were reported to be mainly implicated in this cardioprotective effects of inhaled CO.

4.2 Prolonged CO exposure and ischemic pathology of the heart

All in all, those results mainly suggest that CO possesses some cardioprotective properties. However, this is not in accordance with numerous epidemiological studies reporting the potential toxicological properties of this gas in air pollution (see above). In addition, it was reported in some experimental models, that regular exposure to environmental tobacco smoke, in which CO is one of the main toxic components (CO concentration about 90 ppm), increases infarct size (Zhu et al., 1996, Zhu et al., 1994). Finally, the pathologic phenotypical remodeling of heart contractile cells, as mentioned above, could be taken to suggest that prolonged CO exposure could deleteriously influence heart vulnerability to ischemia-reperfusion. Then, in regard to this phenotypical remodelling of cardiomyocytes, some authors were recently interested in evaluating the influence of prolonged CO exposure on heart sensitivity to ischemia-reperfusion, and the potential link between regular exposure to CO and mortality from cardiac incoherencies during such an ischemic stress. In such experimental work, prolonged CO exposure, simulating urban environmental pollution (30-100 ppm 12 hours/day), was reported to exacerbate rat heart ischemia-reperfusion injuries (Figure 1) (Meyer et al., 2010). This higher vulnerability was characterized in CO rats' myocardium by i) lower recovery of myocardial function and coronary blood flow during post-ischemic reperfusion, ii) higher severity of reperfusion arrhythmias, characterized notably by higher propensity of ventricular fibrillation, and iii) higher infarct size and cells death. This phenomenon is mainly explained in this study by exacerbated oxidative stress. Indeed, increased lipid peroxidation was measured in heart of CO exposed rats after 30 min of reperfusion. This could be logically explained by reduced enzymatic antioxidant defence capacities reported in CO rats' myocardium. Then, it is of interest to note that in this work, at cardiomyocyte level, an antioxidant strategy (N-Acetyl-Cysteine infusion) during anoxia-reoxygenation, was able to normalize post-ischemic functional recovery in CO rat heart cells (evaluated by sarcomere length shortening). These effects seem to be mediated by a normalization of cytosolic Ca^{2+} concentrations. In the same way, in another study, the authors evaluated whether, a cardioprotective strategy, such as exercise, was able to prevent the deleterious effects of CO exposure on cardiomyocytes phenotypical remodelling and then influences heart sensitivity to ischemia-reperfusion (Farah et al., 2010). In this work, it is reported that moderate exercise, specifically designed to follow the recommendation of the World Health Organisation, conducted 4 weeks before CO exposure and all along CO exposure period, prevented the pathological remodelling of the heart, including normalization of myocardial antioxidant status and Ca^{2+} handling. The last result could be notably explained by beneficial effects of exercise training on SERCA-2a expression which restored intra-cellular Ca^{2+} homeostasis. Finally, a main result of this work was that this strategy markedly reduced the vulnerability of CO rat hearts to ischemia-reperfusion.

Figure 1.

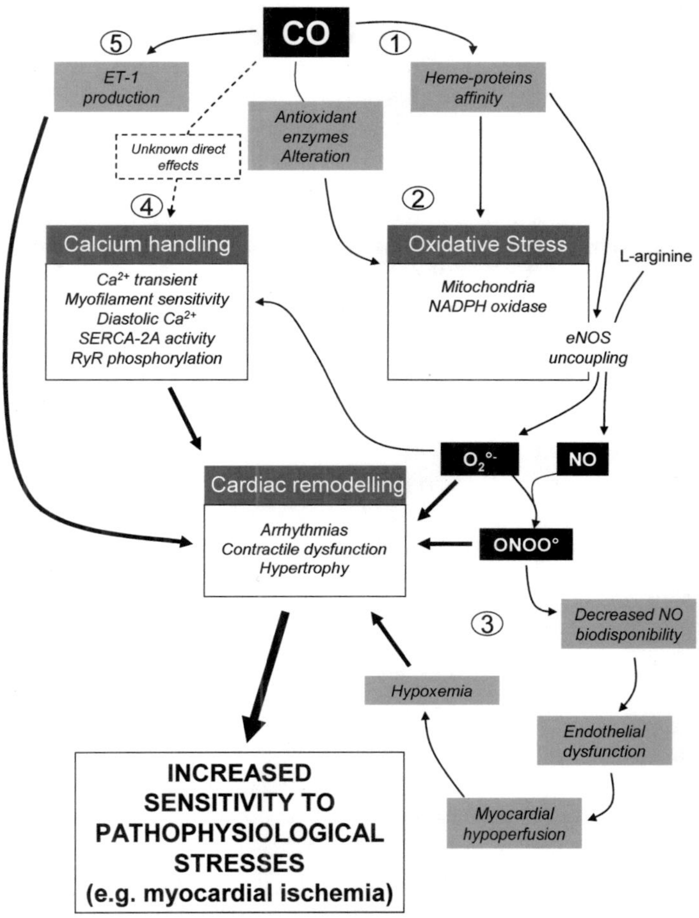

Fig. 1. Potential mechanisms involved in chronic low level CO exposure-induced increased cardiac sensitivity to ischemic stress.

Potential mechanisms involved in chronic low level CO exposure-induced increased cardiac sensitivity to ischemic stress. This figure summarize how as a result of CO effects, the cardiovascular system developed a pathological phenotype which renders the heart more sensitive to myocardial infarction. **1:** CO ability to bound to heme proteins lead to an increased ROS production; **2:** The activation of ROS production associated with reduced antioxidant enzyme defences result in significant CO-induced oxidative stress, leading then to contractile dysfunction and higher occurrence of ventricular arrhythmias; **3:** CO induced potential production of superoxide anion instead of NO (eNOS uncoupling) reduced NO bioavailability. This could lead to coronary artery endothelium dysfunction and then to myocardial hypoxemia; **4:** Ca^{2+} handling play a major role in excitation-contraction coupling. Although today there is no evidence for direct CO effects on Ca^{2+} handling proteins, it is recently demonstrated that prolonged CO exposure markedly altered Ca^{2+}. This could be mediated by CO-induced ROS production; **5:** Probably as a stress signalling pathway, CO induced an increased endothelin (ET-1) production leading then to heart remodelling.

5. Conclusion

Today, among environmental pollutants, CO is less considered, notably because of its very low concentration in urban environment. However, today, such a review of the experimental literature points out that, even at very low concentrations that can be found in urban environment, CO has potential high toxicological properties, and the heart appears to be particularly sensitive to this gas. Indeed, despite during *in-vivo* experiments, at the integrated level, prolonged CO exposure has no major consequence on healthy heart, and induced only modest adaptations with no apparent fatal issue, at the cellular level, those modest events and adaptations hide a compensated pathological remodelling of cardiomyocytes phenotype. Then, one of the main assessments of the present review is that prolonged exposure to low CO level results in a compensated phenotypical remodelling which could render the heart more vulnerable to stress and more particularly to pathological stresses. Therefore, among the numerous environmental air pollutants, exposure to CO pollution seems to be an important risk factor for the development of cardiovascular pathologies.

6. References

Andre, L., Boissiere, J., Reboul, C., Perrier, R., Zalvidea, S., Meyer, G., Thireau, J., Tanguy, S., Bideaux, P., Hayot, M., Boucher, F., Obert, P., Cazorla, O. & Richard, S. (2010). Carbon monoxide pollution promotes cardiac remodeling and ventricular arrhythmia in healthy rats. *Am J Respir Crit Care Med,* Vol. 181, No. 6, pp. 587-95,1535-4970 (Electronic).

Bak, I., Szendrei, L., Turoczi, T., Papp, G., Joo, F., Das, D.K., de Leiris, J., Der, P., Juhasz, B., Varga, E., Bacskay, I., Balla, J., Kovacs, P. & Tosaki, A. (2003). Heme oxygenase-1-related carbon monoxide production and ventricular fibrillation in isolated ischemic/reperfused mouse myocardium. *FASEB J,* Vol. 17, No. 14, pp. 2133-5,1530-6860 (Electronic).

Bak, I., Varadi, J., Nagy, N., Vecsernyes, M. & Tosaki, A. (2005). The role of exogenous carbon monoxide in the recovery of post-ischemic cardiac function in buffer perfused isolated rat hearts. *Cell Mol Biol (Noisy-le-grand),* Vol. 51, No. 5, pp. 453-9

Bell, M.L., Peng, R.D., Dominici, F. & Samet, J.M. (2009). Emergency Hospital Admissions for Cardiovascular Diseases and Ambient Levels of Carbon Monoxide. Results for 126 United States Urban Counties, 1999-2005. *Circulation.*

Bevan, M.A., Proctor, C. J., Baker-Rogers, J., and Warren, N. D. (1991). Exposure to carbon monoxide, respirable syspended particulates, and volatile organic compounds while commuting by bicycle. *Environ. Sci. Technol.,* Vol. 25, pp. 788-79.

Bhatnagar, A. (2006). Environmental cardiology: studying mechanistic links between pollution and heart disease. *Circ Res,* Vol. 99, No. 7, pp. 692-705,1524-4571 (Electronic).

Brook, R.D., Franklin, B., Cascio, W., Hong, Y., Howard, G., Lipsett, M., Luepker, R., Mittleman, M., Samet, J., Smith, S.C., Jr. & Tager, I. (2004). Air pollution and cardiovascular disease: a statement for healthcare professionals from the Expert Panel on Population and Prevention Science of the American Heart Association. *Circulation,* Vol. 109, No. 21, pp. 2655-71,1524-4539 (Electronic).

Burnett, R.T., Cakmak, S., Brook, J.R. & Krewski, D. (1997). The role of particulate size and chemistry in the association between summertime ambient air pollution and hospitalization for cardiorespiratory diseases. *Environ Health Perspect,* Vol. 105, No. 6, pp. 614-20.

Bye, A., Sorhaug, S., Ceci, M., Hoydal, M.A., Stolen, T., Heinrich, G., Tjonna, A.E., Najjar, S.M., Nilsen, O.G., Catalucci, D., Grimaldi, S., Contu, R., Steinshamn, S., Condorelli, G., Smith, G.L., Ellingsen, O., Waldum, H. & Wisloff, U. (2008). Carbon monoxide levels experienced by heavy smokers impair aerobic capacity and cardiac contractility and induce pathological hypertrophy. *Inhal Toxicol,* Vol. 20, No. 7, pp. 635-46.

Chau, C.K., Tu, E.Y., Chan, D.W. & Burnett, J. (2002). Estimating the total exposure to air pollutants for different population age groups in Hong Kong. *Environ Int,* Vol. 27, No. 8, pp. 617-30,0160-4120 (Print).

Clark, J.E., Naughton, P., Shurey, S., Green, C.J., Johnson, T.R., Mann, B.E., Foresti, R. & Motterlini, R. (2003). Cardioprotective actions by a water-soluble carbon monoxide-releasing molecule. *Circ Res,* Vol. 93, No. 2, pp. e2-8,1524-4571 (Electronic).

Cunnington, A.J. & Hormbrey, P. (2002). Breath analysis to detect recent exposure to carbon monoxide. *Postgrad Med J,* Vol. 78, No. 918, pp. 233-7,0032-5473 (Print).

D'Amico, G., Lam, F., Hagen, T. & Moncada, S. (2006). Inhibition of cellular respiration by endogenously produced carbon monoxide. *J Cell Sci,* Vol. 119, No. Pt 11, pp. 2291-8,0021-9533 (Print).

Farah, C., Meyer, G., Andre, L., Boissiere, J., Gayrard, S., Cazorla, O., Richard, S., Boucher, F., Tanguy, S., Obert, P. & Reboul, C. (2010). Moderate exercise prevents impaired Ca2+ handling in heart of CO-exposed rat: implication for sensitivity to ischemia-reperfusion. *Am J Physiol Heart Circ Physiol,* Vol. 299, No. 6, pp. H2076-81,1522-1539 (Electronic).

Favory, R., Lancel, S., Tissier, S., Mathieu, D., Decoster, B. & Neviere, R. (2006). Myocardial dysfunction and potential cardiac hypoxia in rats induced by carbon monoxide inhalation. *Am J Respir Crit Care Med,* Vol. 174, No. 3, pp. 320-5.

Fujimoto, H., Ohno, M., Ayabe, S., Kobayashi, H., Ishizaka, N., Kimura, H., Yoshida, K. & Nagai, R. (2004). Carbon monoxide protects against cardiac ischemia--reperfusion injury in vivo via MAPK and Akt--eNOS pathways. *Arterioscler Thromb Vasc Biol,* Vol. 24, No. 10, pp. 1848-53,1524-4636 (Electronic).

Gautier, M., Antier, D., Bonnet, P., Le Net, J.L., Hanton, G. & Eder, V. (2007). Continuous inhalation of carbon monoxide induces right ventricle ischemia and dysfunction in rats with hypoxic pulmonary hypertension. *Am J Physiol Heart Circ Physiol,* Vol. 293, No. 2, pp. H1046-52.

Guo, Y., Stein, A.B., Wu, W.J., Tan, W., Zhu, X., Li, Q.H., Dawn, B., Motterlini, R. & Bolli, R. (2004). Administration of a CO-releasing molecule at the time of reperfusion reduces infarct size in vivo. *Am J Physiol Heart Circ Physiol,* Vol. 286, No. 5, pp. H1649-53,0363-6135 (Print).

Jones, A.Y. & Lam, P.K. (2006). End-expiratory carbon monoxide levels in healthy subjects living in a densely populated urban environment. *Sci Total Environ,* Vol. 354, No. 2-3, pp. 150-6,0048-9697 (Print).

Loennechen, J.P., Nilsen, O.G., Arbo, I., Aadahl, P., Nilsen, T., Waldum, H.L., Sandvik, A.K. & Ellingsen, O. (2002). Chronic exposure to carbon monoxide and nicotine: endothelin ET(A) receptor antagonism attenuates carbon monoxide-induced myocardial hypertrophy in rat. *Toxicol Appl Pharmacol,* Vol. 178, No. 1, pp. 8-14,0041-008X (Print).

Marx, S.O., Reiken, S., Hisamatsu, Y., Jayaraman, T., Burkhoff, D., Rosemblit, N. & Marks, A.R. (2000). PKA phosphorylation dissociates FKBP12.6 from the calcium release channel (ryanodine receptor): defective regulation in failing hearts. *Cell,* Vol. 101, No. 4, pp. 365-76,0092-8674 (Print).

Meyer, G., Andre, L., Tanguy, S., Boissiere, J., Farah, C., Lopez-Lauri, F., Gayrard, S., Richard, S., Boucher, F., Cazorla, O., Obert, P. & Reboul, C. (2010). Simulated urban carbon monoxide air pollution exacerbates rat heart ischemia-reperfusion injury. *Am J Physiol Heart Circ Physiol,* Vol. 298, No. 5, pp. H1445-53,1522-1539 (Electronic).

Murphy, E. & Steenbergen, C. (2008). Mechanisms underlying acute protection from cardiac ischemia-reperfusion injury. *Physiol Rev,* Vol. 88, No. 2, pp. 581-609.

Piantadosi, C.A. (2002). Biological chemistry of carbon monoxide. *Antioxid Redox Signal,* Vol. 4, No. 2, pp. 259-70,1523-0864 (Print).

Piantadosi, C.A. (2008). Carbon monoxide, reactive oxygen signaling, and oxidative stress. *Free Radic Biol Med,* Vol. 45, No. 5, pp. 562-9,0891-5849 (Print).

Samet, J.M., Dominici, F., Zeger, S.L., Schwartz, J. & Dockery, D.W. (2000). The National Morbidity, Mortality, and Air Pollution Study. Part I: Methods and methodologic issues. *Res Rep Health Eff Inst,* No. 94 Pt 1, pp. 5-14; discussion 75-84,1041-5505 (Print).

Samoli, E., Touloumi, G., Schwartz, J., Anderson, H.R., Schindler, C., Forsberg, B., Vigotti, M.A., Vonk, J., Kosnik, M., Skorkovsky, J. & Katsouyanni, K. (2007). Short-term effects of carbon monoxide on mortality: an analysis within the APHEA project. *Environ Health Perspect,* Vol. 115, No. 11, pp. 1578-83.

Stein, A.B., Guo, Y., Tan, W., Wu, W.J., Zhu, X., Li, Q., Luo, C., Dawn, B., Johnson, T.R., Motterlini, R. & Bolli, R. (2005). Administration of a CO-releasing molecule induces late preconditioning against myocardial infarction. *J Mol Cell Cardiol,* Vol. 38, No. 1, pp. 127-34,0022-2828 (Print).

Stern, F.B., Halperin, W.E., Hornung, R.W., Ringenburg, V.L. & McCammon, C.S. (1988). Heart disease mortality among bridge and tunnel officers exposed to carbon monoxide. *Am J Epidemiol,* Vol. 128, No. 6, pp. 1276-88,0002-9262 (Print).

Stieb, D.M., Szyszkowicz, M., Rowe, B.H. & Leech, J.A. (2009). Air pollution and emergency department visits for cardiac and respiratory conditions: a multi-city time-series analysis. *Environ Health,* Vol. 8, pp. 25.

Thom, S.R., Fisher, D., Xu, Y.A., Garner, S. & Ischiropoulos, H. (1999). Role of nitric oxide-derived oxidants in vascular injury from carbon monoxide in the rat. *Am J Physiol,* Vol. 276, No. 3 Pt 2, pp. H984-92,0002-9513 (Print).

Thom, S.R., Fisher, D., Xu, Y.A., Notarfrancesco, K. & Ischiropoulos, H. (2000). Adaptive responses and apoptosis in endothelial cells exposed to carbon monoxide. *Proc Natl Acad Sci U S A,* Vol. 97, No. 3, pp. 1305-10.

Wright, G.R., Jewczyk, S., Onrot, J., Tomlinson, P. & Shephard, R.J. (1975). Carbon monoxide in the urban atmosphere: hazards to the pedestrian and the street-worker. *Arch Environ Health,* Vol. 30, No. 3, pp. 123-9.

Zhu, B., Sun, Y., Sievers, R.E., Shuman, J.L., Glantz, S.A., Chatterjee, K., Parmley, W.W. & Wolfe, C.L. (1996). L-arginine decreases infarct size in rats exposed to environmental tobacco smoke. *Am Heart J,* Vol. 132, No. 1 Pt 1, pp. 91-100,0002-8703 (Print).

Zhu, B.Q., Sun, Y.P., Sievers, R.E., Glantz, S.A., Parmley, W.W. & Wolfe, C.L. (1994). Exposure to environmental tobacco smoke increases myocardial infarct size in rats. *Circulation,* Vol. 89, No. 3, pp. 1282-90,0009-7322 (Print).

Zuckerbraun, B.S., Chin, B.Y., Bilban, M., d'Avila, J.C., Rao, J., Billiar, T.R. & Otterbein, L.E. (2007). Carbon monoxide signals via inhibition of cytochrome c oxidase and generation of mitochondrial reactive oxygen species. *Faseb J,* Vol. 21, No. 4, pp. 1099-106,1530-6860 (Electronic).

9

Application of the Ultramicro Forward-Mutation Assay to the Monitoring of Indoor and Outdoor Air Mutagenicity-Examples of Chengdu City and Tokyo

Yukihiko Takagi[1], Daisuke Nakajima[2],
Sun Chengjun[3] and Sumio Goto[1]
[1]*Azabu University,*
[2]*National Institute for Environmental Studies,*
[3]*West China School of Public Health,*
[1,2]*Japan*
[3] *China*

1. Introduction

Various chemicals are emitted into the air from factories, offices, incinerators, and vehicles by industrial activity (Alfhei & Mψller, 1981; Mψller et al, 1982; Watanabe & Hirayama, 1997). In addition, indoor air is polluted by chemicals used or exhausted intentionally or unintentionally during heating (use of town gas and fossil fuel), cooking, smoking and building materials (Endo et al, 2000; Koyano et al, 1999; Takagi et al, 1997). People are concerned about the health impacts of the hazardous chemicals contained in those materials. The carcinogens and mutagens detected in air can be classified into two groups: particulate matter and gas/vapor matter. Regarding particulate matter, various substances including inorganic ones such as heavy metals and organic compounds such as polycyclic aromatic hydrocarbons are detected. Such substances and compounds include polycyclic aromatic hydrocarbons (PAHs) like benzo[a]pyrene, which is now attracting attention as a carcinogenic/mutagenic substance, and dinitropyrene, which shows extremely high mutagenicity for *Salmonella* TA98 strain (Watanabe & Hirayama, 1997). It is widely known that PAHs are formed during the incomplete combustion of organic matter (Somenath & Wilson, 1992). PAHs are also formed when fossil fuel is burned by industry and in daily life and so the health hazards of PAHs contained in the environment cannot be avoided. People spend 80 to 90% of their time indoors, and especially infants, elderly people and sick people with a weak immune system spend even longer hours indoors. Therefore, it is important to keep the indoor environment clean because human health is greatly influenced by the environment. However, there have been few studies on the mutagenicity of indoor air because the amount of such substances that can be sampled is limited. A new mutagenicity test that is more sensitive than the existing widely-usedAmes method: "plate incorporation method" and "preincubation method" needs to be developed. We studied use of the ultramicro forward mutation Assay, which is is more sensitive than conventional methods. In this method, a mini pump was used to collect suspended particulate matters (SPMs) onto quartz fiber filters at 1 L/min for 24 hours and the filters were then subjected to sonication. The extracts were used as samples for mutagenicity measurement. We used the ultramicro forward mutation assay with *Salmonella typhimurium* TM677 strain in our mutagenicity test and confirmed that the new test method is sufficiently sensitive to measure indoor air samples. Therefore, we compared the mutagenicity of indoor and outdoor SPMs and that of air samples obtained in Chengdu, China and Tokyo, and report on the measurements of PAHs in those samples.

2. Materials and methods

2.1 Reagents and instruments

We used dichloromethane (Wako Chemical Industries, Ltd.) for the residual pesticides test, methanol (Wako Chemical Industries, Ltd.) for high-performance liquid chromatography, and dimethyl sulfoxide (Dojindo Laboratories) for fluorescence analysis. We used agar (BBL, Nutrient Broth, Difco), D-biotin (Merck), 8-azaguanine (Sigma Chemical), and other commercially available reagents. For counting colonies, we used a Bio Multi Scanner (BMS-400, Ipros Corporation and CA-7, System Science).

2.2 Collection of samples and method

We asked residents in Chengdu and Tokyo (ten families in each) to collect air samples from their kitchen, bedroom, living room and outdoors. Mini pumps (MP-15CF, Sibata Scientific Technology Ltd.) were used to collect the samples onto quartz fiber filters (2500 QAT-UP ϕ25 mm, Pallflex) at the flow rate of about 1 L/min for 24 hours. The samples were collected in Chengdu in summer (July 2000) and winter (Dec. 2000 - Jan. 2001) and in Tokyo in winter (Jan. - Feb. 2001). In each case, indoor and outdoor conditions were recorded when the air samples were collected. The collected quartz filters were stored in deep freezer.

2.3 Extraction of organic matter

To extract organic matter in indoor and outdoor SPMs collected with the mini pumps, the quartz fiber filters were removed from the freezer, cut into small pieces, put into stoppered test tubes and subjected to extraction by sonication. After the test tubes containing the samples with 9 mL of dichloromethane were sealed, they were dipped in an sonication generator and exposed to ultrasonic waves for 15 minutes. Subsequently, 3 mL of the supernatant extract was dispensed into a screw cap test tube for HPLC analysis and a further 6 mL was dispensed into another screw cap test tube for the mutation test. For HPLC analysis, the solvent was distilled away under nitrogen flow, then the dried up extract was redissolved in 1.5 mL of acetonitrile and centrifuged. Four hundred micro liter of the obtained supernatant was used for analysis of PAHs. For the mutagenicity test, the solvent was distilled away from 6 mL of extract and then the supernatant was kept in a freezer at −80°C until the test.

2.4 Preparation of samples

It was necessary to minimize the amount of DMSO, which was used to dissolve the samples in the ultramicro forward mutation assay, because the toxicity of DMSO to bacteria should be restricted as much as possible. Therefore, the medium-exchange procedure was used to prepare solutions of respective concentrations. Namely, 0.2 μL of DMSO was dispensed into sterilized micro vials for test samples in advance and then the solutions of test substances in different additive amounts were added. Nitrogen gas was blown into the mixed solutions in the vials to distill away the solvent and obtain the DMSO solutions of respective concentrations, which were then used for the mutation test. We used the extracts of outdoor SPMs as a positive reference material in the mutation test.

2.5 Mutagenicity test

We conducted this test using the ultramicro forward mutation assay with *Salmonella typhimurium* TM677 strain. The frozen bacteria of the TM677 strain, which had been stored at −80°C, were dissolved at room temperature, the bacteria suspension was stirred well, then 0.3 mL of the suspension was inoculated into an L-shaped test tube with 2.7 mL of minimal E medium (ME). The L-shaped test tube was subjected to culture shake in an incubator shaker (37°C) for 3 hours. (The composition of 1 L of ME was as follows: 20 g of glucose, 2 g of magnesium sulfate heptahydrate, 20 g of citric acid, 100 g of dibasic potassium phosphate, 19.2 g of dibasic potassium phosphate, 6.6 g of sodium chloride, 12.2 mg of D-biotin, and 1000 mL of ion-exchange water.) This culture solution was diluted with ME again ten times. The obtained solution was used as a test bacteria liquid without S9mix. The mutation test in this study was conducted using the ultramicro forward mutation assay without adding S9mix. Namely, 10 μL of bacteria liquid was put into a micro vial that contained the analyte solution and the bacteria were pre-incubated in an incubator at 37°C. In this pre-incubation, a rotator was used to turn the micro vial and to thoroughly mix the analyte solution and the bacteria liquid. After incubation, 90 μL of 0.15 M sterilized phosphate buffer (pH 7.4, PBS) was added into the micro vial and mixed well. Eighty micro liter of the obtained solution was dispensed into each aluminium-capped test tube cap. Then, 2.5 mL of agar containing 8-azaguanine was put into each of these small test tubes, mixed and overlaid on a culture medium (agar plate) to use the plates for measurement of mutagenicity. Ten micro liter of the remaining sample in the micro vial was dispensed into a screw cap bottle, which contained 10 mL of PBS, mixed well, then 33.5 μL of this sample was dispensed into each of three test tubes with an aluminum cap. Different from measuring the mutation, 2.5 mL of soft agar without 8-azaguanine was put into each of these small test tubes, mixed well and overlaid on a culture medium (agar plate) to be used for counting viable bacteria. After incubation, the formed colonies were counted with a colony counter, and with the obtained numbers of mutated colonies and living bacteria colonies, the following formula was used to calculate the mutation frequency.

$$\text{Mutation frequency} = \text{Number of mutated colonies} / (\text{Number of living bacteria colonies} \times 2400)$$

In this study, for the air samples found to be positive or false-positive, the primary regression equation was obtained from the direct part of the dose-response relationship by the least-squares method. The mutation frequency was then obtained per m³ of air (converted from the extract solution) in the primary regression analysis. The control value (spontaneous mutation frequency) was subtracted from this value to obtain the mutagen-specific activity. In addition, the fluctuation of bacteria activity depending on the test date was corrected with the results of mutation tests of the positive reference material, which were conducted simultaneously on the same test dates.

2.6 Analysis of PAHs

The following eight substances were examined in the PAH analysis: pyrene (Py), benz[a]anthracene (BaA), benzo[k]fluoranthene (BkF), benzo[a]pyrene (BaP), dibenz[a,h]anthracene (dBahA), benzo[b]chrysene (BbC), benzo[ghi]perylene (BghiP), and dibenzo[a,e]pyrene (dBaeP). An HPLC provided with a concentrating column/spectral fluorescence detector was used for the analysis. A hundred micro liter of the sample solution was injected into the HPLC and separated into acetonitrile and aqueous mobile phase. After separation, fluorescence was detected at suitable wavelengths for the respective PAHs, and a quantitative determination was conducted from the peak heights of the respective chromatograms.

3. Results

3.1 Mutagenicity of indoor and outdoor SPMs in ordinary family homes in Chengdu in summer and winter

We measured the mutagenicity of the extracts obtained from the samples collected by our collaborators living in Chengdu, and compared the results. Figure 1 shows one example relation between the mutation frequencies and the respective sample amounts for the mutagenicity of the obtained samples. The test results show a good dose-response relationship between the air sample amounts and the mutation frequencies, and mutagenicity was detected in the air samples of Chengdu. As shown, we could detect the

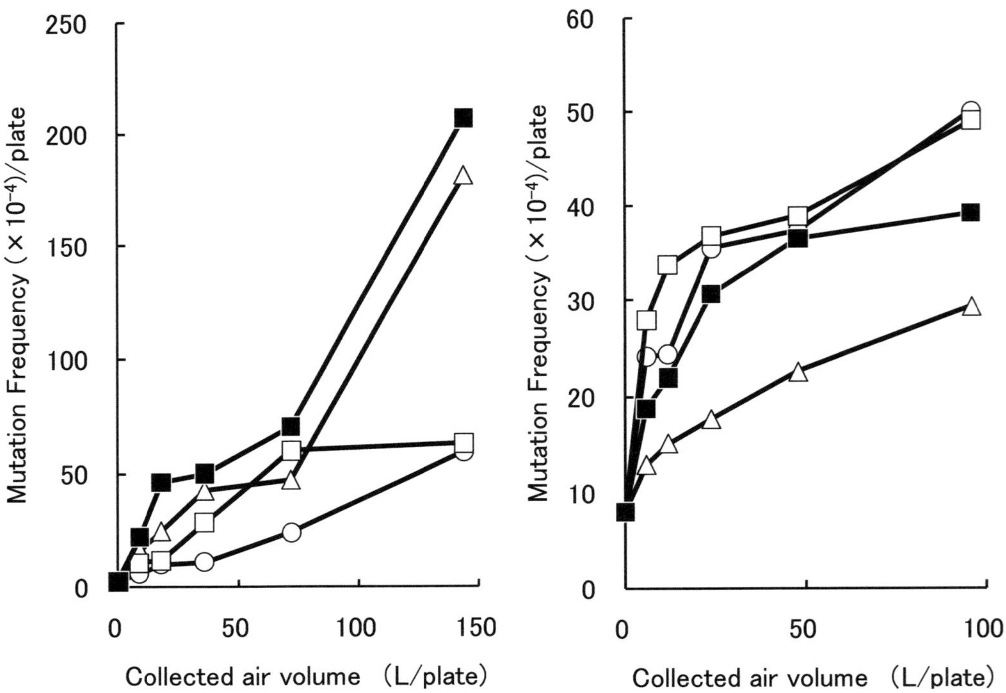

Fig. 1. Mutation test results of indoor and outdoor SPMs in Chengdu (A) winter, (B) summer, circle: kitchen, triangle: living room, open square: bedroom, closed square: outdoors

mutagenicity of indoor air by using the ultramicro forward mutation assay. Figures 2 and 3 show the measurement results of mutagenicity of the SPMs in the kitchen, bedroom, living room and outdoors of the respective collaborators. The results are shown as mutagen-specific activity obtained per m^3 of air converted from the extract solution in two seasons (Fig. 2 - winter and Fig. 3 - summer). Table 1 shows the values in the respective sampling places in both seasons. As shown in Figures 2 and 3 and Table 1, the average values of mutagen-specific

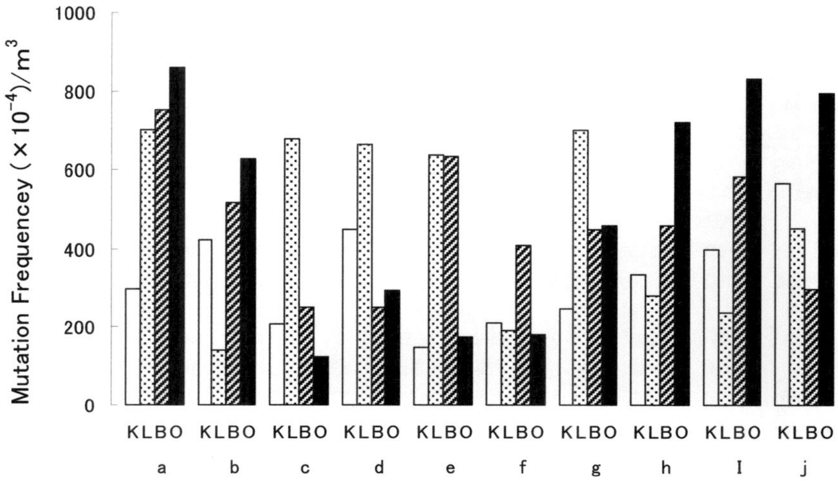

Fig. 2. Mutagenicity of indoor and outdoor SPMs in Chengdu (winter) K: kitchen, L: living room, B: bedroom, O: outdoors

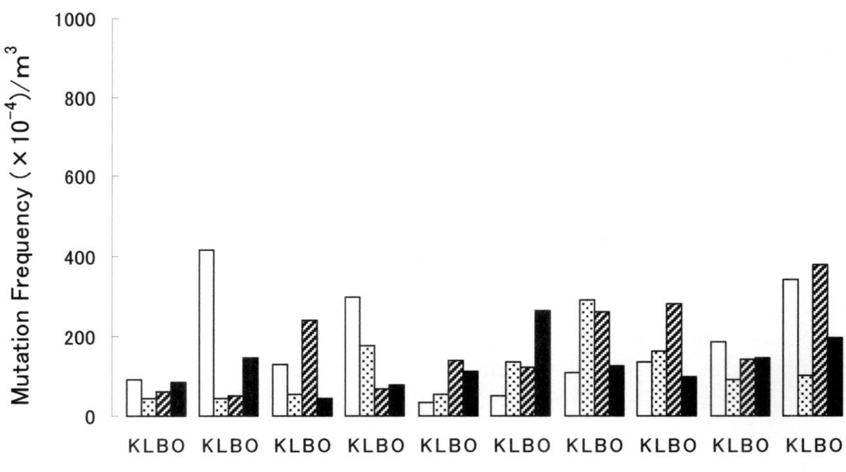

Fig. 3. Mutagenicity of indoor and outdoor SPMs in Chengdu (summer)K: kitchen, L: living room, B: bedroom, O: outdoors

activity in winter were 329 x 10-4/m^3 in the kitchen, 469 x 10-4/m^3 in the living room, 461 x 10-4/m^3 in the bedroom and 507 x 10^{-4}/m^3outdoors, and those in summer were 179 x 10-

$^{4}/m^3$ in the kitchen, 115 x $10^{-4}/m^3$ in the living room, 174 x $10^{-4}/m^3$ in the bedroom, and 129 x $10^{-4}/m^3$ outdoors. Thus, the mutagen-specific activity was higher in winter than in summer. In winter, the values were higher in outdoor air than in indoor air, and in summer were higher in indoor air than in outdoor air. For the sampling places, the value in the kitchen was the lowest in winter, but the highest in summer. There was no specific difference in the values between the different floor levels.

Season	Sampling place	Mutation frequency ($\times 10^{-4}$) $/m^3$										
		a	b	c	d	e	f	g	h	I	j	Average value
Winter	Kitchen	299	423	209	450	149	211	249	336	401	568	329
	Living	702	141	678	664	638	191	702	283	237	452	469
	Bedroom	752	518	250	252	635	411	448	461	583	298	461
	Outdoors	860	626	125	294	173	180	458	722	832	797	507
Summer	Kitchen	91	414	129	299	35	51	110	136	186	342	179
	Living	44	44	54	175	53	137	291	164	90	101	115
	Bedroom	62	50	241	68	137	121	261	282	143	379	174
	Outdoors	83	146	44	79	110	265	126	97	144	197	129
Remarks		7F	6F With smoker	3F	4F	3F	6F	6F	16F With smoker	3F	3F	

Table 1. Mutagen specific activity by sampling places in Chengdu

3.2 Comparison of mutagenicity of indoor and outdoor SPMs in ordinary family homes in Chengdu and Tokyo in winter

We measured the mutagenicity of the SPMs collected by our collaborators living in Tokyo, and compared the results with those in Chengdu. Figure 4 shows one example result of the air sample amounts and the mutation frequencies for the mutagenicity of the obtained SPMs. The results show a good dose-response relationship between the air sample amounts and the mutation frequencies, and mutagenicity was detected in the samples collected in Tokyo. With the dose-response relationship obtained as in Figure 4, Figure 5 shows the mutagen-specific activity by respective collaborators living in Tokyo, which were calculated from the measurement results of the samples collected in the kitchen, bedroom, living room and outdoors. Table 2 shows the mutagen-specific activity for the respective sampling places. Figures 2 and 5 show that the mutagen-specific activity was generally higher in Chengdu than in Tokyo. Tables 1 and 2 show that the average values of mutagen-specific activity per unit air amount (m^3) in Tokyo were77 x $10^{-4}/m^3$ in the kitchen, 127 x $10^{-4}/m^3$ in the living room, 96 x $10^{-4}/m^3$ in the bedroom, and 66 x $10^{-4}/m^3$ in outdoor, which were lower than those in Chengdu. Regarding outdoors and indoors, the values outdoors were higher than indoors in Chengdu while those outdoors were lower than indoors in Tokyo. Regarding the mutagen-specific activity in terms of building structure, generally the values were lower in detached houses than in collective housing. In Tokyo, generally the indoor values in smokers' houses were higher than in non-smokers' houses.

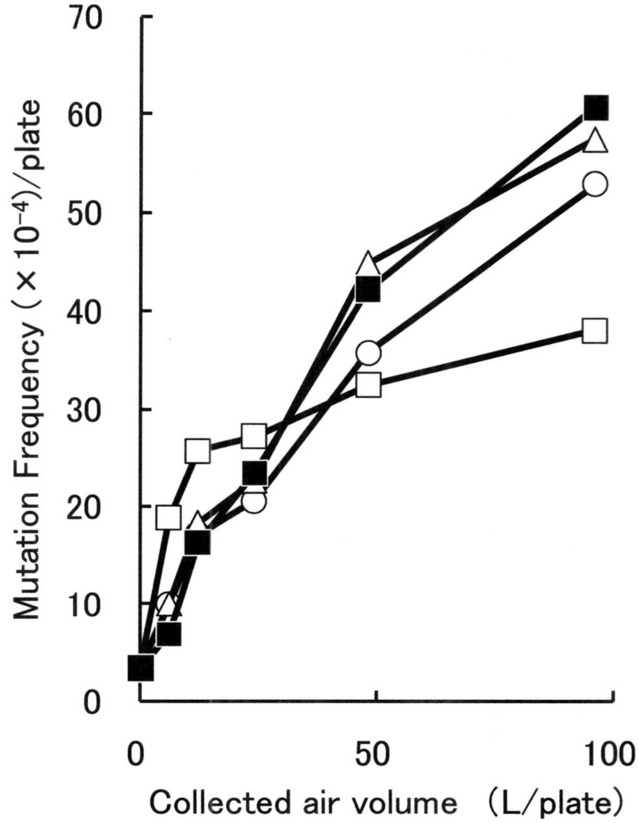

Fig. 4. Mutation test results of indoor and outdoor SPMs in Tokyo (winter) circle: kitchen, triangle: living room, open square: bedroom, closed square: outdoors

Season	Sampling place	Mutation frequency ($\times10^{-4}$) /m^3										
		a	b	c	d	e	f	g	h	I	j	Average value
Winter	Kitchen	8	135	55	33	115	134	172	47	56	16	77
	Living room	45	110	37	55	147	540	169	50	63	54	127
	Bedroom	12	122	41	25	115	319	208	80	11	30	96
	Outdoors	38	110	72	55	54	72	132	24	46	53	66
Remarks		Detached house	Collective housing 14F With smoker	Detached house	Detached house	Collective housing 7F With smoker	Detached house	Detached house With smoker	Collective housing 4F	Detached house	Detached house	

Table 2. Mutagen specific activity by sampling places in Tokyo

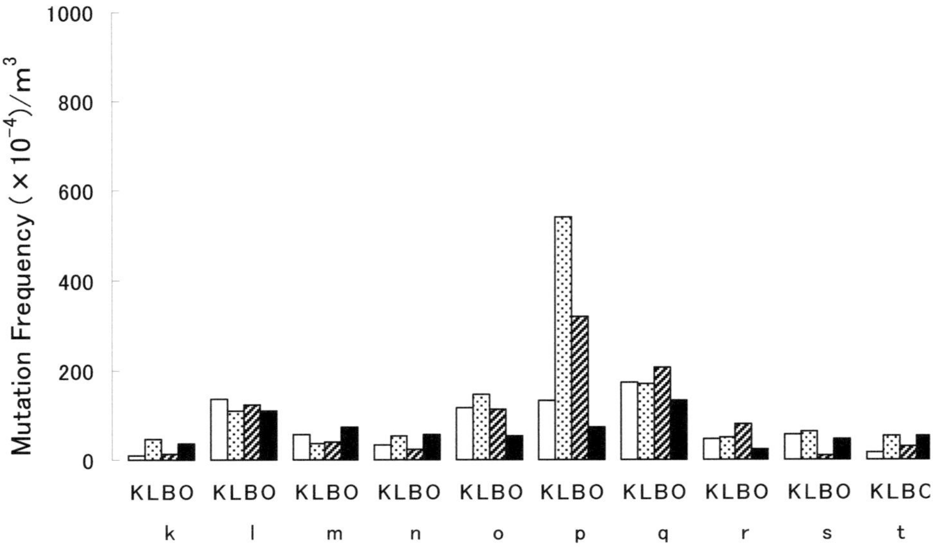

Fig. 5. Mutagenicity of indoor and outdoor SPMs in Tokyo (winter) K: kitchen, L: living room, B: bedroom, O: outdoors

3.3 Comparison of concentrations of polycyclic aromatic hydrocarbons contained in indoor and outdoor SPMs in Tokyo and Chengdu in winter

Figures 6, 7 and 8 show the concentration of BaP, which is a typical carcinogen in PAHs, detected in the kitchen, bedroom, living room and outdoors in Tokyo in winter and in Chengdu in both winter and summer. Tables 3, 4 and 5 show the concentration of the eight target substances (Py, BaA, BaP, dBahA, BdC, BghiP and dBaeP) detected in the respective houses of our collaborators. These figures and tables show the average concentrations of BaP per unit air (m^3) as follows: 10.98 ng/m^3 in the kitchen, 17.06 ng/m^3 in the living room, 16.95 ng/m^3 in the bedroom and 16.01 ng/m^3 outdoors in Chengdu in winter; 3.60 ng/m^3 in the kitchen, 2.06 ng/m^3 in the living room, 3.09 ng/m^3 in the bedroom and 8.39 ng/m^3 in Chengdu in summer; 0.34 ng/m^3 in the kitchen, 0.38 ng/m^3 in the living room, 0.33 ng/m^3 in the bedroom, and 0.52 ng/m^3 in Tokyo. In Chengdu, the values were higher in winter than in summer, whereas those in Tokyo were lower than in Chengdu in any season. The average concentrations of other PAHs showed the same trend. In Chengdu, the living room in summer and the kitchen in winter showed slightly lower values than other rooms in the same seasons. In Tokyo in winter, the value in the bedroom was lower than in other rooms in the same season. In Chengdu in winter, there was only a slight difference in the values between indoors and outdoors. Even in summer in Chengdu and in winter in Tokyo when the concentration of outdoor PAHs was comparatively low, generally the concentration of indoor PAHs in smokers' houses was higher than that of outdoor PAHs.

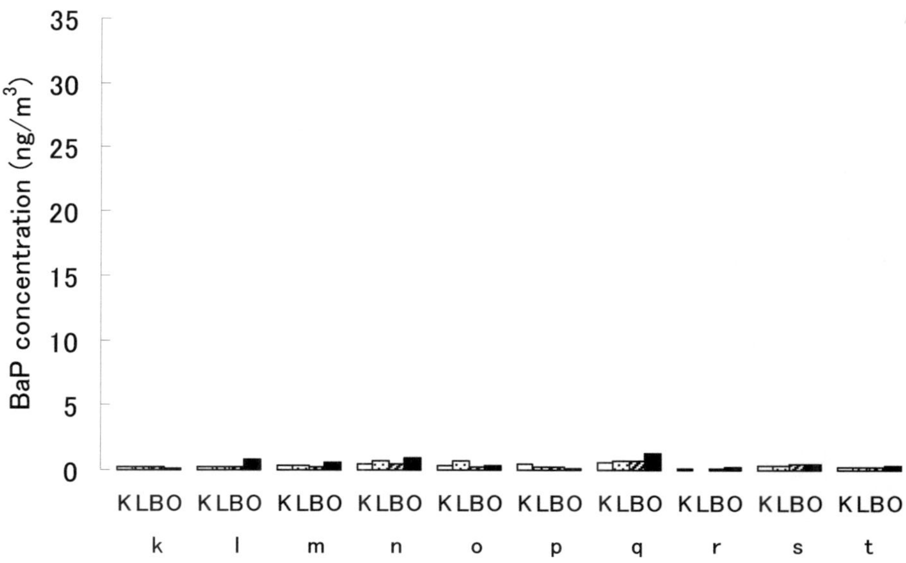

Fig. 6. BaP concentration in indoor and outdoor SPMs in Tokyo (winter) K: kitchen, L: living room, B: bedroom, O: outdoors

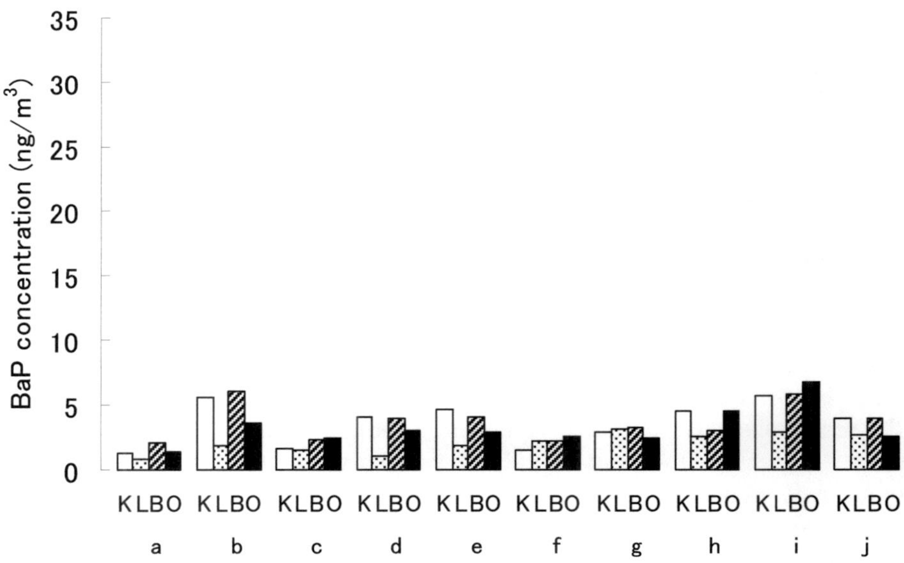

Fig. 7. BaP concentration in indoor and outdoor SPMs in Chengdu (summer) K: kitchen, L: living room, B: bedroom, O: outdoors

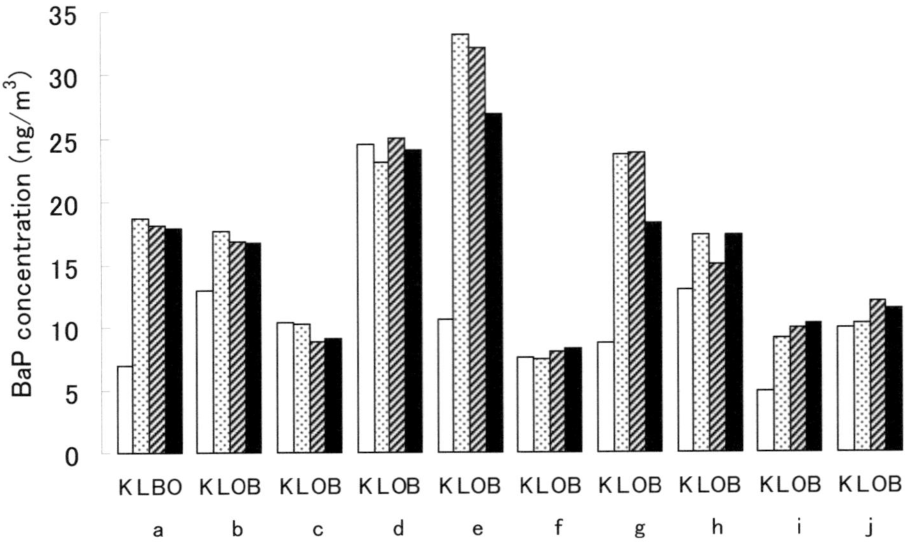

Fig. 8. BaP concentration in indoor and outdoor SPMs in Chengdu (winter) K: Kitchen, L: living room, B: bedroom, O: outdoors

4. Discussion

In the environment including indoor and outdoor air, soil and river water, there are various hazardous chemical substances such as carcinogens and mutagens (Goto et al, 1982; Iwamoto et al, 1990; Kasahara, 1990; Urano et al, 1992; Yamamoto, 1977). Automobiles, factories, offices, heating, cooking, etc. emit hazardous chemicals including benzo[a]pyrene (BaP), PAHs, heavy metals, NOx, nitrosamine, chlorinated hydrocarbons such vinyl chloride, SOx, etc. These substances are now attracting attention as major causes of human respiratory diseases and lung cancer. Especially in city areas, a close relationship has been found between the high incidence of lung cancer and outdoor air pollution. Substances attached to SPMs are inhaled by humans into the lungs. The area of the lung where such particles are deposited varies depending on the particle diameter: the smaller they are, the more hazardous (Broddin, 1977, Pierce & Katz, 1975; Sugita et al, 1996). Especially, particles smaller than 2.5 μm penetrate deep into human lungs (Heyder et al, 1986), and some substances cause asthma and cancer and have immunotoxicity and genetic toxicity. Recently, some substances have been found to be endocrine disruptors, and thus chemical substances can damage the human body in various ways. The amount of SPMs caused directly by incineration is decreasing in advanced countries that are switching energy sources from coal to oil and modifying their facilities. On the other hand, in China and other countries that are growingly rapidly, large amounts of hazardous substances such as SOx are continuously emitted because coal is still a major energy source. Coal, including charcoal and artificial coal, is also used for cooking and heating in ordinary family homes and so indoor and outdoor air pollution caused by gas emissions cannot be avoided. Since people spend most of their time indoors, indoor air pollution can be very hazardous for human

Sampling place		Date of starting sampling (yymmdd)	Quantity of airflow (m^3)	PAH concentration in air (ng/m^3)								
				Pyrene	BaA	BkF	BaP	dBahA	BdC	BghiP	dBaeP	Remarks
a	Kitchen	001218	1.504	6.88	6.08	2.99	6.99	1.29	1.45	9.34	1.15	7F
b		001219	1.539	11.18	10.84	5.42	13.02	2.47	2.69	18.14	2.26	6F
c		001220	1.758	9.73	8.13	3.83	10.38	2.16	2.18	15.56	1.88	3F
d		001222	1.669	23.76	23.80	9.15	24.55	4.19	4.91	32.44	3.87	4F
e		001225	1.680	7.41	7.70	4.70	10.66	2.22	2.52	15.95	1.92	3F
f		001231	1.655	7.30	6.14	3.45	7.60	1.93	1.80	11.78	1.34	6F
g		010101	1.673	6.06	6.67	3.43	8.73	2.02	1.72	11.74	1.26	6F
h		010104	1.639	11.41	12.29	5.55	13.02	3.11	2.74	17.60	2.06	16F
I		010114	1.644	5.69	4.37	2.39	4.87	1.25	1.10	7.70	0.85	3F
j		010115	1.598	7.42	8.08	4.67	9.94	2.41	2.06	14.79	1.70	3F
	Average value			9.68	9.41	4.56	10.98	2.31	2.32	15.50	1.83	
a	Living room	001218	1.483	13.10	15.29	7.81	18.78	3.60	3.92	25.51	3.10	7F
b		001219	1.517	14.18	15.22	7.68	17.64	3.41	3.65	24.58	2.96	6F
c		001220	1.758	8.21	7.90	3.80	10.31	2.04	2.18	15.44	1.96	3F
d		001222	1.656	18.93	21.04	8.97	23.07	3.91	4.87	31.16	3.64	4F
e		001225	1.656	23.17	24.73	15.24	33.17	8.62	7.52	50.21	5.59	3F
f		001231	1.655	5.70	6.12	3.55	7.44	2.11	1.81	11.83	1.36	6F
g		010104	1.673	12.45	17.07	9.06	23.64	5.43	4.86	30.98	3.33	6F
h		010104	1.650	14.47	17.12	7.31	17.28	4.15	3.63	23.53	2.76	16F
I		010114	1.621	5.67	8.15	4.00	9.08	2.11	1.93	13.60	1.37	3F
j		010115	1.621	8.40	8.61	4.90	10.23	2.51	2.17	15.59	1.63	3F
	Average value			12.43	14.13	7.23	17.06	3.79	3.65	24.24	2.77	
a	Bedroom	001218	1.473	12.57	14.62	7.61	18.10	3.44	3.71	24.86	2.95	7F
b		001219	1.512	13.58	14.33	7.25	16.86	3.34	3.54	23.34	2.81	6F
c		001220	1.764	6.99	5.46	2.90	8.84	1.16	2.02	13.07	1.64	3F
d		001222	1.669	24.16	23.97	9.75	24.93	4.22	5.08	32.68	3.85	4F
e		001225	1.680	20.80	20.65	13.32	32.03	6.44	7.48	47.07	5.56	3F
f		001231	1.644	8.52	7.41	3.82	8.07	2.19	1.89	12.36	1.47	6F
g		010104	1.673	14.94	20.46	9.21	23.79	5.36	4.90	30.92	3.44	6F
h		010104	1.627	11.11	13.29	6.36	14.98	3.96	3.11	20.58	2.41	16F
I		010114	1.644	9.79	8.62	4.29	9.86	2.26	2.03	14.40	1.56	3F
j		010115	1.621	10.30	10.70	5.75	12.03	2.88	2.48	17.67	1.98	3F
	Average value			13.28	13.95	7.03	16.95	3.53	3.62	23.70	2.77	
a	Outdoor	001218	1.473	14.26	15.67	7.44	17.91	3.39	3.68	23.90	2.95	7F
b		001219	1.517	13.25	13.58	7.17	16.69	3.25	3.47	22.93	2.78	6F
c		001220	1.796	7.13	5.63	3.11	9.05	1.42	2.02	13.70	1.78	3F
d		001222	1.645	19.80	23.09	9.30	24.07	4.15	4.82	31.88	3.68	4F
e		001225	1.656	17.63	18.12	11.61	26.83	5.20	6.46	39.83	4.79	3F
f		001231	1.668	9.49	8.19	3.95	8.20	2.50	1.90	12.51	1.39	6F
g		010104	1.673	15.13	18.38	7.21	18.31	3.90	3.66	23.26	2.64	6F
h		010104	1.650	14.28	16.68	7.36	17.33	4.21	3.64	23.84	2.79	16F
I		010114	1.644	11.26	9.39	4.49	10.30	2.39	2.15	15.04	1.55	3F
j		010115	1.621	10.88	10.49	5.47	11.45	2.80	2.37	16.97	1.76	3F
	Average value			13.31	13.92	6.71	16.01	3.32	3.42	22.39	2.61	

* With smoker in b and h

Table 3. Analysis of PAH in the outdoor air and indoor air in Chengdu (winter)

	Sampling place	Date of starting sampling (yymmdd)	Quantity of airflow (m^3)	PAH concentration in air (ng/m^3)								Remarks
				Pyrene	BaA	BkF	BaP	dBahA	BdC	BghiP	dBaeP	
a	Kitchen	000710	1.423	1.89	1.03	1.29	1.26	0.68	0.67	4.48	0.42	7F
b		000713	1.489	2.95	3.03	2.57	5.61	1.19	1.53	11.20	0.99	6F
c		000706	1.545	1.94	1.07	0.87	1.68	0.54	0.55	4.29	0.35	3F
d		000707	1.418	3.22	2.32	1.88	4.11	0.91	1.02	7.44	0.60	4F
e		000712	1.437	3.56	3.18	2.47	4.60	1.21	1.32	10.01	0.78	3F
f		000714	1.623	1.80	0.97	1.20	1.54	0.73	0.78	6.20	0.55	6F
g		000715	1.673	2.51	1.51	1.89	2.91	1.33	1.24	9.74	0.95	6F
h		000705	1.531	2.69	2.03	2.18	4.57	1.19	1.30	9.94	0.88	16F
I		000719	1.661	3.38	2.67	3.05	5.74	1.79	1.83	14.46	1.29	3F
j		000720	1.562	3.37	3.02	2.11	3.96	1.64	1.43	11.20	1.06	3F
	Average value			2.73	2.08	1.95	3.60	1.12	1.17	8.90	0.79	
a	Living room	000710	1.504	1.26	0.55	0.45	0.81	0.30	0.26	1.88	0.20	7F
b		000713	1.510	1.32	1.49	0.81	1.86	0.39	0.49	3.70	0.33	6F
c		000706	1.534	1.95	1.29	0.77	1.51	0.40	0.47	3.52	0.30	3F
d		000707	1.418	1.23	0.70	0.57	1.06	0.24	0.28	1.97	0.36	4F
e		000712	1.429	1.89	1.84	0.79	1.84	0.49	0.59	4.08	0.43	3F
f		000714	1.646	2.01	1.57	1.22	2.24	0.75	0.81	6.24	0.51	6F
g		000715	1.611	2.36	1.88	1.86	3.10	1.13	1.15	8.80	0.81	6F
h		000705	1.531	1.97	1.26	1.10	2.53	0.58	0.66	4.99	0.40	16F
I		000719	1.673	1.79	1.30	1.70	2.89	0.96	0.97	7.76	0.79	3F
j		000720	1.562	2.41	2.16	1.57	2.73	1.13	1.01	7.77	0.69	3F
	Average value			1.82	1.40	1.08	2.06	0.64	0.67	5.07	0.48	
a	Bedroom	000710	1.504	1.76	1.05	0.85	1.38	0.43	0.43	3.29	0.34	7F
b		000713	1.489	2.34	2.62	1.64	3.64	0.81	1.00	7.29	0.56	6F
c		000706	1.523	2.83	1.67	1.22	2.46	0.61	0.68	5.43	0.57	3F
d		000707	1.418	3.31	1.86	1.42	3.07	0.69	0.70	5.45	0.45	4F
e		000712	1.437	2.28	1.75	1.43	2.85	0.82	0.84	6.53	0.61	3F
f		000714	1.635	2.50	1.72	1.37	2.51	0.76	0.87	6.62	0.40	6F
g		000715	1.685	1.90	1.39	1.45	2.41	0.77	0.83	6.44	0.58	6F
h		000705	1.542	2.47	1.60	1.30	3.03	0.75	0.74	5.61	0.55	16F
I		000719	1.673	3.69	3.04	3.73	6.70	2.85	2.38	18.82	1.74	3F
j		000720	1.562	2.15	1.85	1.37	2.53	0.93	0.93	5.94	0.63	3F
	Average value			2.52	1.86	1.58	3.06	0.94	0.94	7.14	0.64	
a	Outdoor	000710	1.483	2.24	1.41	1.26	2.07	0.60	0.65	4.98	0.51	7F
b		000713	1.500	3.36	3.47	2.59	6.03	1.23	1.51	11.48	0.97	6F
c		000706	1.523	2.60	1.66	1.09	2.28	0.48	5.05	0.64	0.59	3F
d		000707	1.418	3.22	2.42	1.90	3.92	0.90	1.00	7.14	0.67	4F
e		000712	1.458	2.92	2.43	2.03	4.05	1.10	1.21	8.29	0.89	3F
f		000714	1.623	2.15	1.52	1.23	2.23	0.80	0.77	6.36	1.14	6F
g		000715	1.661	2.42	1.81	1.84	3.25	1.10	1.16	9.02	0.86	6F
h		000705	1.509	3.17	2.45	2.06	4.48	1.15	1.23	9.46	0.89	16F
I		000719	1.685	2.85	2.44	3.13	5.76	1.90	1.94	15.17	1.37	3F
j		000720	1.562	3.04	2.58	2.10	3.92	1.64	1.55	11.07	1.11	3F
	Average value			2.80	2.22	1.92	3.80	1.09	1.61	8.36	0.90	

* With smoker in b and h

Table 4. Analysis of PAH in the outdoor air and indoor air in Chengdu (summer)

Sampling place		Date of starting sampling (yymmdd)	Quantity of airflow (m^3)	PAH concentration in air (ng/m^3)								Remarks
				Pyrene	BaA	BkF	BaP	dBahA	BdC	BghiP	dBaeP	
k	Kitchen	010203	1.99	0.37	0.18	0.10	0.21		0.04	0.37		Detached house
l		010122	1.98	0.26	0.14	0.11	0.27	0.08	0.08	0.54	0.09	14F
m		010119	1.96	0.37	0.28	0.20	0.40	0.10	0.10	1.24	0.09	Detached house
n		010116	2.07	0.55	0.29	0.14	0.44	0.06	0.07	1.13		Detached house
o		010206	1.70	0.46	0.25	0.14	0.34	0.05	0.03	0.52		7F
p		010107	2.06	4.31	1.42	0.29	0.48	0.14		1.29	0.11	Detached house
q		010113	1.70	0.39	0.39	0.16	0.53	0.05	0.08	0.67		Collective housing
r		010118	2.11	0.21	0.04	0.03	0.06		0.02	0.14		4F
s		010111	1.97	0.48	0.20	0.12	0.38	0.03	0.07	0.63	0.06	Detached house
t		010221	2.04	0.31	0.11	0.11	0.28	0.05	0.06	0.50		Detached house
	Average value			0.77	0.33	0.14	0.34	0.07	0.06	0.70	0.09	
k	Living room	010203	1.99	0.35	0.16	0.09	0.21	0.03	0.04	0.30		Detached house
l		010122	1.98	0.37	0.14	0.09	0.27	0.06	0.07	0.47		14F
m		010119	2.03	0.38	0.19	0.15	0.34	0.04	0.08	0.54	0.08	Detached house
n		010116	2.13	0.42	0.40	1.39	0.66	5.68	5.03	3.18	2.83	Detached house
o		010206	1.80	0.57	0.49	0.18	0.66	0.05	0.07	0.76		7F
p		010107	1.94	0.45	0.28	0.14	0.29	0.07	0.07	0.65	0.07	Detached house
q		010113	1.77	0.57	0.49	0.18	0.66	0.05	0.07	0.76		Collective housing
r		010118	2.30	0.16	0.03		0.05		0.01	0.14		4F
s		010111	1.92	0.30	0.15	0.13	0.37	0.04	0.06	0.99	0.06	Detached house
t		010221	1.91	0.57	0.24	0.19	0.26	0.07	0.07	0.60	0.11	Detached house
	Average value			0.41	0.26	0.28	0.38	0.68	0.56	0.84	0.63	
k	Bedroom	010203	2.03	0.30	0.16	0.11	0.22	0.04	0.05	0.37		Detached house
l		010122	1.98	0.37	0.10	0.08	0.19	0.05	0.06	0.34		14F
m		010119	2.09	0.33	0.16	0.11	0.29	0.06	0.05	0.65		Detached house
n		010116	2.13	0.47	0.29	0.17	0.50	0.09	0.12	0.80	0.13	Detached house
o		010206	1.76	0.38	0.15	0.09	0.24	0.05	0.05	0.42		7F
p		010107	0.51	0.51	0.27	0.12	0.29	0.06	0.07	0.66	0.06	Detached house
q		010113	1.77	0.48	0.45	0.21	0.65	0.06	0.10	0.78		Collective housing
r		010118	2.13	0.37	0.13	0.06	0.15		0.03	0.20		4F
s		010111	2.00	0.48	0.26	0.15	0.45	0.13	0.06	0.64	0.04	Detached house
t		010221	2.04	0.52	0.15	0.13	0.29	0.06	0.07	0.51	0.11	Detached house
	Average value			0.42	0.21	0.12	0.33	0.07	0.07	0.54	0.09	
k	Outdoor	010203	2.02	0.62	0.20	0.11	0.17	0.05	0.04	0.37		Detached house
l		010122	1.98	1.57	0.75	0.31	0.77	0.07	0.12	1.22	0.12	14F
m		010119	2.01	1.05	0.58	0.30	0.58	0.10	0.11	1.02	0.11	Detached house
n		010116	2.04	1.90	0.87	0.32	0.90	0.10	0.14	1.76	0.14	Detached house
o		010206	1.74	0.92	0.38	0.18	0.36	0.06	0.08	0.70		7F
p		010107	1.93	0.58	0.19	0.13	0.15	0.05	0.04	0.41		Detached house
q		010113	1.67	2.19	1.28	0.57	1.27	0.15	0.21	1.61	0.17	Collective housing
r		010118	1.93	0.69	0.22	0.09	0.21	0.04	0.03	0.34	0.07	4F
s		010111	1.97	1.09	0.46	0.21	0.45	0.06	0.07	0.73	0.05	Detached house
t		010221	2.01	1.11	0.12	0.13	0.32	0.04	0.06	0.50		Detached house
	Average value			1.17	0.50	0.24	0.52	0.07	0.09	0.87	0.11	

* With smoker in b and h

Table 5. Analysis of PAH in indoor air and outdoor air in Tokyo (winter)

health. Therefore, it is crucial to identify the amounts of various hazardous chemical substances such as carcinogens and mutagens in air, the sources of those substances and the exposure of the human body to them. However, there have been few reports on outdoor and indoor air pollution in China and the actual conditions of air pollution remain largely unknown. Therefore, in this study, we collected indoor and outdoor air samples in Chengdu, one of the biggest cities in China, and measured the mutagenicity of the carcinogens contained in the samples. By using a concentrating column, fast chromatography and spectral fluorescence detector, we simultaneously measured the concentration of PAHs. We used the ultramicro forward mutation assay for measurement of mutagenicity. Mutation tests, which use microbes, are widely conducted to measure environmental samples because the tests can easily measure mutagenicity. However, the Ames method, which is the typical method for mutation tests, is not suitable for measuring small amounts of samples because of insufficient detection sensitivity. Therefore, when measuring small amounts of samples, it is necessary to collect samples many times, accumulate and concentrate them to yield sufficient amounts of sample suited for the detection sensitivity. However, with this approach the time resolution decreases, more solvent is needed for extraction, and the work requires more time, cost and labor. In this study, we had to divide the obtained samples into small amounts because we had to measure and analyze the indoor SPMs at the same time. Therefore, we could only use smaller amounts of samples for measuring mutagenicity than usual. Taking these factors into account, we looked for a test method which had higher detection sensitivity and could detect mutagenicity with small amounts of samples, and decided to use the ultramicro forward mutation method which requires only about one-hundredth of the sample amount compared with the Ames method to measure the mutagenicity of all the samples.

4.1 Measurement and comparison of mutagenicity in indoor and outdoor SPMs in ordinary family homes in Chengdu in summer and winter

In general, regarding measurement results obtained by the Ames method, it is well known that the mutagenicity of SPMs in the metropolitan area is highly influenced by direct mutagens (Matsushita et al, 1990; Takagi et al, 1988, 1994; Tamakawa et al, 1989). Our preliminary measurement results showed that the value was lower when S9mix was not added than when it was added, so we conducted the mutation tests without adding S9mix. It is known that the mutagenicity of outdoor SPMs is generally higher in autumn and winter than in spring and summer (Muramatsu et al, 1983; Ohtani et al, 1985; Watanabe & Hirayama, 1997). In the measurement this time, the mutagen-specific activity was two times higher in the kitchen and bedroom in winter than in summer, and four times higher in the living room and outdoors. We think that this phenomenon was due to the geographical conditions of Chengdu and the type of energy source. In 2000, China's dependence on coal for energy still exceeded 70%. Large trucks and tractors are widely used for distributing goods, and as the number of automobiles increases rapidly, the consumption of oil is increasing dramatically. However, China has no choice but to depend on its abundant coal resources rather than oil for its industrialization. At the time we collected the air samples, large amounts of coal were being used by industry and for producing coke (51.7%), power generation (28.6%), and living such as district heating, indoor heating and cooking (17.7%) . Coal is widely used for indoor heating and cooking, but some houses are not equipped with adequate ventilation systems, and the consumption of coal increases significantly in winter.

Therefore, large amounts of mutagens are formed and emitted into indoor and outdoor air. On the other hand, the value was high in the kitchen in summer when mutagen-specific activity was generally low. This phenomenon was likely caused by contaminants discharged during cooking. The influence of smokers in households was not clear, suggesting that air pollution was so serious that the influence of smokers alone could not be detected. However, the result may also have been influenced by the sampling method (Koyano et al, 1999) such as sampler positions and indoor airflow and so the cause remains unclear.

4.2 Measurement and comparison of mutagenicity of indoor and outdoor SPMs in ordinary family homes in Chengdu and Tokyo

The mutagen-specific activity in Chengdu was about four times higher in the kitchen and the bedroom, about three times higher in the living room and about seven times higher outdoors than in Tokyo. We believe the cause of this phenomenon was as follows. In Tokyo, people use gas heating which is not likely to discharge mutagenic SPMs, air conditioners in their houses (Takagi et al, 1997), and air ventilators in their kitchens, while sophisticated measures are taken to prevent outdoor air pollution. In Chengdu, the mutagen-specific activity was higher outdoors than indoors whereas in Tokyo it was lower outdoors than indoors. Houses in Tokyo are sealed more tightly than those in Chengdu, people ventilate their rooms less in winter and so the contaminants accumulate in their rooms. In Tokyo, the air samples collected in collective housing showed higher values than those in detached houses. The reason is not clear, but since collective housing has fewer windows structurally and is not well ventilated, contaminants are more likely to accumulate. However, more samples and detailed studies are needed. In Tokyo, smokers' houses generally showed high mutagenic activity, and smoking was the major cause of indoor air pollution whereas the influence of heating and cooking was small.

4.3 Measurement and comparison of the concentration of polycyclic aromatic hydrocarbons contained in indoor and outdoor SPMs in Chengdu and Tokyo in winter

In Chengdu, the concentration of BaP was three times higher in the kitchen, eight times higher in the living room, and five times higher in the bedroom and outdoors in winter than in summer. Meanwhile, the concentration of BaP was 40 times higher in the living room, 50 times higher in the bedroom, and 30 times higher in the kitchen and outdoors in Chengdu in winter than in Tokyo in winter. The concentration was five times higher in the living room, six times higher in outdoor air, and 10 times higher in the kitchen and bedroom in Chengdu in summer than in Tokyo even in winter. Similar results were found for PAHs. As stated above, we think that the major causes were the differences between the two cities in geographical conditions, energy sources, ventilation systems and measures for preventing outdoor air pollution. Especially, the PAH concentrations became high in Chengdu in winter due to the increased use of coal for heating, its unique climate and geographical conditions. Most of the collaborators for this study lived in the south of Chengdu and the northwest monsoon may carry polluted air from the city center to the area where they lived. In addition, Chengdu is located in the Sichuan basin where there are many cloudy days in winter and an inversion layer tends to form, which is likely to increase the PAH concentrations in winter. In Chengdu in winter when the outdoor PAH concentrations were high, the indoor PAH concentrations were also high. We think that the significant outdoor air contamination influenced the indoor air due to air ventilation. Meanwhile, comparing the indoor and outdoor PAH concentrations in Chengdu, BghiP > BaP > pyrene in both winter and summer. In Tokyo in winter, BghiP > pyrene > BaP. Therefore, in general, the distributions of respective PAH concentrations are not always the same between areas where the PAH concentrations are high and other areas where the concentrations are low. This time, we measured and studied the mutagenicity of SPMs and concentration of PAHs, but could not measure gas/vapor matter because good standards have not been established for the sampling method. Recently, some studies have focused on gas/vapor matter as hazardous outdoor air contaminants (Watanabe & Hirayama, 1997), and so it is important to identify the actual conditions of indoor and outdoor air pollution caused by gas/vapor matter to better understand environmental pollution. We also must measure and study harmful substances to establish proper countermeasures against general environmental pollution.

5. Conclusion

We studied the evaluation of mutagens for small amounts of indoor air. By using the TM677 strain, which is much more sensitive than the commonly-used Ames method, we confirmed that we could measure the mutagenicity with only about 1440 L of samples (1 L/min × 24 hours). We measured air samples collected from ordinary family homes in Chengdu and Tokyo by using this new method and found that the mutagenicity was higher in Chengdu than in Tokyo and higher in winter than in summer.

6. References

Alfheim, I. & Mψller, M. (1981) Mutagenicity of airborne particulate matter in relation to traffic and meterological conditions, In : *Short-term bioassays in the analysis of complex Environmental mixtures 11*, Waters, M. D. et al eds., pp. 85−99, Plenum Press, New York,

Broddin, G.; Van vaeck, L. & Van Cauwenberghe, K. (1977) On the size distribution of polycyclic aromatic hydrocarbon containing particles from a coke oven emission source, *Atmos. Environ.* 11, pp.1061−1064, ISSN 1352-2310

Endo, O.; Koyano, M.; Mineki, S.; Goto, S.; Tanabe, K.; Yajima, H.; Ishii, T.; & Matsushita, H. (1999) Estimation of indoor air PAH concentration increases by cigarette, incense-stick, and mosquito-repellent-incense smoke, *Polycyclic Aromatic Compounds*, 21, pp.261-272, ISSN 1040-6638

Goto, S; Kato, Y; Orii, A; Tanaka, K.; Hisamatsu, Y. & Matsushita, H. (1982) Daily variation of mutagenicities of airborne particulates, *J. Jpn. Soc. Air Pollut.*, 17 (4) pp. 295−303, ISSN 0386706

Heyder, J.; Debhart, J.; Rudolf, G. & Schiller, C.; & Stahlhofen, W. (1986) Deposition of particles in the human respiratory tract in the size range 0.005-15 μm, *J. Aerosol Sci.* 17, pp. 811−825, ISSN 0021-8502

Iwamoto, S.; Utsunomiya, A.; Ooishi, O. & Shimohara, T. (1990) Behavior of airborne particulates in urban area and its surroundings, *J. Jpn. Soc. Air Pollut.*, 25 (2), pp. 170−179, ISSN 0386706

Kasahara, M. (1990) Air pollution problems by particulate matter analysis of pollution mechanisms and evaluation of pollution level, *J. Environ. Chem.*, 25 (2), pp. 111－122, ISSN 0917-2408

Koyano, M.; Sun, C.-J.; Endo, O.; Goto S.; Watanabe, I.; Machii, K.; Mineki, S. & Matsushita, H. (1999) Mutagenicity and PAH concentration of extracts from airborne particulate sampling with low flow rate cascade impactor, *J. Environ. Chem.*, 9 (4), pp. 955－968, ISSN 0917-2408

Matsushita, H.; Goto, S.; Takagi, Y.; Endo, O. & Tanabe, K. (1990) Human exposure to airborne mutagens indoors and outdoors using mutagenesis and chemical analysis methods, In : *Genetic Toxicology of Complex Mixture*, Waters, M. D. et al. ed., pp. 33－55, Plenum Press, ISBN 978-0306436833, New York

Muramatsu, M.; Umemura, S. & Tomota, H. (1983) Development of a nicotine personal monitor for the quantitative evaluation of tabacco smoke exposure, *J. Jpn. Soc. Air Pollut.*, 18, pp. 291－299, ISSN 0386706

Mψller, M.; Alfheim, I.; Larssen, S.; & Mlkalsen, A. (1982) Mutagenicity of airborne particles in relation to traffic and air pollution parameters, *Environ. Sci. Technol.*, 16 pp. 221－225, ISSN 0013-936X

Ohtani, Y.; Shimada, Y.; Ujiiye, A.; Nishimura, T. & Matsushita, H. (1985) Comparison between mutagenic activities of airborne particulates in Maebashi and in Minato-ku Tokyo, *J. Jpn. Soc. Air Pollut.*, 20 (6), pp. 463－469, ISSN 0386706

Pierce, R. C. & Katz, M. (1975) Dependency of polynuclear aromatic hydrocarbon content on size distribution of atmospheric aerosols, *Enciron. Sci. Technol.*, 9, pp. 347－353, ISSN 0013-936X

Sugita, K.; Chengiun, S.; Goto, S.; Tanabe, K.; Takagi, Y.; Mstyushita, H. & Lewtas, J. (1996) Particle distribution of polycylic aromatic hydrocarbons in the air, *7th intern. Conf. Indoor Air Quality and Climate (Indoor Air '96)* l3, pp. 391－396

Mitra, S. & Wilson, N. K. (1992) Pattern of polynulear aromatic-hydrocarbons in indoor air-exploratory principal component analysis, *Environ. Int.*, 18 (5), pp. 477－487, ISSN 0160-4120

Takagi, Y.; Hatano, A.; Kohzaki, K.; Goto, S. & Matsushita, H. (1994) The study on exposure factors to airborne mutazens -the comparisonk of the mutagenicity between personal exposure and outdoor samples-, *J. Jpn. Soc. Air Pollut.*, 29 (1), pp. 16－23, ISSN 0386706

Takagi, Y.; Goto, S.; Kou, C.-T.; Sugita, S.; Murata, M.; Lewtas, J. & Matsushita, H. (1988) Ultramicro forward-mutation assay and it's application to the survey of indoor air pollution, *J. Jpn. Soc. Air Pollut.*, 24, pp. 244－251, ISSN 0386706

Takagi, Y.; Kan, M.; Koyano, M.; Goto, S.; Kato, Y.; Kaneuchi, C. & Kohzaki, K. (1997) Using kerosene or gas heaters and concentration of polycyclic aromatic hydrocarbons in indoor air particles, *J. Jpn. Vet. Med. Assoc.*, 50 (3), pp. 169－172

Tamakawa, K.; Matsumoto, K.; Takahashi, Y.; Seki, T. & Lewtas, J. (1989) An application of the sensitive ames test (accelerated microsuspension procedure) to assess indoor air pollution-mutagenicity of dust on filters in air conditioners-, *J. Jpn. Soc. Air Pollut.*, 24, pp. 37－44, ISSN 0386706

Urano, K.; Miyamoto, K.; Okuyama K. & Fujiie K. (1992) Harocarbons and aromatic hydrocarbons in urban air of Japan, *J. Jpn. Soc. Air Pollut.*, 27（5,）pp. 227－236, ISSN 0386706

Watanabe, T. & Hirayama, T. (1997) Mutagens and carcinogens in atmospheric environment, *Environ. Mutagen Res.*, 19, pp. 37－41（1997）

Yamamoto, G. (1977) Atomospheric pollution and Climate, *J. Jpn. Soc. Air Pollut.*, 11 (5), pp. 378－387, ISSN 0039900

10

Air Pollution and Urban Morphology: A Complex Relation or How to Optimize the Pedestrian Movement in Town

Gilles Maignant and Jérôme Dutozia
CNRS, UMR ESPACE,
University of Nice-Sophia Antipolis, Nice,
France

1. Introduction

1.1 Understand the air pollution in town - modelling aspect

Urban air pollution is traditionally estimated by using techniques based on geostatistical methods, such as interpolation, applied to a set of data stemming from measures of stations of pollution. Now very often, these stations are in insufficient number or do not measure the same pollutants to allow mapping finely dispersion of air pollution through urban spaces. Numerous studies work then from land registries of broadcasts. Although interesting in a regional scale, these studies bring only not enough information in the understanding of the phenomena to a scale as fine as the intra-urban. So, it is necessary to resort to the fine three-dimensional modelling to dread this intra-urban scale and it is what we describe now. Without this aspect of modelling, we cannot work on the intra-urban scale, because in the hypotheses of modelling of the land registries of broadcasts, (figure 1) we consider the homogeneity of the urban morphology, what, naturally, is not the case. The rule of the urban morphology in the dispersal of pollutants will be described in the following paragraph. Let us be interested here in the phase of modelling of the dispersal of pollutants in urban zones.
From modelling point of view, the three dimensional model allows to solve fluid mechanics equations (Navier-Stockes) for each cell of the model. Space is modelled by small boxes (three dimensional cells: eulerian model) for which we applied the equations (figure 1).

$$(1)\quad \frac{\partial \rho}{\partial t} + \vec{\nabla}.(\rho\vec{v}) = 0$$

$$(2)\quad \frac{\partial(\rho\vec{v})}{\partial t} + \vec{\nabla}.(\rho\vec{v}\otimes\vec{v}) = -\vec{\nabla}p + \vec{\nabla}.\bar{\bar{\tau}} + \rho\vec{f}$$

$$(3)\quad \frac{\partial(\rho e)}{\partial t} + \vec{\nabla}.[(\rho e + p)\vec{v}] = \vec{\nabla}.(\bar{\bar{\tau}}.\vec{v}) + \rho\vec{f}.\vec{v} + \vec{\nabla}.\vec{q} + r$$

Fig. 1. The three Navier-Stokes non-linear equations of fluid mechanics

In the figure 1, the first equation describes the preservation of the mass, the second one is for preservation of the impulse, and the third one is for the conservation of energy. Those three equations depicting the fluid mechanics (Navier-Stokes equations) are coupled with the

advection and diffusion equation. As the Navier-Stokes equations are nonlinear partial differential equations; the nonlinearity makes most problems difficult to solve in an analytical point of view, that's why we use eulerian model to approximate solutions. For this calculus, by successive approximations, the space is indented as elementary cells for which two types of information are calculated (wind speed and direction, pollutants concentrations).
For each cell we affect one value of polluting flow, and the model calculates the effective concentration after dispersion. The dispersion is estimated by two ways. First of all, we implement the wind field in a specific zone which is not perturbed by the urban morphology that is to say at a high level (200 meters high). After implementing the input data, the model starts running. To stop the model we have two choices, we could stop it after a fixed time (number of iterations) or stop it when concentrations begin stable. We choose the second option and we fixed the stability when differences between concentrations calculated for each cell and for two successive iterations are less than 10^{-6}. So the results are that we could estimate with a fine precision all concentrations in a three dimensional space with a five meters horizontally and two meters vertically resolution (figure 2).

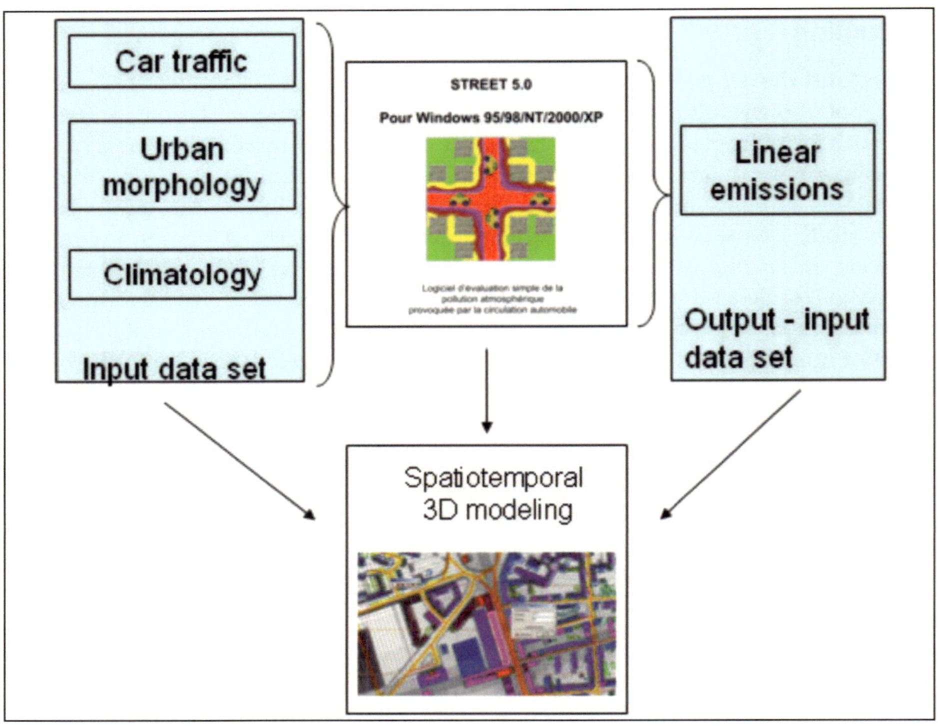

Fig. 2. Air pollution modelling, from sources to maps.

1.2 Why the urban morphology creates spatial differentiations in dispersal of pollutants?

The same broadcasts (emissions) produced in configurations of different streets engender very different polluting loads after dispersal. Now it is indeed these polluting, called immissions loads that interest us within the framework of the problem of the pedestrian routes, because it is about the pollution effectively inhaled by the city-dweller.

Indeed, for the same car traffic, there are spatial configurations of particularly fatal arteries in the dispersal of pollutants (streets canyons) which are "traps with pollutants". It is in these very specific streets that particular attentions in terms of urban planning must be proposed. For example, the "hollow teeth" of the urban morphology should be protected to leave free spaces, useful for a better dispersal of pollutants. In terms of town and country planning, it would be sensible to rethink the filling of these interstitial spaces of a systematic point of view. For example, if the land pressure is such as the filling of these spaces seems to be the only possible alternative, then this measure should be coupled with the institution of a decrease of the traffic on the artery.
The spatial differentiation (gradient of pollution), noticed by a spatial, horizontal point of view, also meets from a vertical point of view (Figure 3). Indeed, spaces near the ground will be more polluted, what will have naturally an influence on the choice of routes particularly at the vulnerable persons whom are the children and the old persons. Furthermore, in the same street, a pavement can be more polluted than the other following one how it is subjected to the wind. All these factors will thus have to take into account for the calculation of an indicator of exposure, which is a function of the length of the chosen arc, the time pasted to go through it (related to the speed of movement of the person) and of the intrinsic vulnerability of the person.

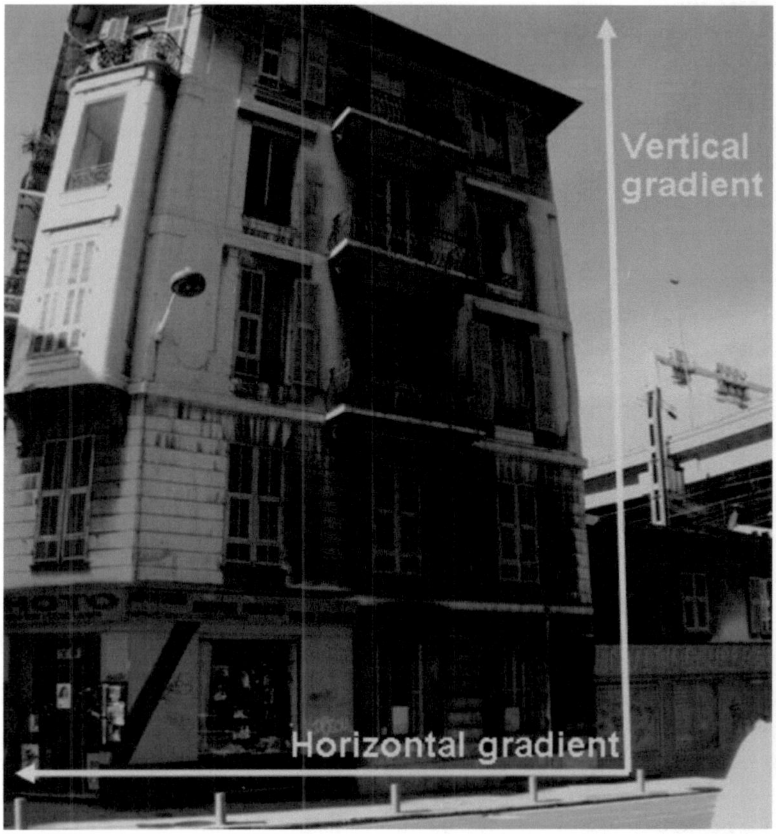

Fig. 3. Building in the centre of Nice, air pollution spatial differentiation (Photo: Gilles MAIGNANT)

2. Optimal pedestrian routes

2.1 Classic vision: from geomarketing approach to societal demand

The problem of itinerary optimization is an old mathematical question, stemming from a problem based on the graphs theory; it knew a new breath thanks to the power of computers. Traditionally, roads are dreaded through software of optimization of type "Chinese post-office employee" or "sales representative", whose purpose is to minimize a cost. These algorithms knew a new breath thanks to the development of strategies of Geomarketing or geo-localization. For instance, the minimisation of emergency services response times (by the Dijkstra or Floyd-Warshall algorithms) and the locating of large infrastructures such as commercial centres, housing developments, leisure centres and transport nodes (train stations, airports etc.) are key considerations in the decision. In the examples which we have dealt with previously, notably in the Geomarketing trend, space is perceived as a constraint in optimisation terminology. This does not mean that it does not play a role, but rather that the objective function is independent from this and could, for example, restore the emergency services response times. This approach is most notably found on online route planning sites such as Via Michelin, Mappy or others on which constraints can be economic, temporal or distance-related; the objective is to find the best possible itinerary which satisfies these user-imposed constraints.

In this approach, the minimization is established on an easily quantifiable criterion (time, outstrips, cost) and does not thus take on character connected to a specific individual. Now in the indicator of exposure which we set up, the subjective vulnerability of the pedestrian is integrated according to three classes at least into the most vulnerable. The more vulnerable is the pedestrian, the more he will be affected by air pollution; that is to say, for the same itinerary, total exposure indicator has to be higher for a pedestrian of vulnerability class 3 than indicator for a pedestrian of vulnerability class 2. This way, attribution of the vulnerability class is very important in our protocol. But this step is also very debatable: why only 3 classes of vulnerability? What should be the more pertinent criterions to allocate the suitable vulnerability class for each pedestrian? As far as we concerned, we consider fuzzy logic could be an interesting methodology to deal with the inherent imprecision related to individual vulnerability evaluation (Bouchon-Meunier, 2007).

The following paragraph has for objective to discuss the foundations of the concept of optimization, its vocabulary and how it is used in this chapter of work.

2.2 Reflection on the optimum

Before question how to applied optimization to the pedestrian movements according to the inhaled polluting load, it seems to us necessary to position the question of the definition of the optimum, particularly in the field of the human and social sciences.

In the *dictionary Larousse*, the definition of *optimum* explicitly refers to a choice between several configurations or fields of possibilities, it is the choice judged most favourable in relation to other solutions or pre-established criteria. This definition, therefore, implicitly demonstrates *optimum* to be a relative term. In other words, the presentation of an *optimum* must not be taken out of context or disassociated from the underlying conditions which have led the modeller to express this *optimum*. The *optimum,* it seems, is always relative to a context or to a particular set of constraints; it is highly dependant on the objective one sets oneself as well as the size and scale of the enquiry. We will now define the notions of context, constraints and objective (Maignant, 2010).

To optimise is to choose the best solution from a spectrum of possible solutions. This supposes a relatively thorough knowledge of the choices available to us (Baquiast, 2007). In the numerous cases presented here, testing all possible configurations is not realistic (too large a number, unknown configurations...); optimisation rests therefore on a selection of choices which seem, in the first instance, to the eyes of those looking to make the optimal choice, the least non-optimal. As soon as we are faced with a choice or with a decision to make, optimisation is present; we look for the best possible solution in relation to one or indeed several fixed objectives as well as to the inherent constraints of the situation (temporal, spatial or financial constraints).

In the case which interests us here, the function "objective" is not directly connected to a cost of economic nature but represents the respiratory hardness to choose a specific urban artery to walk. Here, optimum operates with only one constraint: to minimize pollution exposure during a walking route between point A and point B. Acceptability for this optimal itinerary is relative to individual sensitivity and awareness about air pollution, but also relative to ability of this optimum to not totally take out of distance and travel time constraints.

2.3 Innovative vision

The innovative vision of this chapter lives in the coupling and or the chainage of methods (figure 4). From data of traffic, data of climatology and information on the urban shape, the linear theoretical emissions are calculated in STREET 5.0 (software of estimation of the atmospheric pollution), according to a method of classifications of the various types of vehicles, standards of normalized broadcasts and various cycles of driving including individual behaviour. These theoretical issues are then joined into a three-dimensional model of dispersal of pollutants allowing to produce fine mappings (cartographies) of immissions (precision five meters horizontally and two meters vertically). The model used in this chapter is a three-dimensional model of the fluid mechanics which is non - hydrostatic allowing solving the equations of Navier-Stockes in a space in the complex morphology.

Those average imissions are then joined into a geographical information system to which the module of optimization is applied. The roughness of the route is then modelled through classic spatial constraints (distance, time) and environmental requirements (air pollution) and individual (three classes of vulnerability of the person).

Our system of risk is complex due to considering the vulnerability differentiated by the pedestrians. Indeed, we know that according to the state of health, the age and the biological specificities, the same event will have different impacts on two persons; it is in a sense, a kind of sensibility on the initial conditions. We decided to differentiate three levels of vulnerability, according to which the exposure in the environmental pressure is going to have a more or less strong impact on the health of the pedestrians. For the same route, and thus an exposure amounts, the vulnerable populations, such as the children or the old persons for example, are thus going to be more weakened, than persons not answering particular criteria of vulnerability.

By proposing these comparisons between the environmental optimal routes and the optima in terms of distance, we do not mean there are only two factors influencing the populations in the selection of their pedestrian route. The literature on the behaviour of movements is plentiful, for a state of the recent work on all the criteria which have an influence on the pedestrians in their choices of urban routes, we can refer to Sonya Lavadinho's works and Giuseppe Pini of the University of the mobility of Geneva, who identify more than twenty-five characteristics having a potential impact on the choices of pedestrian routes (Pini, on 2005).

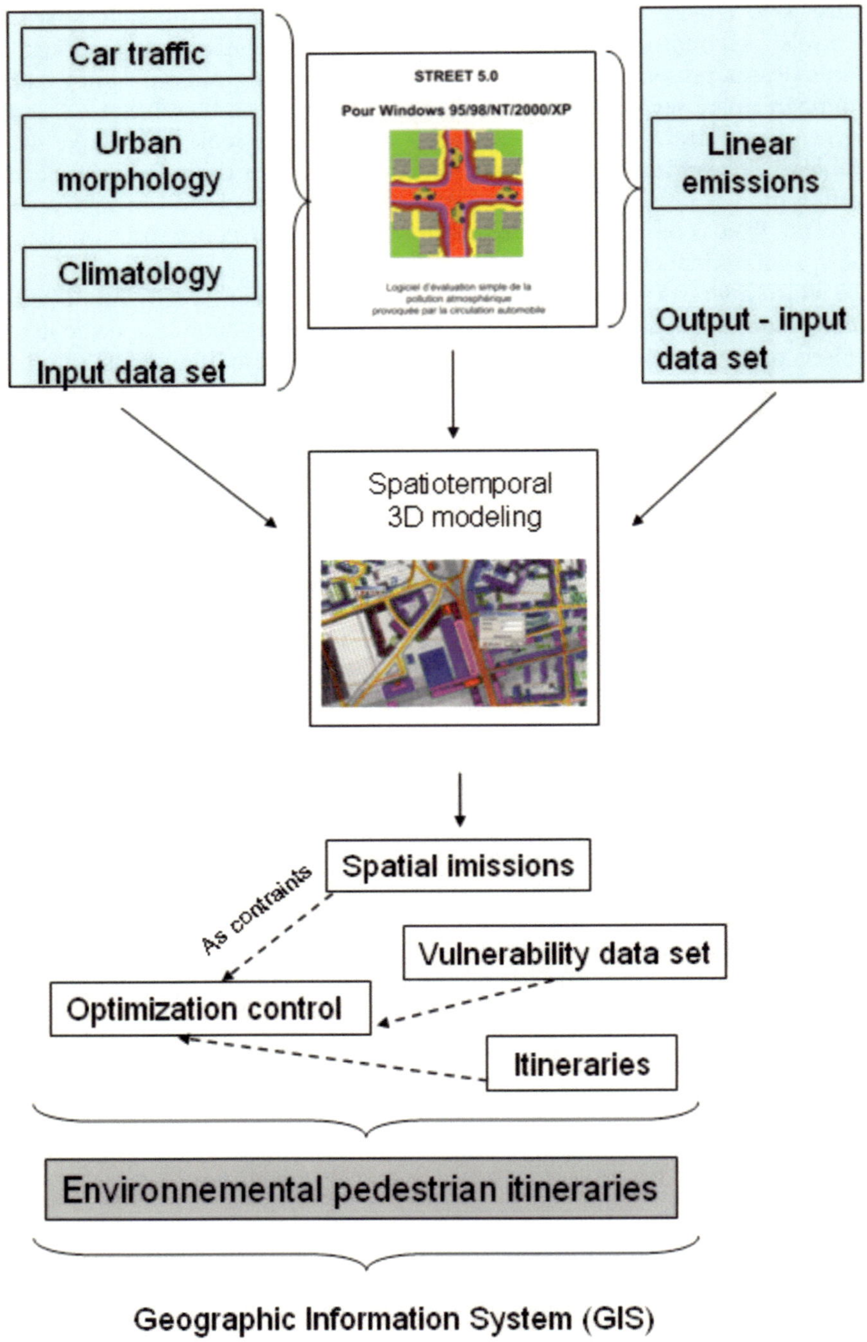

Fig. 4. Scheme of modelization, from air pollution modelling to pedestrian itineraries

To tell the truth, understand what could incite an individual to take an artery rather than the other one is not the subject of our study. We make simply the hypothesis that if a method is able to detect a route minimizing the exposure level in the polluting flows, and if this optimal route is relatively similar to the optimum outstrip time, then this plan will be considered as acceptable for a part of the population. This threshold of acceptability is not fixed but can vary according to the pedestrian, to its practices, characteristics and the purpose of its movement. On the other hand, dealing with of the difference between the plans of the optimal routes in distance (OD) and the optimal routes in terms of environment (OE), we should not neglect the importance of the time of movement (which is also the time of exposure), integrated into the formulation of the indicator of exposure through the factor length of the route.

In this chapter's book, we voluntarily simplified the application by considering that about their levels of vulnerability, the populations move in an identical and constant speed. So, the time of exposure varies only according to the length of arteries. If we had considered various types of pedestrian movements, by distinguishing for example a walking mode and a chasing mode, the modelled system would have been much more complex due to the strong interactions between speed of movement, time of exposure and volume of inhaled air. In running position, an individual moves approximately in 15 kph while he moves only in 5 kph by walking. So, the runner is going to reduce sharply his exposure time; but its global level of exposure in pollutants will not fall inevitably, because decline of the time of exhibition, which could be calculated in our indicator by balancing the distance by a value lower than 1, will be compensated with the sharp rise.

The search for an optimal route consists in identifying the route which minimizes the time, the necessary distance or the economic cost, to connect one point A to one point B. The notion of optimum leans here on the other preoccupations, because the methodology proposed here, aims at the detection of pedestrian routes minimizing the environmental pressure undergone by the pedestrians. In town, various types of routes offer themselves to the pedestrian. More or less consciously and more or less effectively, people select their road according to their constraints. The workers tend to privilege the shortest road at time, whereas the walker will choose more a good quality road environmental especially if he coincides with centres of proprietary (cultural or environmental) interests or spaces offered to the view. One of the preoccupations of the planners could be to conciliate visual interests sites (architectural, landscapes etc.) with routes of better environmental qualities.

From here, for a given route, the time of route is inevitably equal in the time of exposure of the pedestrian to a variable load of pollutants, one of the objectives of the approach is to know if it's better to take the shortest road but very polluted rather than a very long and little polluted road? Several categories of bows occur: long and polluted bow, short and healthy bow, short and polluted bow, long and healthy bow. The first one is not an optimum and it is evident that nobody is going to take it, the second is an absolute optimum but does not exist frequently in the reality (otherwise everybody would take it) ; both last ones constitute the heart of the discussion.

Is it better to take a short arc but polluted rather than a long but healthy arc? If we consider only one of the factors outstrip or environment, it is easy to decide between these two roads. The complexity comes to have to integrate into the indicator two factors which are not of the same order. But the length of the route influences strongly the possibilities of adjournment. It is evident that if the "healthy" route consists in extending the route in a not reasonable factor, the optimal plan of an environmental point of view will be not used due to an excessive loss of the temporal constraint, that is to say: go instead of appointment as quickly as possible.

A pedestrian route consists of bows (streets, boulevards etc.), crossed in any sense or direction and from which the rate of pollution differs between every artery according to the car traffic, local climatic conditions and of the surrounding urban morphology, as we said previously.
The vulnerability of the pedestrian is a qualitative variable which is function of the age, the sex, the state of health, the sports activity of the person. The concentration in pollutants is estimated from complex calculations integrating the urban morphology (network and built), a database of traffic, a database of broadcasts, a database of climatology factors implemented in a model of dispersal of pollutants. The vulnerability of the persons is defined according to the following classes: 1 for little vulnerable, 2 for vulnerable and 3 for very vulnerable.
The method is partially based on construction of indicators, integrating into their formulation the polluting load of the chosen artery but also the length of this one, as well as the vulnerability of the pedestrian. Because, the more the artery is long, the more the fact that it is polluted is binding, the exposure time of the user being globally proportional to the length of the route and conversely proportional to the speed of movement. To inform every arc of the local area, an indicator of exposure was created.
The indicator set up for the calculation of optimization (the function "objective" to minimize) is the product (in constants near) of the present concentration of pollutants on the artery by its length and by the vulnerability of the considered person. Its theoretical formulation is the following one: $E=V.L.[C]$, where V is the vulnerability of the pedestrian, L the length of the borrowed arc, [C] the concentration in pollutants of the arc (for a specific pollutant).
Once this value is calculated and allocated to every bow of the local area, the implementation is made via the interface of the software Chronovia. From a technical point of view, the integration of multifactor constraints in the module of accessibility, implemented in the software of geographical information system (GIS) is not so easy; that why we have to create a specific plug - in. The principle of this type of tool is based on the theory of the graphs and the algorithm of the shortest road (Djkstra, Floyd - Warshall etc.), in distance, time or cost. Thus, the objective is to minimize the sum of the constraints.
Within the framework of a problem of distance, the sum of the distances to go of a knot to another knot must be minimal. It is the same problem for the studied environmental nuisance; it is a question of minimizing the environmental pressure undergone by the pedestrian; in other words minimize the sum of the arterial exposures, the exhibitions which also take into account the time which we need to walk on the axis and, of course the length of the axis.
The add-on Chronovia allows a very precise characterization of a public road network and these various users, this capacity was not used in our example, because our objective was not to reproduce a reality, but to use a theoretical case. The user of the network is configured to be a pedestrian who moves, on average, in a constant speed of five kilometres per hour. From the available information in the majority of the geographical databases on networks, Chronovia models the network in graph and calculates various indicators of accessibility and coherence. The tool is then capable of detecting an optimal route on the network according to the distance, the distance time and the economic cost, by taking into account factors of configuration of the network (structure, curve, flow) of the traffic at various hours; sense of traffic (circulation); traffic lights.
It is possible to attribute a cost of specific passage to every artery. To integrate the exposure indicator, we have planned to use the function of calculation of route according to an economic cost, by having beforehand replacing the cost by artery, by our indicator. But, Chronovia needs a fixed cost which, according to the distance, adds a value representing the cost of the gasoline; this fixed value which would have disrupted the detection of the

optimal routes of an environmental point of view, obliged to us to integrate the indicator of exposure into the place of the distance, which is the only completely independent factor.

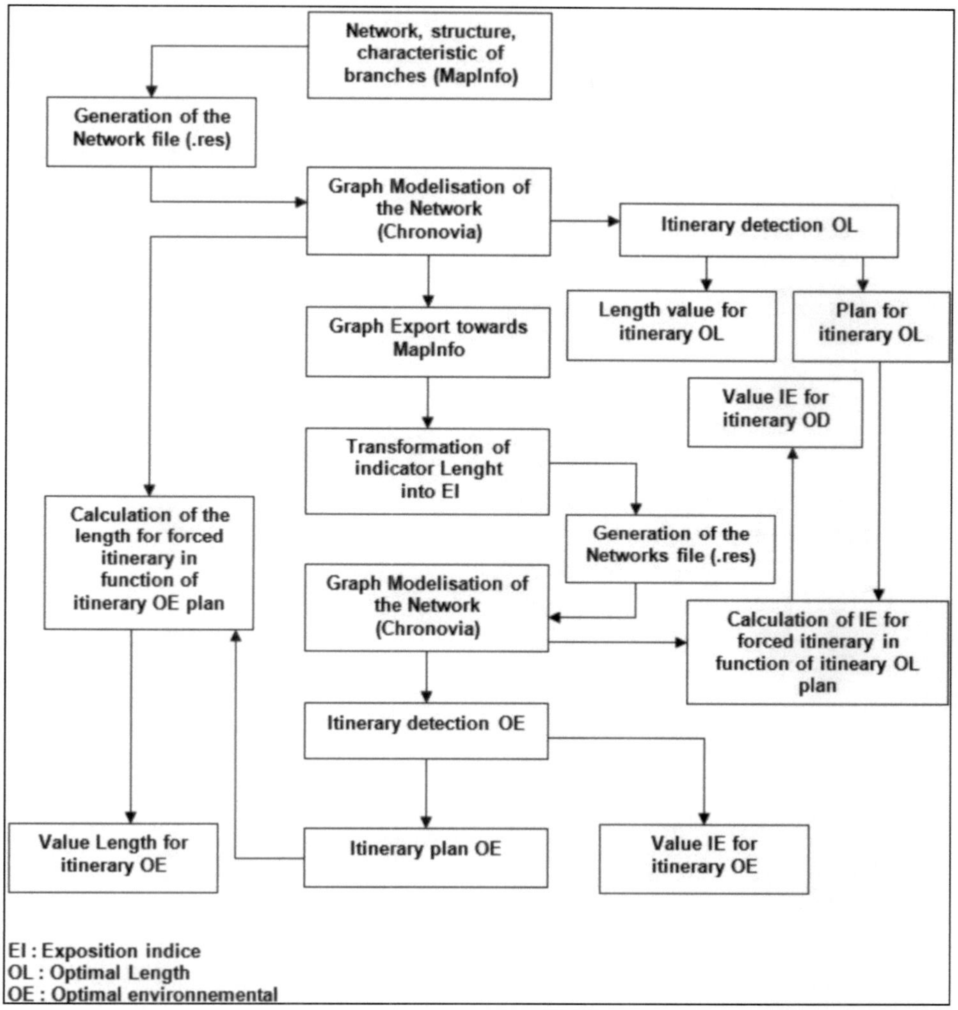

Fig. 5. Protocol of detection of route, calculation of the distances and the total exposure of the optimal plans.

This forced choice (by technical point of view), slightly complicated the protocol of calculation, presented in the figure 4 which follows. For every route [AB], we wished to obtain the plan of the optimal route, according to the distance, and according to the environmental exposure at the various levels of vulnerability; the crossed distance and to the total level of exposure for each of the plans.

In the figure 5, we speak about "calculation of itinerary forced in function of a plan", this expression deserves some precision. We wished to obtain the total value of exposure in pollutants for the optimal routes according to the distance. Now, as we said it previously, we had to replace the indicator outstrip to integrate our own indicator. The optimal routes were calculated from two different graphs, the information available on the one not existing on the other one; from there, the question was how to calculate the value of the environmental exposure according to an optimal plan outstrip (OD)?

The detection of optimal route between A and B can be forced by the passage by some number of points on the network. To resolve our problem we used this function by constraining the itinerary to preselected knots of the network so as to reproduce the plan of the route OD on the graph where we had integrated the indicator of exposure into pollutants. We obtain then the information concerning the total distance and the global level of exposure for every plan of optimal route.

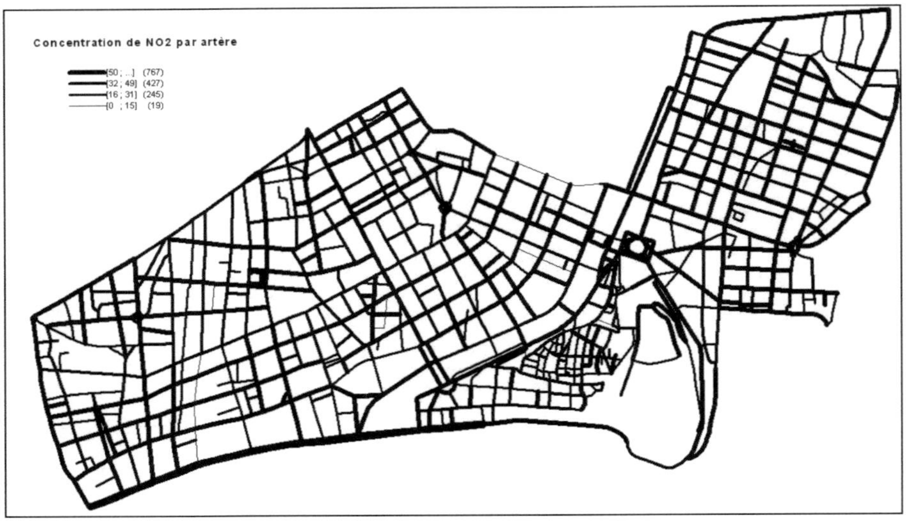

Fig. 6. Network branches and NO_2 concentration

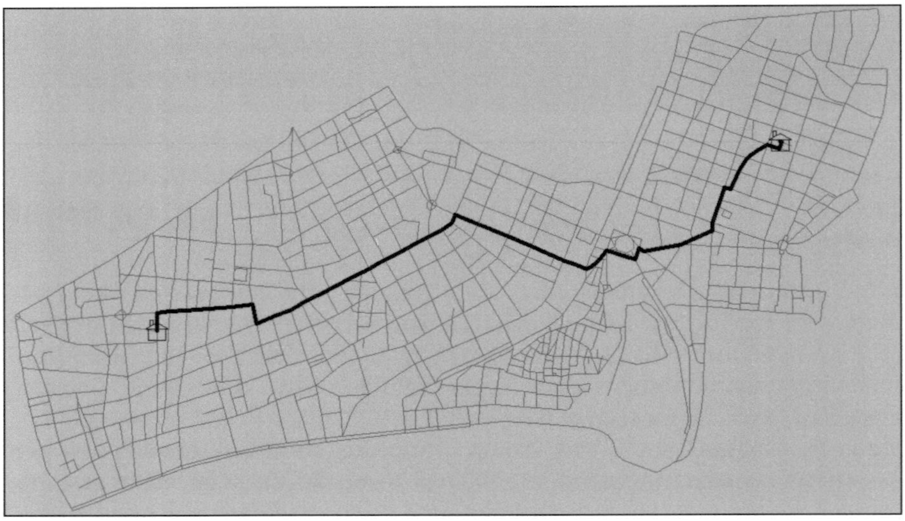

Fig. 7. Optimal itinerary minimizing distance. (2,978km)

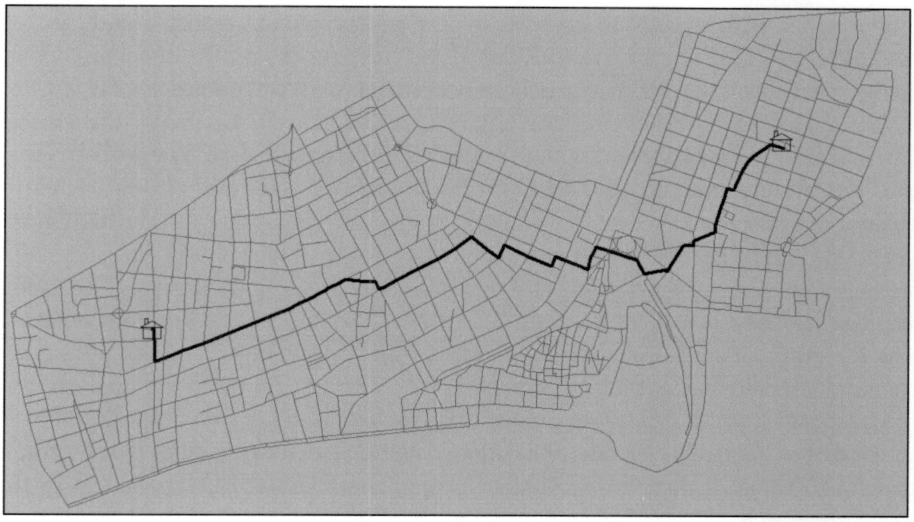

Fig. 8. Optimal itinerary minimizing environmental exposure for level pedestrian of vulnerability 1. (Distance = 3,223km; IE = 0,139)

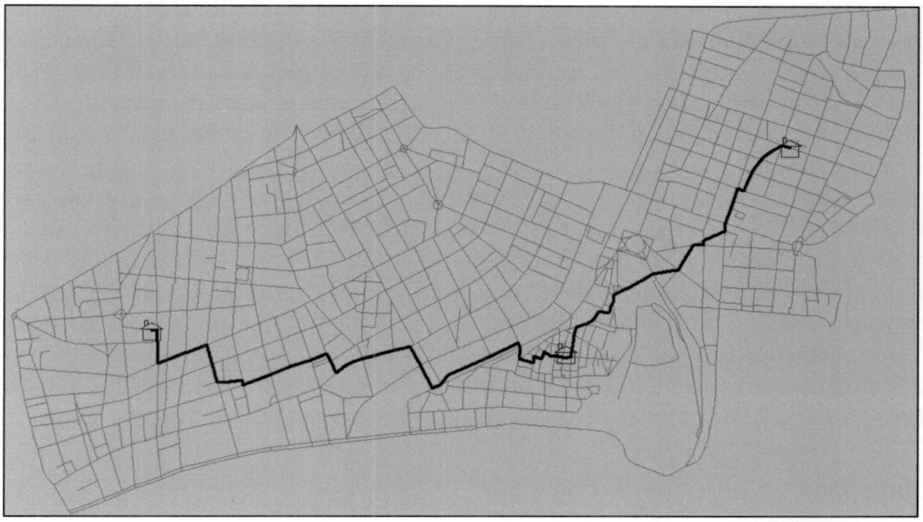

Fig. 9. Optimal itinerary minimizing environmental exposure for level pedestrian of vulnerability 2. (Distance = 3,617km; IE = 0,263)

3. Conclusion

Through the concept of *optimality*; the operational elements of optimisation can be utilised for the construction of a more sustainable world. It must be seen as a key to reinterpreting the world. The notion "better" implicitly entails choosing "non-violence" when it comes to what exists already. This means, particularly in spatial planning, that we cannot simply forget our past actions and start from scratch. On the contrary, we must move already existing elements into a new order with a view to creating a new reality; a new reality which, in terms of complex collective criteria, we expect will be better. In terms of courses of action, this method (reframing what exists already) is much less intrusive and constitutes a new approach in prospective spatial planning. In this way, age-old questions which remain unanswered give life to the scientific activity of the moment. Michel Godet explains that "The world changes, yet problems remain [creating] an advantage for the thoughtful man: past efforts are hardly ever obsolete and in order to rediscover the majority of mechanisms and reports created in the past, all we need to do is bring them up to date using recent data" (Godet, 2000).

The problems of routes try systematically to optimize certain parameters as the time or the distance. We saw that it is possible to introduce new preoccupations into the choice of these routes as for example environmental issues (air quality on axes or still noise pollutions). The various parameters to be optimized can be combined in a multicriteria analysis with the ultimate purpose of which is to save some energy, under whatever forms whether it is. Energy savings are one of the main concerns of a better sustainable management of the environment.

Considering the steady rhythm of broadcasting of the technologies connected to the GPS (henceforth available on the GSM), it is very likely that in court or middle term of new generations of GPS are born. By adapting itself to the new practices of mobility in town, and by taking into account preoccupations of the populations, this new GPS could indeed integrate new among others environmental factors of optimization.

Other interest of the method, proposed in this chapter, lives in the coupling vulnerability of the persons - vulnerability of the urban axes in front of the polluting load. In the objective of a "requalification" of urban areas, in particular by the implementation of new pedestrian areas, or reduced traffic lanes, the quality of life of these spaces tends to improve, the notion of sustainable development underlying this evolution. So, the pedestrian would begin to find a place in town.

By means of feedback, it is going to improve the global quality of life of our cities. Indeed the pedestrian noticing an improvement of the environmental quality of certain taken routes will tend to favor the soft modes of movements and will so contribute to ameliorate the quality of life, the phenomenon similar to the entropy of a closed system. However, in terms of urban planning, we cannot give the whole street to the pedestrian. Some structuring axes of the city must be mainly dedicated to the automobile mobility. In this optics, the problem of environmental optimal routes takes a quite new bend: how is it possible to avoid the structuring axes knowing that these are penalizing from a public health point of view?

4. References

Baquiast, J.P. (2007). *Pour un principe matérialiste fort*, Ed Jean Paul Bayol, 300 p.

Bouchon-Meunier B. (2007). *La logique floue*, Coll. Que sais-je ?, PUF, 128 p.

Godet M. (2000). *De la rigueur pour une indiscipline intellectuelle*, in « La prospective stratégique d'entreprise » Lesourne (dir.), Dunod, 28 p.

Maignant G. (2010). *Reflections on optimisation in Geography, envisaging "Geography for the better"*, Lambert Academic Publishing, And ISBN: 978-3838394886, 113 p.

Pini P., Lavadinho S. (2005). Développement durable, mobilité douce et santé en milieu urbain, *Actes du colloque « Développent urbain durable, gestion des ressources et gouvernance »* Lausanne, 8 p.

Part 2

Environmental Case Studies

11

Air Pollution in Moscow Megacity

Gennady Gorchakov[1], Eugenia Semoutnikova[2],
Aleksey Karpov[1] and Elena Lezina[2]
[1]*Oboukhov Institute of Atmospheric Physics, Russian Academy of Science*
[2]*State Environmental Institution (SEI) Mosecomonitoring*
Russia

1. Introduction

Investigation results of the gas and aerosol air composition over megapolisis are of great interest for the ecology and climate theory. In Moscow statistical regularities can developed from the monitoring data obtained at the Moscow network of automatic stations monitoring air quality (SEI "Mosecomonitoring"). Alternative data are limited essentially.

Monitoring data received in 2003 - 2004 have been analyzed partly in (Gorchakov et al., 2006). Hydrocarbon concentration variations have been studied comprehensively (Gorchakov et al., 2009a). Statistical analysis of the aerosol mass concentration (PM10) variations in 2004 was carried out (Gorchakov et al., 2007). Carbon monoxide and nitrogen oxides concentration profiles in the urban boundary layer according to the data of Ostankino TV Tower measurements during the winter described in (Gorchakov et al., 2009b). Week - long cycle of the air pollution in Moscow was treated in (Gorchakov et al., 2010c). Statistical prediction possibilities of the air pollution in Moscow were analyzed (Gorchakov et al., 2010a, 2010b, 2010c).

Moscow faces a severe atmospheric pollution problem during the smoke haze episodes determined by the forest - peatbog fires (Gorchakov et al., 2003, 2004). Such episodes occurred in July - August 2010. The objective of this chapter is to characterize comprehensively concentration variations of gaseous impurities and aerosol mass concentration (PM10, PM2.5) variations in Moscow. In particular the air pollution in the smoky atmosphere is concerned.

Monitoring system is described in section 2. Temporal variability of the gaseous species of the concentration is discussed in section 3. The results of the statistical analysis are presented in section 4. Aerosol mass concentration variations have been considered in section 5. Section 6 is devoted to the air pollution in the urban boundary layer. The air pollution in the smoky atmosphere is outlined in section 7. Meteorology and the air pollution influence on the health are discussed briefly in section 8. The main results are stated in section 9.

2. Monitoring system

The Air quality monitoring system in Moscow was founded in 1995. The set-up of the air quality monitoring network was designed taking into consideration international

experience, such as experience gained by European cities and Directives of the European Union concerning the selection of controlled pollutants, measurement methods, number and location of automatic stations.
Directive 2008/50/EC sets the requirements for number and location of monitoring stations (sampling points), controlled pollutants, measurement techniques, data capture, time coverage and the accuracy of measurements, gathered data and final information on mean concentrations of pollutants.
Regarding the number and location of automatic stations, monitored parameters, monitoring techniques and assets, Air quality monitoring system in Moscow complies with the EU Directives. The measurement techniques are presented in Table 1.

Pollutant	**measurement method used by Mosecomonitoring**
Carbon monoxide	Electro-chemistry, Non-dispersive infrared spectrometry
Nitrogen oxides	Chemiluminescence, DOAS
Sulfur dioxide	Ultraviolet fluorescence method, DOAS
Ozone	Ultraviolet photometry method, Ultraviolet fluorescence method, DOAS
PM10, PM2.5	Beta-guage, TEOM
VOC, Methane	Flame ionization (gas chromatography)
Ammonia	Chemiluminescence
H2S	Ultraviolet fluorescence method
Formaldehyde, Benzene, Toluene, Xylene, Phenol, etc.	DOAS
CO2	Infrared- absorption

Table 1. Measurement techniques.

At present, the Air quality monitoring system includes 37 automatic monitoring stations situated in all administrative districts of the city and covering typical locations of the city in order to represent exposure of general population to different levels and sources of pollution (Fig. 1). Four stations adjoin major motorways, 14 stations are located in residential areas, two stations - in protected nature areas, six stations – in residential areas adjoining industrial enterprises. In addition to this in 2007 two more monitoring stations were set up outside Moscow, at a distance of around 40-50 km from the borders of the city, on the leeward and windward sides judging by the dominant wind direction.
Furthermore, a multilevel monitoring station, which supplies the system with information on air quality at different altitudes (2 m, 130 m, 248 and 348 m above ground), was set up on Moscow TV tower Ostankino in November 2006 (Table 2).

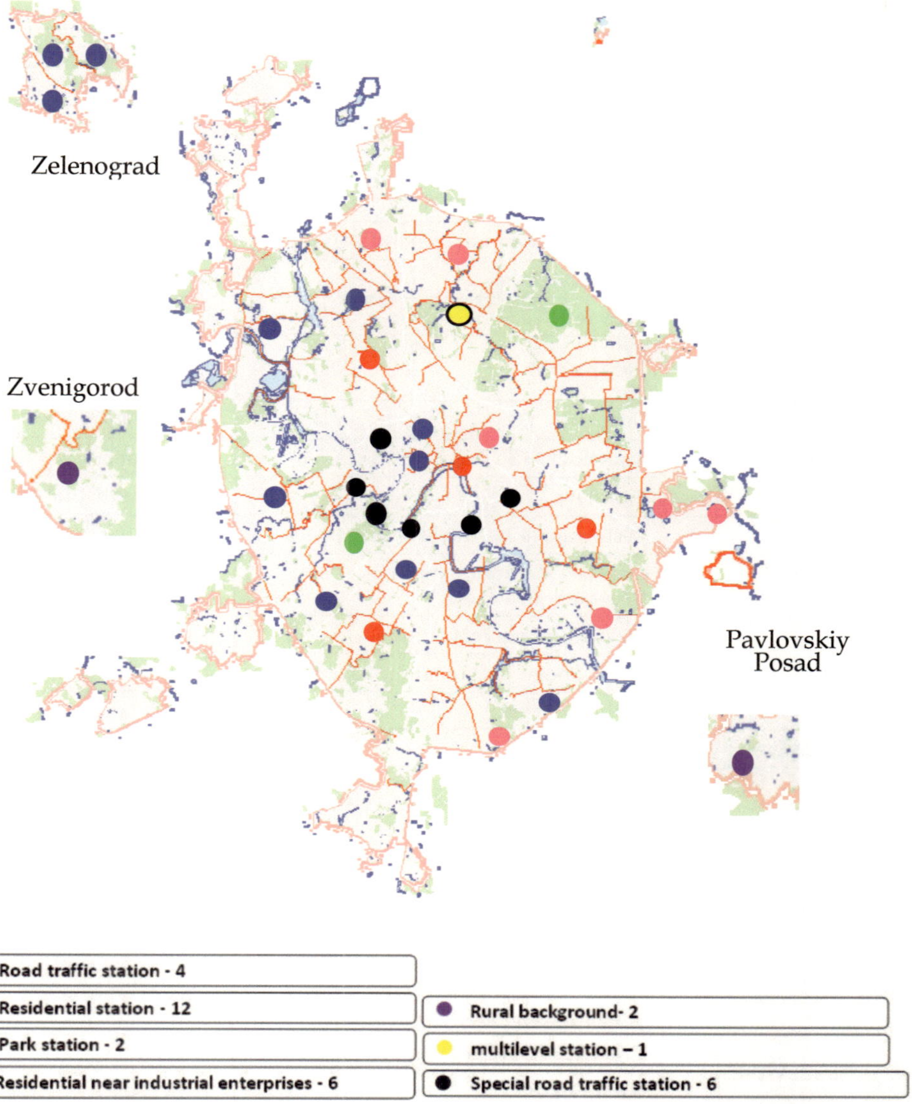

Fig. 1. Location of the automatic stations for the air quality monitoring in Moscow.

Automatic monitoring stations operate twenty-four-hours a day. The complete list of controlled pollutants includes 22 substances, such as CO, NO, NO_2, O_3, SO_2, H_2S, NH_3, CO_2, non - methane hydrocarbons (CH),methane (CH_4), formaldehyde (H_2CO), benzene, toluene, phenol and aerosol (mass concentration PM10 and PM2.5). The list of pollutants, controlled by any particular station, is individual and depends on the type of the territory and emission sources in the area. Still, the concentrations of nitrogen oxides and carbon monoxide are measured by every station. PM10 concentrations are measured at nine stations, ozone concentrations – at 9 and sulfur dioxide – at 10 stations (Table 3).

	Moscow district	Station name	Type of station
1	West	3d Circle ring (Kutuzovskiy pr.)	Special road traffic station
2		3d Circle ring (Kutuzovskiy pr.)	Special road traffic station
3	South West	3d Circle ring (Gagarina sq.)	Special road traffic station
4		3d Circle ring (Hamovnicheskiy Val st.)	Special road traffic station
5	South	3d Circle ring (r. Chura)	Special road traffic station
6	North	3d Circle ring (N. Maslovka st.)	Special road traffic station
7	Central	Balchug (Ovchinnikovskaya nab.)	Road traffic
8		Spiridonovka st.	Residential
9		Chayanova st.	Residential
10		Kazakova st.	Residential (R.) near industrial enterprises
11	South	Gur'evskiy pr.	Residential
12		Shabolovka (Shabolovskaya st.)	Residential
13		Biryulevo	R. near industrial enterprises
14	South East	Veshnyaki (4 Veshnyakovskiy pr.)	Road traffic
15		Marjino (Mar'inskiy park) (Novomarjinskaya st.)	R. near industrial enterprises
16	East	Kosino (Orangerejnaya st.)	R. near industrial enterprises
17		Kozhukhovo (Lukhmanovskaya st.)	R. near industrial enterprises
18		Losiniy Ostrov	Park station
19	North East	Polyarnaya st.	R. near industrial enterprises
20	North	MADI (Leningradsky pr.)	Road traffic
21		Dolgoprudnaya st.	R. near industrial enterprises
22		Koptevskiy bulvar	Residential
23	North West	Turistskaya st.	Residential
24	West	Tolbukhina st.	Residential
25		Vernadskogo pr.	Residential
26		MSU (Moscow State University)	Park station
27	South West	Cheremushki (Cheremushkinskaya st.)	Residential
28		Butlerova st.	Road traffic
29 30 31	Zelenograd (25 km to north west from Moscow)	Zelenograd 11(mikrorajon 11) Zelenograd 6 (mikrorajon 6) Zelenograd 15(mikrorajon 15)	Residential
32	60 km to west from Moscow	Zvenigorod	Rural background
33	60 km to east from Moscow	Pavlovskiy Posad	Rural background
34-37	North East	Ostankino 2m, 130m, 248m, 348m.	Multilevel station

Table 2. Monitoring stations of the SEI Mosecomonitoring

The initial concentration data are averaged over 20- min synchronous intervals, thus allowing a significance decrease in random measurement errors. Then averaged data are automatically introduce into the electronic data base. In accordance with the international standards, the gas analyzers and other instruments are regularly calibrated.

№	Pollutants	Number of stations
1	CO	32
2	NO_2	34
3	NO	28
4	O_3	17
5	PM10	9
6	PM2.5	2
7	SO_2	10
8	NH_3	2
9	H_2S	3
10	Benzene	6
11	Toluene	6
12	Formaldehyde	6
13	Phenol	6
14	Styrene	6
15	Naphthalene	6
16	M-xylene,	6
17	P-xylene,	6
18	Ethyl benzene	6
19	Methane	15
20	Volatile organic compounds VOC)	15
21	VOC without methane	15
22	CO_2	5

Table 3. Pollutants controlled

3. Temporal variability of the gaseous pollutants

Temporal variations of the pollutant concentrations (for example, CO concentration is denoted [CO]) take place over a wide range from minute to years. Some aspects of gaseous species variability are discussed in this section. Fig. 2. gives an idea about the concentration variations of (a) carbon monoxide, (b) nitrogen dioxide, (c) non – methane hydrocarbons, (d) methane, (e) aerosol and (f) ozone. Diurnal variability of the concentration is expressed markedly. The pronounced intradiurnal concentration variations exists. Temporal variations of the concentrations for the variations species and locations diverged considerably. The results presented in this section (Fig. 2) are in an agreement with those obtained previously (Gorchakov et al., 2009a). Some investigation results of the gaseous impurity concentrations presented in (Belikov et al., 2006; Elansky et al., 2007).

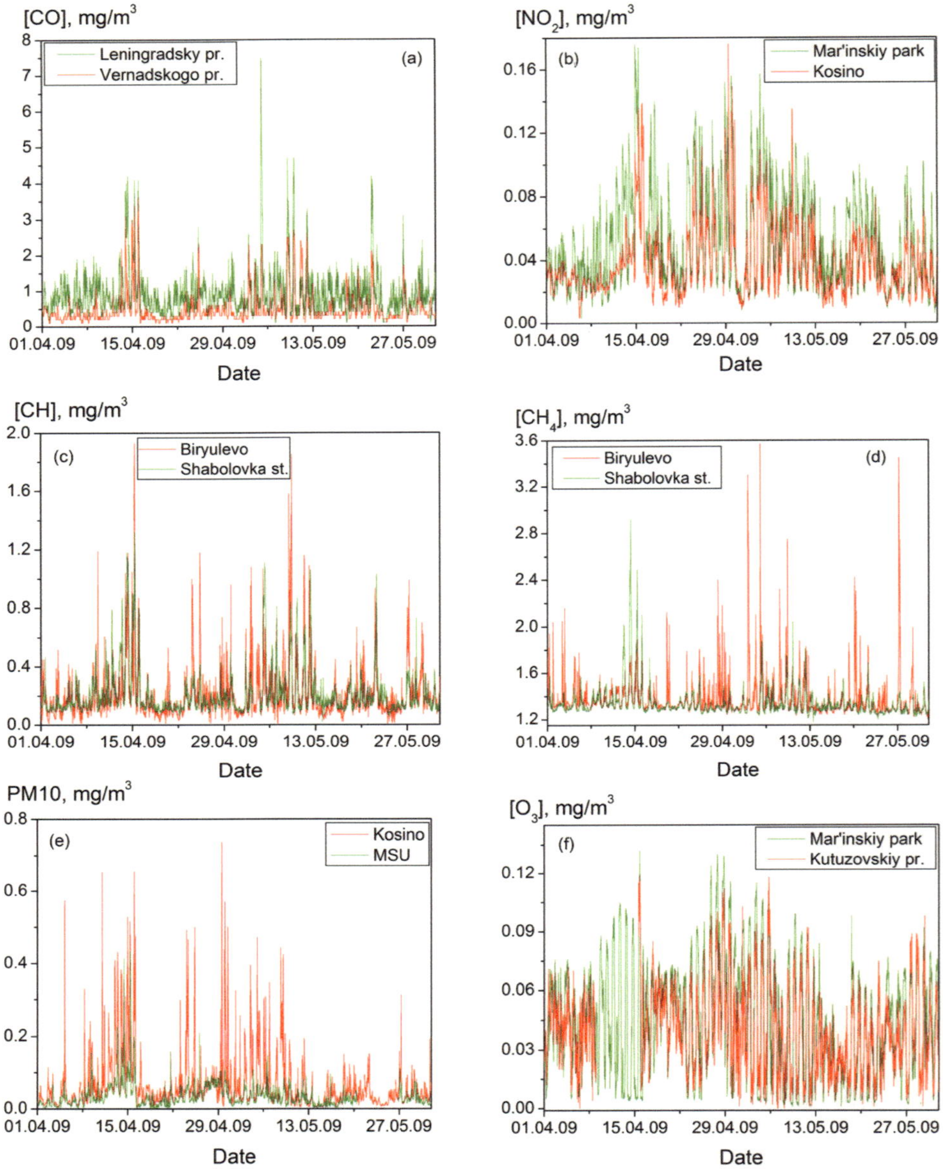

Fig. 2. Concentration variations of (a) carbon monoxide, (b) nitrogen dioxide, (c) non-methane hydrocarbons, (d) methane, (e) aerosol and (f) ozone.

3.1 Diurnal mean cycle of the gaseous species concentrations

Temporal variations of the gaseous species concentrations in 2009 were analyzed. The diurnal mean cycle concentration of carbon monoxide has been shown in Fig. 3 (a - Balchug, b - Kazakova st.). It is evident that the diurnal cycle of the carbon monoxide concentration exhibits the severe seasonal variations. The diurnal mean carbon monoxide various locations are distinguished markedly. Such peculiarities take place for nitrogen dioxide (Fig.

3 c, d), ozone (Fig. 3 e, f) and for other gaseous species. Diurnal concentration variations of carbon monoxide and nitrogen oxides were discussed previously in (Gorchakov et al., 2006). More recently diurnal cycle of non - methane hydrocarbons, methane and toluene was analyzed (Gorchakov et. al., 2009a).

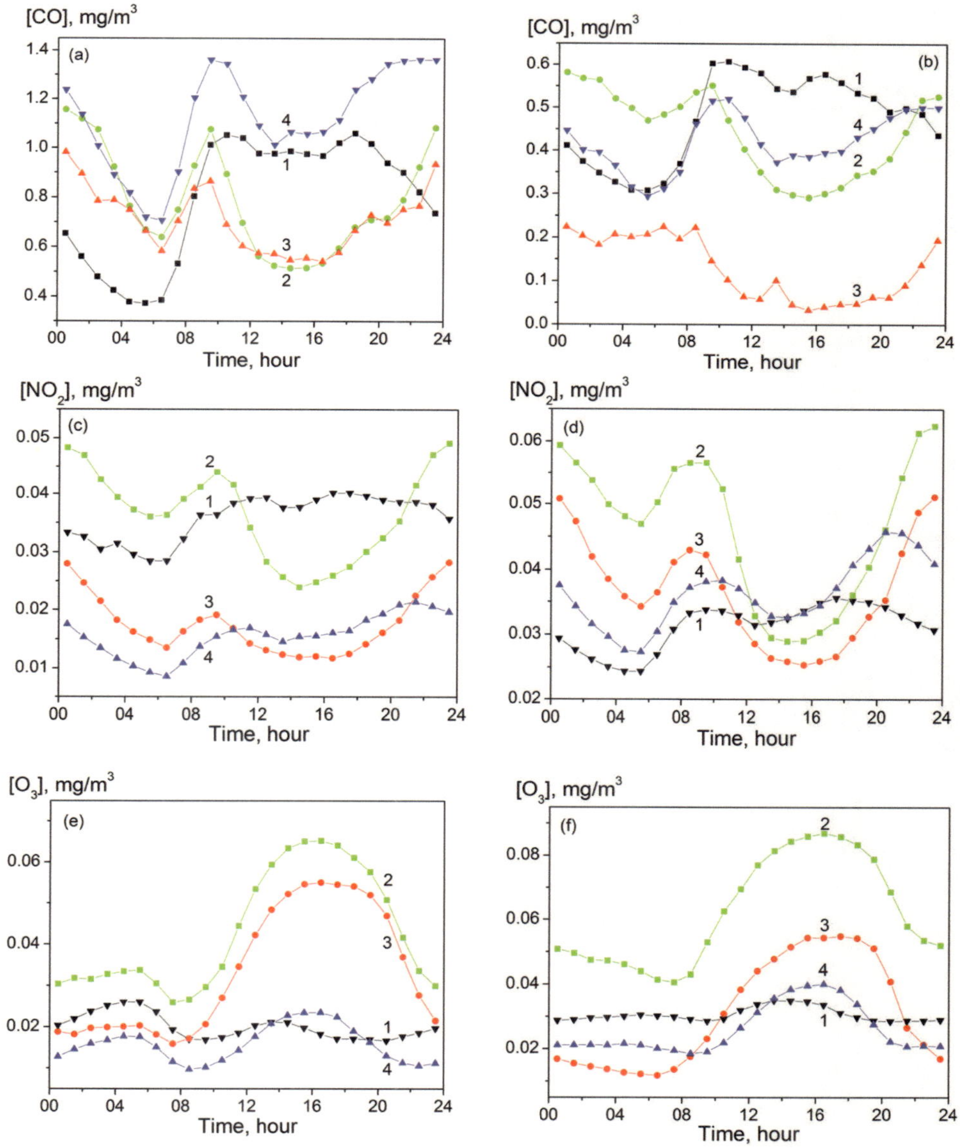

Fig. 3. Diurnal mean cycle (2009) of the carbon monoxide concentration (a - Balchug, b - Kazakova st.), the nitrogen dioxide concentration (c - Balchug, d - Mar'inskiy park) and the ozone concentration (e - Mar'inskiy park, f - Zvenigorod) in (1) winter, (2) spring, (3) summer, and (4) autumn.

As indicated earlier (Gorchakov et al., 2006) the diurnal mean cycle of the carbon monoxide concentration in Moscow changes markedly from the weekdays to the weekends.
Such changes were analyzed on the monitoring data in 2009 (Fig. 4) for (a) carbon monoxide (Balchug), (b) nitrogen dioxide (Mar'inskiy park), (c) ozone (Mar'inskiy park) and hydrogen sulphide (H_2S) (Kosino). Diurnal cycle discussed differ strongly for carbon monoxide, nitrogen dioxide and hydrogen sulphide. The investigation results of the air pollution week - long cycle in Moscow are contained in (Gorchakov et al., 2010) also.

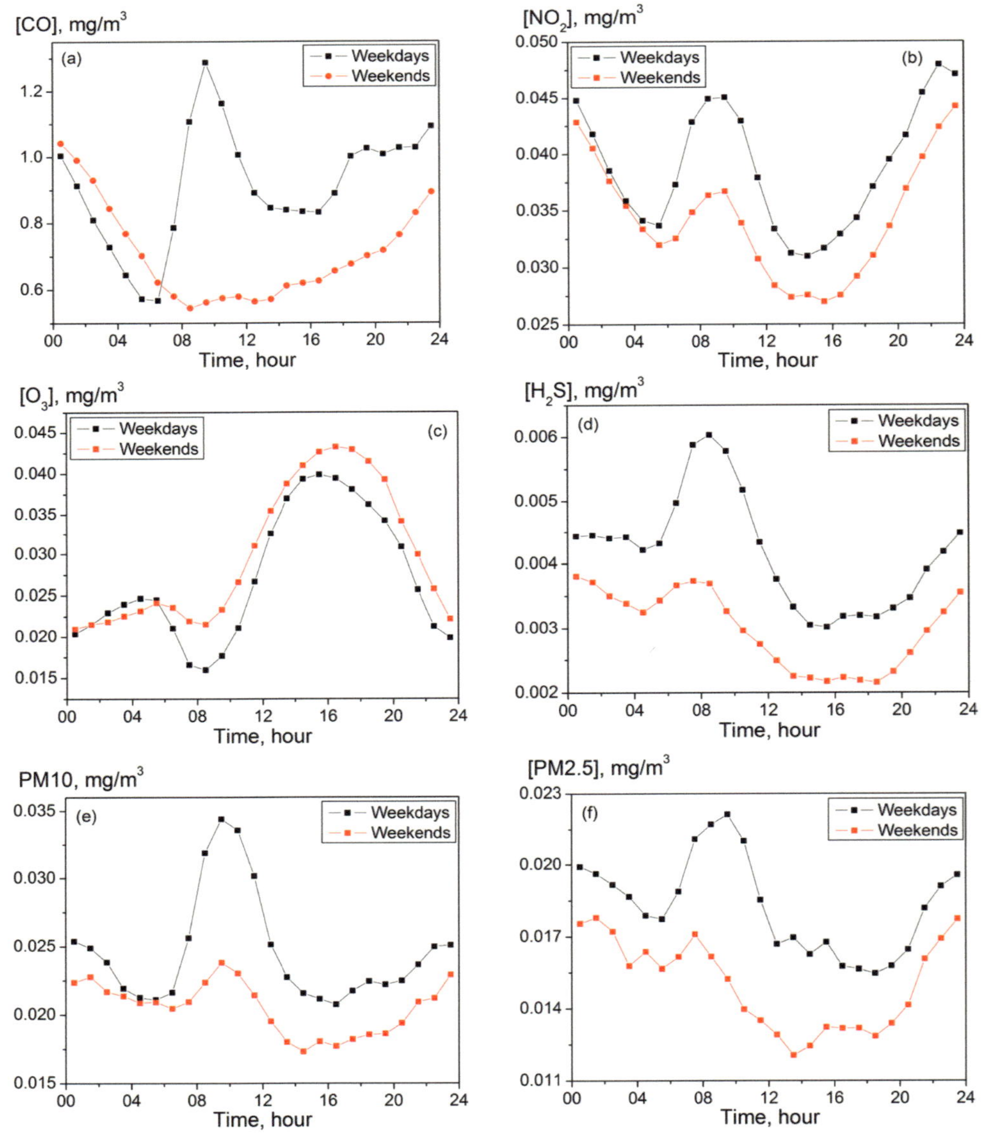

Fig. 4. Diurnal mean concentration cycles (2009) of (a) carbon monoxide (Balchug), (b) nitrogen dioxide (Mar'inskiy park), (c) ozone (Mar'inskiy park), (d) H_2S (Kosino), (e) PM10 (Shabolovka) and (f) PM2.5 (Kosino) at weekdays and at weekends.

3.2 Intraannual variability of the gaseous species concentrations

Intraannual cycles of the gaseous species concentrations (Fig. 5) are of great variety (MSU - Moscow State University). They change from one another for the various species and locations including carbon monoxide (Fig. 5a), nitrogen dioxide (Fig. 5b), non - methane hydrocarbons (Fig. 5c), methane (Fig. 5d) and ozone (Fig. 5f). Intraannual and seasonal concentration variability's for carbon monoxide, non-methane benzene, toluene, metaxylene and formaldehyde has been discussed in (Gorchakov et al., 2009a). Enhanced concentrations

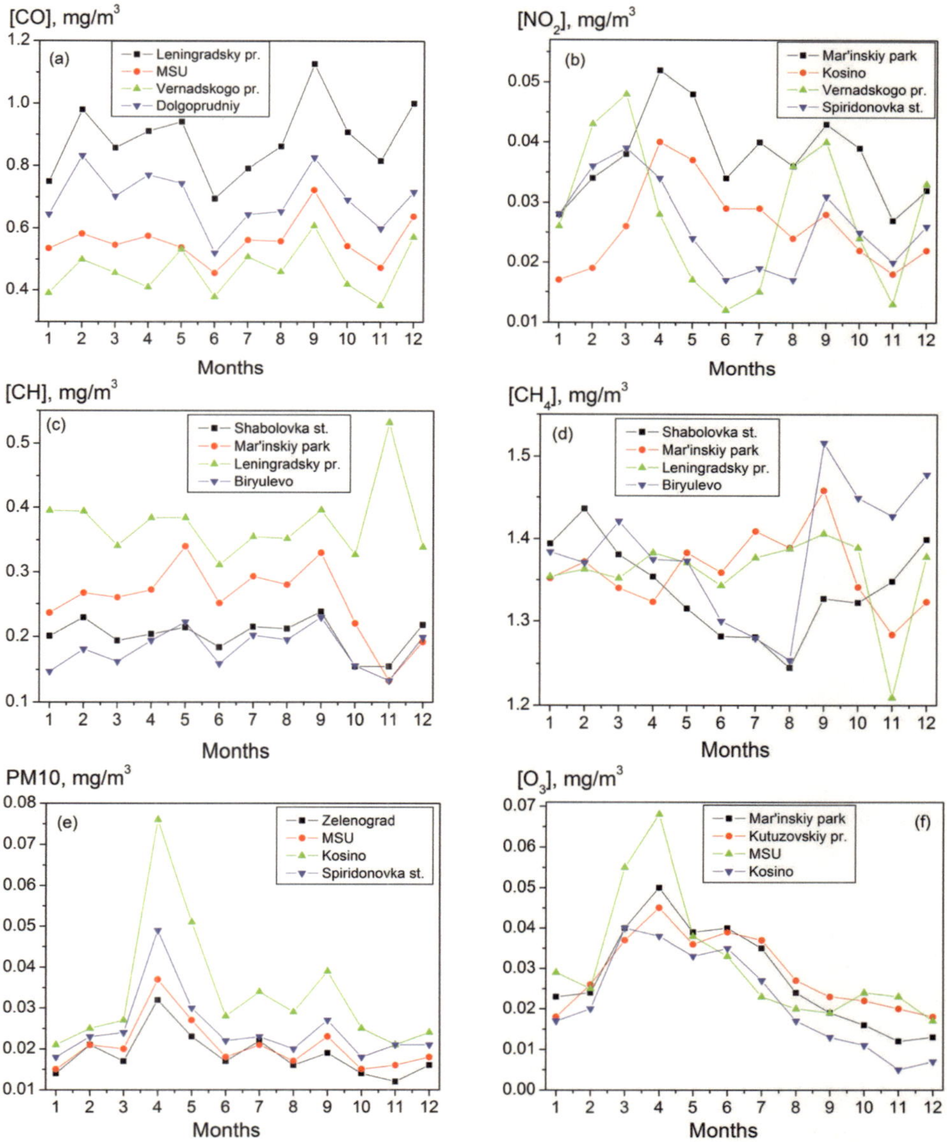

Fig. 5. Monthly average concentration (Moscow, 2009) of (a) carbon monoxide, (b) nitrogen dioxide, (c) non-methane hydrocarbons, (d) methane, (e) PM10 and (f) ozone.

of the gaseous species are observed under adverse weather conditions or smoke invasions during the forest and peatbog fires (section 7).

3.3 Interannual variability of the gaseous species concentrations

In Moscow the gaseous species interannual concentration experience a large variations. As an example we discuss the annual average concentration of the carbon monoxide (Table 4). There are many irregular variations of the carbon monoxide concentrations. It is evident (Table 4) that the average (for station group) concentration of carbon monoxide in 2002 - 2003 was approximately 2.5 times greater than the average concentration in 2008 - 2009.

Station	Year							
	2002	2003	2004	2005	2006	2007	2008	2009
Leningradsky pr.	2.2	2.5	2.4	2.2	1.5	1.3	0.9	0.9
Biryulevo	1.6	1.1	1.4	1.5	1.5	1.3	0.6	0.8
Balchug	1.5	1.7	1.2	1.1	1.0	0.8	0.8	0.9
Mar'inskiy park	1.6	2.1	1.0	0.8	0.7	0.8	0.5	0.5
Kazakova st.	2.0	1.8	1.2	1.6	1.5	0.9	0.5	0.4
Shabolovka st.	1.3	-	0.9	0.8	0.7	0.5	0.4	0.6
Kosino	-	0.7	1.6	0.7	0.8	0.9	0.6	0.5
Losiniy ostrov	-	0.7	0.6	0.6	0.4	0.4	0.4	0.4

Table 4. Annual average concentrations of carbon monoxide (mg/m^3).

3.4 Spectral analysis of the gaseous species concentration variations

The power spectral densities (Bendat & Piersol, 1986) of the gaseous species concentration variations were calculated for a number of stations. As an example, Fig. 6 shows the power spectral density of the nitrogen dioxide concentration variations calculated from the 2004 data obtained at Vernadskogo pr. It is easily seen that the spectral density $S(f)$ (1 in Fig. 7), where f is the frequency in inverse days, contains two components: continuous and quasi - discrete.

The continuous component is satisfactory approximated by a piecewise power spectrum

$$S_{*}(f) = Af^{k},$$

where $A = const$ and $k -$ exponent. Irregular diurnal variations in $[NO_2]$ with a periods of less than 24 h are approximated by the power spectrum (2 in Fig. 7) with the exponent - 2 approximately . It should be noted that there are no grounds to assign this power spectrum to universal spectrum. It was found that, for different stations and different years, the spectrum's exponent varies within a sufficiently wide range, a result which cannot be explained by measurement errors. The day-to-day variations of $[NO_2]$ are also approximated by a power spectrum (3 in Fig. 7). In the case under consideration, the exponent of the second approximating spectrum is approximately - 0.55. This spectrum cannot to universal spectra either. This exponent of spectrum varies within a comparatively wide range from station to station and from year to year. The approximating power spectra are joined together near the frequency $f_0 \cong 1$ day. The quasi - discrete component of the spectrum $S_{**}[NO_2]$ (4, 5 and 6 in Fig. 7) is due to the existence of a regular diurnal cycle containing harmonies with periods of 24, 12 and 8 h. The structure of the spectrum also varies markedly from station to station, this testifying to the spatial variability of the diurnal cycle of $[NO_2]$.

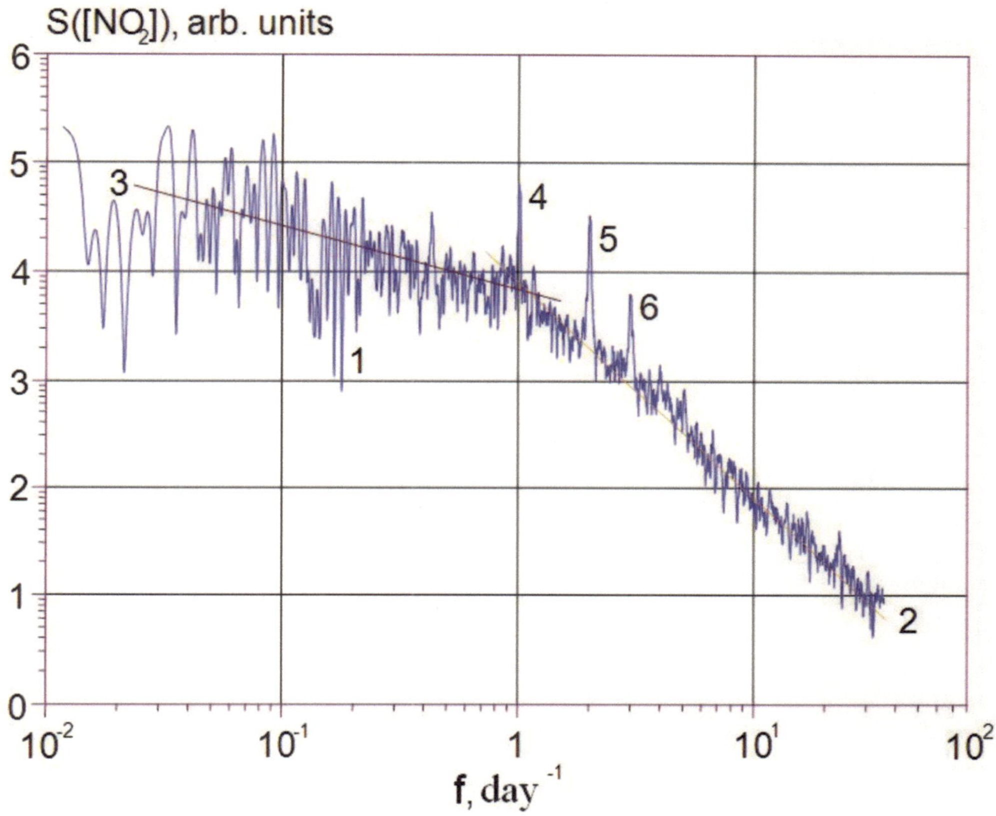

Fig. 6. Spectral power of the nitrogen dioxide concentration variations on the measurement data at Vernadskogo pr. in 2004 (2 and 3 – exponential approximating spectra; 4, 5 and 6 – harmonics with period 24, 12 and 8 hour).

4. Statistical analysis of the gaseous species concentration variations

The average values of the concentrations $\bar{C}_i = n_i^{-1}\sum_k C_{ik}$ (i is the pollutant number, k is the measurement number, and n_i is the number of measurements of the it h pollutant) were determined for the various time intervals. The basic statistical characteristics of concentration variations were calculated: the standard deviations σ_i and the dispersions $\sigma_i^2 = (n_i - 1)^{-1}\sum_k c_{ik}^2$ (for large series, it is convenient to replace n_i -1 by n_i), where

$c_{ik} = C_{ik} - \bar{C}$ - the deviations from average values; the variation coefficients $\gamma_i = \sigma_i / \bar{C}_i$, the skewness parameters $A_i = n_i^{-1} \sum_k c_{ik}^3$, and the excess parameters $E_i = -3 + n_i^{-1} \sigma_i^{-4} \sum_k c_{ik}^4$. In section 4, statistical characteristics of concentration variations were calculated from the monitoring data during 2009.

4.1 Carbon monoxide

Statistical characteristics of the carbon monoxide concentration variations for 8 station presented in Table 5. It is evident that average concentrations in Moscow is 2 - 3 times greater than outside the Moscow city (Pavlovskiy Posad, Losiniy ostrov, Zvenigorod). Carbon monoxide concentrations in 2004 in the average were approximately 2-times larger than the concentrations in 2009 (Gorchakov et al., 2006). As to the variation coefficients γ_i, they were approximately the same. An example of the empirical distribution function w [CO] (Narodnogo Opolcheniya st., 2004) is Fig. 7. This function is satisfactory approximated by log - normal distribution

$$p(x) = \frac{B_1}{\sigma_* \sqrt{2\pi}} \exp\left\{ -\frac{(x - x_0)^2}{2\sigma_*^2} \right\},$$

where $x = \ln([CO])$, $x_0 = 0.4$, $\sigma_* = 0.035$ and $B_1 = 18.5$. The empirical distribution

Station	$\bar{C}$ (mg/m³)	σ (mg/m³)	γ	A	E
Balchug	0.86	0.82	0.96	3.72	22.6
Leningradsky pr.	0.89	0.55	0.62	1.98	8.9
Biryulevo	0.78	0.72	0.92	3.60	19.9
Cheremushki	0.55	0.64	1.17	5.26	39.6
Chayanova st.	0.53	0.44	0.83	3.07	16.2
Pavlovskiy Posad	0.40	0.29	0.72	2.64	14.3
Losiniy Ostrov	0.37	0.29	0.78	3.34	23.5
Zvenigorod	0.28	0.26	0.92	1.78	8.7

Table 5. Statistical characteristics of the carbon monoxide (CO) concentration in 2009.

function w calculated on monitoring data in 2009 is shown in Fig. 8a with the distribution function for the smoke episode (section 7).

4.2 Nitrogen oxides

Statistical characteristics calculation results for nitrogen oxide and nitrogen dioxide are depicted in Table 6 and Table 7. Average annual concentrations of nitrogen oxides in 2009 are 1.5 - 2 times smaller than average concentrations in 2004 (Gorchakov et al., 2006). The empirical distribution function w of the nitrogen dioxide concentration is presented in Fig. 9 (Narodnogo Opolcheniya st., 2004). This distribution function is satisfactory approximated by log - normal distribution

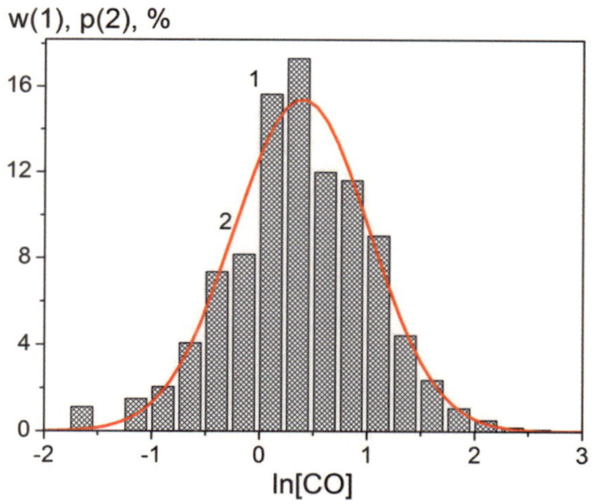

Fig. 7. The empirical distribution function w(1) of the carbon monoxide concentration in 2004 (Narodnogo Opolcheniya st.) and the log-normal approximated distribution p(2).

$$p(y) = \frac{B_2}{\sigma_{**}\sqrt{2\pi}} \exp\left\{-\frac{(y-y_0)^2}{2\sigma_*^2}\right\},$$

where $y = \ln([NO_2])$, $y_0 = -3.7$, $\sigma_{**} = 0.79$ and $C = 31.5$.

Additional examples of the empiric distribution function and NO_2 (2009) are presented in Fig. 8b. Temporal variations of the NO_2 concentration are illustrated in Fig. 3c, Fig. 3d, Fig. 4b and Fig. 5b.

4.3 Ozone

Ozone plays the important role in the atmospheric chemistry (Belan, 2009). The ozone importance in the ultraviolet and infrared radiation transfer is significant. The large ozone concentrations are a potential health hazard. Temporal variations of the ozone concentration is shown in Fig. 2f, the diurnal mean cycle of concentration – in Fig. 3e, Fig. 3f and Fig. 4c. Examples of the monthly average ozone concentration are presented in Fig. 5f.

Statistical characteristics of the ozone concentration variation at 5 stations (Moscow region, 2009) are presented in Table 8. The empirical distribution function of the ozone concentration is depicted in Fig. 8f.

Station	$\bar{C}$ (mg/m³)	σ (mg/m³)	γ	A	E
Cheremushki	0.029	0.055	1.92	5.78	45.0
Kazakova st.	0.030	0.051	1.68	3.78	37.6
Balchug	0.035	0.043	1.22	4.48	31.3
Kozhuhovo	0.020	0.034	1.72	3.95	20.4
Veshnyaki	0.043	0.082	1.92	4.61	30.0
Leningradsky pr.	0.067	0.057	0.85	2.68	13.2

Table 6. Statistical characteristics of the nitrogen oxide (NO) concentration in 2009.

Station	$\bar{C}$ (mg/m³)	σ (mg/m³)	γ	**A**	E
Kutuzovskiy pr.	0.044	0.022	0.50	1.20	2.80
Cheremushki	0.038	0.028	0.75	1.67	5.83
Kazakova st.	0.032	0.022	0.70	1.22	2.56
Balchug	0.026	0.021	0.80	2.30	19.9
Kozhuhovo	0.021	0.016	0.71	1.19	1.74

Table 7. Statistical characteristics of the nitrogen dioxide (NO_2) in 2009.

Station	$\bar{C}$ (mg/m³)	σ (mg/m³)	γ	**A**	E
Zvenigorod	0.038	0.029	0.76	0.72	0.33
Zelenograd	0.038	0.028	0.75	0.72	0.11
Gagarina sq.	0.033	0.022	0.68	0.81	0.35
Mar'inskiy park	0.028	0.023	0.84	0.99	0.48
Hamovniki	0.023	0.018	0.76	1.31	1.23

Table 8. Statistical characteristics of the ozone (O_3) concentration in 2009.

Station	$\bar{C}$ (mg/m³)	σ (mg/m³)	γ	**A**	E
Leningradsky pr.	0.38	0.17	0.45	2.37	11.1
Balchug	0.27	0.15	0.55	3.22	20.5
Pavlovskiy Posad	0.21	0.12	0.56	4.78	48.8
Cheremushki	0.17	0.16	0.93	3.68	18.2
Ostankino	0.16	0.11	0.67	2.95	14.7

Table 9. Statistical characteristics of the hydrocarbon concentration in 2009.

In the average the ozone concentrations is Moscow are markedly less than outside of city. Temporal variations of the ozone concentration in the Moscow region need further concentration.

4.4 Methane and non-methane hydrocarbons

In 2009 the average non-methane hydrocarbon concentration (Table 9) in Moscow were 20 – 30% higher than that in 2004 (Gorchakov et al., 2009 a). Variation coefficients γ of the non - methane concentration variations in 2009 were markedly less than that in 2004. Temporal variations of the non-methane hydrocarbon concentration are depicted in Fig. 2c and Fig. 5c, and temporal variations of the methane concentration – in Fig. 2d and Fig. 5d. It is hard to evaluate the interannual variability of the methane concentration now (Table 10). In the average the statistical parameters A and E in 2009 are markedly larger than that in 2004 (Corchakov et al., 2009 a).

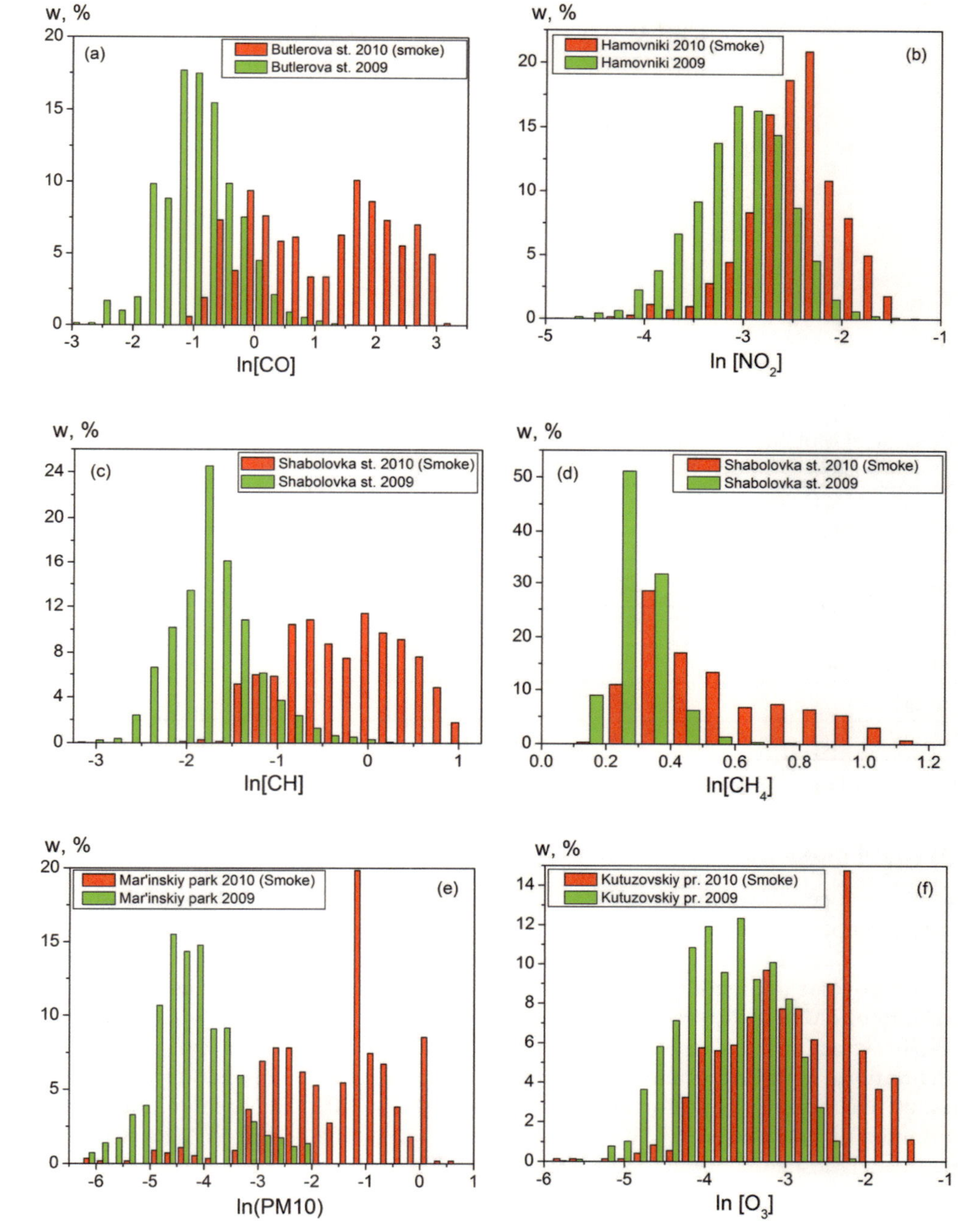

Fig. 8. Empirical distribution function for the concentrations (Moscow, 2009 - green; Moscow 2010, smoke episode - red) of (a) carbon monoxide, (b) nitrogen dioxide, (c) non-methane hydrocarbons, (d) methane, (e) PM10 and (f) ozone.

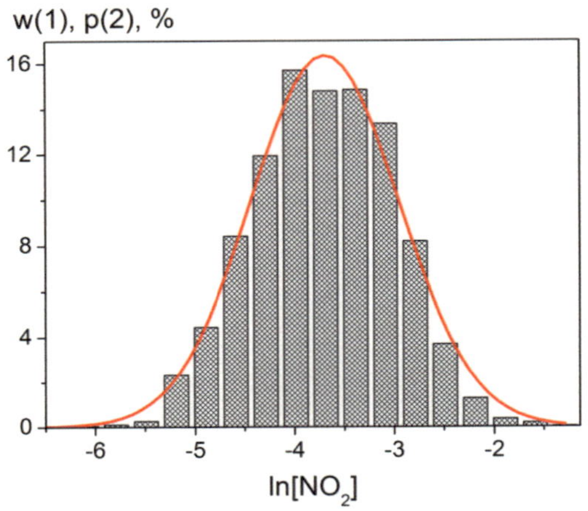

Fig. 9. The empirical distribution function w(1) of the nitrogen dioxide concentration in 2004 (Narodnogo Opolcheniya st.) and the log-normal approximating distribution p(2).

Station	$\bar{C}$	σ	γ	A	E
	mg/m³				
Cheremushki	1.45	0.11	0.078	2.76	35.6
Biryulevo	1.39	0.19	0.73	5.00	58.5
Mar'inskiy park	1.36	0.16	0.12	5.21	40.5
Vernadskogo pr.	1.27	0.25	0.19	7.19	79.3
Ostankino	1.26	0.095	0.076	1.85	9.30

Table 10. Statistical characteristics of the methane (CH_4) in 2009

5. Aerosol mass concentration

Aerosol mass concentration PM10 is measured at 9 stations and PM2.5 - at 2 stations at present. Temporal variability of PM10 is illustrated in Fig 2e. Examples of diurnal cycle of PM10 and PM2.5 at weekdays and weekends are depicted in Fig. 4e and 4f. It is evident that an anthropogenic influence on aerosol mass concentrations in Moscow is large. Intraannual variability of PM10 is illustrated in Fig. 5e. Statistical characteristics of PM10 variations are of PM10 variations are presented in Table 11 (Moscow, 2009). In the average PM10 concentrations in 2009 are markedly less than that in 2004 (Gorchakov et al., 2007) and variation coefficients in 2004 are larger than that in 2009. Example of the empirical distribution on function for PM10 is presented in Fig. 8e. The additional data about PM10 variations in Moscow can find in (Gorchakov et al., 2007).

6. Air pollution in the urban boundary layer

The modern strategy of environmental protection in urbanized territories stimulates the need for data from the monitoring of some pollutant components in the surface atmospheric air for the solutions to problems of the diagnosis and prediction of atmospheric air

Station	$\bar{C}$	σ	γ	A	E
	mg/m³				
Pavlovskiy Posad	0.029	0.030	1.02	5.36	59.3
Ostankino	0.027	0.024	0.87	4.55	41.4
Kozhuhovo	0.026	0.022	0.87	3.19	16.9
Shabolovka st.	0.023	0.020	0.83	4.25	31.9
Zelenograd	0.019	0.015	0.80	2.63	12.4

Table 11. Statistical characteristics of the PM10 in 2009.

pollution. However, the solution of problems of the spread and transformation of gas and aerosol pollutant components of the air basins of big cities presents serious difficulties associated with the lack of information on the meteorological processes in the atmospheric boundary layer over a city, including the formation of low level jet streams; the mechanisms of admixture transport by vertical structures, e.g., in street canyons; the role of the convective process; and the structure of a "multimodal heat island" over a city genetically related with the "pollution cap" and complex air circulation over a city. Hence there is a need for additional experimental studies of the meteorological processes and regularities of the vertical distribution of gas and aerosol admixtures in the urban boundary layer. Therefore, to identify the statistical regularities of pollutant concentration variations in the atmospheric boundary layer, the knowledge of which is necessary in order to create adequate pollutant spread models and to assess the ecologic state under conditions of dense and especially multistorey buildings, these data are clearly insufficient. Therefore, since November 2006 in Moscow, in the framework of an urban system of atmospheric air pollution control, the monitoring of the vertical distributions of certain gas components of atmospheric air pollution from the Ostankino TV Tower has been performed. The monitoring of the vertical profiles of gas components of atmospheric air pollution over the city together with the monitoring of gas and aerosol components at 35 sites in Moscow and two sites outside of the Moscow megapolis provide invaluable information on the complex processes of pollutant transport and transformation in the air basin of a big megapolis.

In this chapter are analyzed the monitoring data of the carbon monoxide and nitrogen dioxide concentrations on 4 levels of the Osnankino TV tower.

Statistical characteristics of the carbon monoxide concentration variations in 2009 (Table 12) are consistent with results presented in (Gorchakov et. al., 2009 b). Vertical profile of the nitrogen dioxide concentration variations are of interest. In the average maximal concentration of nitrogen dioxide is observed at height 130 m (Table 13) and minimal concentration - at height 348 m.

Height, m	$\bar{C}$	σ	γ	A	E
	mg/m³				
2	0.56	0.46	0.82	3.28	17.1
130	0.39	0.29	0.74	2.76	16.7
248	0.40	0.31	0.76	2.64	17.0
348	0.37	0.46	1.23	4.76	40.1

Table 12. Statistical characteristics of the carbon monoxide (CO) concentration (Ostankino, 2009).

Height, м	$\bar{C}$	σ	γ	A	E
	mg/m^3				
2	0.027	0.014	0.54	1.01	1.50
130	0.043	0.025	0.58	2.05	7.22
248	0.025	0.023	0.92	1.70	4.14
348	0.016	0.013	0.81	1.60	4.65

Table 13. Statistical characteristics of the nitrogen dioxide (NO_2) concentration (Ostankino, 2009).

7. Air pollution in the smoky atmosphere

The biomass burning represents a powerful source of the specific aerosol. Large-scale forest, peatbog and steppe fires have long been the subject of geophysical studies, because smoke formation leads to a radical change in the atmospheric radiative regime and, consequently, is capable of causing noticeable regional climatic effects. Characteristic examples of burning of large biomass amounts are the peatbog fires that happened in 1972 and 2002 in central Russia. The extent of the smoke screening of Moscow region in summer 2010 was exceed preceding events (Gorchakov et al., 2011).

7.1 Surface layer contamination

The carbon monoxide concentrations in Moscow during the forest - peat bog fires in the summer season of 2010 reached an extreme large values (Fig. 10). Statistical characteristics of the carbon monoxide concentration variations at 7 stations and maximal concentrations (C_{max}) for during period from 1 August to 11 August are given in Table 14. In this time average concentration of carbon monoxide were 3 – 5 times greater than the annual average concentrations.

Station	$\bar{C}$	σ	C_{max}	γ	A	E
	mg/m^3					
Balchug	7.24	7.34	37.4	1.01	1.48	1.68
Cheremushki	6.84	7.48	33.7	1.09	1.29	0.72
Butlerova st.	5.03	4.88	20.2	0.97	1.13	0.28
Dolgoprudnaya st.	5.02	4.72	23.8	0.94	1.24	1.00
Vernadskogo pr.	4.75	4.57	18.0	0.96	1.13	0.24
Pavlovskiy Posad	4.13	4.15	19.5	1.01	1.52	2.09
Zvenigorod	3.14	3.34	15.4	1.07	1.38	1.22

Table 14. Statistical characteristics of the carbon monoxide (CO) concentration (2010, smoke).

The maximal concentration of carbon monoxide in 2010 was 2.5 times larger than that in 2002 (Gorchakov et al., 2003, 2004). Statistical parameters A and E for the smoky atmosphere were markedly less then that in 2009. The empirical distribution function of [CO] are depicted in Fig. 8a (smoke screening period).

Exceeding probabilities of the some threshold concentration for carbon monoxide in the smoky atmosphere were calculated (Table 15). In 2004 exceeding the level of 15 mg/m^3 are not observed (Gorchakov et al., 2006). Average concentrations of nitrogen dioxide (Table 16) in the smoky atmosphere were approximately 2 - 3 times great as before (in 2009).

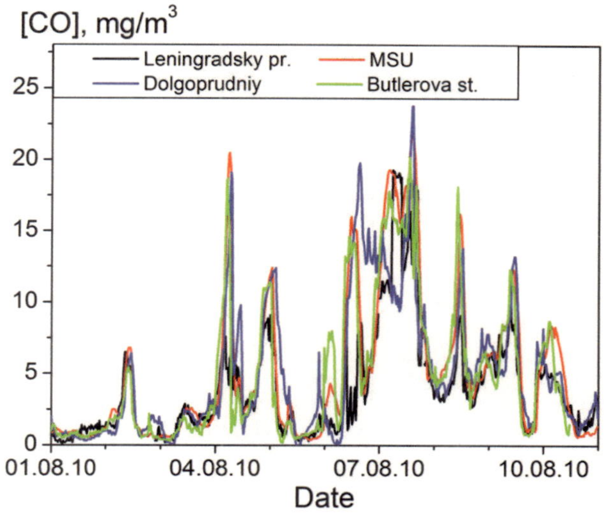

Fig. 10. Temporal variations of the carbon monoxide concentration in the smoky atmosphere.

Ozone concentrations in the Moscow city during the period under review were 1.5 - 2 times greater than the topical concentrations, as a rule (Table 17). Statistical parameters γ, A and E for ozone in the smoky atmosphere differ little from the statistical parameters for ozone in 2009. The empirical distribution functions of [NO_2] and [O_3] are presented in Fig. 8b and Fig. 8f (smoke screening period).

Station	Threshold concentrations						
	5	10	15	20	25	30	35
Balchug	49.2	24.3	15.3	8.5	3.9	1.25	0.14
Cheremushki	44.7	26.6	17.2	9.4	2.8	0.70	-
Gur'evskiy pr.	38.2	9.8	4.0	1.7	0.70	-	-
Biryulevo	29.5	10.2	5.3	1.0	-	-	-
Kazakova st.	25.8	8.3	2.3	1.1	-	-	-
Shabolovka	27.3	12.7	2.0	-	-	-	-

Table 15. Exceeding probabilities (%) of the threshold concentrations (mg/m^3) for carbon monoxide in the smoke screening period.

Statistical characteristics of the concentration variations of non - methane hydrocarbons and methane are presented in Table 18 and Table 19.

The average methane concentration in the smoky atmosphere exceed insignificantly average concentrations in 2009. The empirical distribution function of [CH] and [CH_4] are shown in Fig. 8c and Fig. 8d.

Station	$\bar{C}$	σ	γ	A	E
	mg/m³				
Biryulevo	0.126	0.058	0.46	0.46	- 0.42
Hamovniki	0.094	0.040	0.43	0.90	0.92
Tolbuhina st.	0.073	0.058	0.80	1.36	1.92
MSU	0.068	0.025	0.37	1.88	7.31
Zelenograd	0.058	0.040	0.69	1.10	0.58
Pavlovskiy Posad	0.044	0.026	0.60	1.04	1.12
Cheremushki	0.038	0.021	0.56	0.99	0.93
Zvenigorod	0.032	0.022	0.70	1.17	1.64

Table 16. Statistical characteristics of the nitrogen dioxide (NO_2) concentration (2010, smoke)

Station	$\bar{C}$	σ	γ	**A**	E
	mg/m³				
Kutuzovsky pr.	0.074	0.052	0.70	1.02	0.50
Maslovka	0.063	0.035	0.55	1.20	1.35
Spiridonovka st.	0.049	0.052	1.07	0.96	- 0.04
Mar'inskiy park.	0.045	0.048	1.07	1.31	1.69
Pavlovskiy Posad	0.045	0.036	0.79	0.63	- 0.94

Table 17. Statistical characteristics of the ozone concentration (2010, smoke)

Station	$\bar{C}$	σ	γ	**A**	E
	mg/m³				
Golovacheva st.	1.10	0.73	0.66	1.39	1.88
Tolbukhina st.	1.07	0.73	0.69	0.68	- 0.74
Vernadskogo pr.	0.99	0.60	0.60	1.46	3.90
Cheremushki	0.94	0.72	0.77	1.15	0.79
Mar'inskiy park	0.71	0.78	1.09	1.24	0.70
Biryulevo	0.69	0.56	0.80	1.57	2.23
Zelenograd	0.57	0.41	0.71	0.88	0.02

Table 18. Statistical characteristics of non-methane hydrocarbon concentration (2010, smoke)

Station	$\bar{C}$	σ	γ	A	E
	mg/m³				
Golovacheva st.	1.94	0.69	0.36	1.31	0.84
Cheremushki	1.78	0.42	0.23	1.42	1.58
Biryulevo	1.66	0.45	0.27	2.24	5.81
Zelenograd	1.41	0.26	0.19	1.11	0.53
Tolbukhina st.	1.37	0.31	0.23	1.16	2.62

Table 19. Statistical characteristics of the methane (CH_4) concentrations (2010, smoke)

Temporal variations of the formaldehyde concentrations in the smoky atmosphere are shown in Fig. 11. Statistical characteristics of the formaldehyde concentration variations in 2009 and in the smoky atmosphere (2010) are presented in Table 20.

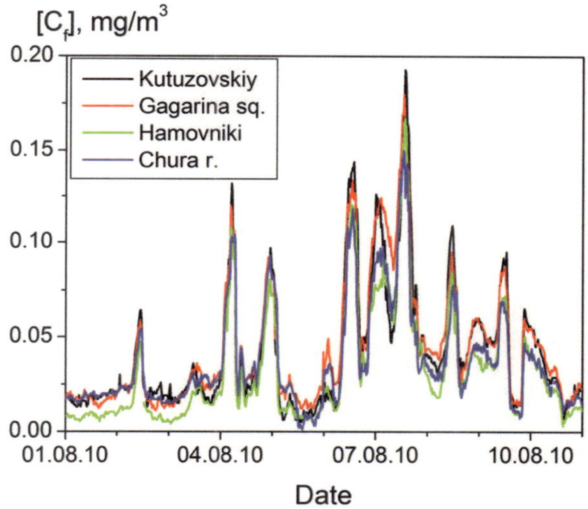

Fig. 11. Temporal variations of the formaldehyde concentration in the smoky atmosphere.

Year	Station	$\bar{C}$	σ	γ	A	E
		mg/m³				
2010 Smoke	Kutuzovskiy pr.	0.042	0.034	0.81	1.60	2.39
	Gagarina sq.	0.044	0.033	0.75	1.48	1.74
	Hamovniki	0.032	0.028	0.73	1.59	2.19
	Chura river	0.038	0.028	0.73	1.58	2.29
2009	Kutuzovskiy pr.	0.0104	0.0079	0.76	1.83	5.11
	Gagarina sq.	0.0143	0.0094	0.66	-0.36	0.19
	Hamovniki	0.0042	0.0030	0.72	0.23	-0.02
	Chura river	0.0106	0.0088	0.82	2.34	9.90

Table 20. Statistical characteristics of the formaldehyde concentrations (2009 and 2010-smoke)

7.2 Urban boundary layer

Extremely large concentrations of carbon monoxide occurred in the boundary layer also. Statistical characteristics of the carbon monoxide concentration variations at heights 2 m, 130 m, 248 m and 348 m are presented in Table 21. The average concentration of carbon monoxide at height of 348 m for less than at the smaller heights.

Statistical characteristics of the nitrogen dioxide concentration variations have been calculated (Table 22). The average profile of the nitrogen dioxide concentration in the smoky atmosphere is similar to the annual average profile. Thus the nitrogen dioxide concentration variations don't associate with the smoke screening of the urban atmosphere.

Height, м	$\bar{C}$	σ	γ	A	E
	mg/m³				
2	3.93	3.90	0.99	1.38	1.42
130	4.27	4.21	0.99	1.22	0.59
248	4.20	3.78	0.90	1.35	1.72
348	1.50	3.14	2.10	3.24	10.7

Table 21. Statistical characteristics of the carbon monoxide (CO) concentration (Ostankino, smoke).

Height, м	$\bar{C}$	σ	γ	A	E
	mg/m³				
2	0.034	0.028	0.84	2.15	11.3
130	0.049	0.029	0.58	0.81	0.07
248	0.025	0.024	0.97	2.20	7.04
348	0.014	0.011	o.77	2.25	7.340

Table 22. Statistical characteristics of the nitrogen dioxide (NO_2) concentration (Ostankino, smoke).

7.3 Aerosol mass concentration

In the smoky atmosphere of Moscow the extreme large aerosol mass concentrations PM10 have been observed (Table 23). Temporal variations of PM10 in the smoky atmosphere are depicted in Fig. 12.

The average mass concentrations in the smoke screening periods were 10 – 15 times greater than the annual average mass concentrations. Statistical parameters A and E in the smoky atmosphere were markedly less than that in 2009.

Station	$\bar{C}$	σ	C_{max}	γ	A	E
	mg/m³					
Kozhuhovo	0.345	0.314	1.68	0.91	1.26	1.25
Mar'inskiy park	0.317	0.303	1.72	0.96	1.40	1.50
Zelenograd	0.288	0.258	1.08	0.90	0.91	- 0.18
MSU	0.280	0.290	1.15	1.03	1.02	- 0.10

Table 23. Statistical characteristics of the aerosol mass concentration PM10 (2010, smoke)

8. Air pollution, adverse weather conditions and pollution health

Sufficiency elevated temperatures took place in July - August 2010 over European part of Russia. The temperature measurement data at Mosecomonitoring stations in the smoke screening period are presented in Fig. 13. "The urban heat island" over Moscow (Spiridonovka st., Ostankino) at the night time is clearly pronounced against a background (Zvenigorod station). The intensity of the temperature inversion reached 10 °C in the lower200 m thick layer. Wind velocity in the lower layer of the atmosphere was moderate

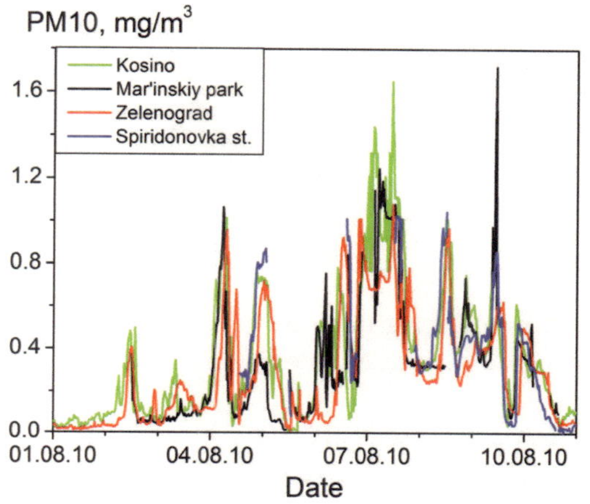

Fig. 12. Temporal variations of PM10 in the smoky atmosphere.

(Kallistratova, 2010). Meteorological conditions in July - August 2010 made for accumulation of the air pollution and containment of the smoke in the urban boundary layer. The joint action of the high temperature and the heavy air pollution impact negatively on the pollution health (Grechko et., 2010). In this period the premature mortality in central Russia has been grown (Revich, 2010).

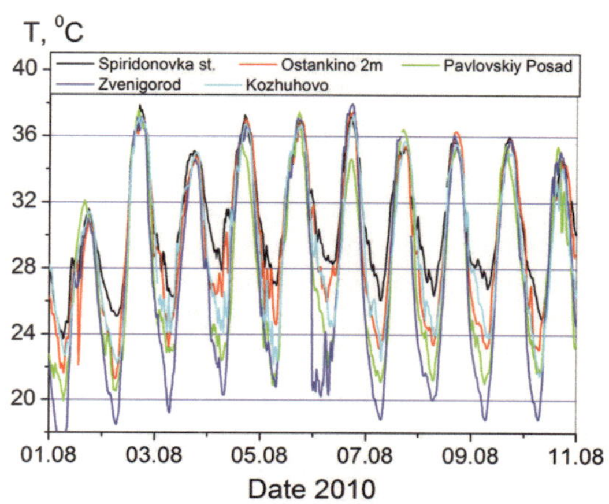

Fig. 13. Air temperature in the atmospheric surface layer at Mosecomonitoring stations (smoke screening period).

9. Conclusion

In this chapter the air pollution monitoring data in the Moscow region have been partly examined. The temporal variation of the gaseous species concentrations were analyzed including the diurnal and annual cycle of abovementioned concentrations. Statistical characteristic of the concentration variations for carbon monoxide, nitrogen oxides, ozone, methane and non - methane hydrocarbons has been calculated.

The aerosol mass concentration variations in Moscow region are discussed. The air pollution investigation results in the urban boundary layer are presented. The gaseous species and aerosol variability in smoky atmosphere is analyzed. It is shown that the aerosol mass concentration and carbon monoxide concentration in the smoke screening period were extremely large. The adverse weather conditions and the heavy air pollution influence on the population health are briefly discussed. It should be noted that the uncontrolled instrumental errors were possible in the smoky atmosphere.

10. Acknowledgment

In the work, the ecological monitoring data performed by State Environmental Institution Mosecomonitoring on the network of automated stations of ambient air quality control were used.

The study was supported by RFBR (project 11 - 05 - 01144).

Authors thank E. Baikova and A. Kolesnikova for the participation in the measurement data processing.

11. References

Belan, B. (2009). Tropospheric Ozone. 6. Components of Main Cycles. *Atmos. Ocean. Opt.* Vol. 22, No. 4. (April 2009), pp. 358 - 370, ISSN 1024 - 8560

Belikov, I.; Brennikmeijer, K.; Elansky, N. & Ral'ko, A. (2006). Methane, Carbon Monoxide, and Carbon Dioxide Concentrations Measured in the Atmospheric Surface Layer over Continental Russia in the TROICA Experiments. *Izv. Atmos. Ocean. Phys.* Vol. 42, No. 1, pp. 46 - 59, ISSN 0001 - 4338.

Bendat, J. & Piersol, A. (1986). *Random Data. Analysis and Measurement Procedures*, Wiley, ISBN 0-471-04000-2, New York, USA

Grechko, E.; Gorchakov, G.; Dzhola, A.; Emilenko, A.; Elokhov, A.; Isakov, A.; Rakitin, V; Sviridenkov, M.; Fokeeva, E.; Teterina, N.; Artamonova, M. & Maksimenkov, L. (2010). Air pollution measurement results in the fire periods (Moscow region, July - August 2010). Preliminary analysis of the fire influence on the population health, *Proceedings of Conference Air basin Moscow city state in extreme weather conditions in summer 2010*, pp. 88 -90, Moscow, Russia, November 25, 2010

Gorchakov, G.; Anikin, P.; Voloch, A.; Emilenko, A.; Isakov, A.; Kopeikin, V.; Ponomareva, T.; Semoutnikova, E.; Sviridenkov, M. & Shukurov, K. (2003). Study of the Composition of the Atmospheric Smoke Screen over the Moscow Region, *Doklady Earth Sciences*, Vol. 390, Part. 2, (May 2003), pp. 562 - 565, ISSN 1028 - 334X.

Gorchakov, G.; Anikin, P.; Voloch, A.; Emilenko, A.; Isakov, A.; Kopeikin, V.; Ponomareva, T.; Semoutnikova, E.; Sviridenkov, M. & Shukurov, K. (2004). Studies of the

Smoked Atmosphere Composition over Moscow during Turf Fires in the Summer - Fall Season of 2002, *Izv., Atmos. Ocean. Phys.*, Vol. 40, No 1, (January 2004), pp. 323 - 336, ISSN 0001 - 4338

Gorchakov, G.; Semoutnikova, E.; Zotkin, E.; Karpov, A.; Lezina, E. & Ul'yanenko, A. (2006). Variations in Gaseous Pollutants in the Air Basin of Moscow, *Izv., Atmos. Ocean. Phys.* Vol. 42, No. 2, (March 2006), pp. 156 - 170, ISSN 0001 - 4338

Gorchakov, G.; Semoutnikova, E.; & Anoshin, B. (2007). Statistical Analysis of the Mass Concentration Variations of the Coarse Aerosol in Moscow. *Atmos. Ocean. Opt.*, Vol.. 20, No. 6, (June 2007), pp. 461 - 464, ISSN 1024 - 8560

Gorchakov, G.; Semoutnikova, E.; Anoshin, B.; Karpov, A.; & Kolesnikova, A. (2009a). Hydrocarbons in an Urban Atmosphere, *Izv., Atmos. Ocean. Phys.*, Vol. 45, No. 3, (May 2009), pp. 314 - 323, ISSN 0001 - 4338

Gorchakov, G.; Semoutnikova, E.; Glyadkov, P.; Karpov,A.; Kolesnikova, A.; & Lezina, E. (2009b). Vertical Profiles of Concentrations of Carbon Monoxide and Nitrogen Oxides in the Urban Atmospheric Boundary Layer, *Atmos. Ocean. Opt.*, Vol. 22, No. 6, (June 2009), pp. 617 - 625, ISSN 1024 - 8560

Gorchakov, G.; Semoutnikova, E.; Anoshin, B.; Karpov, A. & Kolesnikova, A. (2010a). Statistical Prediction of the Urban Atmosphere Contamination. 1. Statistical Regularities of Interdiurnal Variability of the Carbon Monoxide and Nitrogen Oxides Concentrations, *Atmos. Ocean. Opt.*, Vol. 23, No. 4, (April 2010), pp. 309 - 316, ISSN 1024 - 8560

Gorchakov, G.; Semoutnikova, E.; Anoshin, B.; Karpov, A. & Kolesnikova, A. (2010b). Statistical Prediction of the Urban Atmosphere Contamination. 2. Forecasting Method of the Interdiurnal and Intradiurnal Concentration Variability of the Carbon Monoxide and Nitrogen Oxides, *Atmos. Ocean. Opt.*, Vol. 23, No. 5, (May 2010), pp. 396 - 403, ISSN 1024 - 8560

Gorchakov, G.; Semoutnikova, E.; Karpov, A.; Kolesnikova, A.; Baykova, E. & Zadorojnaya, O. (2010c). Air Pollution Week-Long Cycle in Moscow: of Refinement Quantitative Parameters and Statistical Forecasting of Impurity Concentration, *Atmos. Ocean. Opt.*, Vol. 23, No. 9, (September 2010), pp. 784 - 792, ISSN 1024 - 8560

Gorchakov, G.; Kopeikin, V.; Sviridenkov, M.; Semoutnikova, E.; Chubarova, N.; Emilenko, A.; Isakov, A.; Karpov, A. & Lezina, E. (2010d). Optical and microphysical properties of the aerosol in the smoky atmosphere of Moscow region, *Proceedings of Conference Air basin Moscow city state in extreme weather conditions in summer 2010*, pp. 40 -41, Moscow, Russia, November 25, 2010

Gorchakov, G.; Sviridenkov, M.; Semoutnikova, E.; Chubarova, N.; Holben, B.; Smirnov, A.; Emilenko, A.; Isakov, A.; Kopeikin, V.; Karpov, A.; Lezina, E. & Zadorozhnaya, O. (2011) Optical and Microphysical Parameters of the Aerosol in the Smoky Atmosphere of the Moscow Region in 2010, *Doklady Earth Sciences*, Vol. 437, Part 2, (April 2011), pp. 513 - 517, ISSN 1028 - 334X

Elansky, N.; Lokoshenko, M.; Belikov, I.; Skorohod, A. & Schumsky, R. (2007). Variability of Trace Gaseous in the Atmospheric surface Layer from observations in the City of Moscow. *Izv., Atmos. Ocean. Phys.*, Vol. 43, No. 2 (March 2007), pp. 219 - 321, ISSN 0001 - 4338

Kallistratova, M.; Kramer, V.; Kuznetsov, D.; Kulichkov, S.; Kuznnetsova, I. & Ushkov, V. (2010). Wind field and turbulence over Moscow in Summer 2010, *Proceedings of Conference Air basin Moscow city state in extreme weather conditions in summer 2010* , pp. 26 - 28, Moscow, Russia, November 25, 2010

Revich, B. (2010). Hot summer 2010 and population mortality of European part of Russia, *Proceedings of Conference Air basin Moscow city state in extreme weather conditions in summer 2010*, pp.73 - 78, Moscow, Russia, November 25, 2010

12

Impact of Urban Air Pollution on Acute Upper Respiratory Tract Infections

Marcos Abdo Arbex[1,3,4], Silvia Leticia Santiago[3],
Elisangela Providello Moyses[3], Luiz Alberto Pereira[1,2],
Paulo Hilário Saldiva[1] and Alfésio Luís Ferreira Braga[1,2]
[1]*Environmental Epidemiology Study Group,*
Laboratory of Experimental Air Pollution, Pathology Department,
University of São Paulo Faculty of Medical Science,
[2]*Environmental Exposure and Risk Assessment Group,*
Collective Health Post-graduation Program,
Catholic University of Santos
[3]*Internal Medicine Post-graduation Program,*
Federal University of São Paulo Medical School,
[4]*Pulmonology Division, Internal Medicine Department,*
Araraquara University Center Medical School, Araraquara
Brazil

1. Introduction

Epidemiological studies have shown consistent acute adverse health effects of ambient air pollution and in particular, traffic related pollution on the respiratory health system.. Outcomes with different degrees of severity, from sub-clinical lung function changes to respiratory and cardiovascular symptoms, changes in the use of respiratory and cardiovascular medication, impaired activities (e.g., school and work absenteeism), exacerbation of pre-existing diseases such as asthma and chronic obstructive pulmonary disease (COPD), primary care and/or emergency room visits, hospitalizations and mortality have been investigated. Children, the elderly and those with previous cardiorespiratory disease are the most susceptible groups (American Thoracic Society, 2000; Brunekreef & Holgate, 2002; Berstein et al., 2004; Gouveia & Maisonet, 2006; Ko & Huy, 2010; Perez et al., 2010).

In terms of adverse health effects caused by air pollutants, the more severe the clinical manifestation, the less frequent its occurrence. Many people that have been exposed to air pollutants can have sub-clinical effects such as temporary deficits in lung function or pulmonary inflammation while the prevalence of mortality occurs only in a few (Gouveia & Maisonet, 2006). Acute Respiratory Infections (ARIs) is the most frequent and prominent among the respiratory illnesses that affect children and adults due to the morbidity and mortality associated with this illness. ARIs may be classified into upper (URTIs) and lower (LRTIs) respiratory infections, depending on the affected organs (noses, sinuses, middle ear, larynx, and pharynx in the URTIs and trachea, bronchi, and lungs in the LRTIs) (Bellos et al., 2010).

URTIs are generally mild in severity and most often are caused by viruses and sometimes, as in some cases of sinusitis and acute otitis media, with a secondary bacterial infection. Usually more severe than URTis, LRTIs episodes occur in children under 5 , the elderly and the immunocompromised individuals (e.g. HIV-infected). From the estimated 4.2 million of LRTIs annual deaths around the world 1.8 million (43%) occur in children less than 5. Furthermore, these two groups of ARIs are not mutually exclusive. These clinical conditions frequently coexist during the same episode of respiratory infection and besides, URTIs could precede and lead to LRTIs and exacerbation of pre-existing chronic respiratory diseases. (Chauhan et al., 2005; Bellos et al., 2010; Shusterman, 2011)

The nose and the upper airway, play a sentinel role in the respiratory system. Inspired particles of different aerodynamic sizes tend to impact and interact with the upper airway mucosa. Studies have shown that PM_{10} can induce alterations in cells of nasal mucosa promoting inflammatory responses (Brunekreef & Forsberg, 2005). Once trapped in nasal mucous, these particles are transported to the nasopharynx via mucociliary system, being later either swallowed or expectorated. Gaseous/vapor-phase air pollutants can also be removed from inspired air, depending on their water solubility and chemical reactivity (Shusterman, 2011).

Despite growing concerns of ambient air pollution and the burden of URTIs, particularly in major urban centers, research on the effects of pollutants on upper respiratory conditions are relatively sparse. Epidemological studies that have been conducted mainly in children and adolescents, showed in general, effects of pollutants but without evaluating the real impact on different age groups (Jaakkola et al., 1991; von Mutius et al., 1995; Martins et al., 2001; Hajat et al., 2002; Peel et al., 2005; Wong et al., 2006; Larrieu et al., 2009).

In São Paulo, one of the world's most densely populated cities (11.2 million inhabitants), the main source of air pollution is lightweight cars that run on a petrol–ethanol mixture, resulting in the emission of pollutants with a single toxic component. Emergency department (ED) visits related to respiratory disease have been accepted as a sensitive outcome of the short-term effects of air pollution (Peel et al., 2005)

The aim of this study was to estimate the impact of daily air pollution variability on URTIs exacerbation rates, measured via records of daily ED visits, stratifying the analyses by age groups.

2. Methods

We conducted an ecological time-series study. Daily records of UTRIs emergency department (ED) visits for patients were obtained from São Paulo Hospital (SPH), an affiliate of the São Paulo Federal University, from 1 February 2001 to 31 December 2003. The UTRIs cases were defined based on criteria listed in the International Classification of Diseases (ICD) 10th revision and took into consideration the primary diagnosis in each ED visit record. Patients with acute nasopharingytis (common cold) (J00), acute sinusitis (J01), acute pharyngitis (J02), acute tonsillitis (J03), acute laryngitis and tracheitis (J04), acute obstructive laryngitis [croup] and epiglottitis (J05), acute upper respiratory infections of multiple and unspecified sites (J06) were included in the study. The SPH is an accredited teaching hospital and its ED treats approximately 50 000 patients per year. It has, therefore, been used as a sentinel health service centre for epidemiological studies that aims to evaluate the relationship between air pollution and respiratory morbidity.

Daily records of particulate matter with an aerodynamic profile ≤10 µm (PM_{10}), carbon monoxide (CO), sulphur dioxide (SO_2), ozone (O_3) and nitrogen dioxide (NO_2) were obtained for the entire analysis period from the São Paulo State Environmental Agency. Thirteen monitoring stations are distributed throughout the city. For each measured pollutant, the average value among stations was adopted as an estimate of city-wide exposure rates. The measurement adopted for CO (non-dispersive infrared) showed the highest 8 h moving average at five stations. For NO_2 (chemiluminescence) and O_3 (ultraviolet), the highest hourly average was measured at four stations. The highest hourly average over a 24 h period for PM_{10} (beta radiation) was measured at 12 stations and at 13 stations for SO_2 (pulse fluorescence—ultraviolet); 24 h averages were adopted. Small volumes of missing data were replaced by centred moving averages. All pollutants were measured from 00:01 to 00:00. Daily minimum temperatures and daily means of relative air humidity were obtained from the Institute of Astronomy and Geophysics at the University of São Paulo.

The correlations between pollutants and weather variables were estimated using Pearson or Spearman correlation coefficients. The daily number of URTI ER visits was the dependent variable. The independent variables were the daily mean levels of each pollutant (PM_{10}, SO_2, CO, NO_2 and O_3). We also controlled for short-term (ie, days of week) and for long-term (ie, seasonable) and daily climate conditions (minimum temperature and humidity). Counts of daily URTIs ER visits were modeled, for the entire period, using generalized linear Poisson regressions (McCullag & Nelder, 1989). Analysis was stratified by total UTRIs ED visits and by age (younger than 13, between 13-19, 30-39, 40-65 and older than 65). A Poisson regression model was adopted because ED visits are countable events that exhibit a Poisson distribution. We used natural cubic splines (Green & Silverman, 1994) to control for season. Splines were used to account for the non-linear dependence of ED visits on that covariate and to subtract the basic seasonal patterns (and long-term trends) from the data. We used 12 degrees of freedom to smooth the time trend. The number of degrees of freedom for the natural spline of the time trend was selected to minimize the autocorrelation between the residuals and the Akaike Information Criterion (Akaike, 1973). After adjusting for the time trend, no remaining serial correlation was found in the residuals, making the use of autoregressive terms unnecessary.

Indicators for day of the week were included in order to control for short-term trends. Respiratory diseases present a nearly linear relationship with weather. Linear terms for temperature and relative humidity were therefore adopted. Effects of minimum temperature were more relevant from lag 0 to lag 2. Hence, we adopted a 3-day moving average for the minimum temperature. Relative humidity exhibited a short-duration and small-magnitude effect on URTIs ED visits. We adopted a 2-day moving average for relative humidity. To reduce sensitivity to outliers in the dependent variable, we used robust regression (M-estimation).

The lag structures between air pollution and health were analysed using different approaches and time lags. In this study, we tested the lag from the same day to 6 days before the ED visit using a third-degree polynomial distributed lag model (Green & Silverman, 1994). Although this imposes constraints, it also allows for sufficient flexibility to estimate a biologically plausible lag structure that controls for better multicollinearity than an unconstrained lag model. The standard errors of the estimates for each day were adjusted for overdispersion.

Effects of air pollutants were expressed as a percentage increase and as 95% confidence intervals (95% CIs) in URTI ED visits. This was due to increases in pollutant concentrations of a magnitude equal to that of the interquartile range (ie, the variation between the 75% higher and the 25% lower daily concentrations). All analyses were performed using the S-Plus 2000 statistical package for Windows.

3. Results

During the study period, 177,325 visits occurred in the emergency unit of São Paulo Hospital and 137,530 (72%) were due to upper respiratory tract infections.
In terms of age groups, emergency visits of children and adolescents younger than 13 years of age were the most frequent, followed by the groups 40 to 65 years, 30 to 39 years, older than 64 years and adolescents from 13 to 19 years old.
Table 1 presents statistical analyses of the main variables adopted in the study.

Variables	Mean	SD*	Minimum	Maximum	Percentage		
					25	50	75
Acute Upper Respiratory Tract Infections	53.55	23.42	7.00	150.00	37.00	52.00	68.00
POLLUTANTS							
PM_{10} (µg/m³)	48.71	21.87	9.62	168.98	32.29	43.88	60.55
SO_2 (µg/m³)	14.00	6.15	2.14	42.87	9.56	13.18	17.37
NO_2 (µg/m³)	120.34	49.86	30.86	390.78	81.86	113.82	150.17
CO (ppm)	2.71	1.23	0.73	12.09	1.91	2.53	3.16
O_3 (µg/m³)	95.74	44.24	14.52	282.03	63.93	88.62	119.68
WEATHER							
Temperature (°C) †	15.50	3.37	3.70	21.80	13.10	15.80	18.20
Humidity (%) §	79.17	8.43	45.54	96.60	74.50	80.00	85.00

*standard deviation; † minimum temperature; § relative humidity.

Table 1. Descriptive analyses of daily acute upper respiratory tract infections emergency room visits, air pollutants concentrations, and weather variables along study period.

Surpassing of daily air quality standards was rare among primary pollutants (one day for PM_{10}, two days for NO_2, and three days for CO). However, for ozone, the one hour moving average standard was surpassed 52 times along the period.
Low temperature is rare in São Paulo as observed in the studied period. In terms of relative humidity, it was not observed any daily record below 40%.
We explored air pollutants effects on daily number of upper respiratory tract infections ER visits using pollutant-specific models. Figure 1 presents the effects of increases in PM_{10} daily levels on the outcome for the entire group of patients.

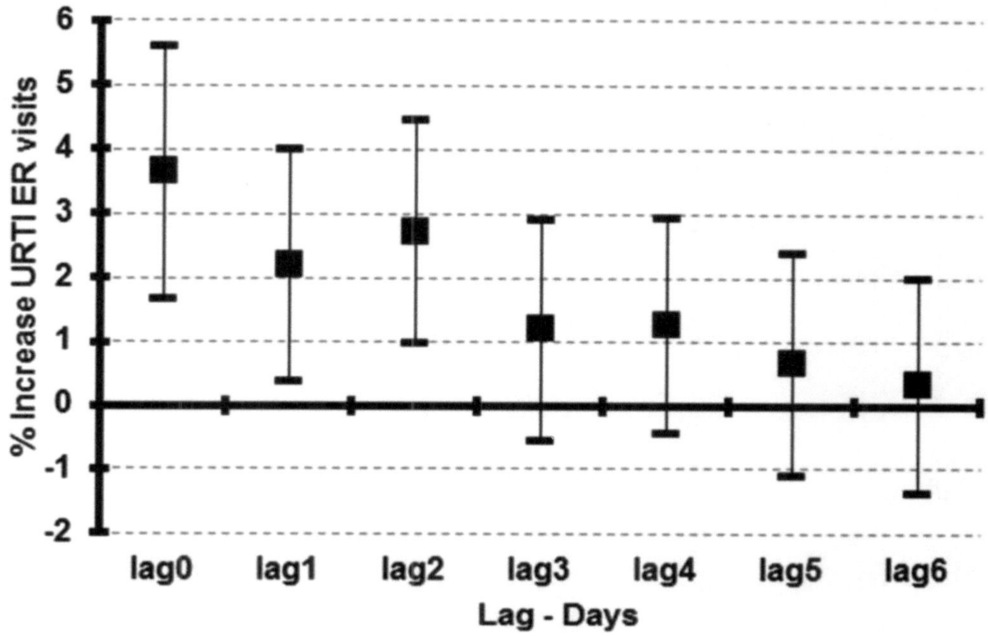

Fig. 1. Percentage increases and 95% confidence intervals on daily upper respiratory tract infections ER visits due to interquartile range increases in PM10 daily concentrations (28.26 μg/m3).

An interquartile range increase in PM_{10} concentration (28.26 μg/m3) led to increases in URTI ER visits. The effect was acute, starting at the same day of exposure (lag0) and remaining for two consecutive days. After that, there was a smooth decline of the effect magnitude until the sixtieth day after the exposure. It was observed a three-day cumulative effect (from lag0 to lag2) of 8.9% (95% CI: 5.7-12.0). When this analysis was stratified by age group it was observed two patterns of lag structure (Figure 2).

The youngest group presented a pattern of effect that was different from the others. Interquartile range increase in PM_{10} (28.26 μg/m3) was associated to an acute effect, starting at the same day of exposure and remaining for three consecutive days. As the most prevalent age group, its effect pattern was determinant for the effect pattern observed for the entire group. The other age groups presented similar lag structures, with acute effects only at the same day of exposure without lagged effects. The four-day cumulative effect observed for the youngest group reached 13.0% (95% CI: 8.3-17.8) increase in URTI ER visits. In the group of people from 45 to 65 years old it was not observed statistically significant effects, although the pattern of the lag structure seems to be similar to those observed for adolescents, adults, and elderly.

Only CO presented a lagged effect (lag 2,3,4) on the outcome for the elderly group. Remaining gaseous pollutants presented similar patterns of acute effects (in the same day of exposure). When the analyses where stratified by age groups the pattern of effect remained the same as observed for the entire group, differently from that observed for PM10 effects. Also, in terms of age groups, it was impossible to define an age-dependent pattern of susceptibility for gaseous pollutants.

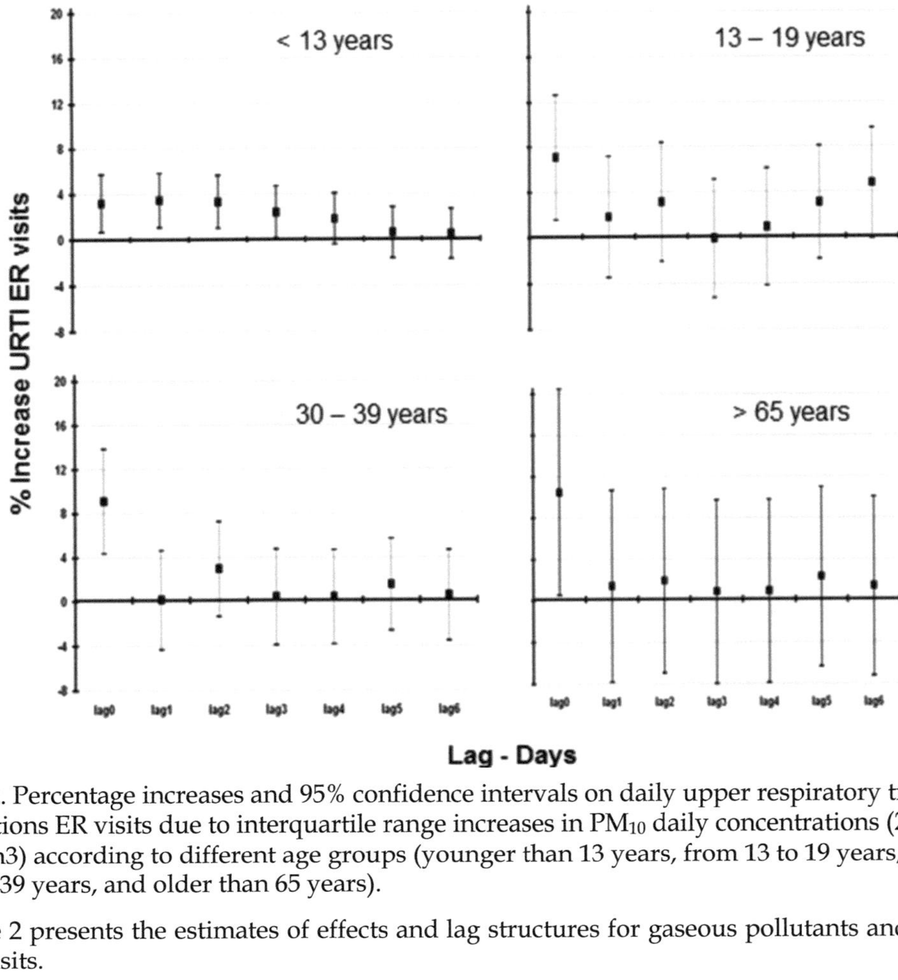

Fig. 2. Percentage increases and 95% confidence intervals on daily upper respiratory tract infections ER visits due to interquartile range increases in PM_{10} daily concentrations (28.26 μg/m3) according to different age groups (younger than 13 years, from 13 to 19 years, from 30 to 39 years, and older than 65 years).

Table 2 presents the estimates of effects and lag structures for gaseous pollutants and URTI ER visits.

Days	URTI ER Visits Percentage Increase (95% Confidence Intervals)			
	CO (1.25 ppm)	NO_2 (68.30 μg/m3)	O_3 (55.76 μg/m3)	SO_2 (7.81 μg/m3)
Lag0	0.8 (-0.6;2.2)	4.3 (2.2;6.4)	3.4 (1.2;5.6)	0.5 (0.2;0.7)
Lag1	0,2 (-1.1;1.5)	0.5 (-1.6;2.6)	-0.3 (-2.3;1.7)	-1.1 (-3.1;1.0)
Lag2	1,5 (0,2;2,8)	0.2 (-1.9;2.2)	-0.2 (-2.0;1.7)	1.5 (-0.4;3.3)
Lag3	0,6 (-0.7;1.9)	-0.2 (-2.2;1.8)	0.5 (-1.3;2.3)	-0.3 (-2.2;1.6)
Lag4	-0.1 (-1.4;1.3)	-0.5 (-2.5;1.5)	0.6 (-1.2;2.4)	0.0 (-1.8;1.8)
Lag5	-0.1 (-1.4;1.2)	0.3 (-1.8;2.3)	1.3 (-0.5;3.0)	0.1 (-1.7;1.9)
Lag6	0.1 (-1.2;1.4)	0.7 (-1.3;2.7)	0.1 (-1.7;1.8)	0.7 (-1.2;2.5)

Table 2. Percentage increases and 95% confidence intervals on daily upper respiratory tract infections ER visits due to interquartile range increases in daily concentrations of CO (1.25 ppm), NO_2 (68.30 μg/m3), O_3 (55.76 μg/m3), and SO_2 (7.81 μg/m3) for the entire patients group.

4. Discussion

We have shown that PM_{10} presented a more consistent adverse effect on respiratory tract evaluated in terms of upper respiratory tract infections ER visits than gaseous pollutants and that this effect has both lag structure and age-dependent magnitude.

In this investigation we adopted the time-series design with the most used regression model to investigate acute effects of air pollutants. Poisson regression and polynomial distributed lag models have been largely tested and they have shown consistent results and less susceptibility to bias.

We adopted upper respiratory tract infection as an endpoint because it is the most common disease in humans that lead patients to medical services. Among them, the emergency departments receive most of those cases (Fendrick et al.,2003; Footitt & Johnston, 2009). The incidence of acute URTIs is inversely proportional to age. On average, the youngest children have 6-8 and adults 2-4 per year (Heikkinen & Jarvinen, 2003).

The effect of air pollutants on health are more demonstrated on children and on the elderly and the evidence of an effect among adults in the general population is more limited (Cesarone et al., 2008). More refined assessment, including analysis of subgroup defined by specific illness or ages, or of air pollutants not routinely monitored, has been limited by study size and available air quality and health outcome data. (Peel et al., 2005). In this study we took advantage of obtaining data at the Federal University Hospital that attends to a considerable number of patients in the most populous city in Brazil with an official network of air monitoring at 14 substations. This fact has allowed us to stratify our results by age group and by air pollutants.

Viruses are the causal pathogens in most upper respiratory tract infection cases, with fewer than 10% of the cases caused by bacteria. The viral pathogens primarily associated with upper respiratory tract infections include picornaviruses (notably, rhinoviruses and enteroviruses), coronaviruses, adenoviruses, parainfluenza viruses, influenza viruses, and respiratory syncytial viruses. (Fendrick et al., 2003; Heikkinen & Jarvinen, 2003) Infections caused by influenza (ICD 10th J10-J11) is not included in the current study and will be presented elsewhere.

Non- influenza viral respiratory tract infection (VRTI) compromises the overall health status of the individual and produce high morbidity. The average length of an episode is about 7 days and one quarter of the cases can reach 14 days. The magnitude of VRTIs impact on public health can be scaled through the study of The National Centre for Health Statistics (USA), which showed that in the United States of America around 500 million non-influenza viral upper respiratory infections occur annually, resulting in a loss of 40 billion US dollar costs and with 40-100 million school and work days lost to absenteeism. (Fendrick et al.,2003; Footitt & Johnston, 2009). In the United Kingdom, treatment of cough, symptom usually associated to viruses, in non-asthmatic pre-school children cost at over 30 million pounds annually. (Hollinghurst et al., 2008).

The airway epithelium acts as the first defense against respiratory pathogens, as a physical barrier, with the mucociliary system and its immunological functions. It initiates multiple innate and adaptive immune mechanisms for efficient antiviral responses. The interaction between respiratory pathogens and airway epithelial cells results in production of substances, including type I and III interferons, lactoferrin, β-defensins, and nitric oxide, and also in the production of cytokines and chemokines, which recruit inflammatory cells and influence adaptive immunity. These defense mechanisms usually result in rapid pathogens clearance. (Becker et al., 2005; Vareilleet et al., 2011). In addition alveolar macrophages (AMs) play a key role in the defense against respiratory infection. At least three properties of AMs play key antimicrobial roles, i.e. the production of inflammatory cytokines, reactive oxidant species (ROS) and interferon (Castranova et al., 2001). Besides macrophages can inhibit viral replication and also limit viral infections by removing the debris of destroyed cells and by presenting viral antigens to T lymphocytes (Mei et al., 2005).

Once installed in the airway epithelium, viral infections can damage the barrier function leading to enhanced absorption of allergens and/or irritants across the airway wall promoting inflammation. Conversely, experimental results have shown that intact epithelium is more resistant to infection of human respiratory viruses. Consequently, external agents such as allergens and pollutants that damage airway epithelium could increase susceptibility to infection and/or lead to more-severe infections. (Gern, 2010)

The mucosa of the upper respiratory (URT) is exposed to almost all of the airborne irritating agents. Depending on both, chemical composition and concentration, these pollutants could alter the morphological patterns of this mucosa at subcellular level and lead to acute and chronic adverse effects that include hypersecretory reaction of the mucous gland and globet cells, decrease of the cilia number and size and loss of the normal pseudo-stratified pattern of the epithelium (Gulisano et al., 1997). Furthermore, experimental evidence suggests that exposures to ambient air pollution may adversely affect lung defense functions such as aerodynamic filtration, mucociliary clearance, particle transport, and detoxification by alveolar macrophages (Mei et al., 2005).

In terms of criteria air pollutants, studies have shown that both particulate and gaseous pollutants can act all over the airways to initiate and exacerbate cellular inflammation. Inflammatory cells have been seen in bronchoalveolar lavage or nasal washes of asthmatics and not-asthmatic patients exposed to diesel exhausts, ozone, sulphur dioxide and nitrogen dioxide in chambers studies or after nasal provocation challenges, respectively (Bernstein et al., 2004).

Coarse particles deposit in the upper airways of the lungs and are associated with increased cytotoxicity and proinflammatory cytokines interleukin-6 and interleukin-8 (Mei et al., 2005). Upon contact with particles AMs are activated, and produce a large quantity of reactive oxygen species (ROS) from various enzymatic sources (Huang et al., 2008). Particulate matter (PM) exposure may also increase or decrease antioxidant defense mechanisms in the lung, which further modulates oxidative stress and enhances pulmonary and systemic inflammation (Huang et al, 2008). Furthemore, PM inhibit the pulmonary production of interferon in response to viral exposure (Castranova et al, 2001). Experimental study showed that exposure to coarse particles significantly exacerbated pulmonary infection in mice (Mei et al., 2005). The suppressive effects of PM on production of antimicrobial agents result in pulmonary susceptibility to both viral and bacterial infection, as demonstrated in animal models. (Castanova et al, 2001).

Inhalation of ozone (O_3) leads to disruption of epithelial barrier, affects the mucociliary clearance and can induce production of proinflammatory factors. O_3 is cytotoxic to macrophages and can modify the macrophage and neutrophil paghocytosis (Hollingsworth et al., 2007). These effects can cause susceptibility to viral and bacterial infections. Two age groups, the children and elderly, are particularly vulnerable to low levels of inhaled O_3 but its effects can be also noted in the other age groups (Hollingsworth et al., 2007). In this study we did not observe lagged effects of ozone or differentiation by age groups.

The health effects of nitrogen dioxide (NO_2) exposure may result from both the direct oxidant effects of the pollutant and from increasing airway susceptibility to other challenges, including respiratory virus infection. NO_2 causes a cascade of events, beginning with injury and inflammation of the distal airway epithelium, recruitment of T lymphocytes from blood to the airways, and increased susceptibility of the injured epithelial cells to viral infection (Frampton et al., 2002). Also, NO_2 cause reduction in ability to macrophage fagocytose and ciliary diskenesis (Chauhan et al., 2005). In this study the NO_2 effects were small and unlikely to be of clinical significance for healthy subjects. Also, effects were acute, on the same day of exposure, without differentiation by age groups. Presence of comorbidities may increase the susceptibility of some age groups to NO_2 effects.

Sulphur dioxide (SO_2) is a respiratory tract irritant that has been shown to cause acute respiratory health effects including cough, bronchoconstriccion and decreased lung function in controlled human exposures. In high concentrations, SO_2 exposure can result in significant airway injury (Chen et al., 2007). Experimental studies have shown that SO_2 causes edema, loss of cilia, epithelial thinning, and epithelial desquamation in the olfactory epithelium in mice (Min et al., 1994), damage to the epithelium of the airways and slowing of ciliary transport of mucus (Lippmann & Ito, 2005) and reduced resistance of female mice to infection by aerosol inoculation with Klebsiella pneumoniae (Azoulay-Dupuis et al., 1982). SO_2 levels have declined in São Paulo over the last decades. However, we have observed adverse effects on health even under this situation (Arbex et al., 2009). In this study, the smallest effect was observed for SO_2 exposure and no effect modification was observed in age groups analyses.

In urban centers carbon monoxide (CO) emissions have declined significantly since the introduction of catalytic converters for motor vehicles (Chen et al., 2007). However, the health risks of exposure to these low levels even below to current standards could produce a considerable public health burden particularly for persons with cardiovascular disease (Bell et al., 2009). Investigators have linked short-and long-term CO exposure mainly with cardiovascular events (Chen et al., 2007; Bell et al., 2009).

Our results have shown that the age group most affected by exposure to particles, NO_2 and O_3 was children.

Three repeated cross-sectional studies of a total of 7,611 East German children aged 5–14 yrs during 1992–1993, 1995–1996, and 1998–1999 found a statistical significant age-adjusted decrease for bronchitis (54.2 versus 38.0%), otitis media (30.7 versus 26.7%), sinusitis (4.6 versus 2.3%), frequent colds (36.7 versus 28.5%) and morning cough (13.4 versus 12.2%) in parallel to an improvement of annual means of SO_2 (60 versus 8 $\mu g\ m^{-3}$) and TSP (56 versus 29%) (Heinrich et al., 2002).

Joaakkola et al. (1991) reported an increased prevalence of URTIs in infants and children living in city polluted by moderate levels of PM_{10}, NO_2 and SO_2 as compared to children of a clean air region and von Mutius et al. (1995) have shown that high concentrations of SO2 and moderate levels of particulate matters and NO_2 are associated with an increase risk of developing upper respiratory symptoms in childhood.

Peel et al. (2005) in a time-series study have shown that URTIs visits, mainly in infants and children, were positively associated with levels of PM_{10}, O_3, NO_2 and CO. Despite our study not showing relationship between CO and URTIs in children the lag structure of studies are very similar.

Study conducted in Finland have demonstrated that higher levels of SO2 and NO2 were associated with an increase number of URTIs (Ponka, 1990) and study conducted in Hong Kong significant association between first visit for URTI and an increase in the concentration of NO_2, O_3, PM_{10}, $PM_{2,5}$ was observed , but not SO_2 (Wong et al., 2006). However the models of the studies have different design from ours since they do not explore lag and age groups.
Our findings are consistent with Hajat et al (2002), who carried out a study in London, UK. They found a stronger association for PM_{10} for upper respiratory diseases on general practitioner: 5.7% for a 31 μg m−3 change in PM_{10} in adults aged 15–64 yrs, and 10.2% in adults aged ≥65 yrs. However, they estimated that a 18 μg m−3 increase in SO_2 resulted in a 3.5% increase in childhood consultations at family practices while in our study the age group more affected by SO_2 exposure was the adults aged between 30 and 65 years.
Similar to our study lag structure, Laurie et al. (2009) have demonstrated the risk of medical home visits in Bordeax, France and upper respiratory diseases was significantly increased by 1.5% (CI 0.3,2.7) during 3 days following a 10-μg/m3 increase in PM_{10} levels.
Cesarone et al. (2008) have shown that indices of exposure to traffic-related air pollution were consistently associated with an increased risk of rhinitis in adults in Rome, Italy. However, different from our study, the authors suggest that the main mechanism was due to allergic process.
Different from previous study, we found an association between increase in CO levels and emergency room visits for URTIs in elderly people at lag 2,3,4. Whereas the main effect of carbon monoxide is on the cardiovascular system, our hypothesis is if the IRTIs could lead to cardiovascular injury in sensitive people.
Despite certain minor differences between our study and those mentioned above, all agree on one major point: urban air pollutants are hazardous and could lead to URTIs. The minor disagreements between age groups and pollutant-specific effects can most likely be attributed to study-specific design characteristics.

5. Conclusion

This study showed that air pollutants exposure in general, and PM_{10} in special, can increase ED visits due to upper respiratory tract infections and that this effect can be modified by age group. Upper respiratory tract infections cannot be considered severe health outcomes. However, it is one of the most frequent groups of respiratory diseases and affects different age groups, increasing cost of medical treatments. Despite the well known susceptibility of the extreme age groups to air pollutants exposure there are other age groups that seem to present pollutant-specific susceptibility, enlarging the burden of air pollutants on health. Despite the observed differences on effects estimates by pollutants, in the outdoor environment people are exposed to a mixture of pollutants and pollutant-specific effects that is really difficult to estimate in the outdoor environment.
We believe that this study may support efforts to limit air pollution emissions to stricter standards than those currently adopted in Brazil. In addition, despite the improvement in car engines and the consequent reduction in emissions, the number of cars has increased over the last decade, bringing more vehicles to the streets every day. Monitoring this scenario will require new studies that evaluate frail population groups and analyzing effect modifiers.

Finally, we identified a clear association between air pollution and daily URTIs-related emergency department visits for individuals with different age groups in the city of Sao Paulo, Brazil. Air pollution remains an under-evaluated cause of URTIs exacerbation. Primary pollutants, which in São Paulo are generated mainly by cars, are among those factors that must be addressed in order to minimize the risks to public health.

5. References

American Thoracic Society. (2000). What constitutes an adverse health effect of air pollution? *American Journal of Respiratory and Critical Care Medicine*, Vol. 165, No. 2, pp. 665-673, ISSN1073-449X

Akaike, H. (1973). Information theory and an extension of the maximum likelihood principal. In: *2nd International Symposium on Information Theory*, Petrov BN, Csaki F, pp. 267-281, Akademiai Kiado, Budapest

Arbex M.A.; de Souza Conceição, G.M.; Cendon, S.P.; Arbex, F.F.; Lopes, A.C.; Moysés, E.P.; Santiago, S.L.; Saldiva, P.H.; Pereira, L.A. & Braga, A.L.F. (2009). Urban air pollution and chronic obstructive pulmonary disease. *Jounal of Epidemiology and Community Health*, Vol. 63, No. 10, pp. 777-783, ISSN 0143-0005X

Azoulay-Depuis, E.; Bouley, G. & Blayo, M.C. (1982) Effects of sulfur dioxide on resistance to bacterial infection in mice. *Environmental Research*, Vol. 29, No. 2, pp. 312-319, ISSN 0013-9351

Becker, S.; Mundandhara, S.; Devlin, R.B. & Madden, M. (2005). Regulation of cytokine prod uction in human alveolar macrophages and airway epithelial in response to ambient air pollution particles: Further mechanists studies. *Toxicology and Applied Pharmacology*, Vol. 207, suppl. 2, pp. S269-S273, ISSN 0041-008X.

Bell, M.L.; Peng, R.D.; Dominici, F. & Samet, J.M. (2009). Emergency hospital admissions for cardiovascular diseases and ambient levels of carbon monoxide. *Circulation*, Vol. 120, No. 11, pp. 949-955, ISNN 0009-7322

Bellos, A.; Mulholland, K.; O'Brien, K.L.; Qasi, S.A.; Gayer, M. & Checci, F. (2010). The burden of acute respiratory infections in crisis-affected populations: a systematic review. *Conflict and Health*, Vol. 4, No. 3, pp. 1-12, ISNN 1752-1505

Bernstein, J.A.; Alexis, N.; Barnes, C.; Bernstein, I.L.; Bernstein, J.A.; Nel, A.; Peden, D.; Diaz-Sanchez, D.; Tarlo, S.M. & Williams, P.B. (2004). Health effects of air pollution. *Jounal of Allergy and Clinical Immunology*, Vol. 114, No. 5, pp. 1116–1123, ISSN 0091-6749

Brunekreef, B. & Holgate, S.T. (2002). Air pollution and health. *Lancet* Vol. 360, No. 9341, pp. 1233–1242, ISSN 0140-6736

Castranova, V.; Ma, J.Y.V.; Yang, H.M.; Antonini, J.M.; Butterworth, L.; Barger, M.W.; Roberts, J. & Ma, J.K.H. (2001). Effect of exposure to diesel exhaust particles on the susceptibility of the lung to infection. *Environmental Health Perspective*, Vol. 109, suppl. 4, pp. 609-612, ISSN 0091-6765

Cesarone, G.; Badaloni, D.P.; Forastieri, F. & Perucci, C.A. (2008). Comparison between various indices of exposure to traffic-related air pollution and their impact on respiratory health in adults. *Occupational and Environmental Medicine*, Vol. 65, No. 10, pp. 683-690, ISSN 1470-7926

Chauhan, A.; Chatterjee, A. & Johnston, S. (2005). Acute respiratory infections. In: *Effects of air pollution on children health and development. A review of the evidence*, European Center of Environmental and Health, pp. 44-69, World Health Organization, Bonn.

Chen, T.M.; Gokhale, J.; Schofer, S. & Kuschner, W.G. (2007). Outdoor air pollution: Nitrogen dioxide, sulfur dioxide, and carbon monoxide health effects. *The American Journal of the Medical Sciences*, Vol. 333, No. 4, pp. 249-256, ISSN 0002-9629

Fendrick, A.M.; Monto, A.S.; Nightengale, B. & Sarnes, M. (2003). The economic burden of non-influenza-related viral respiratory tract infection in the United States. *Archives of Internal Medicine*, Vol. 163, No. 4, pp. 487-494, ISSN 0003-9926

Footitt, J. & Johnston, S.L. (2009). Cough and viruses in airways disease: mechanisms. *Pulmonary Pharmacology and Therapeutics*, Vol. 22, No. 2, pp. 108-113, ISSN 1094-5539

Frampton, M.W.; Boscia, J.; Roberts Jr, N.J.; Azadniv, M.; Torres, A.; Cox, C.; Morrow, P.E.; Nichols, J.; Chalupa, D.; Frasier, L.M.; Gibb, F.R.; Speers, D.M.; Tsai, Y. & Utell, M.J. (2002). Nitrogen dioxide: effects on airways and blood cells. *American Journal of Physiology - Lung Cellular and Molecular Physiology*, Vol. 282, No. 1, pp. L155-L165, ISSN 1040-0605

Gern, J.E. (2010). The ABCs of rhinoviruses, wheezing, and asthma. *Journal of Virology*, Vol. 84, No. 15, pp. 7418-7426, ISSN 0022-538X

Gouveia, N.C. & Maisonet, M. (2005). Health effects of air pollution: an overview. In: *Air quality guidelines. Global Update 2005*, World Health Organization, pp. 87-103, WHO Office for Europe, ISBN 92-890-2192-6, Copenhagen

Green, P.J. & Silverman, B.J. (1994). Non parametric regression and generalized linear models: a roughness penalty approach, Chapman & Hall, London

Gulisano, M.; Marceddu, S.; Barbaro, A.; Pacini, A.; Buiatti, E.A.; Martini, A.P. & Pacini P. (1997). Damage to the nasopharyngeal mucosa induced by current levels of urban air pollution: a field study in lambs. *European Respiratory Journal*, Vol. 10, No. 3, pp. 567-572, ISSN 0903-1936

Hajat, S.; Anderson, H.R.; Atkinson, R.W. & Haines, A. (2002). Effects of air pollution on general practitioner consultations for upper respiratory diseases in London. *Occupational and Environmental Medicine*, Vol. 59, No. 5, pp. 294-299, ISSN 1470-7926

Heikkinen, T. & Jarvigen, A. (2003). The common cold. *Lancet*, Vol. 361, No. 9351, pp. 51-59, ISSN 0140-6736

Heinrich, J.; Hoelscher, B.; Frye, C.; Meyer, I.; Pitz, M.; Cyrys, J.; Wjst, M.; Neas, L. & Wichmann, H.E. (2002). Improved air quality in reunified Germany and decreases in respiratory symptoms. *Epidemiology*, Vol. 13, No. 4, pp. 394–401, ISSN 1044-3983

Hollingwhorst, J.W.; Kleeberger, S.R. & Forster, M.W. (2007). Ozone and pulmonary innate immunity. *Proceedings of the American Thoracic Society*, Vol. 4, No. 3, pp. 240-246, ISSN 1546-3222

Hollinghurst, S.; Gorst, C.; Fahey, T. & Hay, A.D. (2008). Measuring the financial burden of acute cough in pre-school children: a cost of illness study. *BMC Family Practice*, 9:10. ISSN 1471-2296, Available from http://www.biomedcentral.com/1471-2296/9/10

Huang, Y.T.; Li, Z.; Carter, J.D.; Soukup, J.M.; Schwartz, D. & Yang, I.V. (2008) Fine ambient particles; induce oxidative stress and metal binding genes in human alveolar macrophages. *American Journal of Respiratory Cell and Molecular Biology*, Vol. 41, No. 5, pp. 544-552, ISSN 1044-1549

Jaakkola, J.J.K.; Paunio, M.; Virtanen, M. & Heinonen, O.P. (1991). Low-level air pollution and upper respiratory infections in children. *American Journal of Public Health*, Vol. 81, No. 8, pp. 1060-1063, ISSN 0090-0036

Ko, F.W.S. & Hui, D.S.C. (2010). Effects of air pollution on lung health. *Clinical Pulmonary Medicine*, Vol. 17, No. 6, pp. 300-304, ISSN 1068-0640

Larrieu, S.; Lefranc, A.; Gault, G.; Chatignoux, C.F.; Jouves, B. & Filleul, L. (2009). Are the short-term effects of air pollution restricted to cardiorespiratory diseases. American Journal of Epidemiology, Vol. 169, No. 10, pp. 1201-1208, ISSN 0002-9262

Lippmann, M. & Ito, K. (2005). Sulfur dioxide: In: *Air quality guidelines. Global Update 2005*, World Health Organization, pp. 395-420, WHO Office for Europe, ISBN 92-890-2192-6, Copenhagen

Martins, L.C.; Latorre, M.R.D.O.; Saldiva, P.H.N. & Braga, A.L.F. (2001). Air pollution and emergency room visits for upper airway respiratory infection in São Paulo city: evaluation of vehicle restriction. *Revista Brasileira de Epidemiologia*, Vol. 4, No. 3, pp. 220-229, ISSN 1415-790X

McCullag, P. & Nelder, J.A. (1989). *Generalized linear models* (2nd edition), Chapman & Hall, ISBN 0-412-31760-5, London

Mei, L.; Stieb, D.M. & Chen, Y. (2005). Coarse particulate matter and hospitalization for respiratory infections in children younger than 15 years in Toronto: a case-crossover analysis. *Pediatrics*, Vol. 116, No. 2, pp. 235-240, ISSN 0031-4005

Min, Y.G.; Rhee, C.S.; Choo, M.J.; Song, H.K. & Hong, S.C. (1994). Histopathologic changes in the olfactory epithelium in mice after exposures to sulfur dioxide. *Acta Oto-laryngologica*, Vol. 114, No. 3, pp. 447-452, ISSN 0001-6489

Olivieri, D. & Scoditti, E. (2005). Impact of environmental factors on lung defenses. *Eur Respir Rev*, Vol. 14, No. 4, pp. 51-56, ISSN 0905-9180

Peel, J.; Tolbert, P.E.; Klein, M.; Metzger, K.B.; Flanders, D.; Todd, K.; Mulholland, J.A.; Ryan, P.B. & Frumkin, H. (2005). Ambient air pollution and respiratory emergency department visits. *Epidemiology*, Vol. 16, No. 2, pp. 164-174, ISSN 1044-3983

Perez, L.; Rapp, R. & Kunzli, N. (2010). The year of the lung: outdoor air pollution and lung health. *Swiss Medical Weekly*, Vol. 140, pp. E1-E7, ISSN 1424-3997

Ponka, A. (1990). Absenteeism and respiratory disease among children and adults in Helsinki in relation to low-level air pollution and temperature. *Environmental Research*, Vol. 52, No. 1, pp 34-46, ISSN 0013-9351

Shusterman, D. (2011). The effects of air pollutants and irritants on the upper airways. *Proceedings of the American Thoracic Society*, Vol. 8, No. 1, pp. 101-105, ISSN 1546-3222

Vareille, M.; Kieninger, E.; Edwards, M.R. & Regamey, N. (2011). The airway epithelium: soldier in the fight against respiratory viruses. *Clinical Microbiology Reviews*, Vol. 24, No. 1, pp. 210-229, ISSN 0893-8512

von Mutius, E.; Sherril, D.L.; Fritzsch, G.; Martinez, F.D. & Lebowitz, M.D. (1995). *European Respiratory Journal*, Vol. 6, pp. 723-728, ISSN 0903-1936

Wong, T.W.; Tam, W.; Yu, I.T.S.; Wun, Y.T.; Wong, A.H.S. & Wong, C.M. (2006). Association between air pollution and general practitioner visits for respiratory diseases in Hong Kong. *Thorax*, Vol. 61, No. 7, pp. 585-591, ISSN 0040-6376

13

Air Pollutants and Its Effects on Human Healthy: The Case of the City of Trabzon

Yelda Aydın Türk and Mustafa Kavraz
Karadeniz Technical University
Turkey

1. Introduction

Air pollution, both indoors and outdoors, is a major environmental health problem affecting everyone in developed and developing countries alike. Any agent that spoils air quality is called air pollutant. Air pollution can be defined as the presence of pollutants,such as sulphur dioxide (SO2), particle substances (PM), nitrogen oxides (NOX) and ozone (O3) in the air that we inhale at levels which can create some negative effects on the environment and human health (Bayram, 2006). Air pollutants have sources that are both natural and human-based. Now, humans contribute substantially more to the air pollution problem. Though some pollution comes from natural sources, most pollution is the result of human activity. Air pollution is a problem of growing importance. This pollution damages the natural processes in the atmosphere, and affects public health negatively. Currently, several cities stand out as worst cases of air pollution (Kilburn,1992). It was found that until the 1980s, 1.3 billion people lived in cities where pollution was above the air quality standards (Bayram, 2006). Besides, air pollution is a main threat to the vegetation.

Pollutants such as dust, soot, fog, steam, ash, smoke, etc. are introduced into air naturally and as a result of human activities. The athmosphere can neutralize toxic solid, liquid and gaseous substances by melting them; however, due to the production of excessive amounts of such substances and depending on the meteorological and topographic conditions, the atmosphere is in a continuous process of pollution. (Kaypak and Özdilek,2008). There are several main types of pollution. Among the main pollutants in the urban atmosphere are primarily the particle substances (PM), sulphur dioxide (SO_2), nitrogen oxides (NO_x), volatile organic compounds (VOCs), and secondarily ozone (O_3) that is created as a result of photochemical reactions. (Özden et all.,2008).

P**articles** are introduced into the air by burning fuel for energy. The gases produced as a result of burning fuels in automobiles, homes, and industries are a major source of pollution in the air. The exhaust from burning fuels in automobiles, homes, and industries is a major source of pollution in the air. Some believe that even the burning of wood and charcoal in fireplaces and barbeques can release significant quanitites of soot into the air. Another type of pollution is the release of **noxious gases**, such as sulfur dioxide, carbon monoxide, nitrogen oxides, and chemical vapors. These can take part in further chemical reactions once they are in the atmosphere, forming smog and acid rain (URL4).

Air pollution was first seen in Turkey as a serious problem in the early 1970s, and in the following years it spread into other cities mainly Istanbul. The reason for this is that lignite

coal which has a high pollution rate was started to be used as a source of energy (Evyapan, 2008). 41% of the energy sources that are consumed in Turkey is used for heating purposes in houses, and in winters air pollution in the residential areas with intense population reaches levels that threaten human and environmental health.
An air pollutant is any substance which may harm humans, animals, vegetation or material (Kampa and Castanas, 2008). Air pollutants cause adverse effects on human health and the environment. A constant finding is that air pollutants contribute to increased mortality and hospital admissions. Human health effects can range from nausea and difficulty in breathing or skin irritation, to cancer (Kampa and Castanas,2008).
There are studies in literature which report the relationship between respiratory tract diseases and the level of air pollution concentrations (SO_2 and PM). Few scientists found that air pollution is associated with respiratory tract diseases of many sorts, including lung cancer and emphysema.A number of studies have established a qualitative link between air pollution and ill health(Lester and Eugene,1970). In their study, Sardar et al. (2006) investigated the health records and found that there are statistically significant relationships between respiratory tract diseases and rough particles, and that rough particles constitute an important threat for human health. In addition, epidemiological and toxicological research have focused on the role of particles (PM2.5) on the observed health effects (Anderson, 2000, Brown, Stone, Findlay, Macnee, Donaldson, 2000, 1990). In their study, Lipfert et al. (1995) report that there is a statistically significant relationship between atmospheric particle matter size and admissions to hospitals for respiratory tract infections and mortalities. On average, 5% of daily mortality is associated with air pollution.
As is the case of all environmental problems, the two primary causes of air pollution in Turkey are urbanization which has been rapid since the 1950s, and industrialization. Before industrialization, more than 80% of the population lived in rural areas, but now more than 60% live in cities and industrial complexes. Among the developments contributing to air pollution in the cities are incorrect urbanization, low quality fuel, the high content of sulphur and ash in the fuel used for heating and improper combustion techniques, the shortage of green areas, the increase in the number of motor vehicles, inadequate disposal of wastes and meteorological factors (Özer et al,1997).
Combustion of coal and various kinds of oil cause excessive air pollution in Istanbul, Ankara, Bursa, Erzurum and Trabzon. In the Marmara Region, after the introduction of natural gas for heating, the levels of pollution caused by heating was reduced in the cities in this region. However, it has been observed that air pollution is increasing in cities like Gaziantep, Erzurum, Bayburt, Trabzon, Niğde, Kütahya, Isparta and Çanakkale where there is no intense industrialization.
Although air pollution is a serious problem in Turkey, the number of studies on the effects of air pollution on health is rather limited. . In a study that investigated the relationship between air pollution and mortality, Şahin (2000) found a statistically significant correlation between the total suspended particulate matter and daily mortality in Istanbul. In a thesis study, Olgun (1996) concluded that in Istanbul there was an 8% increase in the mortality caused by respiratory system diseases in the children of 0-2 age group during the winters when air pollution is the highest. Another study by Olgun (1996) which again focused on the 0-2 age group investigated the 5-year SO_2 and total suspended particulate matter (PM) values and the admissions to hospitals due to respiratory system diseases. The study found that parallel to the increase in the air pollution, there was an increase in the bronchitis,

sinusitis, laryngitis and pneumonia cases and that there was an increase in the average length of stay in hospitals.

In a study, Keleş et al. (1999) investigated the prevalence of allergic rhinitis and atopy in two quarters of Istanbul, where in one air pollution was intense and where in the other low. They found that allergic rhinitis sympoms were significantly higher in the quarter where there was an intense air pollution.

Ünsal et al. (1999) investigated the admissions to the emergency service of the Eskişehir Public Hospital for symptoms of certain diseases, and they found that parallel to the increase in daily SO_2 levels, there was also an increase in the number of admissions due to lower respiratory tract infections, Chronic Obstructive Pulmonary Disease (COPD) and Cor Pulmonale (Ünsal et al., 1999). Another study carried out in Ankara investigated the relationship between the concentrations of particulate matter (PM), one of the air pollution parameters, and asthma. A correlation was found between emergency asthma admissions and SO_2 and PM concentrations (Evyapan, 2008).

Another study investigated the relationship between air pollution and admissions to hospitals for acute respiratory tract diseases between June 1994 and June 1995 in Istanbul. A positive relationship was found between the PM levels and admissions to hospitals (Dağlı et all, 1996). Similarly, a thesis study that was carried out in Izmit and that covered the years of 1996 and 1997 investigated the relationship between admissions to hospitals due to asthma and air pollution and meteorological parameters. The study found that there is a positive correlation between year-long weekly average smoke concentrations and admissions to hospitals due to asthma (r=0,26; p=0,000001). On the other hand, a weak correlation was found between the SO_2 levels and admissions to hospitals due to asthma in summer times (r=0,22; p=0,002)(Çelikoğlu,1999). Another study that was carried out in Gaziantep investigated the life quality of asthma patients. The study found an increase in the asthma symptoms in times of intense air pollution (Fişekçi et al,2000).

In addition, studies that investigated the relationships between air pollution parameters (SO_2 and PM) and such respiratory tract diseases as COPD and asthma were also carried out in such cities as Gaziantep, Denizli and Diyarbakır. The findings of these studies showed an increase in the admissions to emergency services of hospitals especially in times of intense air pollution.

In the framework of the study, the effects of air pollution on human health were investigated in the city of Trabzon that was chosen as the study area. The time interval of the study was determined to be between 2000-2009, and the possible effects of the air pollution on human health during this time interval were recorded and displayed.

This study aims to investigate the relationship between morbidity (number diseases reported /total population)of the diseases and the air pollution parameters (SO2 and PM concentrations). To this end, the data for diseases caused by air pollutants and air pollution concentrations in the winter months in the city of Trabzon between 2000 and 2009, have been recorded and statistically analyzed.

2. Effects of air pollutants on health

Given the fact that an average person inhales about 13,000-16,000 litres of air daily and 400-500 million litres in his lifetime, then the importance of air quality for human health becomes clearer (Öztürk, 2005). The direct effects of air pollution on human health vary depending on the period of exposure to air pollution, intensity of air pollution, and the general health condition of the population. Although the negative effects of air pollution can also be seen on healthy people, its effects create more serious problems in groups with higher vulnerability. Children and the elderly, those with respiratory tract diseases and cardiocascular diseases, those who are allergic, and those who do exercises are at more risk (URL 9). It has been reported in such studies that air pollution increases the risk of acute respiratory tract diseases in children and leads to an increase in cardiorespiratory morbidity and mortality (Bayram et al., 2006).

As a result of the negative effects of air pollution on health, the following have been observed:

- An increase in lung cancer cases
- An increase in the frequency of chronic asthma crisis
- An increase in the frequency of asthma cases
- An increase in the frequency of coughing/phlegm
- An increase in the acute disorders of upper repiratory system
- An increase in eye, nose and throat irritation cases
- Reduction in respiratory capacity
- An increase in mortality
- A reduction in productivity and production
- An increase in medical treatment expenses

The relationship between air pollution and lung cancer has also been addressed in several case-control. Studies focusing on morbidity endpoints of long-term exposure have been published as well (Cohen,2000, Katsouyannı et al.,1997). Notably, work from Southern California has shown that lung function growth in children is reduced in areas with high PM concentrations (Gauderman et al.,2000 and Guaderman et al.,2002) and that the lung function growth rate changes in step with relocation of children to areas with higher or lower PM concentrations that before (Avol, E.L. et al. 2001).Pollutants in the air cause health defects ranging from unnoticeable chemical and biological changes to trouble breathing and coughing. The ill effects of air pollution primarily attack the cardiovascular and respiratory systems. The severity of a person's reaction to pollution depends on a number of factors, including the composition of the pollution, degree and length of exposure and genetics(URL3).

Health effects of concern are asthma, bronchitis and similar lung diseases, and there is good evidence relating an increased risk of symptoms of these diseases with increasing concentration of sulphur dioxide (SO_2), ozone(O_3) and other pollutants. Moreover, there is increasing evidence to suggest that pollution from particulate matter (PM10 and black smoke) at levels hitherto considered "safe" is associated with an increased risk of morbidity and mortality (disease and death) from heart disease as well as lung disease. This is likely especially in people with other risk factors (such as old age, or pre-existing heart and lung disease). These concerns are the subject of current research throughout the world(URL-1).

The 2005 *WHO Air quality guidelines* (AQGs) are designed to offer global guidance on reducing the health impacts of air pollution.According to WHO; Air pollution is a major environmental risk to health and is estimated to cause approximately 2 million premature deaths worldwide per year. The *WHO Air quality guidelines* represent the most widely agreed-upon and up-to-date assessment of health effects of air pollution, recommending targets for air quality at which the health risks are significantly reduced. By reducing particulate matter (PM_{10}) pollution from 70 to 20 micrograms per cubic metre can cut air quality-related deaths by around 15% and help countries reduce the global burden of disease from respiratory infections, heart disease, and lung cancer (URL2).

Sulphur dioxide (SO_2) and Particulate Matter (PM) are among the most important air pollutants that affect human health negatively. Sulphur dioxide (SO_2) reacts with the moisture content in the nose, nasal cavity and throat and, in this way, it destroys the nerves in the respiratory system and harms human health. (Öztürk, 2005). When the SO_2 concentration is higher than the World Health Organization (WHO) standards, it negatively affects especially those with asthma, bronchitis, cardiac and lung problems (Öztürk, 2005). The studies have shown that air pollution has an important role on the development and progression of lung cancer (URL 10). It was also found that air pollution increases the risk of acute respiratory tract diseases especially in children and that it causes an increase in cardiorespiratory morbidity and mortality (Bayram et al., 2006). The aim of the "Regulations for the Protection of Air Quality" dated 2 November 1986 (published in the official gazette no 19269) is to take under control the soot, smoke, dust, gas, steam and aerosol emissions created by any kind of human activity; to protect human beings and their environment from the dangers caused by air pollution; to prevent and eradicate the negative effects that occur in the environment and that harm the community and neighborhood relations, and itemize the mandatory short- and long-term limit values for various air pollutants (Table1). (Öztürk, 2005). The negative effects of particulate matter on human health increase as the size of the matter gets smaller. Due to the fact that those who do sports especially in areas with high PM concentrations take deeper breaths and more frequently during the activity than those who do not do sports, such matters reaches the lungs more easily and accumulate there (Öztürk, 2005).

SO_2 (ppm)	**Duration of Exposure**	**Effects**
0,037-0,092	Annual Average	With 185 µg m-3 smoke concentration, increase in respiratory track diseases and lung diseases
0,007	Annual Average	With high particulate matter concentration, progression in the respiratory track diseases in children
0,11-0,19	24 hours	In low particle concentration, increase in the respiratory track diseases in the elderly .
0,19	24 hours	Progression in chronic respiratory track diseases in the grown-ups
0,19	24 hours	In low particle concentrations, an increase can be observed in mortality
0,25	24 hours	With 750 µg m-3 smoke concentration, an increase in daily mortality rates may be observed (UK). Sudden increase in morbidity.
0,5	10 minutes	In asthma patients, increase in breathing resistance during exercise (mobility)
5	24 hours	In healthy people, increase in breathing resistance
10	10 minutes	Bronchospasm
20		Eye irritation, coughing

Table 1. Effects of sulphur dioxide (SO_2) on human health (Öztürk, 2005)

SO_2 can affect the respiratory system and the functions of the lungs, and causes irritation of the eyes. Inflammation of the respiratory tract causes coughing, mucus secretion, aggravation of asthma and chronic bronchitis and makes people more prone to infections of the respiratory tract. Hospital admissions for cardiac disease and mortality increase on days with higher SO_2 levels. When SO_2 combines with water, it forms sulfuric acid; this is the main component of acid rain which is a cause of deforestation.

Particulate air pollution is a mixture of solid, liquid or solid and liquid particles suspended in the air. These suspended particles vary in size, composition and origin. It is convenient to classify particles by their aerodynamic properties because: (a) these properties govern the transport and removal of particles from the air; (b) they also govern their deposition within the respiratory system and (c) they are associated with the chemical composition and sources of particles. These properties are conveniently summarized by the aerodynamic diameter, that is the size of a unitEUR/density sphere with the same aerodynamic characteristics. Particles are sampled and described on the basis of their aerodynamic diameter, usually called simply the particle size (URL 11).

The effects of PM on health occur at levels of exposure currently being experienced by most urban and rural populations in both developed and developing countries. Chronic exposure to particles contributes to the risk of developing cardiovascular and respiratory diseases, as well as of lung cancer. In developing countries, exposure to pollutants from indoor combustion of solid fuels on open fires or traditional stoves increases the risk of acute lower respiratory infections and associated mortality among young children; indoor air pollution from solid fuel use is also a major risk factor for chronic obstructive pulmonary disease and lung cancer among adults. The mortality in cities with high levels of pollution exceeds the mortality observed in relatively cleaner cities by 15–20%. Even in the EU, average life expectancy is 8.6 months lower due to exposure to $PM_{2.5}$ produced by human activities. Specifically, the database on long-term effects of PM on mortality has been expanded by three new cohort studies, an extension of the American Cancer Society (ACS) cohort study, and a thorough re-analysis of the original Six Cities and ACS cohort study papers by the Health Effects Institute (HEI) (URL 11).

In view of the extensive scrutiny that was applied in the HEI reanalysis to the Harvard Six Cities Study and the ACS study, it is reasonable to attach most weight to these two. The HEI re-analysis has largely corroborated the findings of the original two US cohort studies, which both showed an increase in mortality with an increase in fine PM and sulfate. The increase in mortality was mostly related to increased cardiovascular mortality. A major concern remaining was that spatial clustering of air pollution and health data in the ACS study made it difficult to disentangle air pollution effects from those of spatial auto-correlation of health data per se. The extension of the ACS study found for all causes, cardiopulmonary and lung cancer deaths statistically significant increases of relative risks for PM2.5. TSP and coarse particles (PM15 - PM2.5) were not significantly associated with mortality (13). The effect estimates remained largely unchanged even after taking spatial auto-correlation into account (URL 11).

Particulate matters can proceed up to the alveoli in the lungs and therefore causes such important problems as asthma and bronchitis (Sloss and Smith,2000).

3. Study area

The City of Trabzon is situated in northeast of Turkey (Figure1), lies on the north sides of the Eastern Black Sea Mountains, between longitudes 38° 30' - 40° 30' E and latitudes 40° 30'

- 41° 30' N (URL 5). The area of Trabzon is about 4.664 km2 and total population of the city is about 293.000. The population density is about 5.000 people per km^2.Trabzon has a typical Black Sea climate, with rainfall throughout the year. Sea climate, with a lot of rainfall throughout the year. Summers are cool and winters are mild and damp. Towards the south, the climate becomes colder. Trabzon has a thick vegetation and receives ample rain [URL 7]. Though, in general, Trabzon has a rainy climate, and rain reaches its peak between September-late June . The average annual rainfall is 800-850 kg/m2, and about 152 days of the year are rainy. Starting from the sea level, the elevation reaches up to 3000 m in the south. The annual average temperature in Trabzon is 14.57 °C [URL 5], and the dominant wind directions are south-southwest in December, southwest in April, south in June, and west-north in the other months. April and especially May are rather foggy, and relative humidity reaches its peaks in May (79%) and June (76%), respectively. The humidity starts to decrease in summer months and reaches 67% in December, which is the minimum level. Sometimes, the humidity reaches 99% (URL-6).

As a result of fast urbanization, there has been quite a dense housing in the city. Residential areas are concentrated on the coastal areas of the city especially in the west of the city (Figure 1). In recent years, the number of high-rise buildings is increasing day by day in the valleys stretching towards the south of the city.

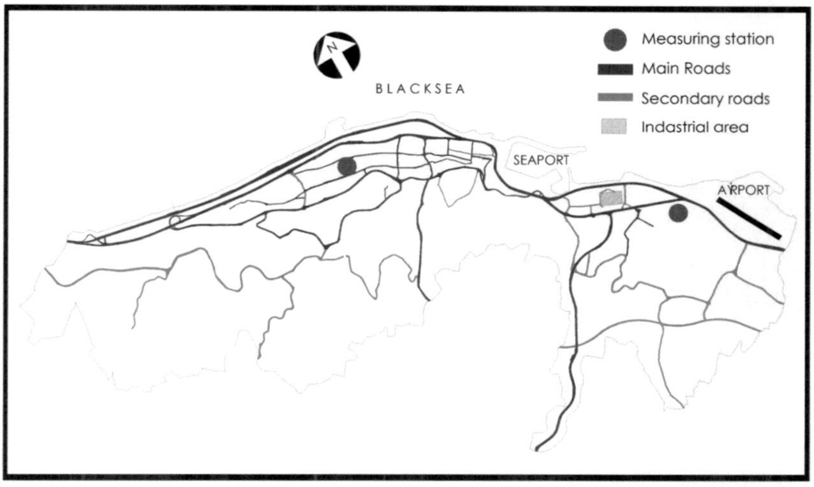

Fig. 1. Trabzon city map.

4. Air pollution in trabzon

Air pollution is an important problem during the winters in Trabzon. The level of SO_2 and PM increases during the winter especially between November and April in Trabzon as it does in the other cities in Turkey. There is a dense air pollution in the residential areas along the coast line in the west of the city. These parts of the city are characterized with high buildings. This prevents the removal of the pollution by the dominant winds in the city (URL 7). Because the pollution is not transported out of the city by the air, a cloud of pollutant particles can easily be seen in winter months (Figure 2).

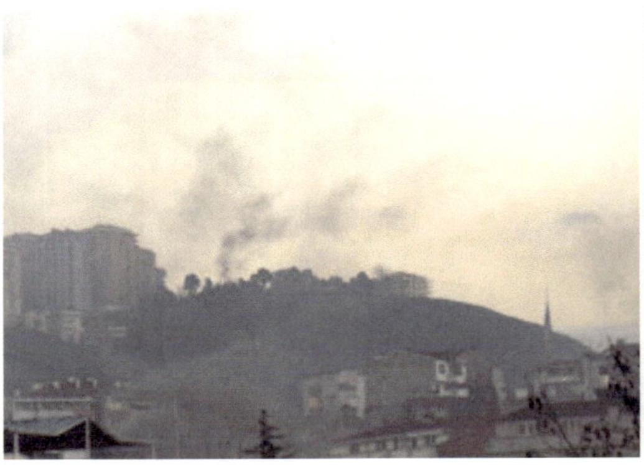

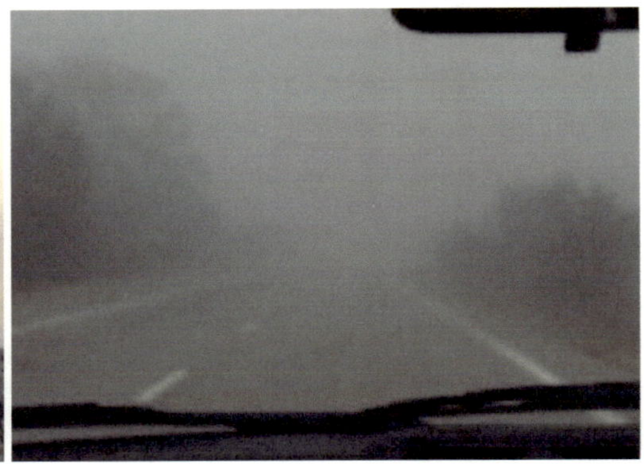

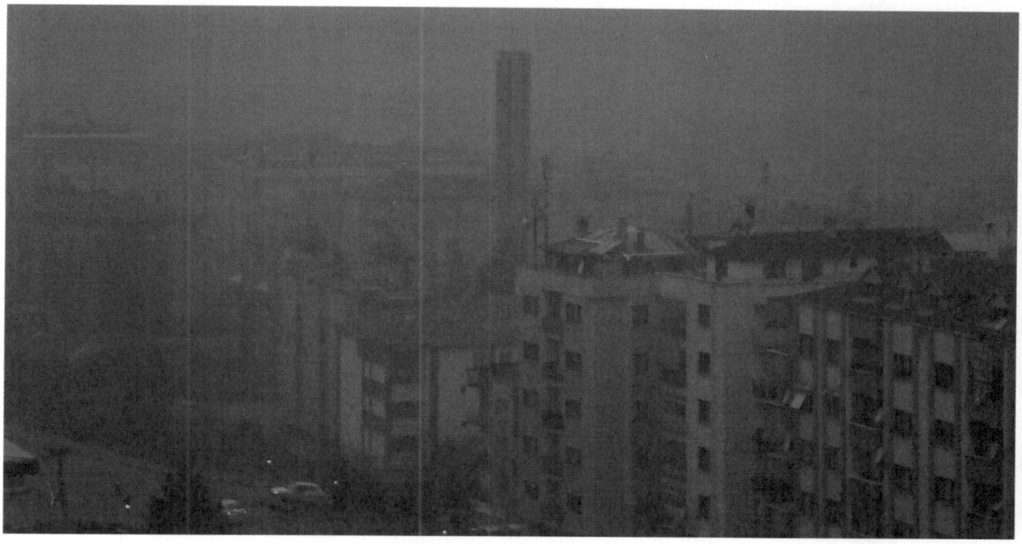

Fig. 2. Air Pollution in Trabzon in Winter Period

According to the data obtained from the Trabzon Local Directorate of Environment and Forest, Trabzon is among the second-level polluted cities in Turkey in terms of air pollution. The geographical and topographical structure of the city, irregular urbanization, and the inadequacy of green areas in the city center are said to be the main causes of air pollution. In addition, the dense housing in the natural air corridors (the valleys) of the city, which would remove air pollution, prevents air circulation especially in winter times, and between 9:00 a.m. and 11:00 a.m., 3:00 p.m. and 6:00 p.m., and 6:00 p.m. and 9:00 p.m. air pollution reaches levels that threatens human health. In addition to dust and gas emissions caused by the burning of solid fuels used for heating purposes, the exhaust gases emitted from motor vehicles at certain times (closing times of schools and shops) increase air pollution.

As in other cities with fast urbanization, many factors such as population growth, irregular and intense urbanization, increase in the number of buildings in the valleys that can be considered as the air corridors of the city, and increase in the number of motor vehicles cause air pollution in Trabzon. The intense air pollution in the city especially between November and April is caused by fuels used for heating purposes in the houses. A study by Uzunali showed that the main factor that causes air pollution is PM and that this was the result of the use of coal for heating purposes in the residences. When we investigate the annual amounts of coal (Kg) used for the purpose of heating in the city, we see that there is a gradual increase in the amount of the consumptiom of this type of fuel (Figure 3).

Natural gas is not yet used in the city for heating purposes. However, the necessary infrastructure works for this have been in progress. The active use of natural gas in the future will decrease the PM pollution. In their study, Akkoyunlu and Ertürk (Akkoyunlu and Ertürk,2002) investigated the effect of the increased share of natural gas in residential areas on air pollution levels. The pollution map indicated that the increased use of natural gas in residential areas significantly improved the air quality.

In addition to the aforementioned factors, the light industrial complexes that may contribute to the air pollution in the city are located in the east of the city. Air pollution in this part of the city where there is a cement plant is high but is lower than the pollution in the west. For there is no residential settlement in this area.

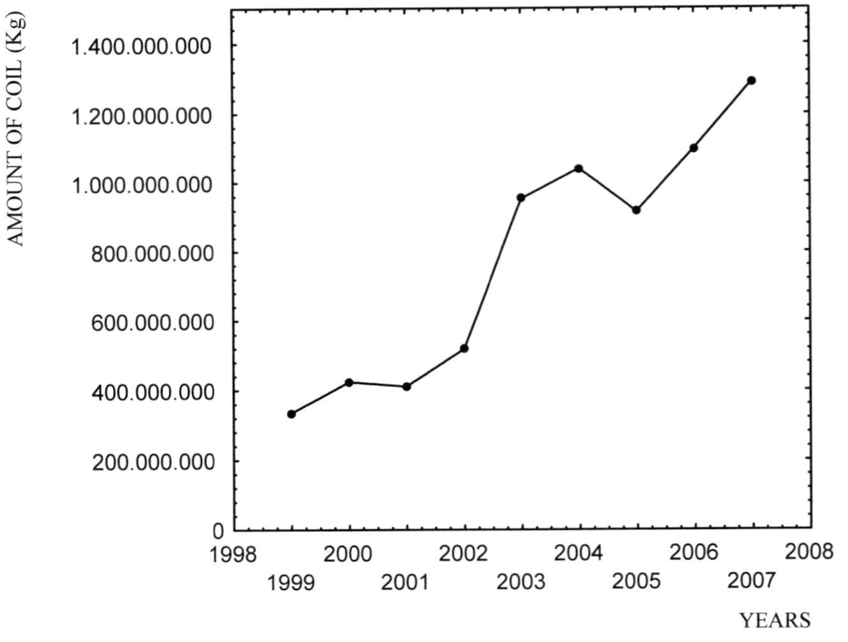

Fig. 3. Annual amounts of coal consumed for the purpose of heating in Trabzon

5. Evaluation of the data(results and discussion)

The air pollution measurements were carried out by the Local Directorate of Environment and Forest in Trabzon for the past 9 years (2000-2009) in the winter months (November-April). Continuous daily observations of SO2 and PM have
been measured in the city at 2 stationary stations at different places in the city as shown in Figure 1. The monthly average APCs were taken into consideration in this study and are presented in Table 2. Data related to the kinds of diseases in statistic documents have been provided by the Medical Board of Trabzon. Figures 4 and 5 show that, in winter seasons until 2009, the limit of Turkish Air Quality Control Regulation (AQCR) was exceeded significantly both for SO2 and PM . But the limits in AQCR are less stringent than the standards recommended by the World Health Organization (Table 3). When compared to the WHO standards, the PM values increased especially in December, January, February and March, after 2003. The limits of air pollutant concentrations recommended by the Turkish Standards and WHO Guidelines are plotted as horizontal lines (URL8).
An evaluation of the air pollution data covering the 2000-2009 period showed that the SO_2 and PM concentrations were higher in winter times than in the summer times (Figure 6). In this context, various studies carried out in different years on the air pollution in Trabzon and this study are important in that they show the variations in air pollutants by years. The aforementioned studies (Çuhadaroğlu, 1994-1995; Topbaş et al., 1994-2000) and the present study have shown that the SO_2 and PM valuses are increasing especially in the winter times. The main reason for this is the use of low quality coal for heating purposes mainly in the residential areas.

Years	APCs	November	December	January	February	March	April
2000-2001	SO2	67	53	63	57	60	41
	PM	38	58	64	58	63	45
2001-2002	SO2	44	63	85	86	72	71
	PM	46	74	93	107	72	71
2002-2003	SO2	79	80	73	59	66	72
	PM	87	90	92	69	74	81
2003-2004	SO2	71	86	109	77	72	67
	PM	90	133	101	73	84	81
2004-2005	SO2	81	98	95	82	88	49
	PM	89	111	79	110	107	58
2005-2006	SO2	79	80	92	64	56	9
	PM	96	127	132	208	119	81
2006-2007	SO2	56	88	100	30	30	19
	PM	77	128	122	100	67	54
2007-2008	SO2	6	8	7	9	4	4
	PM	51	89	80	67	64	58
2008-2009	SO2	20	44	46	26	26	17
	PM	40	94	110	79	66	60

Table 2. The monthly average APCs data in Trabzon.

	Turkish Standards		WHO Standards	
	LTS	STS	Long Term	Short Term
SO2 μg/m³	150	400	50	125
PM μg/m³	150	300	50	120

LTS: long-term standarts STS: short-term standarts (maximum daily average)

Table 3. Air quality limits in Turkey and comparison to WHO Standards

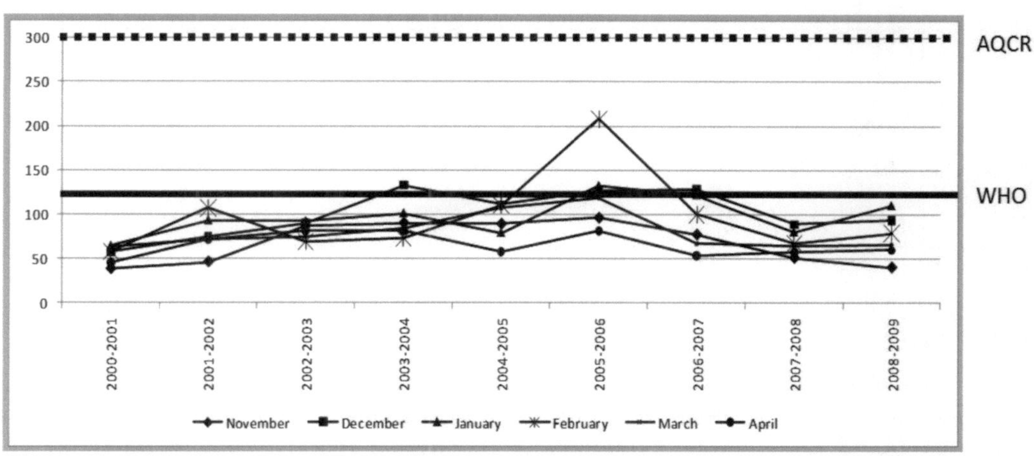

Fig. 4. Measured and calculated monthly mean PM concentrations in winter seasons from 2000 to 2009

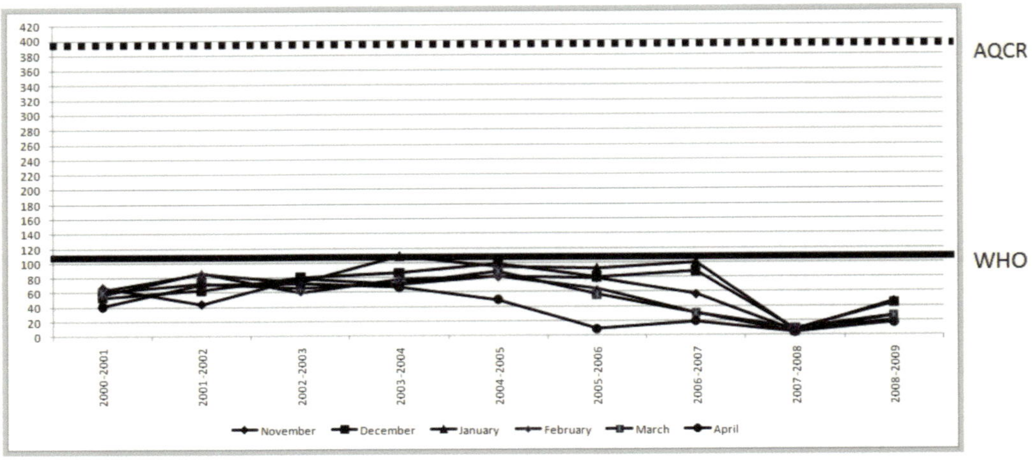

Fig. 5. Measured and calculated monthly mean SO_2 concentrations in winter seasons from 2000 to 2009.

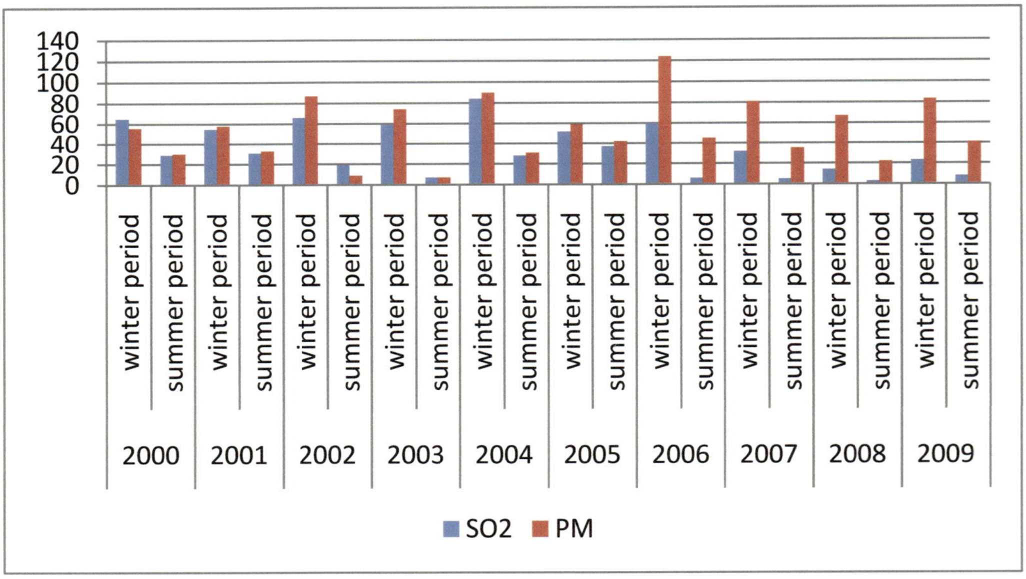

Fig. 6. Distribution in air pollutants in Trabzon in the winter and summer times between 2000 and 2009.

It was found that air pollution in Trabzon has also a serious effect on human health and that there is an increase in the number of air pollution-related diseases. As seen in Figure 7, there is an increase in acute upper respiratory tract infection (URTI), acute tonsilitis, acute bronchitis, and acute pharyngitis in winter times. This increase is a clear indication of the relationship between the air pollutants and respiratory tract infections.

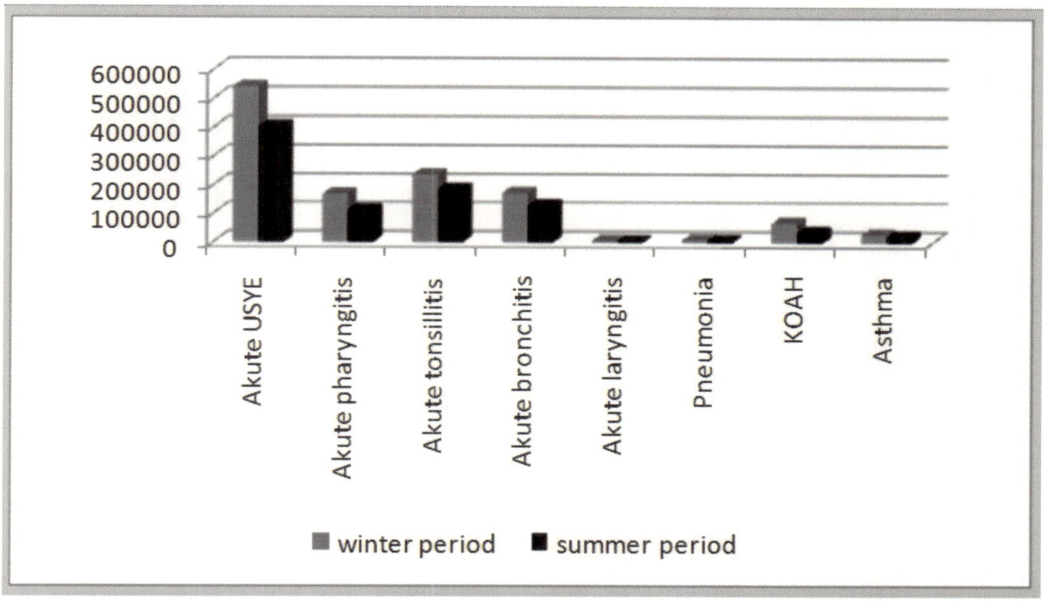

Fig. 7. Distribution in respiratory tract infections in winter and summer times(KOAH:Disease of chronic obstructive lung).

In addition, as seen in Figures 8 and Figure 9, if we examine the distribution of diseases in winter and summer times by years, we see that there is an increase in the number of disesases in the years when the SO_2 and PM values are high (2002-2003, 2004-2005, 2007-2008)).

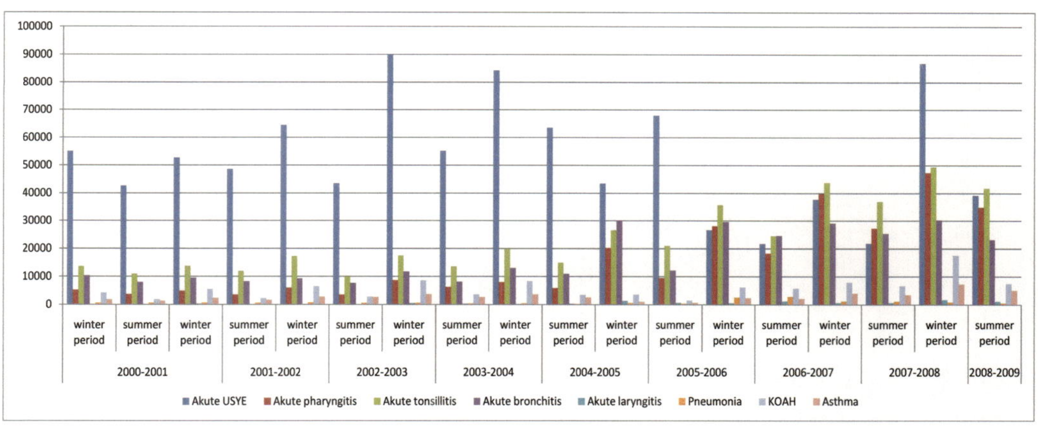

Fig. 8. Distribution in the respiratory tract infections in the 2000-2009 period(KOAH:Disease of chronic obstructive lung).

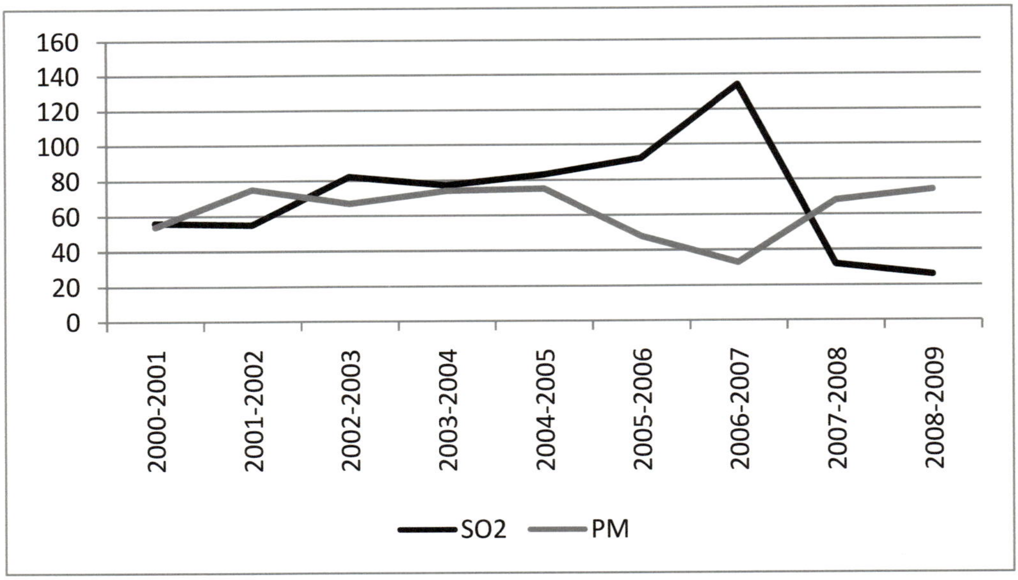

Fig. 9. Distribution in SO_2 and PM values in the 2000-2009 period.

The increase in morbidity that stands out in Figure 10 can be associated with the higher uses of fuels in the years when there was an increase and with the consequent increase in the values of air pollutants (SO_2 and PM).
The increase in the morbidity values of Acute URTI, acute tonsilitis, acute bronchitis, and acute pharyngitis (Figure 11) can be associated with the increasing air pollution in the same years.

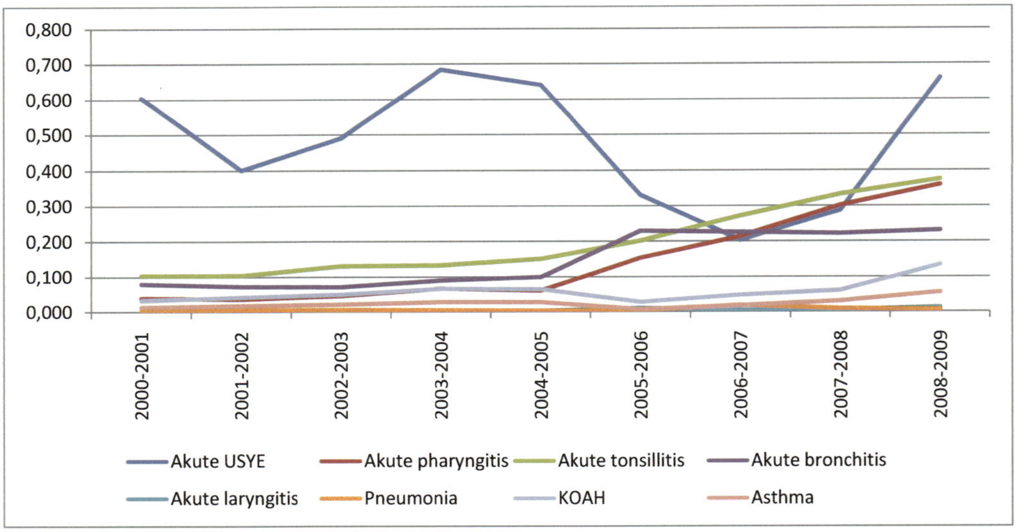

Fig. 10. Distribution in the morbidity values of respiratory tract infections between 2000 and 2009 (KOAH:Disease of chronic obstructive lung).

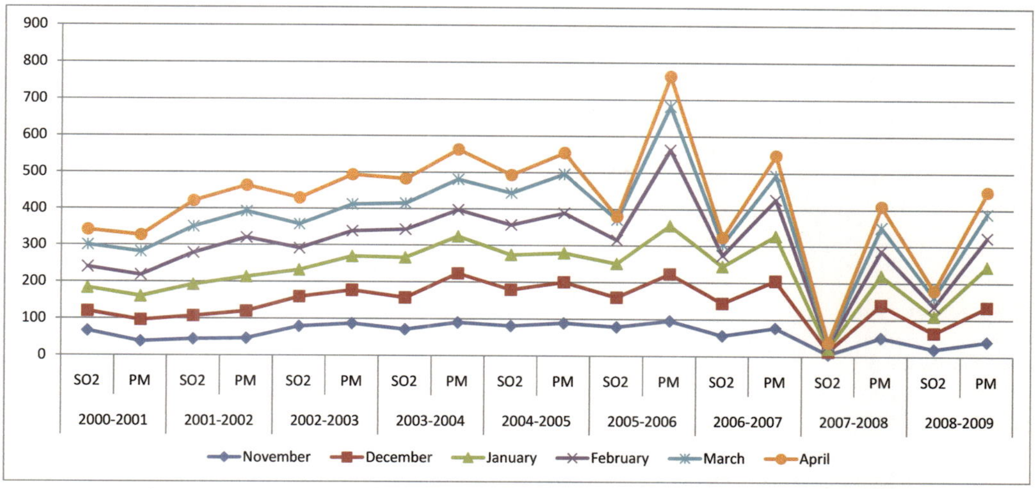

Fig. 11. Distribution in SO_2 and PM values in the winter months between 2000 and 2009.

6. Conclusions

As known, in general, respiratory tract diseases increase with an increase in APCs. According to the results of 9 years obtained from data analysis, as the APCs (SO_2 and PM) increase, so does the morbidity and number of respiratory tract diseases.

The results of this study show that there is a relationship between APCs and respiratory tract diseases.Furthermore, in a study carried out by Topbaş et al. (2004) between 1994-2000, it was found that the SO_2 levels in Trabzon increased especially in the winter months. The other two studies carried out in Trabzon at different times and this study can be considered to be complementary, and are important due to the fact that they show the variations in air pollutants in Trabzon. The aforementioned studies and our study show that the SO2 and PM values increase especially in winter months. Because of the use of low quality coal for the heating of residences, Trabzon has a high level of air pollution in winter months. and APCs in the problem of air pollution can be solved with a multidisciplinary approach. The use of natural gas for the heating, and a reduction in coal particles, should be encouraged by the Official Institutions in Trabzon. For a short-term solution, high quality coal and fuel oil can be used for heating of residences and for energy. In addition, the direction of wind throughout the winter months should be taken into consideration in the urban structure plan. To improve the wind circulation in the city, buildings, streets and heights of buildings should be thoroughly planned, and designed by taking into consideration the direction of the prevailing winds. In this way air pollution can be reduced.

According to the findings of this study, there are relationships between the respiratory tract infections and SO_2 and PM concentrations in Trabzon. Therefore, because those who do exercises take deep breaths and more frequently, sports activities should not be done in the city especially in the streets, roads and squares where pollution is dense. In this way, more pollutant intake into the body can be prevented. Furtheremore, the values regarding the pollutants in the "Air Quality Control Regulation" must be reevaluated and must be gradually aligned with the EU standards. Air pollution has a serious effect especially on the health of the elderly with respiratory problems and children. To this end, the public must continuously be informed of air pollution values. For everyone living in a city has the right to know about the quality of the air that they breathe.

The increases in the diseases associated with the air quality requires more detailed studies on the air quality of the city. If such studies are planned by being based on the already efficient health statistics, they will make significant contributions to the solution of the problem. In this context, it is important from country level in general to city level in particular to adopt sustainable approaches by taking into consideration the total environmental quality.

7. References

Akkoyunlu, A. & Erturk, F. (2002). Evaluation of Air Pollution Trends in İstanbul. *International Journal of Environment and Pollution*, 18(4), pp.388-398.

Anderson, H.R. (2000). Differential epidemiology of ambient aerosols, *Philosophical Transactions of The Royal Society of London Series A-Mathematical Physical and Engineering Sciences*, 358, pp.2771-2785

Avol, E.L. Et al. (2001). Respiratory Effects Of Relocating to Areas Of Differing Air Pollution Levels. *American Journal Of Respiratory And Critical Care Medicine,* 164: pp.2067–2072

Bayram, H., Dörtbudak, Z., Fişekçi, F. E. Kargın, M. & Bülbül, B. (2006). Hava Kirliliğinin İnsan Sağlığına Etkileri, Dünyada, Ülkemizde ve Bölgemizde Hava Kirliliği Sorunu, *Dicle Tıp Dergisi*, 33, pp.105-112.

Cohen, A.J. (2000).Outdoor air pollution and lung cancer. *Environmental health perspectives,* 108: pp.743–750

Çelikoğlu,M., (1999),Kocaeli İli'nde Hava Kirliliği ve Meteorolojik Faktörlerin Astım Bronşiale Üzerine Etkisi *(Thesis),* Kocaeli Üniversitesi Tıp Fakültesi, Kocaeli/Turkey

Çuhadaroğlu, B. (1997).Influence of some meteorogological factors on air pollution in Trabzon City. *Energy and Buildings*, Vol. 25, pp.179-184

Dağlı, E., Erk,M., Tutluoğlu,B., & et al. (1996). Istanbul'da Hava Kirliliği ile Akut Solunum Yolu Hastalıkları Arasındaki İlişki, Toraks Derneği 1. Yıllık Kongresi Nevşehir/Turkey, Kemal Matbaası (Adana),pp.31

Fişekçi,F.,Özkurt,S.,Baser, S., Daloğlu, G. And Hacıoğlu,M.,(2000). Air Pollution and Asthma Attacks, *Eur Respir Journal,* 16 (31),pp. 290s.

Evyapan, F. (2008). Hava Kirliliğinin Solunumsal Morbidite ve Mortalite Üzerindeki Etkileri: Türkiye ve Dünya Verileri. Turkiye Klinikleri *J Pulm Med-Special Topics*, 1(2):pp.48-60

Gauderman, W. J. et al. (2000).Association Between Air Pollution And Lung Function Growth İn Southern California Children. *American Journal Of Respiratory And Critical Care Medicine*, 162: pp.1383–1390

Gauderman, W. J. et al. (2002).Association between air pollution and lung function growth in southern California children. Results from a second cohort. *American journal of respiratory and critical care medicine*, 166:pp.76–84

Kampa,M. & Castanas,E. (2008). Human Health Effects of Air Pollution, *Environmental Pollution*, Vol.151,pp.362-367

Katsouyannı, K. & Pershagen G. (1997).Ambient air pollution exposure and cancer. *Cancer causes & control*, 8: 284–291

Kaypak,Ş.&Özdilek,H.G.(2008).Hatay ve Çanakkale Örneklerinde Dış Hava Kalitesi ile İlgili Seçilmiş Bazı Hastalıkların Morbiditelerinin Zamansal Değişimi Üzerine Bir Ön

Değerlendirme, Hava Kirliliği ve Kontrolü Sempozyumu, Bildiriler Kitabı, pp.471-485, Hatay/Turkey, October 22-25, 2008.

Keleş N, Ilıcalı O.C.& Değer K. (1999).Impact of air pollution on prevalence of rhinitis in İstanbul. *Arch Environ Health;* 54 (1), pp. 48-51.

Kilburn, K.H. (1992).Pulmonary Responses to Gases and Particles. Last, J.M., Wallace, R.B., Eds., *Public Health and Preventive Medicine.* Appleton & Lange, Division of Prentice Hall, pp. 463-477.

Lester,B., and Eugene,P.S. (1970).Air Pollution and Human Health The quantitative effect,with an estimate of the dolar benefit of pollution abatement, is considered, *Science,*Vol. 169,No. 3947, pp.723-733

Lipfert,F.W.,Wyzga,R.E. (1995).Air pollution and mortality:issues and uncertainties, *Journal of Air and Waste Management Association* Vol.45, pp.949-966.

Olgun Ç. (1996).Hava Kirliliğinin 0-2 Yaş Grubunda Solunum Sistemi Enfeksiyonlarında Mortalite ve Morbidite Yönünden Etkisi *(Thesis),* Sağlık Bakanlığı Şişli Etfal Hastanesi, Istanbul/Turkey.

Özden,Ö.,Yay,D.O.,Altuğ,H.,Gaga,E.,Demirel,G.,Döğeroğlu,T.,Örnektekin,S.,Meliefste,K.&Doorn,W.(2008).Hava Kirliliği ve Kontrolü Sempozyumu, Bildiriler Kitabı, pp.631-642, Hatay/Turkey, October 22-25, 2008.

Özer, U., Aydin, R. and Akçay, H. (1997). Air pollution profile of Turkey. *Chemistry International,* 19 (6), pp.190-191.

Öztürk, M. (2005). Şehir İçi Bölgelerde Hava Kirliliğinin Sağlık Üzerine Etkileri, Çevre ve Orman Bakanlığı, Ankara/Turkey.

Özer,U., Aydin, R., & Akçay,H. (1997).Air Pollution Profile of Turkey, *Chemistry International,* Vol. 19, No. 6,pp.190-191

Sloss,L.L. & Smith, I.M., (2000). PM_{10} and $PM_{2.5}$: an international perspective, *Fuel Processing Technology,* 65-66,pp.127-141,

Sardar, S.B., Geller, M.D., Sioutas, C. & Solomon, P.A. (2006). Development and evaluation of a high-volume dichotomous sampler for chemical speciation of coarse and fine particles, *Aerosol Science,* 37, pp.1455 - 1466.

Şahin Ü. (2000). İstanbul'da 1994-1998 Hava Kirliliği Düzeyleri ile Mortalite Arasındaki İlişki *(Thesis)* İstanbul Üniversitesi Tıp Fakültesi

Topbaş, M. Can, G.& Kapucu, M. (2004). Effects of local decisions on air pollution in Trabzon, Turkey during 1994-2000. *Turkish Journal of Public Health,* 2 (2), pp. 80-84 Local Directorate of Environment and Forestry of Trabzon

Uzunali, D. (2004).Air pollution maps based on the data collected between 1998 and 2002 for the center of Trabzon City. *M. Sc. Thesis,* Department of Mechanical Engineering, Karadeniz Technical University

Ünsal,A., Metintaş,S. & İnan, O.Ç., (1999). Eskişehir'de Hava Kirliliği ve Bazı Hastalıklar Nedeniyle Acil Başvurularının İncelenmesi, *Tüberküloz ve Toraks,* 47(4),pp. 449-455

URL-1.Air Quality and Health http://www.agius.com/hew/resource/airqual.htm

URL-2 Air quality and health http://www.who.int/mediacentre/factsheets/fs313/en/index.html, 2008

URL-3 The Effects of Air Pollution on Human Health By Charlotte Mission, How Contributor http://www.ehow.com/about_5397380_effects-air-pollution-human-health.html

URL-4 Indoor & Outdoor Air Pollution, http://www.lbl.gov/Education/ELSI/pollution-main.html,2010
URL5 Devlet Meteoroloji Müdürlüğü, http://www.meteor.gov.tr/2006/tahmin/tahminiller aspx?m=TRABZON, 2009
URL-6 Gezi Yerleri, Trabzon'un İklim Verileri (2007), http://www.geziyerleri.net/gezi/10-trabzonun-iklimverileri html, 2009
URL 7 Coğrafya Dünyası, Trabzon İklim ve Bitki Örtüsü, http://www.cografya.gen.tr/tr/trabzon/iklim.html, 2009
URL 8 World Health Organization, Air Quality Guidelines for Particulate Matter, Ozone, Nitrogen Dioxide and Sulfur Dioxide, Summary of Risk Assessment (2006), http://www.whqlibdoc.who.int/hq/2006/WHO_SDE_PHE_OEH_0 6.02_eng.pdf -, 2009
URL 9 Uçku, R., Karababa, A. O., Ergör, A., Sarıkaya, Ö., Civaner, M., Demiral, Y., 2000,Hava Kirliliği, Türk Tabipleri Birliği Yatağan'da Hava Kirliliğinin Değerlendirilmesi Raporu http://www.ttb.org.tr/eweb/yatagan/icin.html
URL10 Kalkan, O., 2001, Hava Kirliliği, http://www.bsm.gov.tr/makale/20013.asp?donem=Mart%202001&sayi=20013#03
URL 11 Health Aspects of Air Pollution with Particulate Matter, Ozone and Nitrogen Dioxide, 2003. Report on a WHO Working Group.Bonn/Germany(*This document was text processed in Health Documentation Services WHO Regional Office for Europe, Copenhage)* http://www.euro.who.int/__data/assets/pdf_file/0005/112199/E79097.pdf

14

Air Pollution and Its Impacts – The City of Rijeka Case Study

Ana Alebić-Juretić
Teaching Institute of Public Health/ School of Medicine, University of Rijeka Croatia

1. Introduction

During the late sixties and seventies the city of Rijeka underwent second rapid industrialization. Few huge plants (new petroleum refinery facilities, power plant, coke plant) were erected in the industrial zone eastwards from the city. As a consequence, high emission levels resulted in elevated ambient air pollution so that the city was one of the most polluted in Croatia during the mid-eighties. Thus the annual means of sulphur dioxide exceeded double the WHO guideline at some urban sites. The beginning of air pollution monitoring programme dates back to early seventies with first measurements of sulphur dioxide (SO_2), black smoke (BS) and fallout within the city. Due to air pollution from the newly built industrial plants, the programme was extended to more parameters at the beginning of eighties, thus including: nitrogen dioxide (NO_2), ammonia (NH_3), hydrogen sulphide (H_2S), total suspended particulates (TSP), metals and polynuclear aromatic hydrocarbons (PAHs). All these parameters were measured by chemical methods, while first automatic network with only three analyzers (SO_2, O_3 and TSP) was established only in 2000, as the first automatic network in Croatia.

As the ambient levels of air pollutants diminished considerably since mid-nineties, a synthesis of the work done in the last 25 years dealing with long-term air pollution and its effects on materials, plants and humans is presented.

2. Long-term trends of air pollutants

2.1 Emissions

The elevated air pollution since the beginning of eighties was the reason to undertake first steps towards its abatement. Therefore, the first emission inventory including major big sources was done as early as 1989 (MEISA, 1991).

This inventory attributed major emissions of SO_2 and NO_2 to industrial point sources. Reduced production in war/post-war period resulted in approx. 70% lower emissions of SO_2 and 35% of NO_2 in 1995 (Ekonerg, 1997). The recuperation of economic activity and use of cleaner fuel led to their increase in 2001 (Regional Centre, 2002) and 2006 (County, 2009). Contrary to SO_2 , whose total emission remained bellow 50% of that in 1989, the total NO_2 emission is approaching that on 1989, but due to increase of contribution from traffic. In fact, the number of vehicles increased by 60% between 1995 and 2001, with additional increase of 20% in the period 2001-2006. In all these inventories emissions from harbour were missing. The first emission inventory for harbour activities estimated for 2008 SO_2 emission to 425 t $year^{-1}$ and NO_2 to 849 t $year^{-1}$ (ARCADIS, 2011) that is < 5% for SO_2 and approx 20% for NO_x of the total emission in 2006.

	SO_2				NO_2			
Sources	1989	1995	2001	2006	1989	1995	2001	2006
Petroleum refinery Urinj	16000	5651	7795	7127	2019	1501	1918	1552
Rijeka I power plant	8600	3237	7179	6672	1240	943	1172	1335
Petroleum refinery Mlaka	3557	1036	1639	1761	472	283	128	208
Coke plant	4778				955			
Subtotal:	32935	9924	16613	15560	4686	2727	3218	3095
Other industry	1260	411	470	185		76	159	29
Traffic	200	171	163	147	864	705	1100	1400
Other	2035	356	635	422		119	118	200
Total:	36430	10862	17881	16314	5550	3627	4595	4724

Table 1. Emissions of sulphur dioxide and nitrogen oxides (as NO_2) in t $year^{-1}$ in the Rijeka Bay Area

2.2 Ambient levels of some pollutants

Maen daily concentrations of various pollutants were determined by the following methods:

a. sulphur dioxide - standard British acidimetric method (WHO, 1976); since 2000 automatic analyzer Monitorlab 8850 (Monitorlab, USA)
b. black smoke - reflectometry (Perry & Jung, 1977)
c. nitrogen dioxide - modification of Saltzman method (Perry & Jung, 1977); since 2003 analyzer API M 200 (Advanced Pollution Instrumentation, USA)
d. ammonia - spectrophotometrically with Nessler reagent (WHO, 1976)
e. hydrogen sulphide - modification of molibden blue method (Vadic, 1982)
f. ozone - analyzer API M 400 (API, USA)
g. total suspended particulates (TSP) and since 2006 PM_{10} - gravimetrically (WHO, 1976)
h. suspended particulates PM_{10} - since 2003 analyzer TEOM 1400a (Rupprecht &Pataschnik, USA)
i. metals - atomic absorption spectroscopy (van Loon, 1985)
j. polycyclic aromatic hydrocarbons - HPLC with UV detector (Alebic-Juretic, 1994)

Comparing the results of chemical methods with those obtained by analyzers of SO_2 and NO_2, it turned out that there is no significant difference between either methods for SO_2, while NO_x analyzer gave approx 20% higher concentrations relative to chemical method. As the PM_{10} concentrations obtained by analyzer are systematically lower, the corresponding correction factor was employed (EC, 2002). Since 2000 the sulphur dioxide and ozone analyzer from the Institute site together with TSP analyzer in the suburban site above shipyard formed a first automatic Air Quality Network in Croatia with automatic collection and elaboration of the data. Three years later the network was extended to six more automatic sites, with possibility for display of the hourly data in real time on the Institute web-site (www. zzjzpgz.hr). That was also the first such a web site established in Croatia.

2.2.1 Sulphur dioxide and black smoke

Sulphur dioxide (SO_2) is generated by combustion of fossil fuel. Its emission depends on sulphur fuel content. Annual mean concentrations of SO_2 in four urban sites (Fig 1) follow

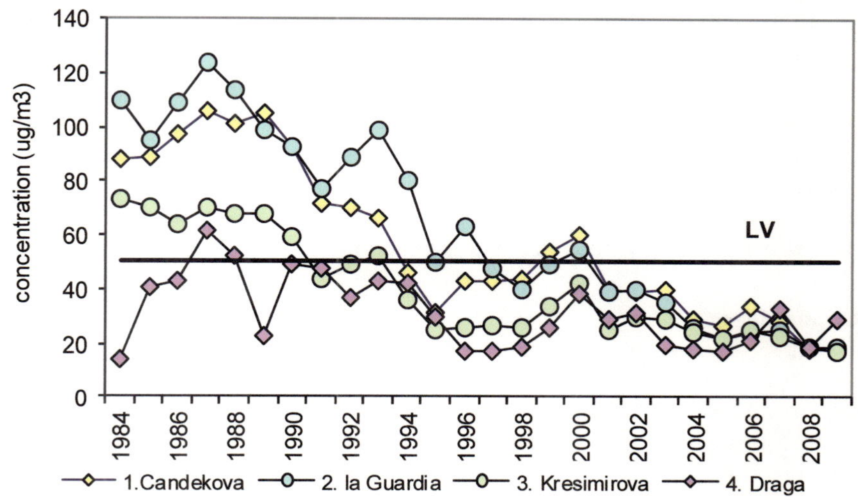

Fig. 1. Annual mean concentrations of sulphur dioxide (limit value LV=50 µg m^{-3})

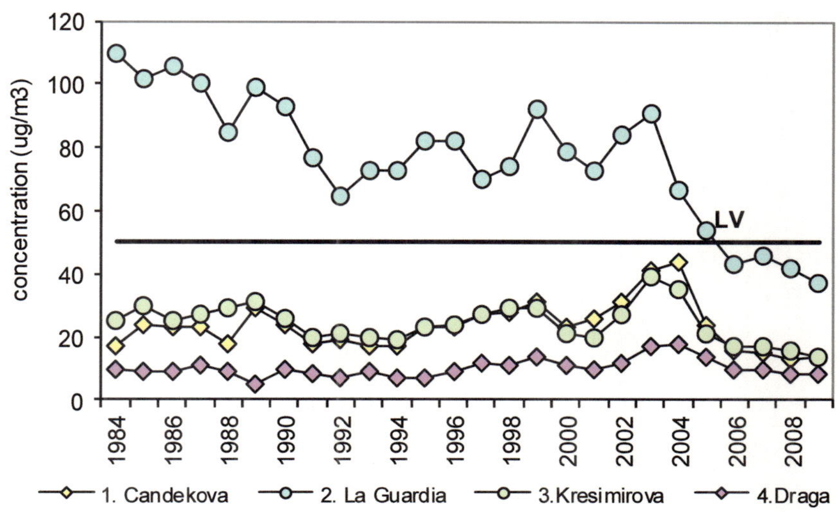

Fig. 2. Annual mean concentrations of black smoke (limit value LV=50 µg m^{-3})

the emission patterns. Sulphur dioxide and black smoke (BS) were blamed for several smog episodes during fifties and sixties in Europe and America that caused increased mortality among exposed population. Because of switch to cleaner fuel, the SO_2 concentrations diminished considerably during early eighties in Europe, with annual means < 100 µg m^{-3} (WHO, 2000) that are presently even lower (20-30 µg m^{-3}). Similar behaviour is observed in Rijeka. Thus, 70% in SO_2 emission reduction resulted in the equivalent decrease in ambient air SO_2 concentrations between 1989 and 1995 (Matkovic & Alebic-Juretic, 1998). Subsequent increase in SO_2 emissions in 2001 followed by slow decrease towards 2006 are reflected proportionally in ambient air concentrations. Since 2001 the limit value for SO_2 is observed at all four urban sites.

Except for urban F. la Guardia street with heavy traffic, the black smoke did not represent critical pollutant. In spite of a slight increase in annual concentrations from 2000 to 2004, the BS at three urban sites obeyed the limit value since the beginning of monitoring. Sharp decrease in BS concentration in 2004 (except at suburban site Draga) is due to introduction of natural gas in the city center for heating, that finally enabled drop of annual BS concentrations bellow limit value in F. la Guardia street in 2006 (Fig. 2).

2.2.2 Nitrogen dioxide

Nitrogen oxides NOx are generated mostly from air by combustion of fossil fuels. Therefore it is more difficult to diminish their emissions and consequently ambient levels. The principal source of NOx is traffic. NO_2 is precursor of photochemical smog. As irritant, NO_2 might affect respiratory system. Urban levels of NO_2 are in the range 20-90 µg m^{-3}, while background level is 10 µg m^{-3} (WHO, 2000). Time trends in annual NO_2 concentrations in Rijeka show a decreasing trend at industrial site (Mlaka) and no significant trend at urban traffic site (Krešimirova St), in spite of the increased emission of NO_2 in the period 2001-2006 (Fig 3).

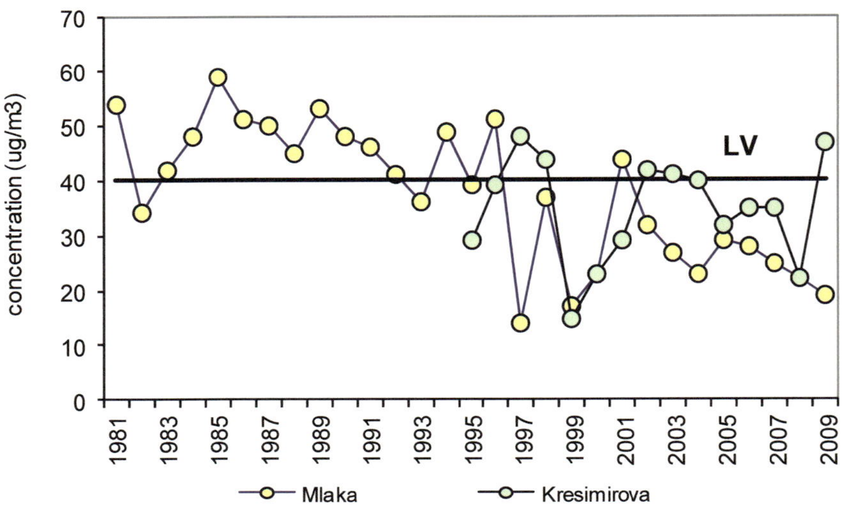

Fig. 3. Annual mean concentrations of nitrogen dioxide (limit value LV=50 µg m^{-3})

2.2.3 Ammonia

Ammonia ambient levels also show a slight decline (Fig. 4). It is interesting to notice that closing up the coke plant in 1994, a major source of ammonia in the area (993-1323 t/year estimated by emission inventory from 1989), did not affect significantly the time trend, not even at the neighbouring site Kraljevica. It is well known that ambient levels of ammonia do not follow its emission. Such a behaviour is explained by high reactivity and/or volatility of airborne ammonia.

Agriculture is generally considered as the main source of airborne ammonia, but it is scarcely present in this karst area. The urban and suburban levels of ammonia are rather high, but they are diminishing in the remote areas, with distance from the city (Alebic-Juretic , 2008). Therefore, urban and industrial sources should be responsible for the observed ammonia levels.

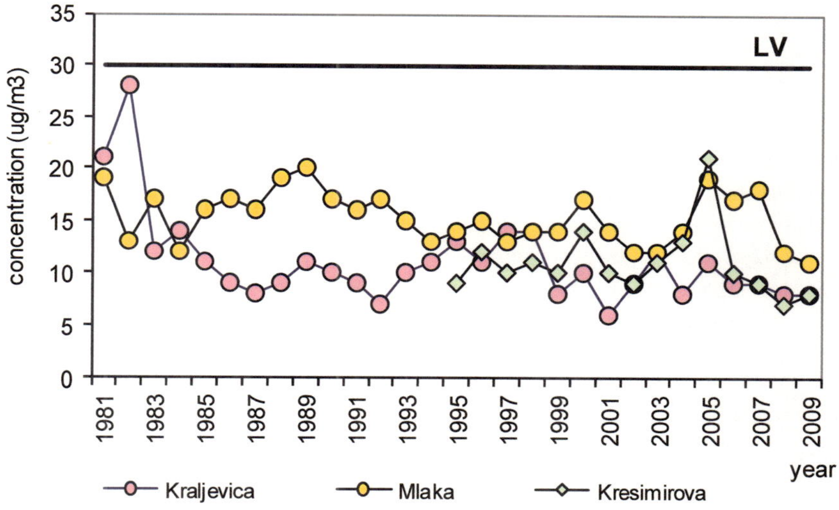

Fig. 4. Annual mean concentrations of ammonia (limit value LV=30 µg m^{-3})

2.2.4 Hydrogen sulphide

Hydrogen sulphide is a gas of unpleasant smell. It is generated from elementary sulphur or sulphur compounds and organic material exposed to elevated temperature. There is no trend in hydrogen sulphide regarding the annual means at the site opposing petroleum refinery, in spite of temporarily high annual values (Fig 5). Such a curve shape reflects the (un)success in control of production processes. In 2008 the production ceased at this location, but in spite of that, the area resulted to be excessively polluted by H_2S due to hourly tolerant limit values (TV=7.6 µg m^{-3} in 2009) exceedances at automatic monitoring station (Trogirska St) during heating season, thus indicating boilers as the H_2S sources (Alebic-Juretic et al, 2009).

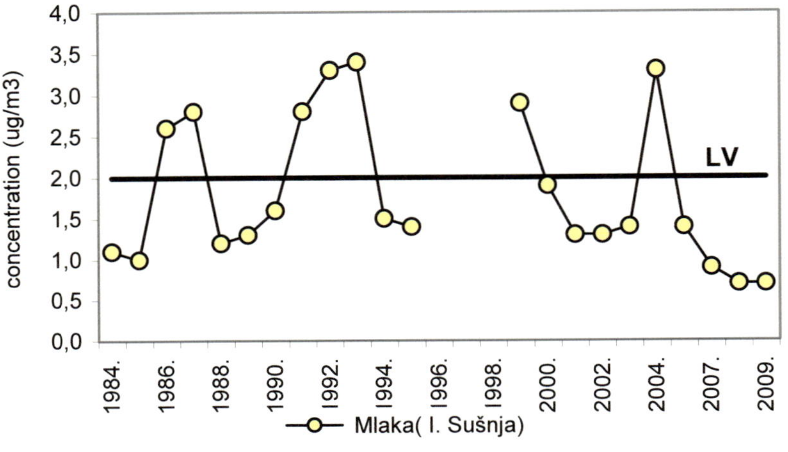

Fig. 5. Annual mean concentrations of hydrogen sulphides (limit value LV=2 μg m-3)

2.2.5 Ozone

Tropospheric ozone is secondary pollutant generated from NOx and reactive hydrocarbons under conditions of high insolation and elevated temperature. Therefore elevated concentrations of tropospheric ozone are registered during summer. Ground levels of ozone are the result of several processes taking place in the boundary layer like local photochemical production, horizontal transport on regional and/or synoptic scale, vertical transport from the stratosphere and ozone sinks like photochemical destruction with NO and deposition on surfaces. Ground level ozone is irritant and might have harmful effects on human health.

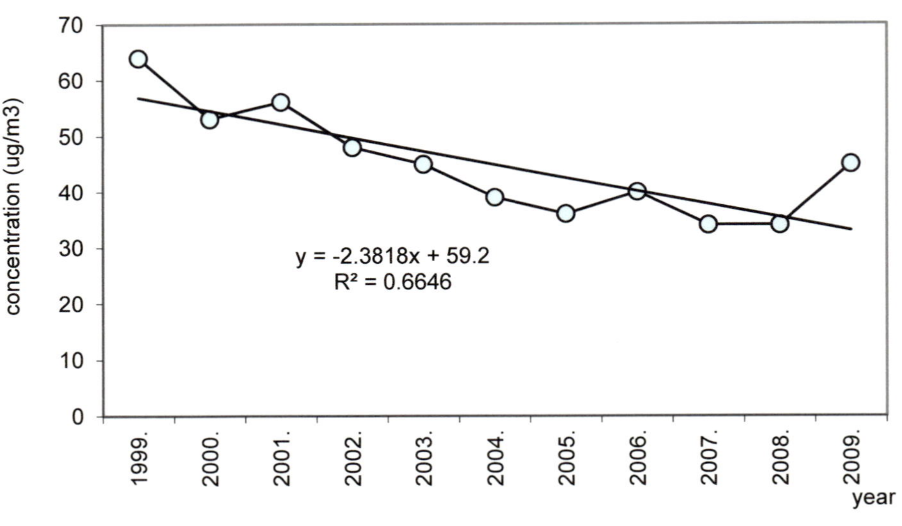

Fig. 6. Annual mean concentrations of ozone

Contrary to some other parts of Europe, the ambient concentrations of ozone show a declining trend in Rijeka since the beginning of measurements in 1999. As the same trend is observed at elevated remote location (Puntjarka) since 1990, this seems to be regional phenomena (Alebic-Juretic, 2008a).

Declining trend of ozone is preserved in spite of higher annual concentration in 2009 relative to several preceding years.Such a high concentration is obtained because an exceptionally high summer temperature and ozone levels in August, with registered hourly means above 200 µg m^{-3}. Similar condition has appeared only in August 2000, and was only recently explained by combination of local ozone production and regional transport.

2.2.6 Suspended particulate matter (TSP and PM_{10})

Suspended particulates are formed of complex mixture of organic and inorganic compounds. According to their dimensions, the suspended particulates are grouped into fine with aerodynamic diameter $d<2.5$ µm, and coarse particulates with $d>2.5$ µm. Fine fraction of particulates contains secondary generated aerosols (from gas-solid conversion), particulates formed by combustion and secondary adsorbed metals and organics. Coarse fraction usually contains soil particles, fugative dust from streets and industrial sources. Suspended particulates are usually divided into: total suspended particulates (TSP), particulate matter with aerodynamic diameter <10 µm (PM_{10}) and particulate matter with aerodynamic diameter <2.5 µm ($PM_{2.5}$). Particulate matter that can reach human respiratory system (PM_{10}) are emitted from various sources: natural (volcanoes or dust storms) or anthropogenic (industry, domestic heating, traffic). The latter sources are more important regarding air pollution (WHO, 2000).

First systematic monitoring of particulates started with discontinuous TSP measurements in Rijeka in 1991. Due to change in legislation, these measurements are switched to PM_{10} in 2006. These are not the first measurements of PM_{10} ever, since three years earlier a continuous monitoring with analyzer started.

2.2.6.1 Discontinous measurements

The grain silo in the harbour was a big source of suspended particulates. Thus, the annual concentrations of total suspended particulates (TSP) were always close to the limit value (Fig.7a), but the daily values were often exceeded (Alebic-Juretic, 2005). Only after installation of the new dust suppression system in the silo in mid 2003, the limit value was finally obeyed. Results of PM_{10}, that replaced TSP measurements in 2006 (Fig 7b), also fulfilled the limit value. The number of exceedances was bellow allowed 35 days per year. This limit was approached only in 2006 (6 month).

2.2.6.2 Continous measurements

Continous measurements of PM_{10} with analyzers started in 2003 in the city of Rijeka. The results are given in Fig.8. The analyzer is a part of a traffic station on the busy street level, thus the results are different from discontinous sampler located on the roof of the Institute, in the same street. Though the annual means were around limit value LV, the number of exceedances was 2-3 times higher than allowed per year (35 times). This number diminished only in 2007, presumably due to introduction of natural gas in the city center.

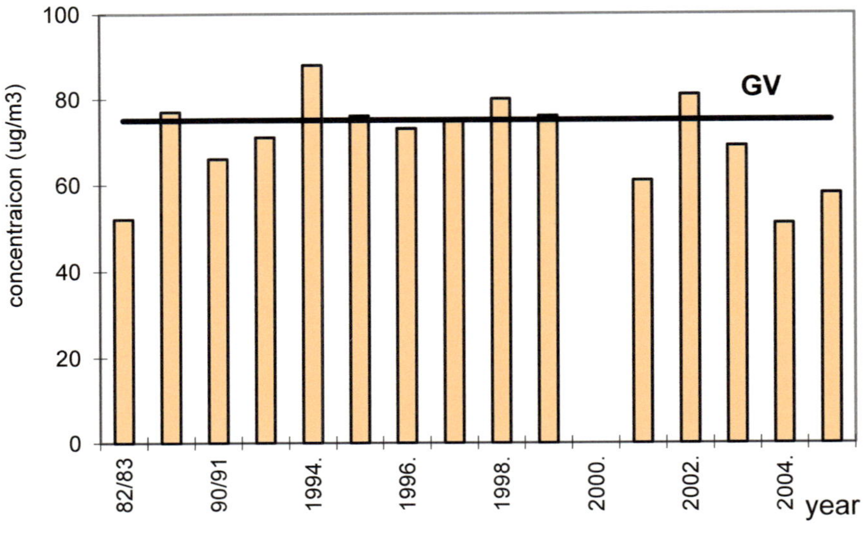

a.

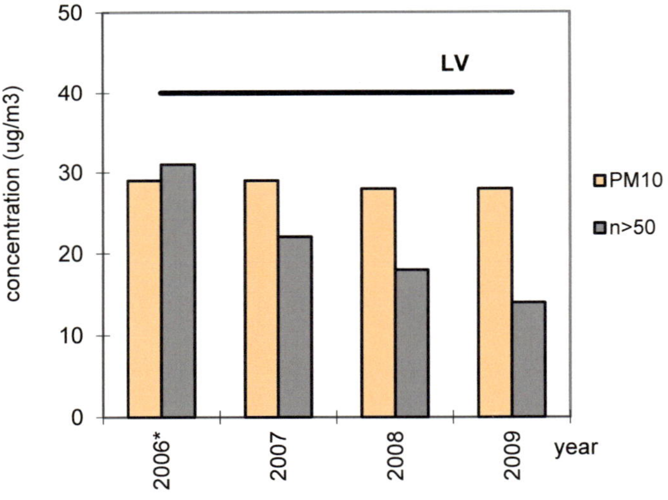

b. * six months data

Fig. 7. Annual means of a. TSP (guideline value GV = 75 µg m^{-3}) and b.: PM_{10} (limit value LV = 40 µg m^{-3}) in the city of Rijeka (n>50 – number of average daily concentrations exceeding daily limit value LV_d = 50 µg m^{-3})

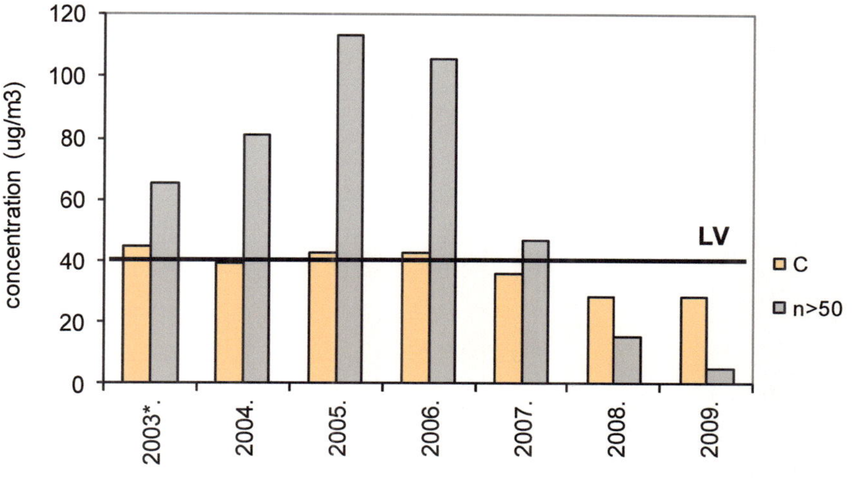

Fig. 8. Annual means (C) of PM_{10} measured with analyzer (n>50- number of exceedances of LV_d =50 μg m^{-3})

2.2.7 Lead in suspended particulate matter (TSP and PM_{10})

Samples of TSP and PM_{10} were analyzed on lead and cadmium content since the beginning of PM measurements. These analyses were extended to iron, zinc and copper, as typical for metal and shipyard industry. The biggest differences in metal concentration over time is found with lead, since traffic was the main source of this metal, and switch to unleaded petrol diminished the airborne lead considerably. Concentrations of lead in TSP were always bellow respective limit value since the beginning of measurements in early nineties. As the traffic was the main source of lead, its airborne concentrations show increase to the end of nineties due to increase in number of vehicles. The subsequent decreasing trend is due to major use of unleaded petrol (Alebic-Juretic, 2005), up to 2006 when the leaded petrol disappeared from the market (Fig 9). Lead content in PM_{10} is also low and bellow the respective limit value.

2.2.8 Polycyclic aromatic hydrocarbons in suspended particulate matter (TSP and PM_{10})

Polycyclic aromatic hydrocarbons (PAHs) are generated by incomplete combustion of organic material (fossil fuel). The main sources of PAHs are coke plants, petroleum refineries, traffic and domestic heating. The most studied PAHs is benzo(a)pyrene , a known carcinogen representing potential threat to public health. Occasional determination of PAHs in TSP dates back to mid eighties, while systematic measurements started only in 2001. Since 2006 PAHs are analysed in the PM_{10} fraction. The highest concentrations of BaP and PaHs were obtained at the beginning of nineties, at the time with the highest pollution with combustion products (SO_2, black smoke). The concentration of BaP was up to 5 ng m^{-3}, while the concentrations of total PAHs were 10-12 times higher. The declining trend of BaP and PAHs started by the end of nineties (Alebic-Juretic, 2005), while in 2005 the concentrations of BaP fell bellow 1 ng m^{-3}. In the PM_{10} fraction of suspended particulates the concentrations of BaP are even lower.

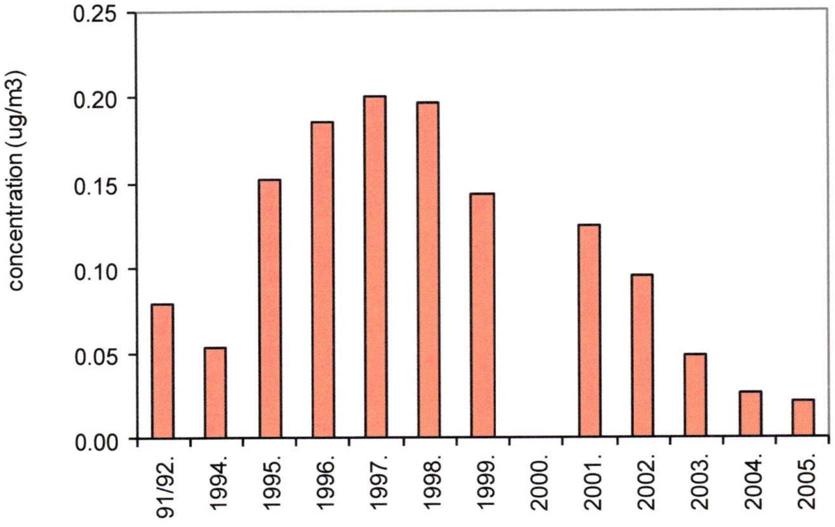

a.

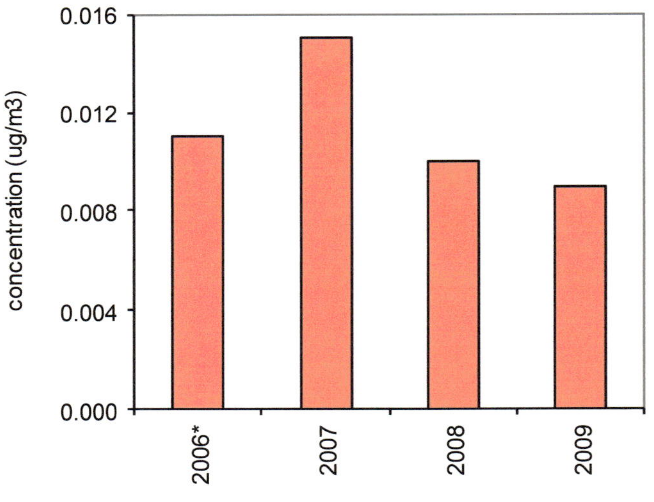

b.

Fig. 9. Lead in suspended particulates in Rijeka, a. TSP (LV=1 µg m^{-3}) and b. PM_{10} (LV=0.5 µg m^{-3}) (* six month value)

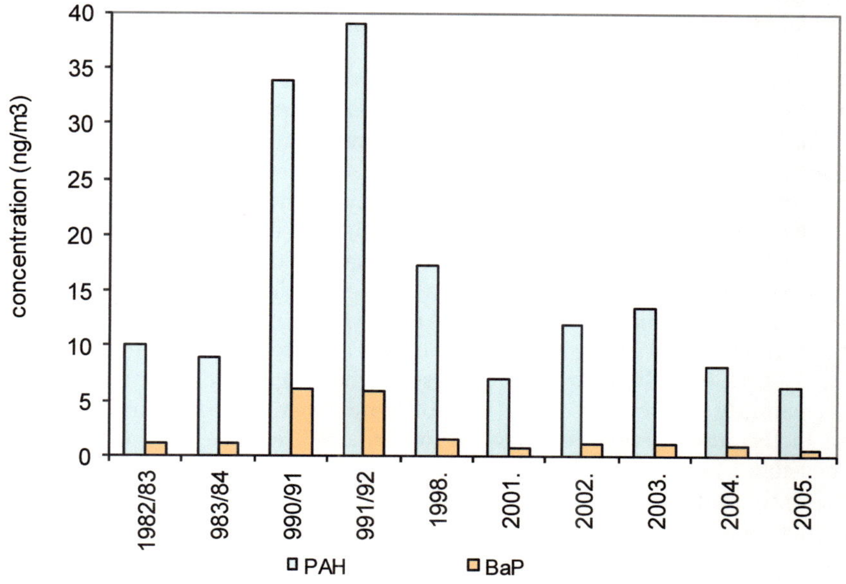

a.

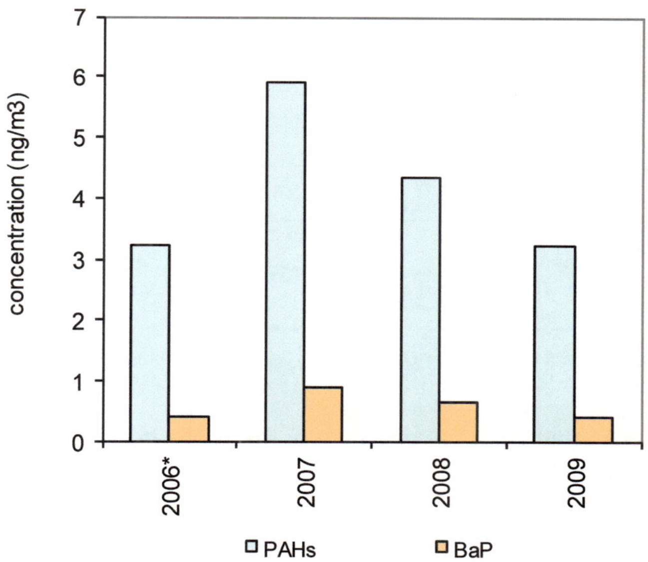

b.

Fig. 10. Concentrations of total PAHs in a. TSP and b. PM_{10} (* six months value)

2.3 Air pollution effects on materials - paintings

High ambient concentrations of SO_2 might deteriorate the buildings and sculptures made of calcite. As a consequence the edges loose their sharpness and the surface is covered by a layer of dirt formed from gypsum (derived from airborne H_2SO_4 and calcite) and soot. Similar process occurs in indoor environment, i.e. interior walls covered with plaster. Therefore, the most abundant aerosol in indoor environment is gypsum, $CaSO_4 \times 2 H_2O$. Indoor gaseous and particulate pollution in museums is often correlated to pollutants outdoor concentrations leading to different conclusions: indicating outdoor pollution as a source for the observed indoor concentrations (Ligocki et al, 1993), pointing out some (un)known indoor sources (Mouratidou & Samara, 2004) or taking as a proof of effectiveness of the installed HVAC system (Salmon et al, 2005).

The Museum of Modern and Contemporary Art (MMCA) in Rijeka is situated on the second floor of a building located in the very center of the city, between two busy city roads. The Museum will move into the new location, also in the city centre, facing another busy city road and apparently worse considering air pollution. Since air pollution is found to be one of the risk factors for preventive conservation of artworks, the aim of the work was to evaluate possible effects of air pollution on paintings already kept in the central depot located within the Museum area. The paintings analyzed were randomly chosen from those that were subjected to restoration prior to be exposed in the exhibition area. Two of the paintings were kept in the central depot, while the other two were stored in the auxiliary depot, and were taken for comparative purposes. The characteristics of the selected paintings are given in Table 2.

No	Author	Title	Year	Technique	Dimension/ cm	Depot/ since	Remark
1.	Butozan M.	Man in the interior	1942	oil/ canvas	138x100	Central/1980	thick paint layers, varnish, mostly smooth surface
2.	Seferov V.	The nude	1933	oil/ canvas	117x170	Central/1974	visible canvas fiber, mostly rough surface
3.	Lusic T.	Imbarco a ferro	1989	acrylic/ canvas	151x249.5	Cent/1993 Auxil/1994	completely smooth surface
4.	Grozdanic Ž.	Kiefer-Knifer	1991	combined	159.5x224	Cent/1991 Auxil/1994	rough structured, uneven wax coated surface

Table 2. The characteristics of the paintings selected for analyses (Alebic-Juretic & Sekulic-Cikovic, 2009)

The central depot is located on the second floor of the Museum's building, in the very centre of the city. The storage rooms were ventilated occasionally just by opening the windows, thus enhancing penetration of the outdoor pollution. Furthermore, the paintings were exposed to considerable seasonal temperature oscillations. The auxiliary depot was located in the basement flat of the building situated on the busy city road. The paintings remained locked in this location until restoration. No exact measurements of air pollution are available for the depots' locations. Due to environmental conditions (sampling point heights approx 15 m above street level, location between two busy roads) the results of such measurements obtained at the Institute building (Site 1) may approximate the outdoor air pollution at the central depot, characterized by higher pollution with SO_2 relative to that of black smoke. The air pollution at the auxiliary depot is very likely to be similar to that of another, poorly ventilated busy street (Site 2) in the city center that is characterized by high black smoke concentrations, exceeding SO_2 since mid-nineties.

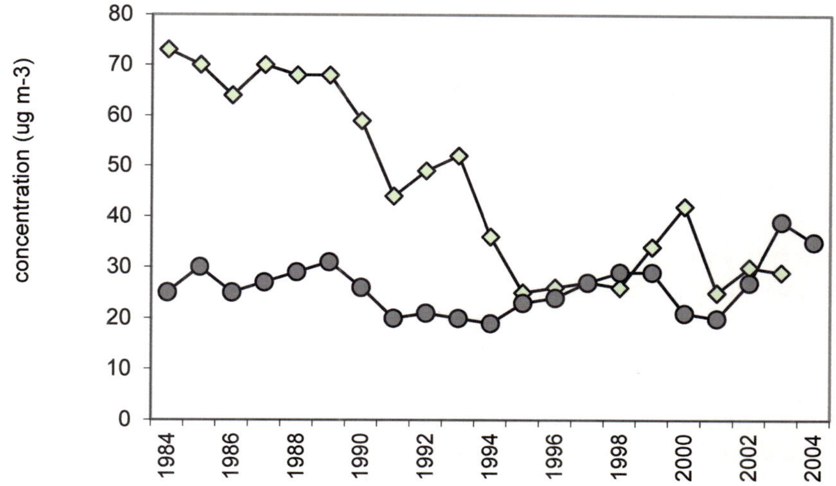

a.

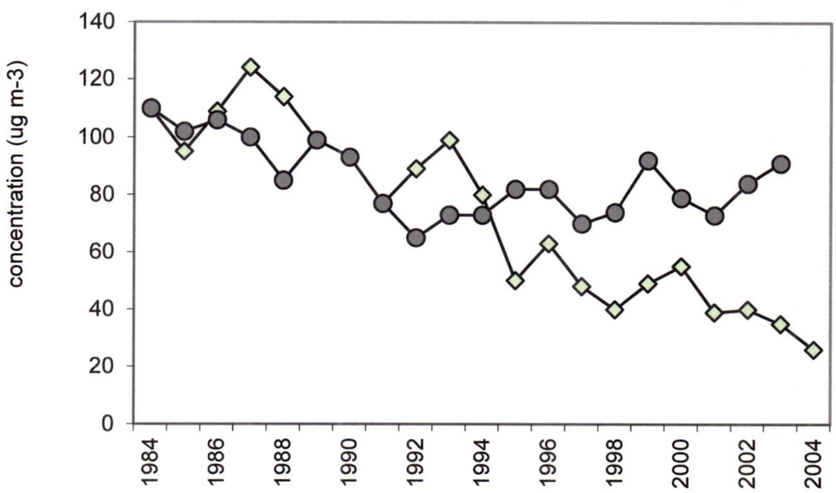

b.

Fig. 11. Annual means of SO_2 (green) and black smoke (grey) at: a. Site 1 representing central depot, and b. Site 2 representing auxiliary depot (from Alebic-Juretic & Cikovic-Sekulic, 2009)

Instead of measuring a set of gaseous and particulate pollutants indoor and outdoor, dirt removed from paintings during restoration works was analysed. Dirt is deposited on the paintings surfaces as the result of soiling process during decades of storage in the depots. The surface dirt was removed from the first painting (No 1: Butozan) by pieces of cotton wool soaked in demineralized water, while subsequently cotton wool was replaced by a synthetic fiber cloth .The parameters determined were those used for ambient air pollution monitoring: total "dirt", soot, lead, individual polynuclear aromatic hydrocarbons (PAHs) and water extract ionic content.

The amount of dirt was determined gravimetrically, as the weight gain of cotton wool/synthetic cloth after cleaning the paintings. To enable the comparison between the obtained results, the total amount of dirt was normalized against the paintings surface area giving the results in mg m^{-2}.The amount of soot is also determined gravimetrically, as the ignition loss at 800°C of ashes obtained by burning the cotton wool/synthetic cloth samples. The lead content was measured by graphite furnace AAS (Perkin-Elmer Z 4001) after dissolving ashes in acidic mixture HNO_3/HCl (van Loon, 1985). The ionic content of the dirt was determined from the water extract obtained by extraction of "dirt" in ultrasonic bath for 60 min. The ionic content was determined by modular Methrom ion chromatography system. The operating conditions are described elsevere (Alebic-Juretic & Sekulic-Cikovic, 2009). The PAHs were extracted from cotton wool/cloth by cyclohexane (100 ml) in ultrasonic bath (60 min). The individual PAHs were determined from the purified cyclohexane extract using HPLC (Helwett Packard 1050) with UV-VIS detector, according to the previously described procedure (Alebic-Juretic, 1994).

The highest amount of total "dirt", soot, lead and total PAHs (Figure 12) are obtained from painting No1 (Butozan). Since this is the second oldest painting in this study, the unknown previous history of keeping, as well as the nature of thick oily paint might be responsible for this result. In the oldest painting No 2 (Seferov) lower values of total "dirt", soot and particularly lead and total PAHs are found, thus indicating better keeping conditions, e.g. more distant from combustion sources, prior to arrival in the Museum's depot. The lowest amount of total "dirt" and total PAHs are found in painting No3 (Lusic), possibly due to incorporation of dust and dirt onto the acrylic film. The (non-polar) wax coated surface of painting No 4 (Grozdanic) collected more total "dirt", soot and total PAHs than painting No 3, that was contemporary kept in the auxiliary depot. Unexpectedly low lead content in water extract from the same painting was found. The possible reasons for were: either the low possibility of sticking the mineral particles onto non-polar wax surface, or the mineral particles were embedded into the wax layers that prevented their efficient extraction. The interesting feature is that the percent content of soot obtained from paintings kept in the auxiliary depot is relatively high (approx. 0,65%) compared to those found on paintings kept in the central depot, in spite of 2-3 times longer exposure times to possible air pollutants. The plausible reason for this finding is the impact of soot emission from heavy traffic, as the auxiliary depot was located beneath the street level. (Alebic-Juretic & Sekulic-Cikovic, 2009). The individual PAH profile (Fig 13) also indicate the possible air pollution impact. The more complete profile is found in paintings kept in the auxiliary depot (No 3 and 4), i.e. in the vicinity of the busy street - the source of PAHs. Lack of some individual PAHs in paintings from the central depot (No1 and 2) suggest their earlier date exposure to exhaust gases containing PAHs and subsequent degradation.

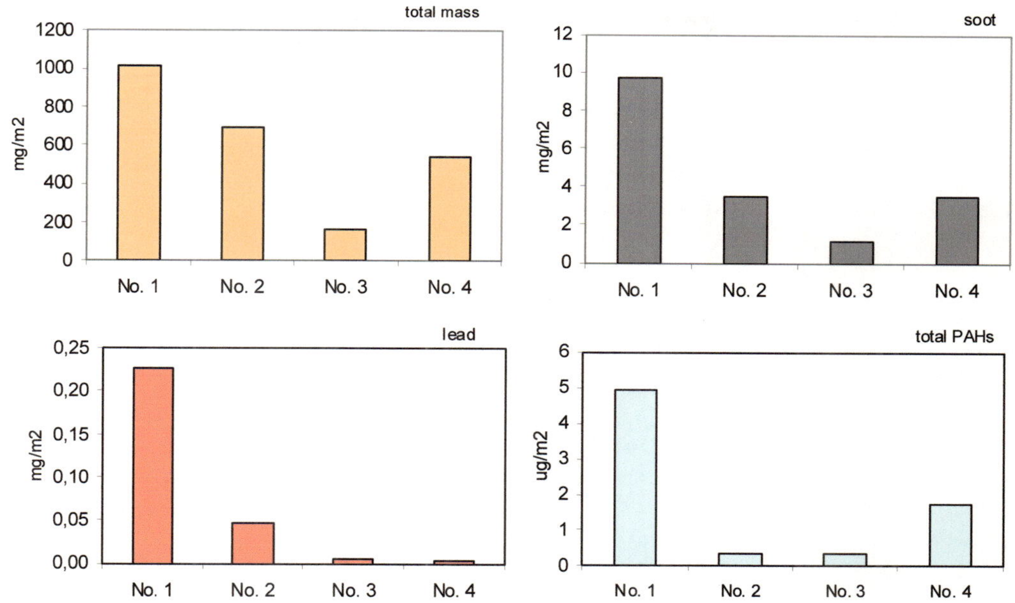

Fig. 12. Total mass, soot, lead and total PAHs deposited on paintings: No1: Butozan, No2: Seferov, No3: Lusic and No4: Grozdanic

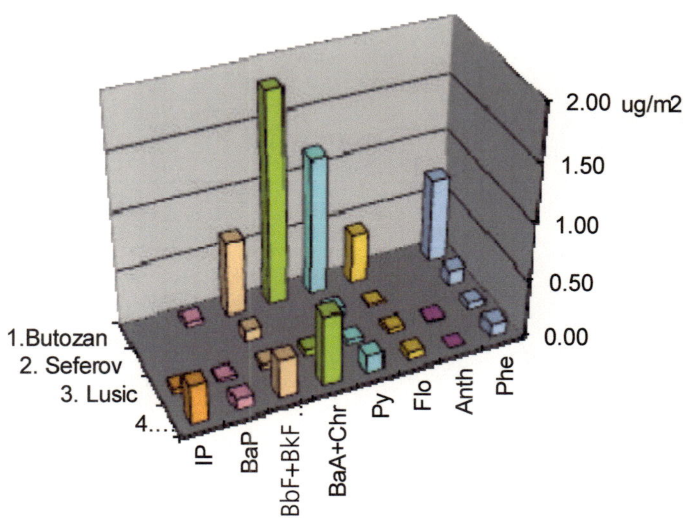

Fig. 13. Individual PAH profile obtained from surface dirt analyses (Phe-phenanthrene, Anth-anthracene, Flo-fluoranthene, Py-pyrene, BaA- benzo(a)anthracene, Chr-chrysene, BbF-benzo(b)fluoranthene, BkF-benzo(k)fluoranthene, BaP-benzo(a)pyrene, IP-indeno(1,2,3-c,d)pyrene)

A common feature of the analysed fractions is the predominance of sulphate and calcium in all paintings (though with different percentage). This is in agreement with findings that Ca rich particles are the most abundant in the indoor museums atmosphere (Camuffo et al., 2001). Higher values of analysed ions are found in older paintings (No 1 and 2) kept in the central depot indicating thus the cumulative effect. Comparing the ionic content expressed in meq m^{-2}, a clear difference between paintings kept in the central and auxiliary depot is evident (Fig 14). The excess of sulphate in paintings from the central depot may indicate the

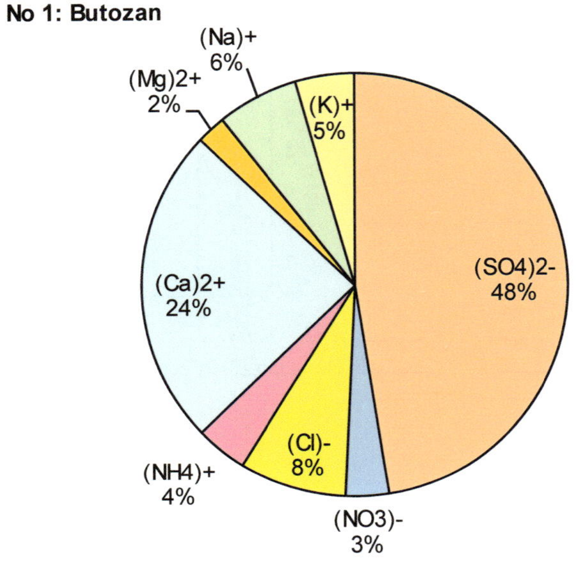

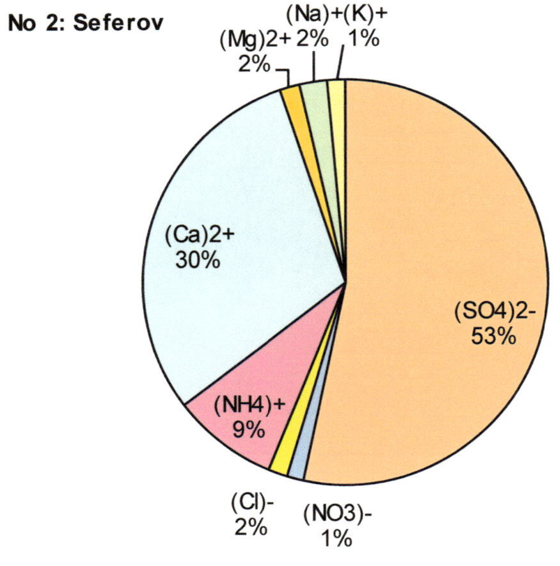

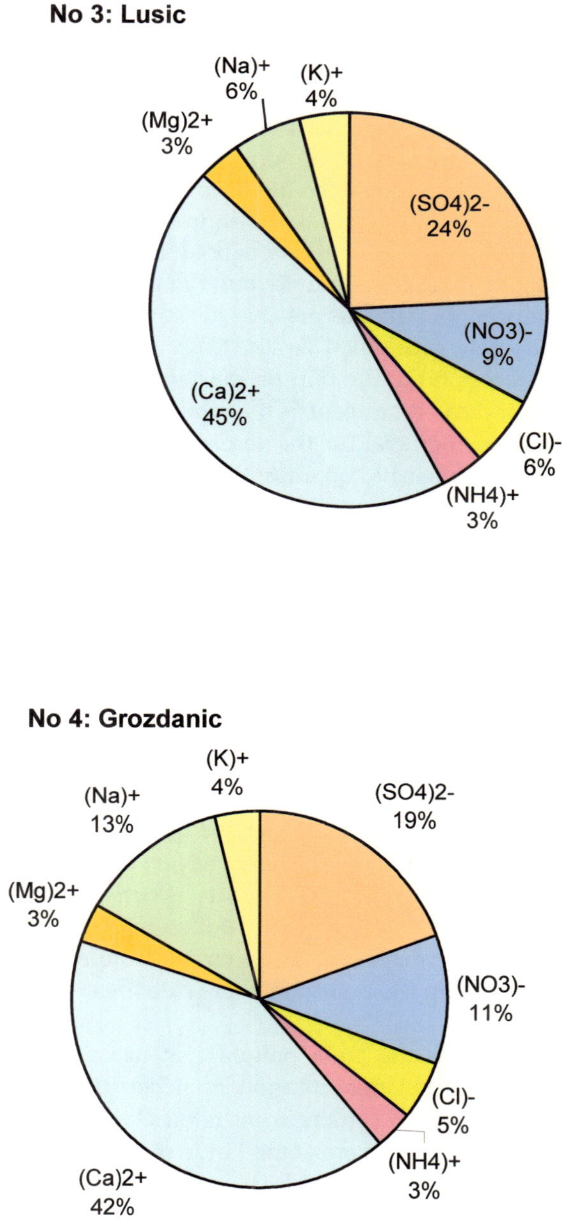

Fig. 14. Percent content of ionic components of dirt on painting analysed given as meq m^{-2} (Alebic-Juretic & Sekulic-Cikovic, 2009).

impact of air pollution by sulphur dioxide during decades of storage, including the eighties with highest air pollution with SO_2 within the city. The excess of sulphate may originate either from the reaction of SO_2 with already deposited calcite on the paintings, or as the result of H_2SO_4 formation via catalitic reaction on the surface of the paintings thus causing damages. Traces of reduced sulphur compounds (sulphides, mercaptans, disulphides), either gaseous or as constituent of pigment (e.g. cinober) might also be the source of SO_2 and sulphates on painting surfaces (Van Grieken et al., 1998). On the contrary, excess of calcium was found on paintings from the auxiliary depot, and could be attributed to dominant pollution by soil and/or plaster wall particles. It is worth to notice that meq m^{-2} amounts of ions are similar in paintings that were contemporary kept in the auxiliary depot (No 3 and 4), thus indicating the cumulative effect of soiling. Higher quantity of nitrate found in the latter paintings might also be in favour of some traffic impact, though bias are due to the fact that some pigments and coatings contain nitrate (Alebic-Juretic & Sekulic-Cikovic, 2009).

In conclusion: the excess of sulfates on a dirt film on paintings kept in depots during the period of highest air pollution indicated ambient SO_2 as the possible source. The nature of pigments, varnish and paints is also crucial for the aerosol deposition and/or surface gas reactions on artworks. Therefore it is hard to quantify their deposition/reaction rates. Since the ambient SO_2 concentrations decreased considerably, the traffic originated pollutants: NOx and particulates will be critical for the artworks to be stored in the new museum building. In spite of the fact that higher museum standard will be achieved, considering the air pollution and high financial cost regarding implementation of HVAC, further efforts for preventive measures are needed. These may include: identification and measuring indoor and outdoor air pollutants, space planning of the storage area, target cleaning, adequate protection of artwork and proper maintenance of the exhibition and storage areas (Alebic-Juretic & Sekulic-Cikovic, 2009).

2.4 Air pollution effects on vegetation – lichens

Lichens are an association of fungi (mycobionts) and green algae or cyanobacteria (photobiont). As they have no cuticle or protective wax layer and no stomata to regulate uptake of gaseous molecules, the exchange of nutrients occurs directly on the lichens surface. Therefore lichens are very sensitive to air pollution and have been used as bioindicators for over a century. Absence of cuticle favours accumulation of toxic metals in thallus and lichens can be used to map the pollution over wide areas (Minganti et al., 2003; Pinho et. al., 2004).

For many years sulphur dioxide was the main pollutant in urban and industrial areas. Elevated concentrations of SO_2 induced deterioration of lichen flora within such areas. Depending on air pollution levels, urban centers were often classified as "lichen desert", surrounded by so called "struggle zone" where some kinds of lichens can survive, though with some morphological changes. It is succeeded by so called "normal zone" with least air pollution and normal abundances of lichens. Though the first study of lichen flora in Rijeka was published already in 1902 (Schuler, 1902), the first classification on zones was done only in 1986 (Figure 15), at the time of highest air pollution within the city (Alebic-Juretic & Arko-Pijavac, 1989).

Except in the city center, two small lichen deserts were found at the elevated areas (>100 m a.s.l) under impact of plumes from paper mill (No 15: Kozala) and new built plant facilities in the east industrial zone (G. Vezica).

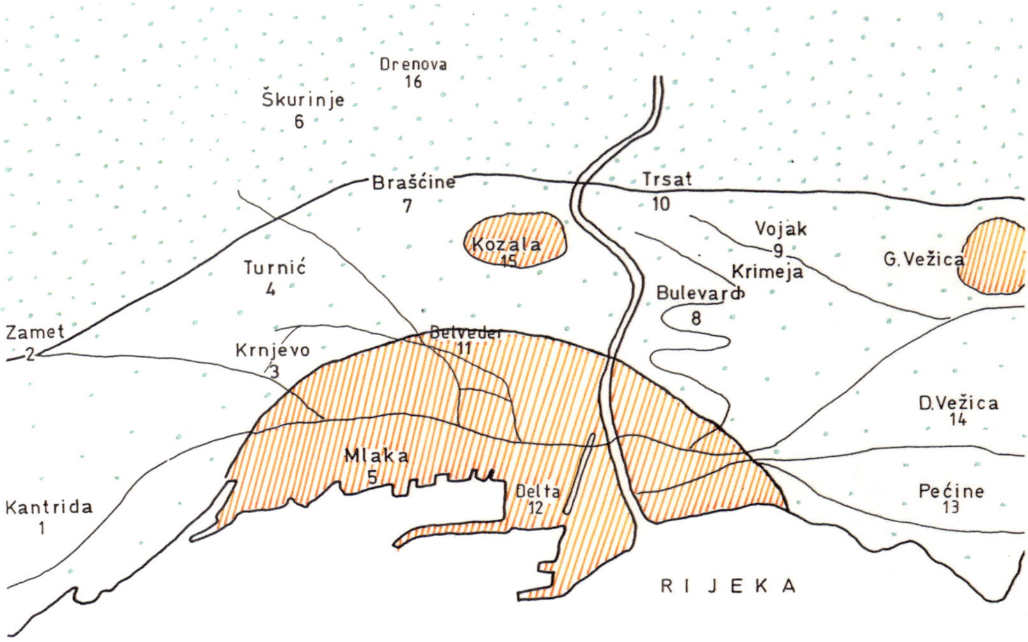

Fig. 15. Lichen zones in the city of Rijeka in 1986: lichen desert- yellow lines; struggle zone- rare green dots; normal zone- green dots (Alebic-Juretic & Arko-Pijavac, 1989)

Samples of two lichen species collected in winter 1985/86 *Parmelia tiliacea* (Hoffm) Ach and *Pannaria testacea* Jørg were used to perform simple biological test sensitive to early stages of membrane damage (Pearson, 1985). After preconditioning in humidity chamber for 2 hours (water temperature 35°C), and rinsing with deionized water for few seconds, pieces of lichen thalli (approx 50 mg weight) were immersed in deionized water (conductivity 1.5-2,.0 µS) for 5 min. The increased conductivity of the solution, caused by electrolyte leakage (mainly K ions) from the tissue, was measured by a conductometer. The lichens were desiccated for 48 h and weighted, and conductivity per mass of lichen and volume of solution were calculated (.µS mL^{-1} g^{-1}). The same solution was used to check the leakage of potassium ions in deionized water by flame photometry and calculate the amount of K per mass of lichen (mg g^{-1}). Measurements were done in triplicate, except in the case when mass of lichen was insufficient for the third measurements. Correlations between K (mg g^{-1}) and conductivity (.µS mL^{-1} g^{-1}) confirmed (r>0.9) leakage of potassium to be the principal cause of the increased conductivity (Alebic-Juretic & Arko-Pijavac, 1989). The results of the Pearson test are given in Fig 16.

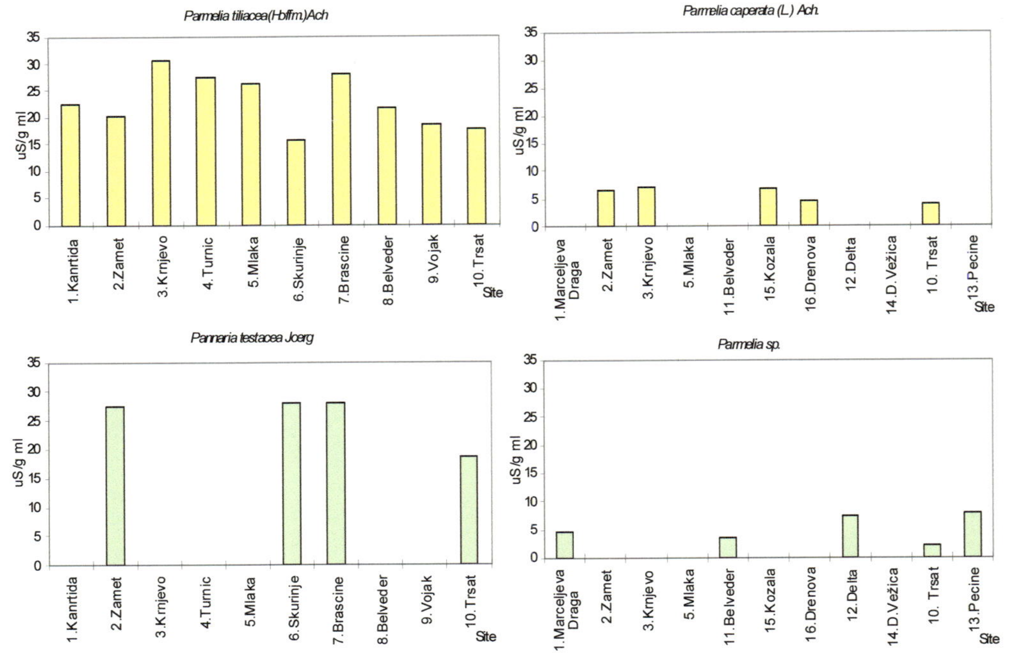

a. winter 1985/86. b. winter 1995/96.

Fig. 16. Results of Pearson biological test applied to lichen specimens collected in a. winter 1985/86 and b. 1995/96 (Alebic-Juretic & Arko-Pijavac, 2005)

In the *Parmelia tiliacea* experiment the largest specific conductivity was found in samples from sites 3, 4, and 5 (above the petroleum refinery facilities) thus indicating that these zones were exposed to higher air pollution levels, with winter concentrations > *70 µg m*$^{-3}$ that were indeed measured in the city centre (Fig. 17). *Panaria testacea* (more susceptible to SO_2 concentrations) collected at Sites 2,6,7 and 10 - where the same test applied to *Parmelia tiliacea* had its lowest values (except site 7) also showed increased specific conductivity implying that these zones had experienced winter average concentrations above 30 µg m^{-3}. There are no data on SO_2 concentrations in these areas, but it is assumed to be the cleanest within the urban area, because of largest distance from the city centre and industrial zones and, being on the elevated terrain, more exposed to dominant winds (mainly from NE directions). The unexpected result obtained with *P. tiliacea* at Site 7 could be explained by the fact that this complex hilly area is on the boundary between the struggle zone and the normal zone, but in the proximity of a small lichen desert (Fig. 15), where *P. testacea* can still be found (Alebic-Juretic & Arko-Pijavac, 1989).

The test on membrane integrity was repeated to specimens of lichens collected randomly within the city area after ten years, in winter 1995/96 (Alebic-Juretic & Arko-Pijevac, 2005). In the meantime, the sulphur dioxide emission within the wider city area was reduced by 70%, due to the switch to lower sulphur content oil, reduced production and/or cessation of activity of some industrial plants, e.g. coke plant. Consequently, the ambient levels of SO_2 were diminished by 50-70%. As a result, the annual means of SO_2 at the most polluted city center dropped from 100-110 to less than 50 µg m^{-3} (Matkovic & Alebic-Juretic, 1998), while the winter means decreased from approx. 80-140 to 30-60 µg/m^3 (Fig. 17).

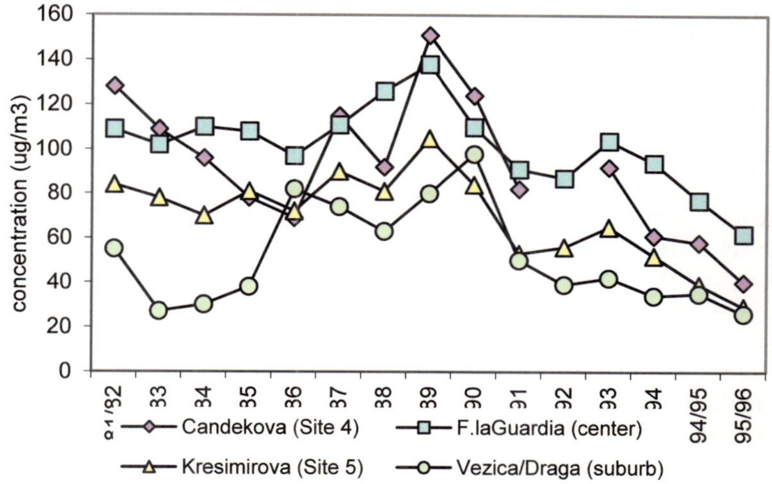

Fig. 17. Winter average (December- February) concentrations of SO_2 in the city of Rijeka (Alebic-Juretic & Arko-Pijevac, 2005).

The lichens collected during this second campaign were: *Parmelia spp., Parmelia caperata (L.) Ach., Parmelia conspensa* and *Physcia sp*. Generally, the values of specific conductivity (Fig. 16 b) are 2-4 times lower compared to the values obtained in the first campaign (Fig.16 a). The maximum values of specific conductivity in *P. caperata* specimens were obtained from samples collected at the same sites (3-Krnjevo) or in their proximity (15-Kozala) where the maximum values were obtained during the 1985/86. study. The same stands for the minimum values obtained in two strains of lichens collected within the park area at Site 10 (Trsat) during the both campaign undertaken. *P. caperata* strain is more sensitive among *Parmelia* species and is known to tolerate ambient SO_2 concentrations up to 40-50 $\mu g/m^3$ (Ferry, 1973).The highest specific conductivity in *Parmelia sp.* strains were found in samples collected at Site 12 (Delta), a former lichen desert zone, and Site 13 (Pecine) area (Fig 16.b). The largest specific conductivity was obtained in specimens of *P. conspensa* (18.6 $\mu S\ g^{-1}\ ml^{-1}$) collected at Site 14 (Donja Vežica), situated close to the former small lichen desert. Another species that gave high specific conductivity was *Physcia spp.* (8.6 $\mu S\ g^{-1}\ ml^{-1}$) collected within the park area at Site 5 (Mlaka), but close to the petroleum refinery (Alebic-Juretic & Arko-Pijevac, 2005).

In conclusion, the lower specific conductivity, the predominance of more sensitive *P. caperata* among the collected samples and reappearing of lichens in the areas classified earlier as lichen desert (city center and a small lichen desert zone in the upper part of the city) indicated recovering of their natural habitat due to decrease of SO_2. Similar situation with new lichen species found and disappearance of "lichen desert" subsequent to reduction in SO_2 emission was observed in central Italy during mid-nineties. Even earlier, during the eighties, the decrease of SO_2 levels in Paris caused the reappearance of lichen species from the previous century in the Luxemburg Gardens (Conti & Cecchetti, 2001).

2.5 Air pollution effects on human health

2.5.1 Respiratory system

Air pollution affects primarily human respiratory and cardiovascular, and indirectly reproductive system. During the period of high air pollution in the eighties several studies were conducted to estimate the air pollution effect on human health. The first of this study dates back in early eighties (September 1981-August 1982) and investigated occurrence of respiratory disease among preschool children (n=1299) in the city of Rijeka and its suburban communities affected by air pollution from SO_2 and black smoke. The level of air pollution varied significantly between selected six locations, except for SO_2 in summer. The city centre suffered the highest air pollution with annual means twice as much as WHO guideline values for SO_2 and black smoke. Maximum levels of both pollutants were found in winter at all sites. Spearman rank correlation indicated that incidence of overall acute respiratory diseases, acute diseases of lower respiratory system and acute non-obstructive bronchitis were in correlation to black smoke ($p<0.05$). The incidence of non-obstructive bronchitis correlated also with ambient SO_2 concentrations ($p<0.05$). Other correlations were not statistically significant. In spite of the good correlations between air pollution and respiratory diseases in preschool children, the authors could not eliminate infectious diseases as a possible cofounding factor, since there was no significant difference in incidence of respiratory diseases in six communities with different level of air pollution (Bartonicek-Brgic and Matkovic, 1989).

The second investigation was carried out during late eighties regarding ventilatory functions in non-smoking woman (n=176) living in two settlements in/or close to the industrial zone (Bakar, Krasica) with higher level of air pollution comparative to women (control group, n=58) living in the community on the west side of the city of Rijeka (Viškovo) without direct impacts from the industrial plants. Relative values of forced vital capacity (FVC), forced respiratory volume in one second (FVC_1), and values of FEV_1/FVC ratio, i.e. Tiffeneau index (TT) as absolute and relative in relation to normal population according to CECA norms were analysed. During the period 1986-1990 annual SO_2 concentrations exceeded WHO guideline of 50 $\mu g\ m^{-3}$ at Bakar and Krasica. While the annual concentrations were in the narrow range (67-74 $\mu g\ m^{-3}$) in Bakar, after initial increase up to 78 $\mu g\ m^{-3}$ in 1988, the annual values in Krasica decreased approaching the WHO guideline in 1990. The annual means of SO_2 remained approx. 40 $\mu g\ m^{-3}$ during the whole 5 year period. In the first measurements in 1986, women from Bakar and Krasica showed considerably lower values of all ventilatory functions, except for the Tiffeneau index, than did the controls from Viškovo. In the repeated measurements five years later, the values of all pulmonary functions, except for Tiffeneau index were again lower in Bakar, but not in Krasica, where no statistical difference regarding control group (Viškovo) was found. These observed effects might indicate the long-term exposure to air pollution (Matkovic et al, 1998).

2.5.2 Reproduction

The adverse effects of environmental exposure to air pollution on reproductive events are less investigated. There are several studies regarding associations between air pollution by and low birth weight. Air pollution with SO_2 and TSP, or more complex mixture of these pollutants were associated to excess risk for low birth (Wang et al., 1997) and preterm delivery (Xu et al., 1995). In the Czech study both, low birth weight and prematurity were associated to SO_2, and to less extent to TSP pollution, while there was no such an association for IUGR (Bobak, 2000). Since the town of Rijeka suffered from high air pollution during the eighties, a retrospective control study was performed in order to evaluate possible impact on the outcome of pregnancies.

Sulphur dioxide was chosen as an indicator of air pollution because of the most abundant data available, i.e. the longest time series and the largest number of monitoring stations. Maternal residence during pregnancy was taken as the exposure variable: the city of Rijeka being the high exposure and the rest of the region forming the low exposure zone (≤ 40 μg/m³. Based on the birth records from the Clinic, a retrospective cohort study was carried out. The "preterm cohort" comprised all preterm births (gestational age <37 weeks) registered during 1987-1996. IUGR newborns, defined as those having birth weights bellow 10th percentile, formed "IUGR cohort" (not shown here). A common "reference cohort" comprised eutrophic term newborns. An increase in preterm incidence since 1993, in spite air pollution decline (Fig. 18), was the reason to analyze the periods 1987-1992 and 1993-1996 separately (Alebic-Juretic et al., 2001).

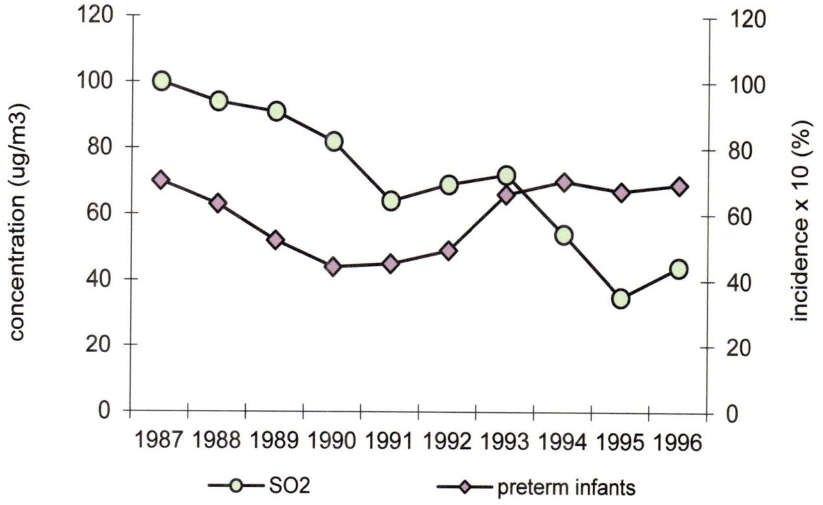

Fig. 18. Annual means of SO_2 concentrations within the city with incidence of preterm deliveries among mothers-city residents

For the overall period we found an increase of 11% in risk of preterm delivery among mothers-city residents (Table 3).

Zone	Preterm cohort	Reference cohort	OR	95% CI
1987-1996				
Region	714	11591	1	
City	1110	16188	1.11	1.01-1.23
1987-1992				
Region	352	7253	1	
City	662	11016	1.24	1.08-1.41
1993-1996				
Region	362	4338	1	
City	448	5172	1.04	0.90-1.20

Table 3. Risks of preterm birth within the city area relative to the rest of the region (Alebic-Juretic et al., 2001)

During the years of higher pollution this risk is even higher, while in the subsequent period a slightly elevated, but not statistically significant risk is observed. The calculated Mantel-

Haenszel estimator of the common odds ratio (OR), controlled for two periods studied, was OR_{MH}= 1.14 (95%CI=1.03-1.25) suggesting a 14% higher relative risk for preterm deliveries within the city. The Breslow-Day test for the homogeneity of the ORs was boundary significant (p=0.055), suggesting the possible difference in ORs between analyzed periods. Considering each socio-demographic parameter (maternal age, education, martial status, smoking habits and newborns sex) and two periods, an increase from 12 to 16% in relative risks is observed within the city (Table 4). Ambient concentrations of SO_2 were taken as an index of air quality. Breslow-Day tests for homogeniety of the ORs were insignificant in all cases for the two periods and levels of socio-demographic factors, these factors could not account for the elevated relative risks for preterm births observed in Rijeka vs. the region. Thus, elevated ambient air pollution may be considered as a possible cause. No association regarding IUGR births was found in this study (Alebic-Juretic et al., 2001).

	Preterm births		IUGR births	
Parameter	OR	95% CI	OR	95%CI
Mothers' age	1.12	1.02-1.24	1.08	0.97-1.20
Education	1.15	1.04-1.27	1.07	0.96-1.19
Martial status	1.13	1.03-1.25	1.06	0.95-1.01
Smoking habits	1.14	1.03-1.25	1.06	0.95-1.18
Newborns' sex	1.16	1.05-1.27	1.08	0.97-1.20

Table 4. Estimate of common relative risk adjusted for two periods considered and each of the listed parameters

3. Conclusion

This work gave synthesis of air pollution problem in the city of Rijeka. Due to early identification, a lot of work has been done for its abatement. Therefore, Rijeka had a leading role in many aspects regarding air pollution monitoring and management. Thus, Rijeka is the only town in Croatia with 25 year experience in providing emission inventories, one of the few places with long term data of nitrogen pollutants (NH_3 and NO_2), and the first town to establish automatic network for air quality monitoring and providing information to public of real time data on the web site. All these actions resulted in significant reduction of air pollution due to combustion processes (SO_2, black smoke, lead, PAHs, H_2S, fallout, TSP). Though, there is still to work on air pollution by traffic (NO_2, VOC, particulates), traffic related secondary pollutants (O_3, nitrate, sulphates), and long range transport (wet and dry deposition, PM_1, ozone).

4. Acknowledgment

Financial contribution from the University of Rijeka Foundation (Contract No: SN-IZ 1/2001) was used for open-access publishing. Opinions given within this chapter are solely the author's and do not express neccessarily the statements from the University of Rijeka Foundation.

5. References

Alebic-Juretic, A. Matković, N., Crvelin, G. Zubak, *V* (2009) New Regulations on Air Quality – The Case of the Petroleum Refinery Mlaka. *Proceedings of 6th Croatian Meeting Air*

Protection '09, pp. 376-382, ISBN 978-953-6609-06-2, Zadar, Croatia, September 14-19, 2009 (in Croatian)

Alebic-Juretic, A. (2008) Airborne Ammonia and Ammonium within the Northern Adriatic Area, Croatia. *Environmental Polution*, Vol. 154, n.d., pp. 439-447, ISSN 0269-7491

Alebic-Juretic, A. (2008a) Ozone levels in the Rijeka Bay Area, Northern Adriatic, Croatia. Proceedings of HARMO12 Conference, *Hrvatski meteorološki časopis (Croatian meteorological Journal)*, Vol. 43, n.d., pp.397-400, ISSN 1330-0083

Alebic-Juretic, A. (2005) Polycyclic Aromatic Hydrocarbons and Metals in Total Suspended Particulates Collected in Rijeka, 1982-2004. *Proceedings of 4th Croatian meeting Air Protection '05*, pp.184-189, ISBN 953-6609-04-05, Zadar, Croatia, September 12-16, 2005

Alebic-Juretic, A. (1994) Polycyclic Aromatic Hydrocarbons in the Urban Atmosphere of Rijeka (Croatia*), Fresenius Environmental Bulletin*, Vol.3, n.d. ,pp. 89-94., ISSN 1018- 4619

Alebic-Juretic, A. & Arko-Pijevac, M. (2005) Lichens as Indicators of Air Pollution in the City of Rijeka, Croatia. *Fresenius Environmental Bulletin*, Vol. 14, No. 1, pp. 40-43, ISSN 1018-4619

Alebic-Juretic, A. & Arko-Pijevac, M. (1989) Air Pollution Damage to cell Membranes in Lichens- result of Simple Biological test Applied in Rijeka, Yugoslavia. *Water, Air and Soil Pollution*, Vol. 47, n.d., pp. 25-33, ISSN 0049-6979

Alebic.Juretic, A., Frkovic, A. & Simic,D. (2001) The Effects of Air Pollution on the Outcome of Pregnancies. *International Journal of Gynecology&Obstetrics*, Vol.75, n.d., pp. 315-316. ISSN 0020-7292

Alebic-Juretic & Sekulic-Cikovic (2009) The Impact of air Pollution on the Paintings in Storage at the Museum of Modern and Contemporary Art, Rijeka, Croatia. *Studies in Conservation*, Vol. 54, No. 1 , (March 2009), pp. 49-57., ISSN 0039-3630

ARCADIS (2011) *Technical Assistance on the Development of Cost-Efficient Emission Reduction Measures for the Port of Rijeka*, Project Report (draft final) , ARCADIS, Project number- 11-004750/Version B/24-01-2011, Antwerp (Belgium), pp. 66/141

Bartonicek-Brgic, V. & Matkovic, N.(1989) Sulphur Dioxide and Black Smoke Air Pollution Impact on Incidence of Respiratoryy Diseases among Preschool Children in Rijeka. Proceedings of the First Yugoslav Clean Air Congress, Book II, pp.734-747, ISBN Zenica, Yugoslavia, June 14-16., 1989 (in Croatian)

Bobak, M. (2000) Outdoor Air Pollution, Low Birth Weight, and Prematurity. *Environmental Health Perspective*, Vol. 108, No. 2, (February), pp. 173-176, doi:10.1289/ehp.00108173

Camuffo, D., Brimblecombe, P., Van Grieken, R., Busse, H-J., Sturaro, G., Valentino, A., Bernardi, A., Blades, N., Shooter, D., De Bock, L., Gysels, G., Wieser, M. & Kim, O. (1999) Indoor Air Quality at the Correr Museum, Venice, Italy. *The Science of the Total Environment*, Vol. 236, n.d., pp. 135-152, ISSN 0048 9697

Conti, M.E. & Cecchetti, G. (2001) Biological Monitoring: Lichens as Bioindicators of Air Pollutin Assessment- A Review. *Environmental Pollution*, Vol.114, n.d., pp. 471-492, ISSN 0269-7491

County (2009) *Programme for Air Quality Protection and Improvement in the Littoral-Highlands County in the Period 2009-2012*, Littoral-highlands County, ISBN 978-953-7221-33-1, Rijeka, pp. 23-28.

EC (2002) Guidance to Member States on PM_{10} Monitoring and Intercomparisons with the Reference Method, EC Working Group on Particulate Matter, January 2002

EKONERG (1997) *Air Quality menagement- Basis for spatial planning of the Littoral-highlands County*, Ekonerg, Zagreb, pp. 10/43-21/43 (in Croatian)

Ferry, B.W., Baddeley, M.S. & Hawksworth, D.L., Eds (1973) *Air Polution and Lichens*, The Althone Press, London, UK

Ligocki, M. P., Salmon, L. G., Fall, T., Jones, M.C., Nazaroff, W.W. and Cass G.R. (1993) Characteristics of airborne particles inside southern California museums, *Atmospheric Environment*, Vol. 27, n.d., pp. 697-711, ISSN 1352-2310

Matkovic, N. & Alebic-Juretic, A. (1998) Emissions and Ambient levels of Sulphur Dioxide in the Rijeka bay Area, *Arhiv za higijenu rada i toksikologiju*, Vol. 49, No.2, pp. 155-1263, ISSN 0004-1254

Matkovic, V., Matkovic, N., Kontosic, I., Jonjic, A. & Matkovic, V. (1998) The Effect of air Pollution on ventilatory Function in Nonsmoking Women. *Arhiv za higijenu rada i toksikologiju*, Vol. 49, No.1, pp. 19-25, ISSN 0004-1254

MEISA (1991) Project *Proposal of Monitoring Air Pollutants and Odours Emitted by Petroleum refinery Rijeka, Iron works Sisak-Coke plant Bakar and TPP Rijeka I* , Environmental Protection Centre, Maribor, pp. 3-11 , 3-63, 3-90, 3-100, 3-108 (in Croatian)

Mingati, V., Capelli, R., Drava, G., de Pellegrini, D., Brunialti, G., Giordani, G. & Modenesi, P. (2003) Biomonitoring of Trace Metals by Different Species of Lichens (Parmelia) in North-West Italy. *Journal of Atmospheric Chemistry*, Vol. 45, n.d., pp. 219-229, ISSN 1573-0662

Mouratidou, Th. & Samara, C. (2004) $PM_{2.5}$ and Associated Ionic Component Concentrations Inside the Archeological Museum of Thessaloniki, N. Greece. *Atmospheric Environment*, Vol. 38, n.d., pp. 4593-4598, ISSN 1352-2310

Pearson, L.C. (1985) Air Pollution Damage to Cell Membranes in Lichens. I Development of a Simple Monitoring Test. *Atmospheric Environment*, Vol. 19, n.d. ,209-212, ISSN 1352-2310

Perry, R. & Young, R.J. Eds. (1977) *Handbook of Air Pollution Analysis*", Chapmam and Hall, ISBN 0 412 12660 5, London

Pinho, P., Augusto, S., Branquinho, C., Bio, A., Pereira, M.J., Soares, A. & Catarino, F.(2004) Mapping Lichen Diversity as a First Step for Air Quality Assessment, *Journal of Atmospheric Chemistry*, Vol. 49 , n.d., pp. 377-389, ISSN 1573-0662

Regional Centre (2002) *Report on Environmental Conditions within the Littoral-highlands County*, Regional Centre for Sustainable Development and Environmental Protection, Rijeka, pp. 43-47 (in Croatian)

Salmon, L.G., Mayo, P.R., Cass, G.R. and Christoforou, C.S. (2005) Airborne particles in new museum facilities. *Journal of Environmental Engineering*, Vol. 131, n.d., pp. 1453-1461, ISSN 1573-0662

Schuler, J. (1902) *Zur Flechtenflora von Fiume*. Separat-Abdruck aus Mittheilungen des Naturwissenschaftlichen Clubs in Fiume., 1901, Jahrgang VI, Buchdrukerei P. Battara, Fiume (Rijeka)

Vadic , V. (1982) Method for Hydrogen Sulphide Measurements in the Atmosphere, *Zaštita atmosfere*, Vol.10, No. 3, 116-118. YU ISSN 0350-1973

van Loon J.E.: *Selected Methods of Trace Analysis: Biological and Environmental Samples*, John Wiley& Son, New York, 1985. ISBN 0-471-89634-9

Wang, X., Ding, H., Ryan, L. & Xu, X. (1997) Association between Air Polution and Low Birth Weight: A Community based Study. *Environmental Health Perspective*, Vol. 105, No.5., (May), pp.514-520, doi:10.1289/ehp.97105514

WHO (1976) *Selected Methods for Measuring Air Pollutants*, WHO offest Publication No 24, ISBN 92 4 170024 6I, Geneva , Switzerland

WHO (2000) *Air Quality Guidelines for Europe*, 2nd Ed., WHO Regional Publications, European series, No. 91, ISBN 13583, Copenhagen, Denmark

Xu, X., Ding, H. & Wang, X. (1995) Acute Effects of Total Suspended Particulates and Sulphur Dioxides on Preterm Delivery: A Community Based Cohort Study. *Archive of Environmental Health*, Vol. 50, No.6 , pp. 407-415 ISSN 0003-9896

15

Air Pollution with Asbestos in Several Cities in Romania

Anca Maria Moldoveanu
University of Medicine and Pharmacy" Carol Davila" Bucharest
Romania

1. Introduction

The general population is exposed to low levels of asbestos primarily by inhalation. Small quantities of asbestos fibers are ubiquitous in air. They may arise from natural sources (e.g., the effect of weathering on asbestos containing minerals), from windblown soil from hazardous waste sites where asbestos is not properly stored, and from deterioration of automobile clutches and brakes or breakdown of asbestos-containing (mainly chrysotile) materials, such as insulation.

Because of these properties, asbestos fibers have been used in a wide range of manufactured goods. In 1989, EPA identified the following asbestos product categories. Many of these materials may still be in use (EPA, 2010).

asbestos-cement corrugated sheet	asbestos-cement flat sheet	asbestos-cement pipe	asbestos-cement shingle
roof coatings	flooring felt	pipeline wrap	roofing felt
asbestos clothing	non-roof coatings	vinyl/asbestos floor tile	automatic transmission components
clutch facings	disc brake pads	drum brake linings	brake blocks
commercial and industrial asbestos friction products	sheet and beater-add gaskets (except specialty industrial)	commercial, corrugated and specialty paper	millboard
rollboard			

Table 1. Representatives asbestos product categories

The exposure of the general population to asbestos has been found to be very low. The concentrations of asbestos fibers in outdoor air are highly variable, ranging from below 0.1 ng/m^3 (equivalent to 3x10^{-6} f/mL measured by phase contrast microscopy [PCM]) in rural areas to over 100 ng/m^3 (3x10^{-3} PCM f/mL) near specific industrial sources such as asbestos mines. Typical concentrations are 1x10^5 PCM (phase contrast microscopy) f/mL in rural areas and up to an order of magnitude higher in urban areas. In the vicinity of an asbestos mine or factory, levels may reach 0.01 f/mL or higher. The concentration of fibers in indoor air is also highly variable, depending on the amount and condition of asbestos-containing materials in the building 1 to 200 ng/m^3 ($3x10^{-5}$ to $6x10^{-3}$ PCM f/mL), (Nicholson 1987). For a human exposed for a lifetime (70 years), this range of exposures corresponds to cumulative doses of approximately 0.002–0.4 PCM f-yr/mL (PCM fiber-years/mL).

2. Units of airborne asbestos levels

Numerous measurements have been performed to determine the concentration of asbestos fibers in environmental media, primarily air. The results were reported in a variety of units, including ng/m^3 (measured by midget impinger counting analysis), TEM f/mL (fibers measured by transmission electron microscopy), and PCM f/mL (fibers measured by phase contrast microscopy). The most accurate and sensitive method for measuring asbestos fiber content in air is electron microscopy, and preferably transmission electron microscopy (TEM) must be used. Phase contrast microscopy cannot distinguish between asbestos and non-asbestos fibers or between different types of asbestos. However, in certain occupational settings where the predominant fiber is asbestos, PCM should give an adequate measure of asbestos concentration. In non-occupational environments where a large fraction of the fibers are not asbestos (e.g., wool, cotton, glass), PCM may greatly overestimate the asbestos levels in air.

Regulations regarding asbestos determine what fibers are counted in the analysis. Established methods define fiber material having a length >5 µm and a length to diameter ratio of >3:1. In the same air sample, the fibers counted by TEM can be 50–70 times higher than those counted by PCM. This relates to the fact that PCM cannot detect fibers less than about 0.20–0.30 µm in diameter while TEM is capable of detecting fibers with diameters as small as 0.01 µm. Therefore, PCM may miss thin fibers as well as include nonasbestos fibrous material. The conversion factors between fibers counted by PCM and those counted by TEM are highly variable. In 1984, the NRC (1984) recommended that a conversion be used to measure asbestos fibers. It was suggested that crude approximations could be achieved by assuming that 1 PCM f/mL is equal to 60 TEM f/mL. Both 1 PCM f/mL and 60 TEM f/mL are approximately equal to a mass concentration of 30 µg/m^3. Since the health effects data regarding inhalation exposure to asbestos are usually expressed in terms of PCM f/mL(fibre/mL), ambient air data reported in units of ng/m^3 or TEM f/mL (fibre/mL) are converted to units of PCM f/mL (fibre/mL) using the factors suggested by NRC (1984).

For a good understanding of the measurement units used it can be stipulated that 10 fibers are typically present in a cubic meter (fibers/m^3) of outdoor air in rural areas. (A cubic meter is about the amount of air that you breathe in 1 hour). Health professionals often report the number of fibers in a milliliter (mL) (equivalent to a cubic centimeter [cm^3]) of air rather than in a cubic meter of air. Since there are one million cm^3 (or one million mL) in a cubic meter, there typically would be 0.00001 fibers/mL of asbestos in air in rural areas. Typical levels found in cities are about 10-fold higher.

Close to an asbestos mine or factory, levels may reach 10,000 fibers/m^3 (0.01 fibers/mL) or higher. Levels could also be above average near a building that contains asbestos products and that is being torn down or renovated or near a waste site where asbestos is not properly covered up or stored to protect it from wind erosion.

In indoor air, the concentration of asbestos depends on whether asbestos was used for insulation, ceiling or floor tiles, or other purposes, and whether these asbestos-containing materials are in good condition or are deteriorated and easily crumbled. Concentrations measured in homes, schools, and other buildings that contain asbestos range from about 30 to 6,000 fibers/m^3 (0.00003–0.006 fibers/mL).

3. Asbestos biomarkers

Biomarkers are broadly defined as indicators signaling events in biologic systems or samples. They have been classified as markers of exposure, markers of effect, and markers of susceptibility (NAS/NRC 1989).

Principal biomarkers of exposure to asbestos fibers include the detection and counting of fibers or asbestos bodies in bronchoalveolar lavage fluid samples (De Vuyst et al. 1982, 1988, 1997; Dumortier et al. 1990, 1998; Roggli et al. 1994a; Sebastien et al. 1988a; Teschler et al. 1994; 1996, Tuomi et al. 1991b),sputum samples (McDonald et al. 1988, 1992; Sebastien et al. 1988b), or in autopsied or surgically resected lung tissue samples (Case 1994; Churg 1982; Churg and Warnock 1981; Churg and Wright,1994; Churg et al. 1993; de Klerk et al. 1996; Dodson et al.,1999; Dufresne et al. 1995, 1996a, 1996b; Sebastien et al. 1989). Asbestos bodies are collections of fibers (usually of length >8 µm) with a protein -iron coating (also known as ferruginous bodies) that, when observed in lung tissue sections in conjunction with fibrosis, have been proposed to be used in the diagnosis of asbestosis (Churg 1989; Craighead et al.,1982). Whereas light microscopy can be used to detect and count asbestos bodies, most uncoated fibers in tissue or fluid samples are too small to be visible (Dodson et al. 1999). Transmission or scanning electron microscopy is used to detect and count uncoated asbestos fibers in lung tissue or fluid samples, and electron diffraction or energy-dispersive x-ray analysis is used to determine asbestos type (e.g. chrysotile, anthophyllite, tremolite) (NIOSH 1994b). These biomarkers provide indicators of retained internal dose, the cumulative net result of deposition and clearance of inhaled asbestos fibers.

Counting asbestos bodies in human tissue, BAL fluid and sputum is easy and reproducible. However, not all fiber types and lengths form asbestos bodies. Therefore, the technique of counting ferruginous bodies in tissue sections is not sensitive, especially for short fibers and chrysotile. The sensitivity increases when a digested sample is evaluated by light microscopy for the presence of ferruginous bodies combined with the evaluation of the digested material for core identification of ferruginous bodies as well as characterization of the uncoated asbestos burden.

Advantages to counting asbestos bodies in human tissue, BAL (bronchoalveolar lavage) fluid, or sputum: Asbestos bodies are easy to identify with light microscopy. The results are easy to reproduce. Asbestos bodies correlate well with the concentration of amphibole fibers, which are the fibers that correlate best with mesothelioma. Counting asbestos bodies in BAL fluid could be used as a screening technique to indicate that exposure to amphibole fibers has occurred.

Disadvantages to counting asbestos bodies in human tissue, BAL fluid, or sputum: Chrysotile does not readily form asbestos bodies. The presence of ferruginous bodies in any sample only represents a population of the longer fibers in that sample. These numbers tell us nothing about the actual numbers of uncoated fibers of any length or type. Counting asbestos bodies may underestimate exposures to fibers that are greater than 5 microns in length and less than 20 microns in length.

Other Considerations: The study should combine analyses of asbestos bodies by light microscopy and fibers by electron microscopy. Electron microscopy can also be used to find

smaller ferruginous bodies and define the presence and types of uncoated asbestos fibers in a sample. The presence of asbestos bodies is a marker of exposure, not of disease.
Pleural plaques and pleural calcification are markers of exposure and may develop 10 to 20 years after initial exposure. Plaques are opaque patches visible on chest x-rays that consist of dense strands of connective tissue surrounded by cells. All commercial types of asbestos induce plaques. Plaques can occur even when fibrosis is absent and do not seem to reflect the severity of pulmonary disease.

4. Asbestos health effects

Asbestos exposure can cause a number of disabling and fatal diseases. The principal rout of exposure is by inhalation through the nose and mouth. Asbestos, traditionally valued for its indestructibility, is especially resistant to the internal defenses of the human body. Once lodged inside the lungs, most fibers will not break up or dissolve, and they cannot be neutralized or removed.
Asbestosis is a disease which is characterized by pulmonary fibrosis, a progressive scarring of the lungs caused by the accumulation of asbestos fibers. Asbestosis is associated exclusively with chronic, occupational exposure. The buildup of scar tissue interferes with oxygen uptake through the lungs and can lead to respiratory and heart failure. Often, asbestosis is a progressive disease, even in the absence of continued exposure.
Asbestos is known to be a human carcinogen. The EPA has determined that asbestos is a human carcinogen (Group A). In addition, the International Agency for Research on Cancer (IARC) has determined that asbestos is carcinogenic to humans (Group 1). These conclusions are based primarily on the evidence that asbestos causes lung cancer and mesothelioma. The World Health Organization Task Group on Environmental Health Criteria for Chrysotile Asbestos (WHO, 1998) concluded that "asbestotic changes are common following prolonged exposures of 5 to 20 f/mL(fibre/mL,)"[these correspond to cumulative exposures of 50–200 f-yr/mL (PCM fiber-years/mL) for a 10-year exposure] and that "the risk at lower exposure levels is not known."
Mesothelioma, a malignant nodular type cancer of the membranes which line the lung cavity, is another disease related to asbestos exposure. Malignant mesotheliomas of these membranes (the pleura and the peritoneum) are extremely rare in persons with no history of asbestos exposure, but may account for 10% to 18% of excess deaths in workers exposed to asbestos. Generally, a latency period of at least 25 to 30 years is required in order to observe mesotheliomas, and some victims have had a latency period of forty years since their initial exposure to asbestos. This form of cancer is incurable and is usually fatal within a year after diagnosis. Mesothelioma has been associated with short term, incidental exposure.
Some health studies have observed increases in esophageal, stomach, colo-rectal, kidney, and possibly ovarian cancers as well as cancers in the nose and throat from exposure to asbestos. While the magnitude of increased cancer risk for these sites is not as great as for lung cancer and mesothelioma, the increased risk may be of considerable importance because of the high background rates of some of these tumors in the general population.
There are many factors which complicate studies of non-occupational exposure, including a lack of data on incidental exposures which may occur, lack of data on non-occupational levels (f/cc) of exposure, and the lack of a control group (zero, or at least known "near zero" exposure). Confounding variables such as migration into and from communities and multiple exposures to other toxic chemicals and carcinogens consistently frustrate attempts

to generalize about the risk of low level exposure. At low levels of exposure, for example, asbestos may serve only as a "cancer promoter", acting as a co-factor along with other substances and carcinogens to elevate the risk of developing cancer above normal. Because asbestos fibers do accumulate in the lungs, and because the risk of developing disease does increase as the ***cumulative*** dose increases, exposure to asbestos should be controlled or eliminated whenever possible. Even a relatively minor source of airborne asbestos fibers should be abated, avoided, or minimized in order to maintain the cumulative dose at a minimum.

5. Purpose of the present study

The aim of the study was to assess the presence of asbestos fibers in the air of several towns in Romania. The main source is traffic and only a single town has traffic and an industrial source. The second purpose of the study was to investigate the presence of asbestos bodies in the lung tissue as biomarkers of the environmental exposure to asbestos through air.

6. Material and methods

The study was carried out in 9 towns in Romania including the capital city, Bucharest. The presence of asbestos bodies in the lung tissue of deceased people was investigated in Bucharest. The study was performed in first year of the new millennium.

6.1 Assessment of air pollution with asbestos

For measuring the levels of air contamination with asbestos fibers, the method used was phase contrast microscopy. Phase contrast microscopy (PCM) accurately assesses fiber exposure levels for fibers >5 μm in length and >0.25 μm in diameter. PCM cannot differentiate between asbestos and nonasbestos fibers. The standard method for the determination of airborne asbestos particles in the workplace is by phase contrast microscopy (NIOSH Method 7400). In the study, air samples were taken with a pump with a flow rate of 2 l/min for 2 hours. Asbestos was collected on a 25 mm cellulose ester filter. The filter was treated to make it transparent and then it was analyzed by microscopy at 400-450x magnification, with phase contrast illumination. A fiber is defined as any particle with a length>5 μm and a length-to-diameter ratio >3:1. The PCM method is relatively fast and inexpensive but it does not distinguish between asbestos and nonasbestos fibers and, it cannot detect fibers thinner than 0.25 μm. Consequently, this method is most useful for the analysis of samples that are composed mainly of asbestos, but only where a significant fraction of the fibers are large enough to be counted. If samples are grossly contaminated by nonasbestiform fibers, then transmission electronmicroscopy (NIOSH Method 7402) should be used for positive identification. Due to some technical problems, we used in the study only the phase contrast microscopy (PCM).Concentrations are reported as fibers/cm^3.
The levels of air pollution with asbestos were measured twice, in the spring and in the fall.

6.2 Assessment of the presence of asbestos bodies in the lung tissue

For assessing the presence of biomarkers of exposure in human body, samples of lung tissues were taken to routine autopsies in a pathology service in one of the important hospitals in Bucharest. The subjects included in the group of investigation were people with different causes of death. All subjects did not have occupational exposure during the life. The group of subjects was made of 25 bodies, 11 female and 14 male. The average value of age was 63.9

years of age. The youngest subject was 47 years old and the oldest 82. The occupational history of the subjects showed that none of them were exposed during their active life to asbestos.
The causes of death were: myocardial infarction, hypertension, arrhythmia, rupture of heart with haemopericardium, heart failure, COPD, chronic bronchitis, acute pulmonary edema, pulmonary thromboembolism, upper gastrointestinal bleeding, gastric ulcer, intestinal infarction, liver cirrhosis, intestinal obstruction.
5 of 25 subjects had died from cancer, 3 cases of pulmonary metastases from breast cancer, 1 case of intestinal metastases of rectal cancer and 1 case of liver cancer.
The identification of the presence of asbestos bodies in the lung tissue was made using light microscopy.

7. Results

7.1 The levels of asbestos in air in the investigated cities

In Bucharest the level of asbestos in air was measured in 21 points.

Measuring point nr.	**Summer (fiber/cm^3)**	**Autumn (fiber/cm^3)**
1	0.0418	0.0498
2	0.0393	0.0398
3	0.0411	0.0378
4	0.0489	0.0500
5	0.0350	0.0367
6	0.0182	0.0237
7	0.0169	0.0168
8	0.0229	0.0126
9	0.0149	0.0177
10	0.0132	0.0202
11	0.0145	0.0158
12	0.0139	0.0325
13	0.0181	0.0104
14	0.0181	0.0088
15	0.0146	0.0108
16	0.0200	0.0220
17	0.0126	-
18	0.0305	0.0280
19	0.0390	0.0430
20	0.0250	0.0260
21	0.0280	0.0240

Table 2. Levels of asbestos in air in Bucharest

Levels of asbestos in air	Summer (fiber/cm^3)	Autumn (fiber/cm^3)
Average value	0.0288	0.0250

Table 3. Levels of asbestos in air in Bucharest - Average values

The levels of asbestos in air of Bucharest had a variation between 0.0126 fiber/cm^3 and 0.0489 fiber/cm^3 with an average value equal to 0.0288 fiber/cm^3 in the summer and a variation between 0.0088 fiber/cm^3 and 0.0500 fiber/cm^3 with an average value equal to 0.0250 fiber/cm^3 in the autumn. The main source in Bucharest is the traffic and demolition of old buildings containing asbestos in their structure.
In Râmnicu Sărat city the level of asbestos in air was measured in 7 points.

Measuring point nr.	Summer (fiber/cm^3)	Autumn (fiber/cm^3)
1	0.0201	0.0271
2	0.0102	0.0358
3	0.0152	-
4	0.0130	-
5	0.0127	0.0340
6	0.0080	0.0143
7	-	0.0239

Table 4. Levels of asbestos in air in Râmnicu Sărat city

Levels of asbestos in air	Summer (fiber/cm^3)	Autumn (fiber/cm^3)
Average value	0.0132	0.02702

Table 5. Levels of asbestos in air in Râmnicu Sărat – average values

The levels of asbestos in air of Râmnicu Sărat had a variation between 0. 0080 fiber/cm^3 and 0.0201 fiber/cm^3 with an average value equal to 0.0132 fiber/cm^3 in the summer and a variation between 0.0143 fiber/cm^3 and 0.0358 fiber/cm^3 with an average value equal to 0.02702 fiber/cm^3 in the autumn. The source in this relatively little town is traffic but the main source is an industrial source.
In the summer, the minimum value was measured in the city of Târgu Jiu, the highest value was measured in the city of Ploieşti followed by the city of Bucharest and the highest average value was measured in Bucharest.
In two towns (Brăila and Alexandria) the minimum level was equal to 0. The maximum value was measured in Bucharest and the highest average value was measured in Râmnicu Sărat during the autumn.
In all 9 investigated towns the source of asbestos is traffic. Only the city of Râmnicu Sărat has an industrial source.
Traffic has the greatest contribution to air pollution with asbestos in Bucharest, town with a heavy traffic.

Name of the city	Minimum Value (fiber/cm³)	Maximum value (fiber/cm³)	Average value (fiber/cm³)
București	0.0126	0.0489	0.0288
Constanța	0.0132	0.0249	0.0164
Rm. Sărat	0.0080	0.0201	0.0132
Ploiești	0.0050	0.0720	0.0060
Brăila	0.0060	0.0130	0.0097
Alexandria	0.0050	0.0080	0.0063
Craiova	0.0028	0.0120	0.0048
Tulcea	0.0028	0.0053	0.0037
Tg.Jiu	0.0010	0.0020	0.0140

Table 6. Levels of asbestos in air in 9 cities in Romania in summer

Name of the city	Minimum Value (fiber/cm³)	Maximum value (fiber/cm³)	Average value (fiber/cm³)
București	0.0088	0.0500	0.0250
Constanța	0.0092	0.0398	0.0159
Rm. Sărat	0.0143	0.0130	0.0270
Ploiești	0.0090	0.0130	0.0110
Brăila	0.0000	0.0180	0.0077
Alexandria	0.0000	0.0070	0.0035
Craiova	0.0090	0.0014	0.0011
Tulcea	0.0037	0.0061	0.0021
Tg.Jiu	0.0010	0.0020	0.0104

Table 7. Levels of asbestos in air in 9 cities in Romania in autumn

An interesting approach will be, if the air pollution level with asbestos will be assess today especially in Bucharest taking into account the fact that the traffic is more intense in comparison with other towns and to the previous period. Also, some technical modification to the disc brake pads and other brake components or clutch plates of cars were made especially to the new cars, trying to reduce the levels of air contamination with asbestos fibers.

The asbestos bodies were present in 4 of 25 investigated bodies.

Name	**Age**	**Sex**	**Occupation**	**Clinical diagnosis**	**Pathology diagnosis**	**Cause of death**	**Presence of asbestos bodies in the lung tissues**
D.A.	59	female	pensioner	lung cancer, breast cancer, respiratory failure	breast cancer, lung cancer – metastases, acute myocardial infarction	metastases, acute myocardial infarction	asbestos bodies present
M.A.	50	male	pensioner	COPD, renal failure	COPD, pulmonary thrombo-embolism cor pulmonale, pulmonary edema, upper gastrointestinal bleeding	-	asbestos bodies present
A.I.	59	female	pensioner	hart failure, liver cirrhosis	pulmonary edema, liver cirrhosis	intestinal obstruction	asbestos bodies present
J.E.	58	male	pensioner (former miner)	liver cancer, paralysis of the left side of the body	COPD cor pulmonale, silicosis, respiratory failure	respiratory failure	asbestos bodies present

Table 8. Presence of asbestos bodies in lung tissue in the investigated bodies in Bucharest

7.2 The presence of asbestos bodies in the lung tissue of the investigated bodies

Assessing the proportion of the presence of asbestos bodies in the subjects' bodies, the result showed that in 16% of investigated subjects the exposure markers were presents due to the environmental exposure.

8. Conclusions

Even if the method used overestimates the level of air pollution with asbestos fibers by including in the same category other types of fibers, the biological marker present in the lung tissue showed the risk of exposure to asbestos and risk to induce a specific morbidity due to the environmental exposure. The presence of asbestos bodies in the lung tissue of persons without occupational exposure shows that human health can be negatively affected by environmental exposure to asbestos and the efforts to reduce and even eliminate this pollutant from the environment may be beneficial for human health.

9. References

ATSDR (Agency for Toxic Substances and Disease Registry (2001),*Toxicological Profile for Asbestos*. Update. Department of Health and Human Services, Public Health Service, Atlanta, GA: U.S.,

ATSDR *Report on the Expert Panel on Biomarkers of Asbestos Exposure and Disease* , May 9-10, (2006), Atlanta, Georgia,

Case BW. (1994), Biological indicators of chrysotile exposure, *Ann Occup Hyg* 38:503-518,

Craighead JE, Abraham JL, Churg A, et al. (1982) The pathology of asbestos-associated diseases of the lungs and pleural cavities: Diagnostic criteria and proposed grading schema. *Arch Pathol Lab Med*106:544-597,

Craighead JE, Mossman BT. (1982) The pathogenesis of asbestos-associated diseases. *N Engl J Med* 306:1446-1455.

Churg AM, Warnock ML. (1981). Asbestos and other ferruginous bodies: Their formation and clinical significance. *Am J Pathol* 102:447-456.

Churg A. (1982) Fiber counting and analysis in the diagnosis of asbestos-related disease. *Hum Pathol* 13(4):381-392.

Churg A. (1989). The diagnosis of asbestosis. *Hum Pathol* 20(2):97-99.

Churg A, Wright JL, Vedal S. (1993) Fiber burden and patterns of asbestos-related disease in chrysotile miners and millers. *Am Rev Respir Dis* 148:25-31.

Churg A, Wright JL. (1994) Persistence of natural mineral fibers in human lungs: An overview.*Environ Health Perspect* 102(Suppl. 5):229-233.

de Klerk NH, Musk AW, Williams V, et al. (1996). Comparison of measures of exposure to asbestos in former crocidolite workers from Wittenoon Gorge, W. Australia. *Am J Ind Med* 30:579-587.

De Vuyst P, Dumortier P, Gevenois PA. (1997). Analysis of asbestos bodies in BAL from subjects with particular exposure. *Am J Ind Med* 31:699-704.

De Vuyst P, Dumortier P, Moulin E, et al. (1988) Asbestos bodies in bronchoalveolar lavage reflect lung asbestos body concentration. *Eur Resp J* 1:362-367.

De Vuyst P, Jedwab J, Dumortier P, et al. (1982) Asbestos bodies in bronchoalveolar lavage. *Am Rev Resp Dis* 126:972-976.

Dodson RF, Williams MG, Huang J, et al. (1999). Tissue burden of asbestos in nonoccupationally exposed individuals from east Texas. *Am J Ind Med* 35:281-286.

Dufresne A, Harrigan M, Masse S, et al. (1995). Fibers in lung tissues of mesothelioma cases among miners and millers of the township of Asbestos, Quebec. *Am J Ind Med* 27:581-592.

Dufresne A, Begin R, Churg A, et al. (1996a), Mineral fiber content of lungs in patients with mesothelioma seeking compensation in Quebec. *Am J Respir Crit Care Med* 153:711-718.

Dufresne A, Begin R, Masse S, et al. (1996b). Retention of asbestos fibres in lungs of workers with asbestosis, asbestosis and lung cancer, and mesothelioma in Asbestos township. *Occup Environ Med* 53:801-807.

Dumotier P, De Vuyst P, Strauss P, et al. (1990). Asbestos bodies in bronchoalveolar lavage fluids of brake lining and asbestos cement workers. *Br J Ind Med* 47:91-98.

Dumortier P, Cöplü L, de Maertelaer V, et al. (1998) Assessment of environmental asbestos exposure in Turkey by bronchoalveolar lavage. *Am J Respir Crit Care Med* 158:1815-1824.

McDonald JC, McDonald AD, Sebastien P, et al. (1988). Health of vermiculite miners exposed to trace amounts of fibrous tremolite. *Br J Ind Med* 45:63-634.

McDonald JC, Sebastien P, Case B.(1992). Ferruginous body counts in sputum as an index of past exposure to mineral fibers. *Ann Occup Hyg* 36(3):271-82.

NAS/NRC (1989) Biologic markers in reproductive toxicology. National Academy of Sciences/National Research Council. Washington, DC: National Academy Press, 15-35.

Nicholson WJ.(1987), Airborne levels of mineral fibres in the non-occupational environment. New York, NY: City University of New York, Mount Sinai School of Medicine, Division of Environmental and Occupational Medicine.

NIOSH. (1989a) Fibers - method 7400. In: *NIOSH manual of analytical methods. 3rd ed. Supplement.* Cincinnati, OH: National Institute for Occupational Safety and Health, 7400-1 - 7400-13.

NIOSH. (1989b) Asbestos fibers - method 7402. In: *NIOSH manual of analytical methods. 3rd ed. Supplement.* Cincinnati, OH: National Institute for Occupational Safety and Health, 7402-1 - 7402-8.

NIOSH. (1994b), Asbestos by TEM. In: *Manual of analytical methods, 4th ed.* Cincinnati, OH: U.S.Department of Health and Human Services, National Institute for Occupational Safety and Health.

NRC. 1984. National Research Council. Asbestiform fibers: nonoccupational health risks. Washington, DC: National Academy Press.

Roggli VL, Coin PG, MacIntyre NR, et al. (1994a) Asbestos content of bronchoalveolar lavage fluid: A comparison of light and scanning electron microscopic analysis. *Acta Cytol* 38:502-510,

Sebastien P, Armstrong B, Monchaux G, et al. (1988b). Asbestos bodies in bronchoalveolar lavage fluid and in lung parenchyma. *Am Rev Respir Dis* 137:75-78.

Sebastien P, McDonald JC, McDonald AD, et al, (1989) Respiratory cancer in chrysotile textile and mining industries: Exposure inferences from lung analysis. *Br J Ind Med* 46:180-187.

Teschler H, Friedrichs KH, Hoheisel GB, et al. (1994) Asbestos fibers in bronchoalveolar lavage and lung tissue of former asbestos workers. *Am J Resp Crit Care Med* 149:641-645.

Teschler H, Thompson AB, Dollenkamp R, et al. (1996). Relevance of asbestos bodies in sputum. *EurResp J* 9:680-686.

Tuomi T, Oksa P, Anttila S, et al. (1991b). Fibres and asbestos bodies in bronchoalveolar lavage fluids of asbestos sprayers. *Br J Ind Med* 49:480-485.
WHO (1998) Chrysotile asbestos: *Environmental Health Criteria*. Geneva: Switzerland: World HealthOrganization.
www.epa.gov/*asbestos*/ Environmental Protection Agency, June 2010,

16

Adverse Effect of Air Pollution on Odor Perception

Marco Guarneros[1], René Drucker-Colín[1],
José Esquivelzeta[2] and Robyn Hudson[3]
[1]*Instituto de Fisiología Celular,*
[2]*Facultad de Medicina,*
[3]*Instituto de Investigaciones Biomédicas,*
Universidad Nacional Autónoma de México
Mexico

1. Introduction

The Mexico City metropolitan area has a population of more than 20 million people (Consejo Nacional de Población, 2009) which makes it one of the largest agglomerations in the world. Mexico City lies at an altitude of 2240m above sea level, and is surrounded by mountains to the south, west, and east. Air pollution driven by local emissions can affect large areas within closed valleys, where restricted air movement concentrates the suspended pollutants. Due to its altitude and latitude, Mexico City receives intense solar radiation, a condition that together with less efficient combustion promotes photochemical formation of secondary pollutants such as ground level ozone and particulate matter (Molina & Molina, 2002) which remain above the Mexican standard for many days of the year in certain city zones (Secretaría de Medio Ambiente del Distrito Federal, 2007).

A great number of studies have reported negative effects of air pollution on health, above all among the most susceptible groups of the population; children, aged persons, and asthmatic patients (review in Rosales-Castillo et al., 2001). Among the many adverse effects that have been attributed to air pollution are dermatological pathologies (Goldsmith, 1996), damage to the eyes (Versura et al., 1999), allergic manifestations (Schierhorn et al., 1999), increased levels of stress (Evans et al., 1988), possible triggering of neurodegenerative conditions such as Alzheimer's disease (Calderón-Garcidueñas et al., 2004) and others related to locomotor behavior (Rivas-Arancibia et al., 2003), as well as a list of harmful effects on the cardiovascular system including problems in the myocardium, deficiencies in the vasoconstriction system and cardiac arrest (Bhatnagar, 2006; Zanobetti & Schwartz, 2006). Consequently, air pollution is also associated with higher levels of hospitalization (Zanobetti & Schwartz, 2006) and mortality (Loomis et al., 1999). However, effects on the respiratory system have received the most clinical and epidemiological attention. For example, it has been demonstrated that air pollutants can cause inflammation and a greater susceptibility to infections in the respiratory tract, worsening of asthma, decrements in peak expiratory flow and increased mortality related to chronic exposure to photochemical pollutants and particulate matter (Romieu et al., 1996; Gold et al., 1999; Borja-Aburto et al., 1997; Loomis et al., 1999; Tovalín et al., 2010). Chronic exposure to environmental toxicants, even below the recommended limits, also plays an important role in the outbreak of respiratory diseases (Lippmann, 1989). The damage inflicted on the respiratory system may affect the bronchia and the bronchioles, produce chronic inflammation of the lung parenchima, abnormal lung growth, delay in the maturation of the lungs and alveolar edemas. Also of concern is the possible increase in the frequency of lung diseases in populations of children exposed to Mexico City air pollution, given that these exposed populations have a higher potential risk of developing chronic respiratory diseases in their future life (Castillejos et al., 1995; Calderón-Garcidueñas et al., 2000, 2001, 2003a).

Despite the extensive literature reporting harmful effects on the sense of smell from chronic exposure to potentially harmful substances in different work environments (e.g., Cometto-Muñiz & Cain, 1991; Berglund et al., 1992; Smeets & Dalton, 2002; Smeets et al., 2002; Hastings & Miller, 2003; Chen et al., 2004; Vent et al., 2004; Zibrowski & Robertson, 2006; Heiser et al., 2010) and considerable evidence of pathological effects of chronic exposure to everyday ambient air pollution on the cellular structure of the nasal epithelium (Calderón-Garcidueñas et al., 1996, 1998, 2000, 2003b, 2009), until recently (Hudson et al., 2006), effects of big city air pollution on odor perception had remained undescribed.

2. Standardized tests

In a recent study (Guarneros et al., 2009) we compared the olfactory function of 30 young subjects from Mexico City and 30 from the neighboring but markedly less polluted state of Tlaxcala. Subjects were tested using an internationally validated olfactory test battery, the Sniffin' Sticks (Fig. 1) (Hummel et al., 1997). In a first test, we presented subjects with a series of dilutions of the odorant molecule 2 phenyl-ethanol, which has a characteristic rose smell, dissolved in an odorless solvent (propylene-glycol) to determine the minimum concentration needed for each subject to detect the presence of the odor (threshold). Subjects from Tlaxcala outperformed subjects from Mexico City on this task (Fig.1a). The results showed that the difference represented a 2- to 4-fold increase in the concentration needed by Mexico City subjects to detect the presence of the stimulus.

Tlaxcala subjects also obtained higher scores in a discrimination test than subjects from Mexico City. In this test, subjects were presented with different pairs of odorants (Table 1), and for each pair, the subjects' ability to distinguish one odor from the other was assessed. All odorants were presented at concentrations that were sufficiently high for every subject to detect. For each pair of odors, the blindfolded subjects were presented two of three times with one stimulus, and one of three times with the other (different) stimulus. The subjects' task was to indicate which stimulus was the different one. The results showed that differences between the two groups of subjects on this test were small but significant; on a scale of 1 to 16 points (correct answers), subjects from Tlaxcala scored an average of 13, more than one point above subjects from Mexico City who scored an average of 11.8 (Fig.1b).

We also evaluated odor identification, which refers to subjects' ability to correctly associate odor stimuli with their names. Subjects were presented with 16 substances that resemble odors from everyday life (Table 2) and had to correctly select each odor's name from a list of four options. It is generally accepted that higher brain functions (such as memory, speech and thought) are implicated in tasks of odor recognition to a greater extent than in other measures of olfactory performance such as odor threshold (minimum concentration for detection) (Lötsch et al., 2008). This might account for the fact that no significant differences were found between the groups in the identification test (Fig. 1c), possibly revealing the ability of the brain to compensate the impairment observed in the threshold and discrimination tests (Hudson et al., 2006).

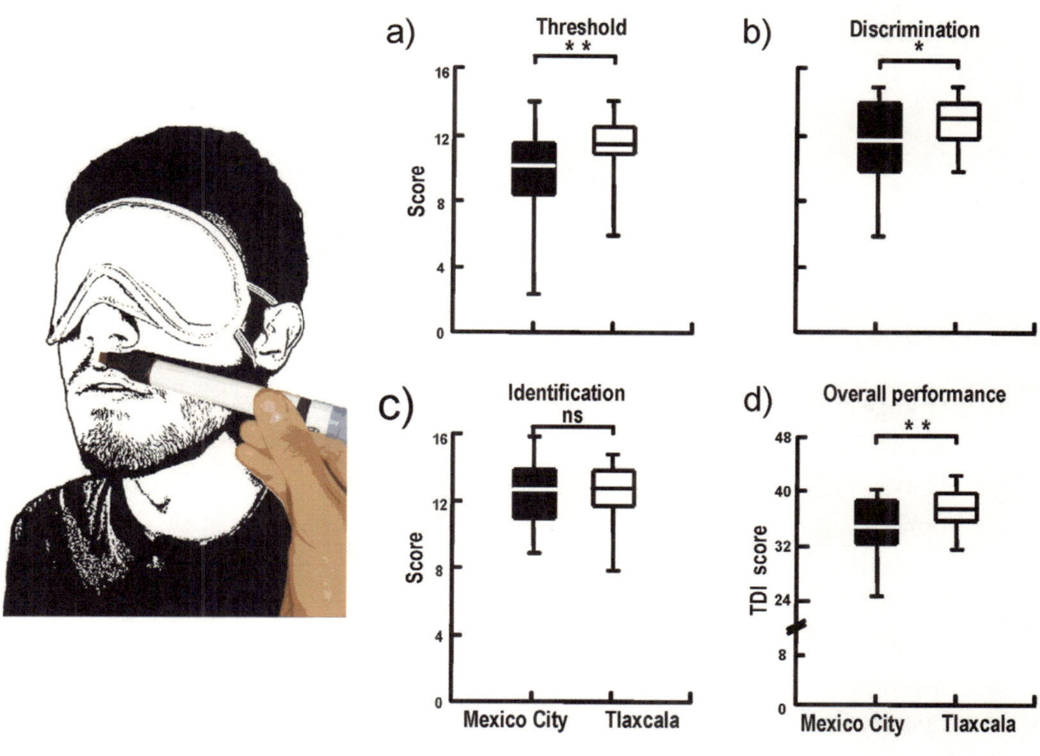

Fig. 1. Performance of subjects from Mexico City and Tlaxcala on the three tests of olfactory performance (a-c) as well as their TDI scores representing the sum of their scores on these (threshold, detection, and identification) tests (d). For each of the tests, subjects could obtain a maximum score of 16 correct responses and consequently a maximum TDI score of 48. Box plots: horizontal lines within boxes give medians, boxes' horizontal limits give the interquartile ranges, and vertical bars give the absolute ranges. *p<0.05, **p<0.01, ns = not significant (Mann-Whitney U tests). (Adapted from Guarneros et al., 2009).

	Target stimuli	Non-target stimuli
1	Butanol	2-phenylethanol
2	Isoamyl acetate	Anetol
3	Anetol	Eugenol
4	Limonene	Fenchone
5	(-) Carvone	(+) Carvone
6	Eugenol	Cinnamon aldehyde
7	Dihydro rosenoxide	Menthol
8	Acetaldehyde	Isoamylacetate
9	Citronellal	Linalool
10	Pyridine	Limonene
11	Limonene	Citronellal
12	Eucalyptol	Dipiridyl
13	Dipiridyl	Cyclopentadecanoate
14	Butanol	Fenchone
15	Octylacetate	Cinnamon aldehyde
16	Carvone	Acetaldehyde

Table 1. Stimuli used in the discrimination test.

1	**Orange**	Blackberry	Strawberry	Pineapple
2	Smoke	**Shoe-leather**	Glue	Grass
3	Honey	Vanilla	Chocolate	**Cinnamon**
4	Garlic	Spruce	**Peppermint**	Onion
5	Coconut	**Banana**	Walnut	Cherry
6	Peach	Apple	**Lemon**	Grapefruit
7	**Licorice**	Gummy bears	Chewing-gum	Cookies
8	Mustard	Rubber	Menthol	**Turpentine**
9	Onion	Cabbage	**Garlic**	Carrot
10	Cigarette	**Coffee**	Wine	Candle smoke
11	Melon	Peach	Orange	**Apple**
12	**Clove**	Pepper	Cinnamon	Mustard
13	Pear	Plum	Peach	**Pineapple**
14	Camomile	Strawberry	**Rose**	Cherry
15	**Anise**	Rum	Honey	Pinetree
16	Bread	**Fish**	Cheese	Ham

Table 2. Identification test. For each of the 16 trials, the target odorant stimulus is indicated in bold to distinguish it from the three distractors showed in the same row.

3. Tests using everyday products

In tests of olfactory performance, monomolecular substances are usually preferred for reasons of stimulus control and experimental convenience. However, tests using the molecular mixtures typical of real life can be considered to provide a more ecologically relevant approximation (Ayabe-Kanamura et al., 1998; Distel et al., 1999; Hudson, 1999; Distel & Hudson, 2001).

We therefore tested a different set of subjects from Mexico City (n=82) and Tlaxcala (n=86) with ascending concentrations of an orange juice preparation and of an instant coffee preparation to determine their thresholds (minimum concentration for detection). In this study (Hudson et al., 2006) subjects were also asked to discriminate between the odors of different dilutions of commercially available powdered preparations of two popular Mexican beverages, horchata (rice-based) and atole (maize-based). The stimuli were presented in polyethylene squeeze bottles (Fig.2) previously used in a number of studies of chemosensory perception (Hudson et al., 1994; Laska et al., 1997, 2000; Laska & Teubner, 1999; Laska & Hubener, 2001). We chose these substances to maximize the ecological validity of the stimuli and the ability of subjects to describe and to accurately name them (cf. Ayabe-Kanamura et al., 1998; Distel et al., 1999; Distel & Hudson, 2001). Again, Tlaxcala residents performed significantly better than Mexico City residents on tests of odor detection and discrimination (Fig. 2 a-c), but the two groups performed equally well on description and naming. Deficits in olfactory performance among Mexico City subjects were apparent even for young, otherwise healthy adults.

In addition, further groups of subjects from Mexico City and Tlaxcala (30 subjects from each location) were compared for their ability to detect, describe and identify the smell of a milk preparation (Guarneros & Hudson, 2009). Again, subjects from Tlaxcala detected and described the odor of milk at lower concentrations than subjects from Mexico City (Fig.2 d-e) but no significant differences were found for the frequency and concentrations for correct identification between the two groups.

4. Are these findings relevant for everyday life?

Our sense of smell plays an important role in a wide range of functions. In a recent systematic review, Stevenson (2010) classified olfactory function into three main categories: 1) functions relating to ingestive behavior, 2) avoidance of environmental hazards, and 3) social communication. For example, the human sense of smell can detect (Porter et al., 2007) and identify foods suitable for eating (Fallon & Rozin, 1983). Also, smelling can modulate appetite, dietary behaviors, and nutritional status (Duffy et al., 1995; Aschenbrenner et al., 2008; Seo & Hummel, 2009). Moreover, olfaction warns of possible microbial threat (e.g., from feces, vomit, or organic decay), evoking disgust (Stevenson et al., 2010), and of nonmicrobial hazards including gas leaks, smoke, and toxic materials, eliciting fear (Cain & Turk, 1985; Cain et al., 1987; Miwa et al., 2001; Santos et al., 2004).

We therefore tested the ability of the last-mentioned subjects to detect, describe and judge the smell of dimethyl-disulfide (DMDS) (Guarneros & Hudson, 2009), a byproduct of the decomposition of various foods which has a characteristic smell of rotten cabbage and is largely responsible for the smell of different decaying or putrefying foods including milk (van Aardt et al., 2005). The subjects from Tlaxcala could detect and give a description of DMDS at lower concentrations than the Mexico City subjects. However, the concentrations at which subjects indicated the smell to be disgusting were not statistically significant between the two groups (Fig.3a). Again, this might be explained by the additional recruitment of higher order mechanisms in the brain involved in attentional capture and enhancement (Grabenhorst et al., 2011).

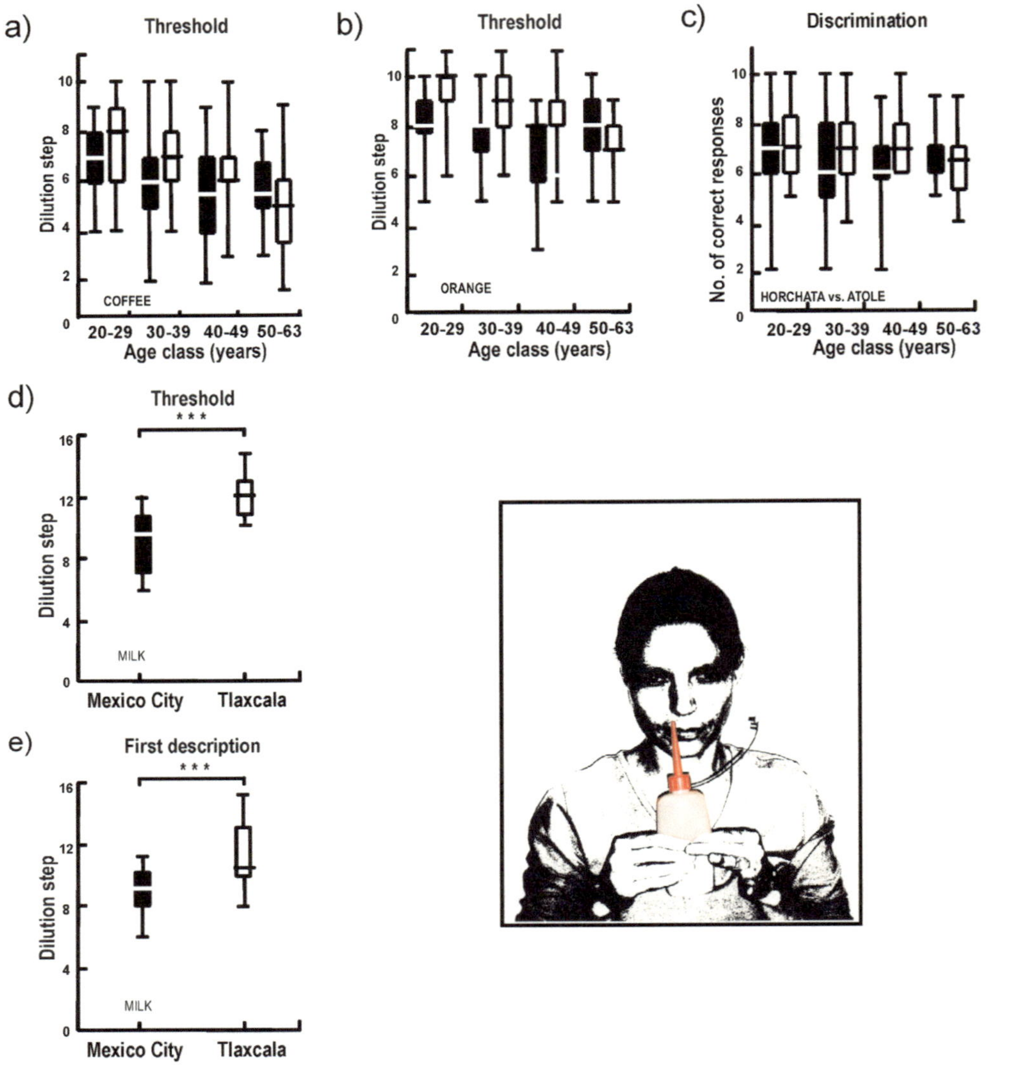

Fig. 2. Responses of subjects from Mexico City and Tlaxcala to the odor of different everyday products. The subjects from Tlaxcala outperformed the subjects from Mexico City in the following tasks a) Thresholds for detection of coffee. b) Thresholds for detection of orange. c) Discrimination task between two different Mexican beverages. d) Thresholds for detection of milk. e) First descriptions for the odor of milk. "Dilution steps" refer to the bottle numbers in the ascending order in which they were presented. Box plots: horizontal lines dividing the boxes = medians, horizontal limits of the boxes = interquartile ranges, vertical bars = percentiles 10 and 90. ***p<0.001, Mann-Whitney U tests. (Adapted from Hudson et al., 2006 and from Guarneros & Hudson, 2009).

Finally, subjects were presented with the powdered milk preparation at the concentration commercially recommended for human consumption but containing ascending concentrations of the contaminant DMDS. The concentration of DMDS at which subjects could discriminate the contaminated milk from milk without the contaminant was registered as the detection threshold for contaminated milk. Subjects from Tlaxcala not only presented lower thresholds (higher sensitivity) for DMDS in milk, but were also able to describe the odor and report it as being unpleasant (more unpleasant than milk alone) at lower concentrations than the Mexico City subjects (Fig.3). It is important to note that differences in scores were more marked for this test than for the previous one, which implies that olfactory impairment might be even more marked for complex olfactory tasks such as detecting a "target" odor when embedded in a "background" odor.
These results thus further warn of the dangers of big city air pollution by providing evidence of damage to the sense of smell and the relevance that this could have for everyday life.

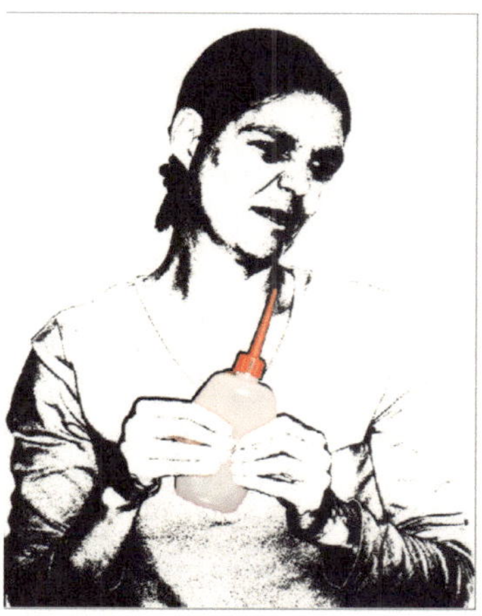

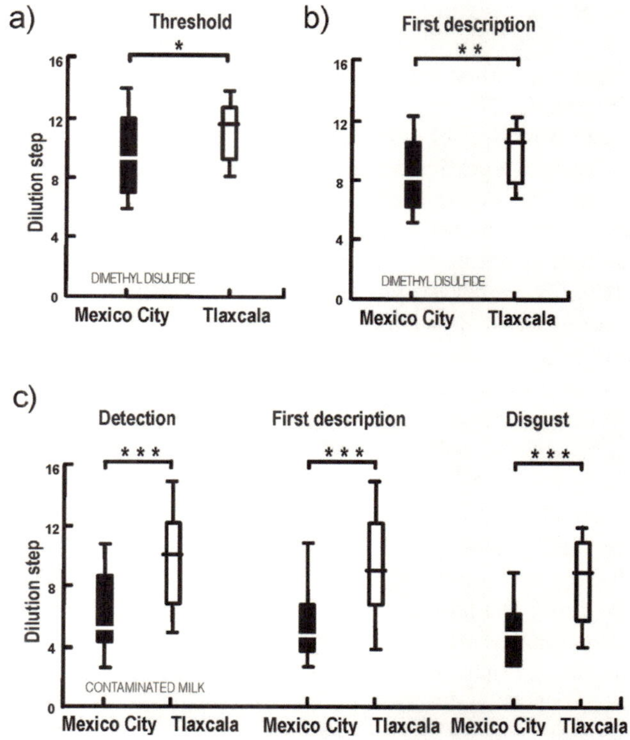

Fig. 3. Responses of subjects from Mexico City and Tlaxcala to the unpleasant stimulus dimethyl-disulfide. a) Thresholds for detection of dimethyl-disulfide. b) First descripton of dimethyl-disulfide. c) Thresholds for detection, first description and disgust (concentration at which subjects reported the stimulus to be disgusting) for milk with increasing concentrations of the contaminant dimethyl-disulfide. "Concentration" refers to the bottle numbers in the ascending order in which they were presented. Box plots: horizontal lines dividing the boxes = medians, limits of the boxes = interquartile ranges, vertical bars = percentiles 10 and 90. *p<0.05, **p<0.01, ***p<0.001, Mann-Whitney U tests. (Adapted from Guarneros & Hudson, 2009).

5. Trigeminal sensitivity

What is commonly known as the sense of smell is composed of multiple sensations predominantly mediated by two distinct but functionally connected neural pathways, the olfactory and the trigeminal systems (Hudson et al., 1994; Laska et al., 1997). In fact, the great majority of chemosensory stimulants produce both olfactory and trigeminal activation (von Skramlik, 1925; Doty et al., 1978; Cometto-Muñiz & Cain, 1991, 1998; Hummel, 2000). Tingling, burning, pungent, prickling, cooling and fresh are common descriptors of intranasal sensations mediated by the trigeminal system. The anterior third of the nasal cavity is provided with trigeminal nerve endings sensitive to chemical substances. These project to the central nervous system including to the amygdala which processes emotional responses such as fear (Hacquemand et al., 2010).

Despite being so closely integrated, the olfactory and the intranasal trigeminal systems appear to have evolved as distinct functional adaptations. An important function of the intranasal trigeminal system is to prevent inhalation of potentially life-threatening substances by reflexively stopping inhalation (Walker et al., 2001; Scheibe et al., 2006) and triggering other protective reflexes, including sneezing, local neurogenic inflammation of the mucosa (Tizzano et al., 2010), and production of tears (Kjaergaard et al., 2004), whereas a major function of the olfactory system is to enable the learning of odors relevant to an individual's particular life experiences and environment (Hudson, 1999).

Given the contribution of both the olfactory and trigeminal systems to odor perception via the intranasal sensory surface, and notable pathological effects of air pollution on the cellular structure of the intranasal epithelium (Calderón-Garcidueñas et al., 1996, 1997, 1998, 2000, 2003b, 2009), we expected that residents of Mexico City would show significantly poorer performance than residents of Tlaxcala on a trigeminal task.

For this, the subjects tested above with Sniffin' Sticks were presented with two 250-mL polyethylene squeeze bottles with Teflon nosepieces that fit into the nostrils (Guarneros et al., 2009). The nosepieces were covered with disposable plastic caps that were replaced for each subject. Whereas the target bottle contained 30 mL of 98% eucalyptol (Fluka, Germany), a stimulus that elicits both olfactory and nasal trigeminal responses in humans (Doty et al., 1978), the odorless control bottle contained only ambient air. The headspace of the bottles was used to stimulate both sides of the nose independently but simultaneously during the same inspiration, and the subject's task was to identify the side of the nose receiving the stimulus. The side of stimulation was pseudorandomized across trials in the same manner for all subjects. Stimuli were presented using a hand-held squeeze device that simultaneously delivered a constant volume (15 mL) of air to each nostril (Fig. 4). Subjects received 40 trials (20 deliveries of eucalyptol to each nostril) from which we calculated the percent of correct responses. This previously described method (Hummel et al., 2003; Dalton et al., 2006) is based on the well-established finding that although subjects have difficulty identifying the nostril receiving a purely olfactory stimulus, they can readily do this for stimuli with a trigeminal component (Cometto-Muñiz & Cain, 1998; Hummel et al., 2003; Wysocki et al., 2003; Dalton et al., 2006).

The Tlaxcala subjects again performed significantly better than the Mexico City subjects (Fig. 4). Whereas subjects from Mexico City scored an average of 70.5% of correct answers, the subjects from Tlaxcala scored 81% of correct answers (Guarneros et al., 2009). This is potentially important given the contribution of the trigeminal system to the perception of odors (Hudson et al., 1994; Laska et al., 1997; Boyle et al., 2007; Frasnelli et al., 2009) and to warning of the presence of toxic substances or other stimuli associated with situations that represent a threat to survival, such as smoke (Silver, 1991).

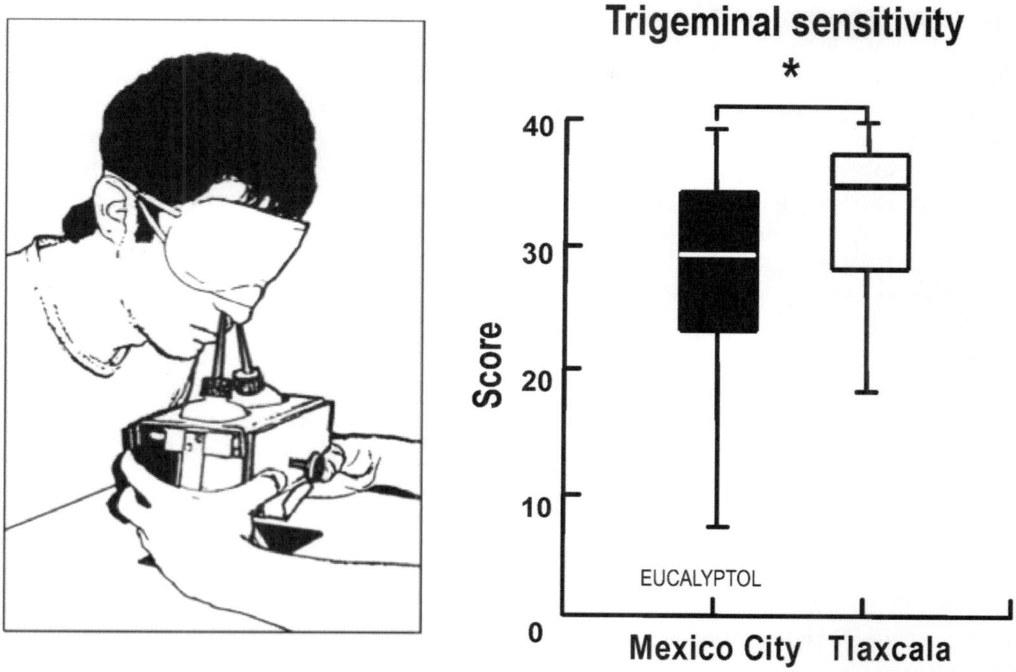

Fig. 4. Ability of subjects from Mexico City and Tlaxcala to correctly identify the nostril receiving the trigeminal stimulus eucalyptol when presented as shown in the drawing. Subjects could obtain a maximum score of 40 correct responses. Box plots: horizontal lines within boxes give medians, boxes' horizontal limits give the interquartile ranges, and vertical bars give the absolute ranges. *$p<0.05$ (Mann-Whitney U test). (Adapted from Guarneros et al., 2009).

6. Mechanisms of intranasal damage and defense

To avoid the olfactory neurons of the nasal mucosa coming into direct contact with toxic agents contained in inspired air, both the respiratory and olfactory systems have evolved an array of defense mechanisms. The first is formed by the trigeminal nerve endings that detect and respond to irritants transmitted by the air. If it is not possible to escape the source of danger, the rhythm of breathing is altered and sneezing and coughing may occur so as to minimize the entry of irritants to the respiratory airways. Second, in addition to the olfactory epithelium, the nasal cavity contains squamous and respiratory epithelia. Both produce antibodies and antimicrobial proteins that protect the system against damaging agents, thereby limiting the effect of these on the olfactory epithelium. A third defense consists in increased production of mucous, which retains many of the agents that could damage the system. However, the efficiency of these defense mechanisms depends to a considerable extent on an individual´s local environment. Chronic exposure to atmospheric contaminants can seriously damage the respiratory and olfactory epithelia, even to the point of causing the development of tumors (Harkema et al., 1987; Berglund et al., 1992; Calderón-Garcidueñas et al., 1994, 1998, 1999; Lewis & Dahl, 1995; Hastings & Miller, 2003).

Although cells of the nasal cavity are able to limit damage to the nasal mucosa when exposure to contaminants is brief, in the case of chronic exposure the mucosa may develop abnormal characteristics that reduce its defense capabilities, causing discomfort and disease. The most common forms of damage within the nasal cavity produced by exposure to air pollution are shortening and partial or total loss of the olfactory cilia, which arise from the dendritic knobs of the olfactory neurons and along which the olfactory receptors are located, necrosis, displasias, metaplasias and hyperplasias of the basal cells from which the olfactory receptor neurons arise during the life-long process of neuronal regeneration characteristic of the olfactory system, and loss of cohesion among cells (Calderón-Garcidueñas et al., 1998, 2001; Schierhorn et al., 1999).

When the mucociliar system is affected, the retention of toxic particles by the mucosa is reduced, thus affecting the rest of the system (Halpern, 1982). With the loss of cilia the canals of the Bowman´s glands, which produce the mucous that baths the nasal cavity, cleans the cilia and is indispensable for efficient regeneration of the olfactory epithelium, are directly exposed to the environment. When these glands are affected, the epithelium regenerates more slowly and eventually may even cease to do so (Morrison & Constanzo, 1990; Hastings & Miller, 2003).

Ozone is one of the most damaging oxidative contaminants among the atmospheric toxic agents, and is probably the one that has received the most attention (Tyler et al., 1988). It is highly reactive and interacts with a great variety of organic molecules, including non-saturated fats, proteins and nucleic acids. Both in humans and laboratory animals, acute or chronic exposure to ozone produces significant damage in the epithelium and the olfactory bulbs (Harkema et al., 1987; Calderón-Garcidueñas et al., 1996, 1998, 1999, 2002, 2009; Colín-Barenque et al., 1999).

Sulfur compounds also produce pathological changes in the respiratory epithelium. Whereas at lower concentrations they cause an increase in the secretion of mucous, at high concentrations they may cause a reduction in the flow of nasal secretions (Halpern, 1982). Other toxic substances such a formaldehyde and carbon dioxide may cause an abnormal structural and functional formation of the cilia, reducing their movement and thus their capacity to eliminate toxic particles (Boat & Carson, 1990). Whereas formaldehyde and acetaldehyde may induce nasal tumors, irritants such as ammonia cause inflammation, hyperplasias, metaplasias and displasias in the nasal epithlium (Hakema et al., 1987).

7. Discussion and future directions

The olfactory system resembles a finely tuned engine. The wrong fuel, containing contaminants, will generally impair the engine's performance and eventually just shut it down. Although the system might be able to cope with toxic agents to a certain degree and remain clinically healthy for prolonged periods in the face of poor air quality, as time passes and toxicity persists, disease will manifest itself. Here it should be noted that some of the deleterious effects of air pollutants on the respiratory cells lining the nasal cavity appear as soon as 15 days after the start of exposure (arrival to the city) to pollutants such as ozone, which induces acute nasal inflammatory responses and significant epithelial lesions in humans (Calderón-Garcidueñas et al., 1994). It would not be surprising to find an associated sensory effect just as soon, although this remains to be investigated.

Conditions and the time necessary for recovery of olfactory function are also unknown, but are likely to depend on the extent of damage. The capacity of the olfactory epithelium to regenerate and recover from environmental insults might be overridden by the rate of damage caused by chronic toxic exposure leading to a loss of the equilibrium and finally a functional collapse resulting in either diminished or the complete loss of olfactory function (hyposmia and anosmia, respectively) (Crews & Hunter, 1994; Smith et al., 2009).

Functional alterations to the olfactory system caused by exposure to toxic agents constitute a problem that has only received attention quite recently despite being known for a long time. For example, at the beginning of the 20th century zinc sulfate was used to irrigate the nasal cavity, with the aim of preventing attacks by viruses and bacteria on the brain. In patients treated with this substance the development of anosmia was observed (Menco & Morrison, 2003). Also, many of the first cases of impaired olfactory function and nasal discomfort were reported in people chronically exposed to high ambient levels of substances in industrial use such as sulfur dioxide, cadmium, lead, and chromium, among others (Cone & Shusterman, 1991; Schiffman & Nagle, 1992; Hastings & Miller, 2003). Unfortunately, there are as yet no available treatments able to reverse the damage caused by the exposure to such agents, although sometimes removal of the source allows repair of the olfactory system and the recovery of normal function (Upadhyay & Holbrook, 2004).

There are very few reports regarding deficiencies in trigeminal sensitivity. However, one of the most important findings is the relation between the decline in olfactory sensitivity and a reduction of trigeminal sensitivity; there is increasing evidence that an acquired loss of the sense of smell results in a reduction in trigeminal sensitivity due to the lack of interaction centrally (Hummel & Livermore, 2002). Both the orbitofrontal cortex and the rostral insula seem to be important in the amplification of trigeminal information, and this amplification is not found in anosmic patients and is reduced in hyposmic patients (Frasnelli & Hummel, 2007). On the other hand, patients suffering from inflammatory processes such as allergic rhinitis (which is frequently worsened by chronic exposure to environmental pollutants) usually present nasal itching and sneezing after toxicant exposure, clinical correlates of the activation of trigeminal nerve endings due to local inflammatory mechanisms (Doerfler et al., 2006). Aging is also associated with impaired trigeminal sensitivity and although it is not known to what extent this reduction is due to central processes, it is known that, at least in part, a reduction in sensitivity occurs in the periphery of the system (Frasnelli & Hummel, 2007).

Many toxic agents cause inflammatory processes that can affect the epithelium of the nasal cavity, and eventually can destroy trigeminal nerve endings. Tobacco smoke and alcohol are among the substances that have been observed to affect the epithelium (Vent et al., 2003; 2004), while acrolein, which is used as a herbicide, produces inflammation and tumors in the nasal cavity (Dorman et al., 2008). However, the effect of environmental toxic agents on the trigeminal system has still been little studied.

The results of previous studies indicate that subjects who are constantly exposed to the high levels of ambient air pollution of Mexico City present a significant reduction in olfactory sensitivity but not in the ability to identify common odorant stimuli (Hudson et al., 2006; Guarneros & Hudson, 2009; Guarneros et al., 2009). The similarities in the findings of these studies and despite the differences in the test methods and stimuli employed suggest the reliability of these conclusions. Furthermore, these findings are extended by the report of an adverse effect of big city air pollution on trigeminal function. This is potentially important given the contribution of the trigeminal system to the perception of odors and to detecting the presence of toxic substances that could inflict damage on the respiratory system (Guarneros et al., 2009).

The subjects in our studies described above were healthy non-smokers and from socio-economical backgrounds characterized by good nutrition, good hygiene and a high standard of medical care. It would not be surprising if among less favored sectors of the heterogeneous population of Mexico City, impairment of chemosensory function would be even greater. This is particularly likely given that people from less favorable socioeconomic backgrounds are typically at a higher health risk associated with often greater exposure to air pollution (O'Neill et al., 2008).

Apart from a study associating the high levels of air pollution of Mexico City with pathological changes in the appearance of the olfactory bulbs and a reduction in the perception of odors (Calderón-Garcidueñas et al., 2009), little is known about the precise nature of the damage that air pollution inflicts on the olfactory and trigeminal systems. However, evidence of notable negative effects on the tissue of the nasal cavity (e.g. Calderón-Garcidueñas et al., 1996, 1997, 1998, 2001; Valverde et al., 1997) suggests that deficits in perception are mainly due to damage in the periphery of the system. Consistent with this we repeatedly found that performance on odor identification tests was equally good for subjects from Mexico City and the control population from Tlaxcala. This may be explained by the fact that the identification of odorants presented at suprathreshold concentrations involves more central cognitive functions based on associative memory processes to a greater extent than simply detecting or discriminating between them when presented at low concentrations (Hudson et al., 2006; Lötsch et al., 2008), thereby compensating the peripheral deficiencies once the concentration of stimuli are above the threshold of perception (Hudson et al., 2006). The equally good performance of the two groups on the tests of odor identification also suggests that subjects were equally motivated and equally able to manage the test situation.

Evidence of deficits in olfactory function and trigeminal sensitivity in young subjects exposed to high levels of urban air pollution raises other questions of relevance to public health. At what age do symptoms first appear? To what extent do certain common activities such as participating in sports in the open worsen such effects, and to what extent is impairment of chemosensory function reversible?

In addition, we do not know to what extent the impairment in olfactory sensitivity could be due to chronic inflammatory disorders of the mucosa and of the paranasal sinuses. These forms of chronic disease can cause nasal obstruction and are a common cause of diminished olfactory function (Doty, 1999; Cullen & Leopold, 1999; Seiden & Duncan, 2001; Welge-Lüssen, 2009). The possibility that, at least in part, olfactory impairment caused by air pollution is due to chronic inflammation seems plausible given that the incidence of inflammatory disorders is especially high in cities with air pollution problems (Arnedo-Peña et al., 2009; Liao et al., 2009; Lindgren et al., 2009; Wichmann et al., 2009), including Mexico City (Meza-Morales et al., 1998).

Although in the last years there has been a reduction in air pollution in Mexico City, air quality standards are still being exceeded for ozone and for particulate matter with an aerodynamic diameter of less than 10 micrometers (PM_{10}) (Instituto Nacional de Ecología, 2007). It is interesting that the authorities have given particular importance to particles less than 2.5 micrometers in diameter ($PM_{2.5}$) that according to various studies have considerable negative effects on health (Borja-Aburto et al., 1997, 1998) because they can reach the periphery of the lungs, the bronchial tubes and the alveoli. On the other hand, the larger PM_{10} particles principally affect the upper airways of the head and neck and only rarely reach the lungs. For this reason, they have been considered comparatively less damaging than finer particles (revision in Molina & Molina, 2002). However, it is very likely that the olfactory epithelium is directly affected by high concentrations of PM_{10}. Consistent with this, there have been several studies of the relation between high atmospheric levels of PM_{10} and health. These studies reveal that the levels of these larger particles are associated with daily mortality and indeed also represent a health risk (Rosales-Castillo et al., 2001; O'Neill et al., 2004).

A more complete view of the risk to public health might be obtained in future studies by investigating the relation between subjects' performance on olfactory and trigeminal tests and levels of air pollution at different study sites on the days that tests are actually conducted. Also, the historical record of air pollution in the areas of study and the degree of individual subjects' exposure could provide additional information resulting in a better understanding of how air pollution affects the olfactory and trigeminal systems, including to what extent effects are due to acute or to chronic exposure to contaminants, and with what possible implications for behavior and treatment.

Notably, while the development of neurodegenerative diseases has also been related to exposure to high levels of air pollution (e.g. Campbell, 2004; Villarreal-Calderon et al., 2010) and to diminished olfactory capabilities (Doty et al., 1991; Fernández-Ruiz et al., 2003; Velazquez-Pérez et al., 2006; Haehner et al., 2007), the relation between these seemingly intertwined elements has only started to be investigated recently (Calderón-Garcidueñas et al., 2009). Thus, further research in this respect might also shed light on the origins and early diagnosis of neurodegenerative diseases that represent important public health issues such as Parkinson's disease.

8. Concluding summary

Mexico City air pollution is associated with impaired olfactory function. Different aspects of odor perception are altered to varying degrees, olfactory sensitivity being the most affected. This is shown by the higher detection thresholds both for monomolecular substances and complex mixtures common in everyday life observed for Mexico City subjects compared to subjects from cleaner-air environments, but equally good performance in describing and naming odor stimuli. Also, air pollution seems to be related to an impaired ability in assessing food edibility. The adverse effects of air pollution on olfactory function appear to result mainly from peripheral damage to this system rather than from effects on more central, cognitive processes. This is supported by an extensive literature reporting the harmful effects of airborne contaminants on the nasal cavity, including to the respiratory and olfactory epithelia. People from air-polluted areas also showed poorer performance in a test of intranasal trigeminal function, which mediates the sensations of freshness, spiciness and pungency via free nerve endings that innervate the nasal cavity, and warns of the presence of potentially dangerous substances in the environment. Important topics for future research include how early in life such impairments are manifested, how they relate to different life circumstances, when and under what conditions they might be reversible, and of particular importance, to what extent they are related to the appearance of neurodegenerative diseases in the increasingly aging populations characteristic of many large urban areas.

9. Acknowledgement

MG gratefully acknowledges the Posgrado en Ciencias Biológicas, UNAM and CONACYT for a doctoral fellowship (CVU 228879).

10. References

Arnedo-Peña, A.; Gacía-Marcos, L.; Carvajal-Ureña, I.; Busquets-Monge, R.; Morales-Suárez-Varela, M.; Miner-Canflanca, I.; Batlles-Garrido, J.; Blanco-Quirós, A.; López-Silvarrey-Varela, A.; García-Hernández, G.; Aguinaga-Ontoso, I. & González-Díaz, C. (2009). Air pollution and recent symptoms of asthma, allergic rhinitis, and atopic eczema in school children aged between 6 and 7 years. *Archivos de Bronconeumología*, Vol.45, No.5, pp. 224-229, ISSN 0300-2896

Aschenbrenner, K.; Hummel, C.; Teszmer, K.; Krone, F.; Ishimaru, T.; Seo, H-S. & Hummel, T. (2008). The influence of olfactory loss on dietary behaviors. *Laryngoscope*, Vol.118, No.1, pp. 135–144, ISSN 0023-852X.

Ayabe-Kanamura, S.; Schicker, I.; Laska, M.; Hudson, R.; Distel, H.; Kobayakawa, T. & Saito, S. (1998). Differences in perception of everyday odors: a Japanese-German cross-cultural study. *Chemical Senses*, Vol.23, No.1, pp. 31–38, ISSN 0379-864X.

Berglund, B.; Lindvall, T. & Nordin, S. (1992). Environmentally induced changes in sensory sensitivities. *Annals of the New York Academy of Sciences*, Vol.64, pp. 304-321, ISSN 0077-8923.

Bhatnagar, A. (2006). Environmental cardiology: studying mechanistic links between pollution and heart disease. *Circulation Research*, Vol.99, No.7, pp. 692-705, ISSN 0009-7330.

Boat, T. & Carson, J. (1990). Ciliary dysmorphology and dysfunction – primary or acquired? *The New England Journal of Medicine*, Vol.323, No. 24, pp.1700-1702, ISSN 0028-4793.

Borja-Aburto, V.H.; Loomis, D.P.; Bangdiwala, S.I.; Shy, C.M. & Rascon-Pacheco, R.A. (1997). Ozone, suspended particles, and daily mortality in Mexico City. *American Journal of Epidemiology*, Vol.145, No.3, pp. 258-268, ISSN 0002-9262.

Borja-Aburto, V.H.; Castillejos, M.; Gold, D.F.; Bierzwinski, S. & Loomis, D. (1998). Mortality and ambient fine particles in southwest Mexico City 1993-1995. *Environmental Health Perspectives*, Vol.106, No.12, pp. 849-855, ISSN 0091-6765.

Boyle, J.A., Frasnelli, J.; Gerber, J.; Heinke, M. & Hummel, T. (2007). Cross-modal integration of intranasal stimuli: a functional magnetic resonance imaging study. *Neuroscience*, Vol.149, No.1, pp. 223-231, ISSN 1873-7544.

Cain, W.S. & Turk, A. (1985). Smell of danger: an analysis of LP-gas odorization. *American Industrial Hygiene Association Journal*, Vol.46, No.3, pp.115–126, ISSN 0002-8894.

Cain, W.S.; Leaderer, B.P.; Cannon, L.; Tosun, T. & Ismail, H. (1987). Odorization of inert gas for occupational safety: psychophysical considerations. *American Industrial Hygiene Association Journal*, Vol.48, No.1, pp. 47–55 ISSN 0002-8894.

Calderón-Garcidueñas, L.; Rodríguez-Alcaraz, A.; García, R.; Sánchez, G.; Barragán, G.; Camacho, R. & Ramírez, L. (1994). Human nasal mucosal changes after exposure to urban pollution. *Environmental Health Perspectives*, Vol.102, No.12, pp. 1074-1080, ISSN 0091-6765.

Calderón-Garcidueñas, L.; Osnaya, N.; Ramírez-Martínez, L. & Villarreal-Calderón A. (1996). DNA strand breaks in human nasal respiratory epithelium are induced upon exposure to urban pollution. *Environmental Health Perspectives,* Vol.104, No.2, pp. 160-168, ISSN 0091-6765.

Calderón-Garcidueñas, L.; Osnaya, N.; Rodríguez-Alcaraz, A. & Villarreal-Calderón, A. (1997). DNA damage in nasal respiratory epithelium from children exposed to urban air pollution. *Environmental and Molecular Mutagenesis,* Vol.30, No.1, pp. 11-20, ISSN 0893-6692.

Calderón-Garcidueñas, L.; Rodríguez-Alcaraz, A.; Villarreal-Calderón, A.; Lyght, O.; Janszen, D. & Morgan K. (1998). Nasal epithelium as a sentinel for airborne environmental pollution. *Toxicological Sciences,* Vol.46, No.2, pp. 352-364, ISSN 1096-6080.

Calderón-Garcidueñas, L.; Rodríguez-Alcaraz, A.; García, R.; Barragán, G.; Villarreal-Calderón, A. & Madden, M.C. (1999). Cell proliferation in nasal respiratory epithelium of people exposed to urban pollution. *Carcinogenesis,* Vol.20, No.3, pp. 383-389, ISSN 1460-2180.

Calderón-Garcidueñas, L.; Devlin, R.B. & Miller, F.J. (2000). Respiratory tract pathology and cytokine imbalance in clinically healthy children chronically and sequentially exposed to air pollutants. *Medical Hypotheses,* Vol.55, No.5, pp. 373-378, ISSN 0306-9877.

Calderón-Garcidueñas, L.; Valencia-Salazar, G.; Rodríguez-Alcaraz, A.; Gambling, M.T.; García, R.; Osnaya, N.; Villareal-Calderón, A.; Devlin, R. & Carson, J. (2001). Ultrastructural nasal pathology in children chronically and sequentially exposed to air pollutants. *American Journal of Respiratory Cell and Molecular Biology,* Vol.24, No.32, pp. 132-138, ISSN 1535-4989.

Calderón-Garcidueñas, L.; Azzarelli, B.; Acuña, H.; García, R.; Gambling, T.; Osnaya, N.; Monroy, S.; Tizapantzi, M.; Carson, J.; Villarreal-Calderón, A. & Rewcastle, B. (2002). Air pollution and brain damage. *Toxicologic Pathology,* Vol.30, No.3, pp. 373-389, ISSN 1533-1601.

Calderón-Garcidueñas, L.; Mora-Tiscareño, A.; Fordham, L.A.; Valencia-Salazar, G.; Chung, C.J.; Rodríguez-Alcaraz, A; Paredes, R.; Variakojis, D.; Villarreal-Calderón, A.; Flores-Camacho, L.; Antúnez-Solís, A; Henríquez-Roldán, C. & Hazucha, M.J. (2003a). Respiratory damage in children exposed to urban pollution. *Pediatric Pulmonology,* Vol.36, No.2, pp.148-161, ISSN 8755-6863.

Calderón-Garcidueñas, L.; Maronpot, R.R.; Torres-Jardón, R.; Henríquez-Roldán, C.; Schoonhoven, R.; Acuña-Ayala, H.; Villareal-Calderón, A.; Nakamura, J.; Fernando, R.; Reed, W.; Azzarelli, B. & Swenberg, J.A. (2003b). DNA damage in nasal and brain tissues of canines exposed to air pollutants is associated with evidence of chronic brain inflammation and neurodegeneration. *Toxicologic Pathology,* Vol.31, No.5, pp. 524-538, ISSN 0192-6233.

Calderón-Garcidueñas, L.; Reed, W.; Maronpot, R.R.; Henríquez-Roldán, C.; Delgado-Chávez, R.; Calderón-Garcidueñas, A.; Dragustinovis, I.; Franco-Lira, M.; Aragón-Flores, M.; Solt, A.C.; Altenburg, M.; Torres-Jardón, R. & Swenberg, J.A. (2004). Brain inflammation and Alzheimer's-like pathology in individuals exposed to severe air pollution. *Toxicologic Pathology,* Vol.32, No.6, pp. 650-658, ISSN 1533-1601.

Calderón-Garcidueñas, L.; Franco-Lira, M.; Henríquez-Roldán, C.; Osnaya, N.; González-Maciel, A.; Reynoso-Robles, R.; Villarreal-Calderón, R.; Herrit, L.; Brooks, D.; Keefe, S.; Palacios-Moreno, J.; Villarreal-Calderón, R.; Torres-Jardón, R.; Medina-Cortina,

H.; Delgado-Chávez, R.; Aiello-Mora, M.; Maronpot, R.R. & Doty R.L. (2009). Urban air pollution: Influences on olfactory function and pathology in exposed children and young adults. *Experimental and Toxicologic Pathology,* Vol. 62, No.1, pp. 91-102, ISSN 0940-2993.

Campbell, A. (2004) Inflammation, neurodegenerative diseases, and environmental exposures. *Annals of the New York Academy of Sciences,* Vol.1035, pp. 117-123, ISSN 1749-6632.

Castillejos, M.; Gold, D.R.; Damokosh, A.I.; Serrano, P.; Allen, G. & McDonnell, W.F. (1995). Acute effects of ozone on the pulmonary function of exercising schoolchildren from Mexico City. *American Journal of Respiratory and Critical Care Medicine,* Vol.152, No. 5 pt.1, pp. 1501-1507, ISSN 1073-449X.

Chen, J.; Shi, J.; Wang, S.; Yang, S.; Lou, J. & Liu, Z. (2004). Environmental mycological study and respiratory disease investigation in tussah silk processing workers. *Journal of Occupational Health,* Vol. 46, No.5, pp. 418-422, ISSN 1341-9145.

Colín-Barenque, L.; Ávila-Costa, M.R.; Fortoul, T.; Rugerio-Vargas, C.; Machado-Salas, J.P.; Espinosa-Villanueva, J. & Rivas-Arancibia, S. (1999). Morphologic alterations of the olfactory bulb after acute ozone exposure in rats. *Neuroscience Letters,* Vol.274, No.1, pp. 1-4, ISSN 1872-7972.

Cometto-Muniz, J.E. & Cain, W.S. (1991). Influence of air-borne contaminants on olfaction and taste in health and disease. In: *Smell and Taste in Health and Disease,* T.V. Getchell; R.L. Doty; L.M. Bartoshuk; and J.B. Snow. (Eds.), pp. 765-785, Raven, ISBN 0881677981, New York, USA.

Cometto-Muñiz, J.E. & Cain, W.S. (1998). Trigeminal and olfactory sensitivity: comparison of modalities and methods of measurement. *International Archives of Occupational and Environmental Health,* Vol.71, No.2, pp. 105–110, ISSN 0340-0131.

Cone, E.J. & Shusterman, D. (1991). Health effects of indoor odorants. *Environmental Health Perspectives,* Vol. 95, pp. 53-59, ISSN 0091-6765.

Consejo Nacional de Población. (2009). Mexico City Metropolitan Area, Government of the State of Mexico. 3.03.2011
http://www.edomex.gob.mx/poblacion/docs/2009/PDF/ZMVM.pdf.

Crews, L. & Hunter, D. (1994). Neurogenesis in the olfactory epithelium. *Perspectives on Developmental Neurobiology,* Vol.2, No.2, pp. 151-161, ISSN 1064-0517.

Cullen, M.M.; Leopold, D.A. (1999). Disorders of smell and taste. *Medical Clinics of North America,* Vol.83, No.1, pp. 57-74, ISSN 1557.9859.

Dalton, P.; Dilks, D. & Hummel, T. (2006). Effects of long-term exposure to volatile irritants on sensory thresholds, negative mucosal potentials, and event-related potentials. *Behavioral Neuroscience,* Vol.120, No.1, pp.180–189, 0735-7044.

Distel, H.; Ayabe-Kanamura, S.; Martínez-Gómez, M.; Schicker, I.; Kobayakawa, T.; Saito, S. & Hudson, R. (1999). Perception of everyday odors—correlation between intensity, familiarity and strength of hedonic judgement. *Chemical Senses,* Vol.24, No.2, pp. 191–199, ISSN 379-864X.

Distel, H.; & Hudson, R. (2001). Judgement of odor intensity is influenced by subjects' knowledge of the odor source. *Chemical Senses,* Vol.26, No.3, pp. 247-251 ISSN 379-864X.

Doerfler, H.; Hummel, T.; Klimek, L. & Kobal, G. (2006). Intranasal trigeminal sensitivity in subjects with allergic rhinitis. *European Archives of Otorhinolaryngology,* Vol.263, No.1, pp. 86-90, ISSN 1434-4726.

Dorman, D.C.; Struve, M.F.; Wong, B.A.; Marshall, M.W.; Gross, E.A. & Willson, G.A. (2008). Respiratory tract responses in male rats following subchronic acrolein inhalation. *Inhalation Toxicology,* Vol.20, No.3, pp. 205-216, ISSN 1091-7691.

Doty, R.L.; Brugger, W.P.E.; Jurs, P.C.; Orndorff, M.A.; Snyder, P.J. & Lowry, L.D. (1978). Intranasal trigeminal stimulation from odorous volatiles: psychometric responses from anosmic and normal humans. *Physiology and Behavior,* Vol. 20, No.2, pp. 175-185, ISSN 0031-9384

Doty, R.L.; Perl, D.P.; Steele, J.C.; Chen, K.M.; Pierce, J.D.Jr.; Reyes, P.; Kurland, L.T. (1991). Olfactory dysfunction in three neurodegenerative diseases. *Geriatrics,* Vol. 46 (August). Suppl 1, pp. 47-51, ISSN 1936-5764.

Doty, R.L. (1999). Olfaction. In: *Nasal polyposis: An inflammatory disease and its treatment.* N. Mygind & T. Linholdt (Eds.), pp. 153-159, Wiley Blackwell, ISBN 8716119681, Copenhagen, Denmark.

Duffy, V.B.; Backstrand, J.R. & Ferris, A.M. (1995). Olfactory dysfunction and related nutritional risk in free-living, elderly women. *Journal of the American Dietitic Association,* Vol. 95, No.8, pp. 879–884, ISSN 0002-8223.

Evans, G.W.; Colome, S.D. & Shearer, D.F. (1988). Psychological reactions to air pollution. *Environmental Research,* Vol.45, No.1, pp. 1-15, ISSN 0013-9351.

Fallon, A. & Rozin, P. (1983). The psychological bases of food rejection by humans. *Ecology of Food and Nutrition,* Vol.13, No.1, pp. 15–26, ISSN 0367-0244.

Fernández-Ruiz, J.; Díaz, R.; Hall-Haro, C.; Vergara, P.; Fiorentini, A.; Núñez, L.; Drucker-Colín, R.; Ochoa, A.; Yescas, P.; Rasmussen, A. & Alonso, M.E. (2003). Olfactory dysfunction in hereditary ataxia and basal ganglia disorders. *NeuroReport,* Vol.14, No.10, pp. 1339-1341, ISSN 1473-558X.

Frasnelli, J. & Hummel, T. (2007). Interactions between the chemical senses: trigeminal function in patients with olfactory loss. *International Journal of Psychophysiology,* Vol.65, No.3, pp.177-181, ISSN 1872-7697.

Frasnelli, J.; Charbonneau, G.; Collignon, O. & Lepore, F. (2009). Odor localization and sniffing. *Chemical Senses,* Vol.34, No.2, pp.139-144, ISSN 0379-864X.

Gold, D.R.; Damokosh, A.I.; Pope, C.A. III.; Dockery, D.W.; McDonnell, W.F. & Serrano, P. (1999). Particulate and ozone pollutant effects on the respiratory function of children in southwest Mexico City. *Epidemiology,* Vol.10, No.1, pp. 8-16, ISSN 1044-3983.

Goldsmith, L.A. (1996). Skin effects of air pollution. *Otolaryngology and Head and Neck Surgery,* Vol.114, No.2, pp. 217-219. ISSN 0194-5998.

Grabenhorst, F.; Rolls, E.T. & Margot, C. (2011). A hedonically complex odor mixture produces an attentional capture effect in the brain. *Neuroimage,* Vol.55, No.2, pp. 832-843, ISSN 1053-8119.

Guarneros, M. & Hudson, R. (2009). La contaminación del aire deteriora la función olfativa cotidiana en residentes de la Ciudad de México. *El Residente,* Vol.4 No. 3, pp. 81-86.

Guarneros, M.; Hummel, T.; Martínez-Gómez, M. & Hudson, R. (2009). Mexico City air pollution adversely affects olfactory function and intranasal trigeminal sensitivity. *Chemical Senses,* Vol.34, No.2, pp.819-826, ISSN 379-864X

Hacquemand, R.; Jacquot, L. & Brand, G. (2010). Comparative fear-related behaviors to predator odors (TMT and natural fox feces) before and after intranasal $ZnSO_4$ treatment in mice. *Frontiers in Behavioral Neuroscience,* Vol.4, (December), pp.188. ISSN 1662-5153.

Haehner, A.; Hummel, T.; Hummel, C.; Sommer, U.; Junghanns, S. & Reichmann, H. (2007). Olfactory loss may be a first sign of idiopathic Parkinson's disease. *Movement Disorders,* Vol.22, No.6, pp. 839-842.

Halpern, P.B. (1982). Environmental factors affecting chemoreceptors: an overview. *Environmental Health Perspectives,* Vol.44, pp.101-105, ISSN 0885-3185.

Harkema, R.J.; Plopper, C.; Hyde, D.; George, J.; Wilson, D. & Dungworth, D. (1987). Response of the macaque nasal epithelium to ambient levels of ozone. *The American Journal of Pathology,* Vol.128, No.1, pp. 29-44, ISSN 1525-2191.

Hastings, L. & Miller, M.L. (2003). Influence of environmental toxicants on olfactory function, In: *Handbook of olfation and gustation,* Second Edition, R.L. Doty (Ed.), pp. 575-592, ISBN 978-0-8247-0719-4, Marcel Dekker, Philadelphia, USA.

Heiser, C.; Grupp, K.; Hörmann, K. & Stuck, B.A. (2010). Loss of olfactory function after exposure to barbituric acid. *Auris Nasus Larynx,* Vol.37, No.1, pp. 103-105, ISSN 0385-8146.

Hudson, R. (1999). From molecule to mind: the role of experience in shaping olfactory function. *Journal of Comparative Physiology A.* Vol.185, No.4, pp. 297-304, ISSN 0340-7594.

Hudson, R.; Laska, M.; Berger, T.; Heye, B.; Schopohl, J. & Danek, A. (1994). Olfactory function in patients with hypogonadotropic hypogonadism: an all-or-none phenomenon? *Chemical Senses,* Vol.19, No.1, pp. 57-69, ISSN 379-864X .

Hudson, R.; Arriola, A.; Martínez-Gómez, M. & Distel, H. (2006). Effect of air pollution on olfactory function in residents of Mexico City. *Chemical Senses,* Vol.31, No.1, pp. 79-85, ISSN 379-864X.

Hummel, T.; Sekinger, B.; Wolf, S.; Pauli, E. & Kobal, G. (1997). 'Sniffin' Sticks': olfactory performance assessed by the combined testing of odor identification, odor discrimination and olfactory threshold. *Chemical Senses,* Vol.22, No.1, pp. 39–52, ISSN 379-864X.

Hummel, T. (2000). Assessment of intranasal trigeminal function. *International Journal of Psychophysiology,* Vol.36, No.2, pp.147–155, ISSN 0167-8760.

Hummel, T. & Livermore, A. (2002). Intranasal chemosensory function of the trigeminal nerve and aspects of its relation to olfaction. *International Archives of Occupational and Environmental Health,* Vol.75, No.5, pp.305-313, ISSN 1432-1246.

Hummel, T.; Futschik, T.; Frasnelli, J. & Hüttenbrink, K.B. (2003). Effects of olfactory function, age, and gender on trigeminally mediated sensations: a study based on the lateralization of chemosensory stimuli. *Toxicology Letters,* Vol.140-141, pp. 273-280, ISSN 378-4274.

Kjaergaard, S.K.; Hempel-Jørgensen, A.; Mølhave, L.; Andersson, K.; Juto, J.E. & Stridh, G. (2004). Eye trigeminal sensitivity, tear film stability and conjunctival epithelium damage in 182 non-allergic, non-smoking Danes. *Indoor Air,* Vol.14, No.3, pp.200-207, ISSN 0905-69-47.

Laska, M.; Distel, H. & Hudson, R. (1997). Trigeminal perception of odorant quality in congenitally anosmic subjects. *Chemical Senses,* Vol.22, No.4, pp. 447-456, ISSN 379-864X.

Laska, M. & Teubner, P. (1999). Olfactory discrimination ability for homologous series of aliphatic alcohols and aldehydes. *Chemical Senses,* Vol.24, No.3, pp. 447-456. ISSN 379-864X.

Laska, M.; Ayabe-Kanamura, S.; Hubener, F. & Saito, S. (2000). Olfactory discrimination ability for aliphatic odorants as a function of oxygen moiety. *Chemical Senses,* Vol. 25, No.2, pp. 189-197. ISSN 379-864X.

Laska, M. & Hubener, F. (2001). Olfactory discrimination ability for homologous series of aliphatic ketones and acetic esters. *Behavioural Brain Research,* Vol.119, No.2, pp. 193-201. ISSN 379-864X.

Lewis, J.L. & Dahl, A.R. (1995). Olfactory mucosa: composition, enzimatic localization, and metabolism. In: *Handbook of olfation and gustation,* Second Edition, R.L. Doty (Ed.), pp. 33, ISBN 978-0-8247-0719-4, Marcel Dekker, Philadelphia, USA.

Liao, M.F.; Liao, M.N.; Lin, S.N.; Chen, J.Y. & Huang, J.L. (2009). Prevalence of allergic diseases of school children in central Taiwan: From ISAAC surveys 5 years apart. *Journal of Asthma,* Vol.46, No.6, pp. 541-545, ISSN 0277-0903.

Lindgren, A.; Stroh, E.; Nihlén, U.; Montnémery, P.; Axmon, A. & Jakobsson, K. (2009). Traffic exposure associated with allergic asthma and allergic rhinitis in adults: A cross-sectional study in southern Sweden. *International Journal of Health Geographics,* Vol.8, pp.25, ISSN 1476-072X.

Lippmann, M. (1989). Effective strategies for population studies of acute air pollution health effects. *Environmental Health Perspectives,* Vol.81, pp. 115-119, ISSN 0091-6765.

Loomis, D.; Castillejos, M.; Gold, D.R.; McDonnell, W. & Borja-Aburto, V.H. (1999). Air pollution and infant mortality in Mexico City. *Epidemiology,* Vol.10, No.2, pp. 118-123, ISSN 1044-3983.

Lötsch, J.; Reichmann, H. & Hummel, T. (2008). Different odor tests contribute differently to the diagnostics of olfactory loss. *Chemical Senses,* Vol.33, No.1, pp. 17-21, ISSN 379-864X.

Menco, B.P. & Morrison, E.E. (2003). Morphology of the mammalian olfactory epithelium: form, fine structure, function and pathology. In: *Handbook of olfation and gustation,* Second Edition, R.L. Doty (Ed.), pp. 17-49, ISBN 978-0-8247-0719-4, Marcel Dekker, Philadelphia, USA.

Meza-Morales, A.; Arreguín-Osuna, L.; Navarrete, F.; Huerta-López, J.G. & Medina, G. (1998). Morphological features of the nasal mucosa in healthy children exposed to different concentrations of atmospheric pollution. *Revista Alergia México,* Vol.45, No.1, pp. 22-26, ISSN 0002-5151.

Miwa, T.; Furukawa, M.; Tsukatani, T.; Costanzo, R.M.; DiNardo, L.J. & Reiter, E.R. (2001). Impact of olfactory impairment on quality of life and disability. *Archives of Otolaryngology - Head and Neck Surgery,* Vol.127, No.5, pp. 497–503, ISSN 0886-4470.

Molina, L.T. & Molina, M.J. (2002). Air quality impacts: local and global concern. In: *Air quality in the Mexico megacity. An integrated assessment,* L.T. Molina & M.J. Molina (Eds.), pp. 1-19, Kluwer Academic Publishers, ISBN 978-1-4020-0452-0, Dordrecht, Netherlands.

Morrison, E.E. & Costanzo, R.M. (1990). Morphology of the human olfactory epithelium. *The Journal of Comparative Neurology*, Vol.297, No.1, pp. 1-13, ISSN 0021-9967.

O'Neill, M.S.; Loomis, D.; Borja-Aburto, V.H.; Gold, D.; Hertz, Piccioto, I. & Castillejos, M. (2004). Do associations between airborn particles and daily mortality in Mexico City differ by measurement method, region, or modeling strategy? *Journal of Exposure Analysis and Environmental Epidemiology*, Vol.14, No.6, pp. 429-439, ISSN 1476-5519.

O'Neill, M.S.; Bell, M.L.; Ranjit, N.; Cifuentes, L.A.; Loomis, D.; Gouveia, N. & Borja-Aburto, V.H. (2008). Air pollution and mortality in Latin America: the role of education. *Epidemiology*, Vol.19, No.6, pp. 810-819, ISSN 1044-3983.

Porter, J.; Craven, B.; Khan, R.; Chang, S-J.; Kang, I.; Judkewitz, B.; Volpe, J.; Settles, G. & Sobel, N. (2007). Mechanisms of scent tracking in humans. *Nature Neuroscience*, Vol.10, No.1, pp. 27–29, ISSN 1097-6256.

Rivas-Arancibia, S.; Dorado-Martínez, C.; Colín-Barenque, L.; Kendrick, K.M.; de la Riva, C. & Guevara-Guzmán, R. (2003). Effect of acute ozone exposure on locomotor behavior and striatal function. *Pharmacology, Biochemistry and Behavior*, Vol.74, No.4, pp. 891-900, ISSN 0091-3057.

Romieu, I.; Meneses, F.; Ruiz, S.; Sierra, J.J.; Huerta, J.; White, M.C. & Etzel, R.A. (1996). Effects of air pollution on the respiratory health of asthmatic children living in Mexico City. *American Journal of Respiratory and Critical Care Medicine*, Vol.154, No.2, pt.1, pp. 300-307, ISSN 1073-449X.

Rosales-Castillo, J.A.; Torres-Meza, V.M.; Olaiz-Fernández, G. & Borja-Aburto, V.H. (2001). Los efectos agudos de la contaminación del aire en la salud de la población: evidencias de estudios epidemiológicos. *Salud Pública de México*, Vol.43, No.6, pp. 544-555, ISSN 0036-3634.

Santos, D.V.; Reiter, E.R.; DiNardo, L.J. & Costanzo, R.M. (2004). Hazardous events associated with impaired olfactory function. *Archives of Otolaryngology Head and Neck Surgery*, Vol.130, No.3, pp. 317–319, ISSN 0886-4470.

Scheibe, M.; Zahnert, T. & Hummel, T. (2006). Topographical differences in the trigeminal sensitivity of the human nasal mucosa. *NeuroReport*, Vol.17, No.1, pp.1417–1420, ISSN 0959-4965.

Schierhorn, K.; Zhang, M.; Matthias, C. & Kunkel, G. (1999). Influences of ozone and nitrogen dioxide on histamine and interleukin formation in a human nasal mucosa culture system. *American Journal of Respiratory Cell and Molecular Biology*, Vol.20, No.5, pp. 1013-1019, ISSN 1044-1549.

Schiffman, S. & Nagle, T. (1992). Effect of environmental pollutants on taste and smell. *Otolaryngology and Head and Neck Surgery*, Vol.106, No.6, pp. 693-700, ISSN 0194-5998.

Secretaría del Medio Ambiente del DF. (2007). La calidad del aire en la Zona Metropolitana del Valle de México 1986-2006. Informe del estado y tendencias de la contaminación atmosférica. Gobierno del Distrito Federal, México DF.

Seiden, A.M. & Duncan, H.J. (2001). The diagnosis of a conductive olfactory loss. *Laryngoscope*, Vol.111, No.1, pp. 9-14, ISSN 1531-4995.

Seo, H-S. & Hummel, T. (2009). Effects of olfactory dysfunction on sensory evaluation and preparation of foods. *Appetite*, Vol.53, No.3, pp. 314–321, ISSN 0195-6663.

Silver, W.L. (1991). Physiological factors in nasal trigeminal chemoreception. In : *Chemical senses, vol. 2, Irritation.* B.G. Green; J.R. Mason & M.R. Kare (Eds.), pp. 21-37, Marcel Dekker. ISBN 0-8247-8323-9, New York.

Smeets, M. & Dalton, P. (2002). Perceived odor and irritation of isopropanol: a comparison between naïve controls and occupationally exposed workers.*International Archives of Occupational and Environmental Health,* Vol.75, No.8, pp.541–548, ISSN 0340-0131.

Smeets, M.; Mauté, C. & Dalton, P. (2002). Acute sensory irritation from exposure to isopropanol (2-propanol) at TLV in workers and controls: objective versus subjective effects. *Annals of Occupational Hygiene,* Vol.46, No.4, pp.359–373, ISSN 0003-4878.

Smith, W.M.; Davidson, T.M. & Murphy, C. (2009). Toxin-induced chemosensory dysfunction: A case series and review. *American Journal of Rhinology and Allergy,* Vol.23, No.6 (Nov-Dec), pp. 578-581, ISSN 1945-8924.

Stevenson, R.J. (2010). An initial evaluation of the function of human olfaction. *Chemical Senses,* Vol. 35, No.1, pp.3–20, ISSN 379-864X.

Stevenson, R.J.; Oaten, M.; Case, T.I.; Repacholi, B.M. & Wagland, P. (2010). Children's response to adult disgust elicitors: development and acquisition. *Developmental Psychology,* Vol.46, No.1, pp.165–177, ISSN 0012-1649.

Tizzano, M.; Gulbransen, B.D.; Vandenbeuch, A.; Clapp, T.R.; Herman, J.P.; Sibhatu, H.M.; Churchill, M.E.; Silver, W.L.; Kinnamon, S.C. & Finger, T.E. (2010). Nasal chemosensory cells use bitter taste signaling to detect irritants and bacterial signals. *Proceedings of the National Academy of Sciences,* Vol.107, No.7, pp.3210-3215. ISSN 027-8424.

Tovalín, H.; Herbarth, O.; Sierra-Vargas, M.; Strandberg, B.; Blanco, S.; Vega, L.; Sioutas, C.; Hicks, J.J.; Marroquín, R.; Acosta, G.; Guarneros, M.; Hernández, V.; Estrada-Muñiz, E.; Olivares, I.; Pérez, D.; Torres-Ramos, Y.; Ulrich, F.; Hudson, R.; Reyes, E.; Rodríguez, T.; Elizondo, G. & Cantellano, E. (2010) Air pollutants exposure and health effects during the MILAGRO-MCMA 2006 Campaign. In: *Air pollution: health and environmental impacts,* B. Gurjar; L.T. Molina & C.S.P. Ojha, (Eds.), pp. 203-227, CRC Press, Taylor & Francis Group, ISBN 978-1-4398-0962-4, Boca Raton, Florida, USA.

Tyler, W.S.; Tyler, N.K.; Last, J.A.; Gillespe, M.J. & Barstow, T.J. (1988). Comparison of daily and seasonal exposures of young monkeys to ozone. *Toxicology,* Vol.50, No.2, pp. 131-144, ISSN 1879-3185.

Upadhyay, U.D. & Holbrook, E.H. (2004). Olfactory loss as a result of a toxic exposure. *Otolaryngologic Clinics of North America,* Vol.37, No.6, pp. 1185-1207, ISSN 0030-6665.

Valverde, M.; López, M.C.; López, I.; Sánchez, I.; Fortoul, T.I.; Ostrosky-Wegman. P. & Rojas, E. (1997). DNA damage in leukocytes and bucal and nasal epithelial cells of individuals exposed to air pollution in Mexico City. *Environmental and Molecular Mutagenesis,* Vol.30, No.2, pp. 147-152, ISSN 0893-6692.

Van Aardt, M.; Duncan, S.E.; Marcy, J.E.; Long, T.E.; O'Keefe, S.F. & Nielsen-Sims, S.R. (2005). Aroma analysis of light-exposed milk stored with and without natural and synthetic antioxidants. *Journal of Dairy Science,* Vol.88, No.3, pp.881-890, ISSN 1525-3198.

Velázquez-Pérez, L.; Fernández-Ruiz, J.; Díaz, R.; González, R.P.; Ochoa, N.C.; Cruz, G.S.; Mederos, L.E.; Góngora, E.M.; Hudson, R. & Drucker-Colín, R. (2006).

Spinocerebellar ataxia type 2 olfactory impairment shows a pattern similar to other major neurodegenerative diseases. *Journal of Neurology*, Vol.253, No.9, pp.1165-1169, ISSN 1432-1459.

Vent, J.; Bartels, S.; Haynatzki, G.; Gentry-Nielsen, M.J.; Leopold, D.A. & Hallworth, R. (2003). The impact of ethanol and tobacco smoke on intranasal epithelium in rat. *American Journal of Rhinology*, Vol.17, No.4, pp. 241-247, ISSN 1050-6586.

Vent, J.; Robinson, A.M.; Gentry-Nielsen, M.J.; Conley, D.B.; Hallworth, R.; Leopold, D.A. & Kern, R.C. (2004). Pathology of the olfactory epithelium: smoking and ethanol exposure. *Laryngoscope*, Vol.114, No.8, pp. 1383–1388, ISSN 0023-852X.

Versura, P.; Profazio, V.; Cellini, M.; Torreggiani, A.; Caramazza, R. (1999). Eye discomfort and air pollution. *Ophthalmologica*, Vol.213, No.2, pp.103-109, ISSN 0030-3755.

Villarreal-Calderon, R.; Torres-Jardon, R.; Palacios-Moreno, J.; Osnaya, N.; Pérez-Guille, B.; Maronpot, R.; Reed, W.; Zhu, H. & Calderón-Garcidueñas, L. (2010). Urban air pollution targets the dorsal vagal complex and dark chocolate offers neuroprotection. *International Journal of Toxicology*, Vol.29, No.6, pp. 604-615, ISSN 1091-5818.

von Skramlik, E. (1925). Über die Lokalisation der Empfindungen bei den niederen Sinnen [On the localization of sensation in the lower senses]. *Zeitschrift für Sinnesphysiologie*, Vol.56, pp.69-140. ISSN 0233-2906.

Walker, J.C.; Kendal-Reed, M; Utell, M.J. & Cain, W.S. (2001). Human breathing and eye blink rate responses to airborne chemicals. *Environmental Health Perspectives*, Vol.109, Suppl.4, pp.507–512, 0091-6765.

Welge-Lüssen, A. (2009). Psychophysical effects of nasal and oral inflammation. *Annals of the New York Academy of Sciences*, Vol.1170, pp.585-589, ISSN 1749-6632.

Wichmann, F.A.; Müller, A.; Busi, L.E.; Cianni, N.; Massolo, L.; Schlink, U.; Porta, A. & Sly, P.D. (2009). Increased asthma and respiratory symptoms in children exposed to petrochemical pollution. *Journal of Allergy and Clinical Immunology*, Vol.123, No.3, pp. 632-638, ISSN 1097-6825.

Wysocki, C.J.; Cowart, B.J. & Radil, T. (2003). Nasal trigeminal chemosensitivity across the adult life span. *Perception and Psychophysics*, Vol.65, No.1, pp.115-122, ISSN 0031-5117.

Zanobetti, A. & Schwartz, J. (2006). Air pollution and emergency admissions in Boston, MA. *Journal of Epidemiology and Community Health*, Vol.60, No.10, pp. 890-895, ISSN 0143-005X.

Zibrowski, E.M. & Robertson, J.M. (2006). Olfactory sensitivity in medical laboratory workers occupationally exposed to organic solvent mixtures. *Occupational Medicine (Lond)*, Vol.56, No.1, pp.51–54, ISSN 0962-7480.

17

Distribution of Indoor Concentrations and Emission Sources of Formaldehyde in Japanese Residences

Naohide Shinohara[1], Atsushi Mizukoshi[2,3], Toshiyuki Kataoka[4], Koichi Takamine[4], Masashi Gamo[1] and Yukio Yanagisawa[2]
[1]*National Institute of Advanced Industrial Science and Technology (AIST)*
[2]*The University of Tokyo*
[3]*The Tokyo Metropolitan Industrial Technology Research Institute*
[4]*The Chemicals Evaluation and Research Institute, Japan (CERI)*
Japan

1. Introduction

Since the 1990s, tight sealing of buildings to save energy and new types of building materials have caused air pollution problems inside many houses in Japan. Many people are suffering from sick building syndrome (SBS), sick house syndrome (SHS), and multiple chemical sensitivity (MCS) in such houses. Formaldehyde has been reported to be one of the chemical substances responsible for causing SBS, SHS, and MCS symptoms, such as eye irritation, respiratory tract irritation, dizziness, fatigue, and neurotoxicity (Kim et al., 2000; Paustenbach et al., 1997; Shinohara et al., 2004). In addition, formaldehyde was reported to be a human carcinogen (IARC 2006).

Formaldehyde has been commonly used in a raw material for synthetic resins such as urea resin, melamine resin, phenolic resin, and synthetic rubber. These resins were used as adhesives in plywood, particle board, and wallpapers in building materials and furniture. The resins react with water to form formaldehyde due to hydrolysis. Formaldehyde has also been used as a bleaching agent and fungicide in wallpaper and curtains. Residual and formed formaldehyde can be emitted from building materials and furniture to the indoor environment of buildings.

Indoor concentrations of formaldehyde are higher in summer than in winter. In Japan, concentration levels were reported to be 39.9 ± 33 μg m^{-3} (Amagai et al., 2000), 34.7 ± 23 μg m^{-3} (Tokyo Metropolitan Government Bureau of Public Health, 2002), and 78.9 ± 22 μg m^{-3} (Shinohara et al., 1999) in summer, while concentrations in winter were 21.7 ± 14 μg m^{-3} (Tokyo Metropolitan Government Bureau of Public Health, 2002), 58.6 ± 20 μg m^{-3} (Shinohara et al., 1999), and 17.6 ± 1.8 μg m^{-3} (Sakai et al., 2004). The formaldehyde concentrations are higher in new houses than those in older houses. The geometric means (GM) of indoor formaldehyde concentrations in new houses were 64.9 μg m^{-3} (Tokyo Metropolitan Institute of Public Health, 2002) and 84.2 μg m^{-3} (Tateno et al., 1999), while those in old houses were 37.7 μg m^{-3} (Tokyo Metropolitan Institute of Public Health, 2002)

and 63.6 μg m^{-3} (Tateno et al., 1999). Most of these data, however, were the results of 30-min average or 24-hour average levels.
Following the increase of SHS, an indoor guideline for 30-min average levels of formaldehyde was published by the Japanese Ministry of Health, Labor and Welfare (MHLW) in 1997 in which the level was set at 100 μg m^{-3} (0.08 ppm) based on the level that has been shown to cause nose and throat irritation in humans (MHLW, 2000). This guideline value is the same as that for chronic exposure published by the World Health Organization (WHO, 1999). In addition, plywood and particleboard in Japan is classified into four categories (F one-star to F four-star) depending on their formaldehyde emission rates, which are measured by using an emission chamber or desiccator methods. In the Japanese Building Codes revised in 2003, the areas in which these materials can be used in house construction are limited by their classification and by the ventilation capacity of the house (MLIT, 2003). The guidelines and law have been successful in reducing the mean indoor concentration of formaldehyde in new houses from 89 μg m^{-3} in 2000 to 32 μg m^{-3} in 2004 (MLIT, 2005).
Since the law applies only to new houses, older houses and furniture are not affected. Hence, when indoor formaldehyde levels are high, the major emission sources have to be identified and removed from older houses. Although it is desirable to remove the major emission sources of formaldehyde, it is difficult to determine which sources significantly affect indoor air quality because there are several possible sources, such as flooring, doors, closets, desks, beds, etc. An emission chamber method (IHCP, 1999; ASTM, 1996; 1997; JISC, 2003; Tichenor, 1989) and a desiccator method (JISC, 2001) have been used to measure the emission rates of chemical compounds from building materials. However, it is impossible or impractical to use these methods on-site in actual rooms because the emission sources to be measured must be placed in a desiccator or a chamber. Recently, field and laboratory emission cells (FLEC) (Risholm-Sundman et al., 1999; Uhde et al., 1998; Wolkoff et al., 1991), a passive flux sampler (PFS) (Fujii et al., 2003; Shinohara et al., 2001; Shinohara et al., 2007; Blondel & Plaisance, 2011), a passive emission colorimetric sensor (PECS) (Shinohara et al., 2008), and an advanced diffusive sampling emission cell (ADSEC) (Akutsu et al., 2000; Aoki et al., 2000) have been proposed and applied to measure the emission rates in the field.
In this study, the 24-h average levels of indoor formaldehyde were measured for 7 days over five seasons in 26 houses to obtain the chronic exposure levels of formaldehyde. In addition, the emission sources identification of formaldehyde in several Japanese houses are reported.

2. Method

2.1 Distribution of indoor formaldehyde concentrations

2.1.1 Survey and analysis

Twenty-four-hour average indoor and outdoor formaldehyde concentrations were measured for 7 days in three rooms of 26 Japanese residences over five seasons: the summer and autumn of 2005, and the winter, spring, and summer of 2006. To include a diverse section of residences, volunteers were solicited on the Internet bulletin boards of some corporations and selected according to family composition, residence architecture, and residence age. Thus, each residence had a different family composition, architecture, and age. The living room, bedroom, and one other room such as a child's room or the dining room/kitchen were selected in each residence for this study.

Formaldehyde was passively sampled for 24 hours with a DNPH (2,4-Dinitrophenylhydrazine)-coated silica gel cartridge (DSD-DNPH; Sigma-Aldrich Japan K.K., Japan) at the center of each room at a height of 1.8 m. Carbonyl compounds, extracted with 5 mL of acetonitrile (Wako Pure Chemical Industries, Ltd., Japan) from the sampling cartridge, were analyzed by HPLC (LC-10A, Shimadzu Co.).

The temperature and humidity were measured in each room and outdoors using a thermohygrometer (HL3631, AS ONE Co.). As part of the survey, the residents were asked in a questionnaire to record the durations for which windows were kept open and ventilation fans were run in each room every day. The air exchange rates were also measured using the perfluorocarbon tracer (PFT) method. The results of the air exchange rates were published previously (Shinohara et al., 2011).

2.1.2 Sampling rates, detection limit, recovery rates, and precision

To obtain the sampling rates of formaldehyde for the DSD-DNPH, the cartridges were left in a chamber, in which the concentrations of formaldehyde were controlled with diffusion tubes, for 24 h (N = 3). The lower limit of detection (LOD) and lower limit of quantitation (LOQ) were defined as 3σ and 10σ of the absolute amount of the analyte (N = 5). To evaluate the recovery efficiencies of absorbed formaldehyde from the DSD-DNPH cartridge, 1.0 μg of formaldehyde was spiked to the adsorbent of the DSD-DNPH in a closed vessel (N = 3) and was allowed to stand for 1 h. Then, the compounds were extracted and analyzed as described above. The obtained sampling rate, LOD and LOQ for 24-h sampling, and the recovery efficiency were 46.4 mL min^{-1}, 0.09 μg m^{-3} and 0.27 μg m^{-3}, and 98.3% ± 0.28%.

2.1.3 Statistics

Statistical analysis was conducted using SPSS 15.0 (SPSS Japan Inc., Japan). Two-way repeated analysis of variance (ANOVA) with a Scheffe test was employed for the statistical comparison of the logarithm of formaldehyde concentrations for different seasons and different residences.

The contribution of factor i (inter-residence variability, seasonal variability, and interaction of seasonal and inter-residence variabilities) to the air exchange rates and the contribution of the daily variability can be expressed with the adjusted variance, V_i and V_{daily}.

$$V_i = \left(SS_i - f_i * SS_{daily}\right) / f_i$$

$$V_{daily} = \left(SST - \sum V_i\right) / f_{daily}$$

where SS_T, SS_i, SS_{daily}, f_i, and f_{daily} are the total sum of squares, sum of squares due to factor i, sum of squares due to the daily variation and other errors, the degree of freedom associated with factor i, and the daily variability, respectively.

In addition, multiple linear regression analysis was conducted to determine the contribution of the architecture of the residence, climate, and human behavior, such as the air exchange rates, building age, construction materials, temperature, and humidity. Because the distribution of the indoor formaldehyde concentration had a log-normal distribution, the dependent variable was the log-transformed data on the daily formaldehyde concentrations in each season and the independent variables were the architecture of the residences (wooden or reinforced) (which was expressed by a dummy variable [1, 0]), air exchange rates, temperature, relative humidity, and other factors associated with the building's age (which was expressed by a dummy variable [1, 0, 0] for age < 1 year, [0, 1, 0] for 1-10 years, and [0, 0, 1] for >10 years). A step-down procedure was conducted under $p < 0.05$ of populated F and $p > 0.10$ of eliminated F.

2.2. Indoor emission sources of formaldehyde

The emission rates of formaldehyde were measured in 8 Japanese houses in 2007 as well as the indoor/outdoor concentrations and the air exchange rates. The 30-min average emission rates of formaldehyde from all emission sources were measured with PECS (Fig. 1; Yanagisawa sensor, Nippon Living Co. Ltd., Japan), developed by Shinohara et al. (2008), in 8 Japanese houses. The indoor formaldehyde was sampled for 30 min using a DNPH cartridge (Supelco Lp DNPH S10, Sigma-Aldrich Co., USA) at 200 mL/min with a pump (Pocket pump, SKC Inc., USA), extracted with acetonitrile (Wako Pure Chemical Industries, Ltd., Japan) and analyzed by HPLC (Agilent1100, Agilent Technologies Co., USA). The air exchange rates were measured by the CO_2 concentration-decay method.
The indoor concentrations of formaldehyde were estimated by the following equation, and the estimated value was compared with the measured one.

$$C_{in\_est} = \frac{\Sigma E_a \times A_a}{N \times V} + C_{out}$$

where C_{in_est} [μg m^{-3}] denotes the estimated indoor formaldehyde concentration; E_a [μg m^{-2} h^{-1}], the emission rate from source a; A_a [m^2], the surface area of source a; N [h^{-1}], the air exchange rate; V [m^3], the room volume; and C_{out} [μg m^{-3}], the outdoor concentration of formaldehyde.

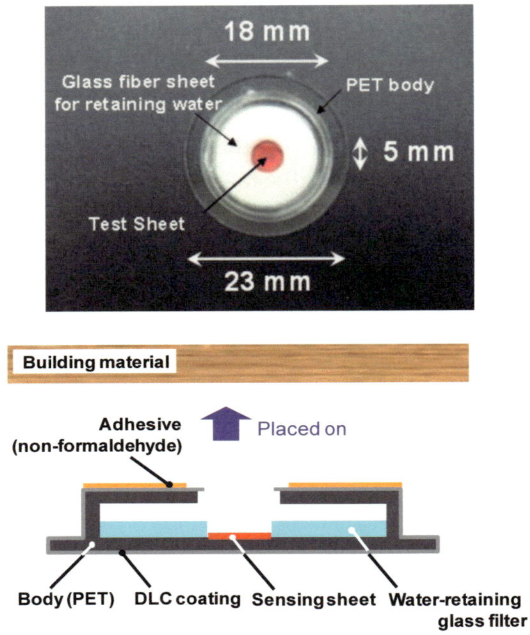

Fig. 1. Picture of PECS (Left) and structure of PECS (Right).

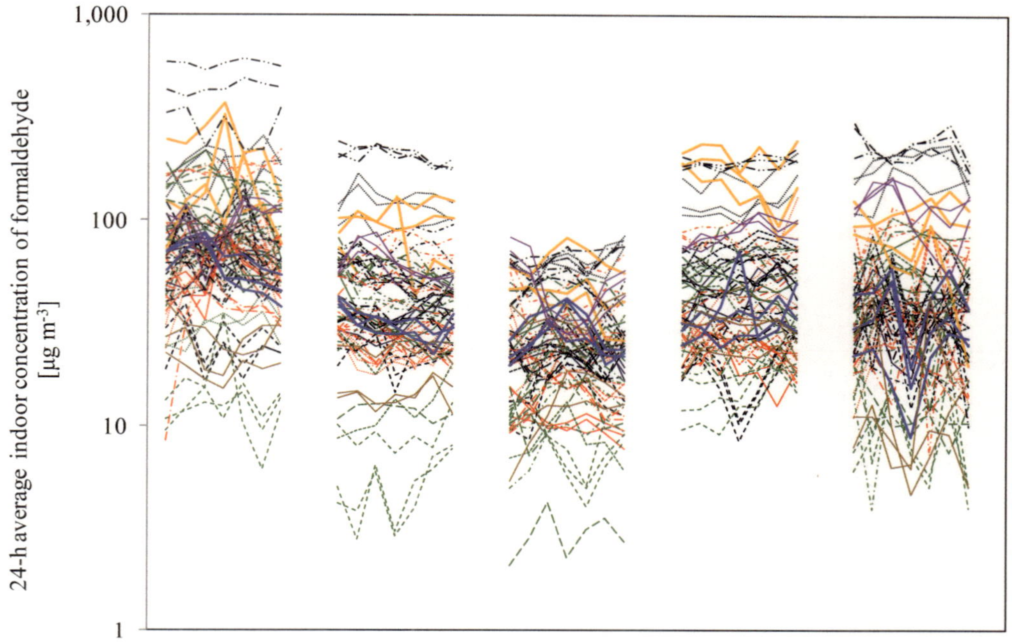

Fig. 2. 24-h average indoor formaldehyde concentrations during the survey. The same line shows data from three rooms of the same residence.

3. Results and discussion

3.1 Distribution of indoor formaldehyde concentrations

3.1.1 Average levels

The geometric mean (GM) of the weekly average indoor formaldehyde levels was 72.8, 38.4, 23.4, 45.4, and 41.1 μg m^{-3} in each of the 5 seasons mentioned in sec. 1.1.1, respectively, and those of the outdoor levels were 6.79, 4.11, 2.49, 4.69, and 3.88 μg m^{-3} (Fig. 2, Table 1). The GM of the yearly average indoor and outdoor formaldehyde concentrations (summer 2005 to spring 2006 and autumn 2005 to summer 2006) was 46.9 and 36.8, and 4.70 and 4.12 μg m^{-3}, respectively.

The percentage of rooms in which the weekly average concentrations were higher than the 30-min average Japanese indoor guideline were 24%, 8.1%, 0%, 12%, and 14% in each season, respectively. The percentage of rooms in which the 24-h average levels were higher than the 30-min average Japanese indoor guideline more than once a week were 43%, 12%, 0%, 19%, and 19% in each season, respectively. Although we did not measure the 30-min average levels of indoor formaldehyde, the 30-min average levels might be higher than the guideline levels in more rooms considering the diurnal variation.

A two-way repeated measures ANOVA revealed that the indoor formaldehyde concentrations differed significantly with respect to seasons, residences, and interaction of seasons and residences ($p < 0.01$). The Scheffe test revealed that the indoor formaldehyde concentrations in both summers and spring were significantly higher than those in winter ($p < 0.05$).

The indoor formaldehyde concentrations in the less than one-year-old residences (yearly average (summer 2005 to spring 2006 and autumn 2005 to summer 2006): 40.7 and 33.6 μg m-3) were lower than those in one-year-old to ten-year-old residences (yearly average: 72.9 and 56.9 μg m-3). The reason for this has been suggested that the revised Building Code in which formaldehyde emission rates and air exchange rates were set in 2003. Those in the more than ten-years-old residences (yearly average: 48.1 and 43.5 μg m-3) were also lower than those in one-year-old to ten-year-old residences. This could be because of the natural decrease of formaldehyde emissions over time.

		Weekly average concentrations					Yearly average concentrations	
		Summer 2005	Autumn 2005	Winter 2006	Spring 2006	Summer 2006	Summer 2005 - Spring 2006	Autumn 2005 - Summer 2006
Indoor	Mean [μg m-3]	94.4	49.4	27.8	58.2	56.7	57.3	46.2
	SD [μg m-3]	88.6	42.3	17.5	48.6	56.0	44.0	37.1
	GM [μg m-3]	72.8	38.4	23.4	45.4	41.1	46.9	36.8
	GSD [-]	2.0	2.0	1.9	2.0	2.2	1.9	1.9
Outdoor	Mean [μg m-3]	7.46	4.68	2.82	4.80	5.05	4.92	4.29
	SD [μg m-3]	3.36	2.38	1.53	1.05	3.70	1.51	1.20
	GM [μg m-3]	6.79	4.11	2.49	4.69	3.88	4.70	4.12
	GSD [-]	1.6	1.7	1.6	1.2	2.3	1.4	1.4

Table 1. Weekly average and yearly average indoor formaldehyde concentrations. (Mean: Arithmetic mean, SD: Standard deviation, GM: Geometric Mean, GSD: Geometric standard deviation)

3.1.2 Variability of the indoor concentrations

The percentage contribution of inter-residence variability, seasonal variability, interaction of seasonal and inter-residence variabilities, and the daily variability to the total variability of the 24-h average air exchange rates in the present survey were 35%, 63%, 1.2%, and 0.12%, respectively. The daily variability was much lower than the other variabilities, inter-residence variability and seasonal variability. Therefore, it is considered that the yearly average levels of formaldehyde could be obtained by a 24-h measurement once every season.

3.1.3 Multiple linear regression analysis

The results of the multiple linear regression analysis (standardized regression coefficients β, and the probability p) are presented in Table 2. The indoor concentration of formaldehyde was strongly associated with temperature. This is because the activity of the hydrolysis reaction increases with temperature and water content, and the vapor pressure increases with temperature. However, the relative humidity was statistically eliminated in this analysis. This might be due to the colinearity. Therefore, the strong association between the temperature and the indoor formaldehyde concentrations can be considered to include the association between the humidity and indoor formaldehyde concentrations. The indoor concentration of formaldehyde was strongly and negatively associated with the air exchange rates. The air exchange can decrease the indoor formaldehyde levels because the outdoor levels were much lower than the indoor levels. In addition, the indoor concentration was negatively associated with wooden buildings and building age (< 1 or > 10 years old). The reasons for this were described above – the Building Code revised in 2003 and the natural decrease of emissions.

	Standardized regression coefficients β	Probability p
Ventilation rate	-0.385	<0.01
Temperature	0.523	<0.01
Wood house	-0.151	<0.01
Building age <1	-0.063	<0.05
Building age >10	-0.130	<0.01

Table 2. Results of multiple linear regression analysis.

3.2 Indoor emission sources of formaldehyde

Fabric furniture and covers, such as curtains, sheets and carpets, were the major source of formaldehyde in many houses. Although formaldehyde is used for permanent-press treatment or bleaching of clothes, the emission/use for clothes is not regulated. On the other hand, the emissions from interior building materials, such as flooring, walls, and ceilings were low. The low emission from the building materials could be because the newly built houses were regulated by the building code.

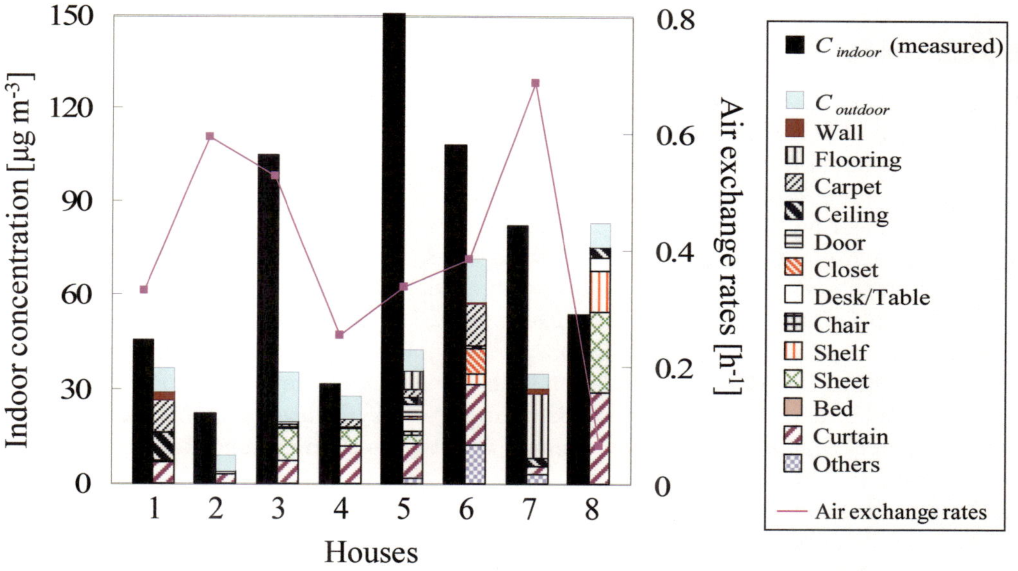

Fig. 3. Measured and calculated indoor concentrations of formaldehyde and the air exchange rates in 8 houses. House 1 and 2 are wooden houses, House 3, 4 and 5 are light-gauge steel houses, while Houses 6, 7 and 8 are reinforced concrete buildings.

In some houses (House 2, 3, 5, and 7), the measured indoor concentrations were significantly different from the calculated concentrations using the emission rates and the air exchange rates. This suggested that there were other emission sources of formaldehyde. Therefore, additional measurements of formaldehyde concentrations were carried out in closets and formaldehyde emission rates were measured around joint gaps on the ceiling and electric outlets on the wall. In the results, the in-closet concentrations were high in House 3 and 7 (> 150 μg m^{-3}). In house 2 and 5, the emission rates were high at the joint gaps. These results suggest that the spaces inside the closet, inside the wall, or under the roof were highly polluted because there are no strict regulations for these materials and spaces, and from there the polluted air could be introduced into the indoor living environment.

4. Conclusions

Formaldehyde has been often used in indoor environments in Japan. The weekly average indoor formaldehyde levels (GM) were 72.8, 38.4, 23.4, 45.4, and 41.1 μg m^{-3} in the summer 2005, autumn 2005, winter 2006, spring 2006, and summer 2006, respectively, and those of the outdoor levels were 6.79, 4.11, 2.49, 4.69, and 3.88 μg m^{-3}, respectively. The indoor formaldehyde concentrations in both summers and in spring were significantly higher than those in winter. The indoor concentration of formaldehyde was strongly associated with temperature, and negatively associated with the air exchange rates, building structure (wooden), and building age (< 1 and > 10 years old). High emission rates of formaldehyde were observed from the cloth furniture and fixtures, such as curtains, sheets and carpets, while low emission rates were observed from building materials. The effect of the intake of formaldehyde from inside closets, inside walls, and under roofs on the indoor formaldehyde levels cannot be ignored.

5. References

Akutsu, T., Aoki, R., Kumagai, K. & Tanabe, S. (2000). Development of Measurement Device (ADSEC) for Aldehydes Emission Rate Using a Diffusive Sampler: Part 2 Examination of the Size of ADSEC and Comparison with FLEC, *Summaries of technical papers of Annual Meeting Architectural Institute of Japan*. D-2, Environmental engineering II, pp. 721-722. (Japanese).

Amagai, T., Ohura, T., Sugiyama, T., Fusaya, M. & Matsumura, H. (2000). A Survey of Indoor and Outdoor Air Pollution by Aldehydes in Summer in Fuji, Shizuoka, *Journal of Society of Indoor Environment, Japan*. 3(1): 35-43. (Japanese)

Aoki, R., Akutsu, T., Kumagai, K. & Tanabe, S. (2000). Development of Measurement Device (ADSEC) for Aldehydes Emission Rate Using a Diffusive Sampler: Part1 Scheme of ADSEC and Examination of Sampling Period, *Summaries of technical papers of Annual Meeting Architectural Institute of Japan*. D-2, Environmental Engineering II, pp. 719-720. (Japanese)

ASTM (American Society for Testing and Materials). (1996). E1333-96, Standard Test Method for Determining Formaldehyde Concentrations in Air and Emission Rates from Wood Products Using a Large Chamber.

ASTM (American Society for testing and materials). (1997). D5116-97, Standard Guide for Small-Scale Environmental Chamber Determinations of Organic Emissions from Indoor Materials/Products.

Blondel, A. & Plaisance, H. (2011). Screening of formaldehyde indoor sources and quantification of their emission using a passive sampler. *Building and Environment* 46: 1284-1291.

Fujii, M., Shinohara, N., Lim, A., Otake, T., Kumagai, K. & Yanagisawa, Y. (2003). A study on emission of phthalate esters from plastic materials using a passive flux sampler. *Atmospheric Environment* 37: 5495-5504.

IHCP (Institute for Health and Consumer Protection). (1999). ENV717-1, WOOD-BASED PANELS. Determination of Formaldehyde Release, Formaldehyde emission by the chamber method.

IARC (International Agency for Research on Cancer). (2006). IARC Monographs on the Evaluation of Carcinogenic Risks to Humans Volume 88: Formaldehyde, 2-Butoxyethanol and 1-tert-Butoxypropan-2-ol. Retrieved October 5, 2010.

URL: http://monographs.iarc.fr/ENG/Monographs/vol88/index.php.

JISC (Japanese Industrial Standards Committee). (2001). JIS A1460, Building boards -- Determination of formaldehyde emission - Desiccator method, Tokyo.

JISC (Japanese Industrial Standards Committee). (2003). JIS A1901, Small chamber method - Determination of the emission of volatile organic compounds and aldehydes for building products. Tokyo.

Kim, W.J., Terada, N., Nomura, T., Takahashi, R.., Lee, S.D., Park, J.H. & Konno, A. (2000). Effect of formaldehyde on the expression of adhesion molecules in nasal microvascular endothelial cells: the role of formaldehyde in the pathogenesis of sick building syndrome. *Clin. Exp. Allergy* 32: 287-295.

MHLW (Ministry of Health, Labour and Welfare, Japan). Interim report of Panel on sick house (indoor air pollution) problem, Environmental Health Bureau, Planning Division: Tokyo, 2000.

MLIT (Ministry of Land, Infrastructure and Transport), Japan. Notice No. 1113 of the Ministry of Land, Infrastructure and Transport, Japan, Tokyo, 2003.

MLIT (Ministry of Land, Infrastructure and Transport). Results of a field survey to measure the concentration of chemicals in indoor environments in 2004 (Advance report), Tokyo, 2005.

Paustenbach, D., Alarie, Y., Kulle, T., Schachter, N., Smith, R., Swenberg, J., Witschi, H. & Horowitz, S.B. (1997). A recommended occupational exposure limit for formaldehyde based on irritation. *J. Toxicol. Env. Health* 50: 217-263.

Risholm-Sundman, M. & Wallin, N. (1999). Comparison of different laboratory methods for determining the formaldehyde emission from three-layer parquet floors. *Holz Als Roh-und Werkstoff* 57: 319-324.

Sakai, K., Norback, D., Mi, Y.H., Shibata, E., Kamijima, M., Yamada, T. & Takeuchi, Y. (2004). A comparison of indoor air pollutants in Japan and Sweden: formaldehyde, nitrogen dioxide, and chlorinated volatile organic compounds. *Environmental Research* 94(1): 75-85.

Shinohara, N., Yanagisawa, Y., Nakai, S., Takagi, Y, Nishioka, Y. ､ Vallarino, J., Spengler, J., Kawai, R., Maeda, M. & Ikeda, K. (1999). Measurement of indoor air in Hokkaido：multi-year aldehyde study, *Journal of Society of Indoor Environment, Japan* 2(1): 84-85. (Japanese).

Shinohara, N., Fujii, M. & Yanagisawa, Y. (2001). Development of passive type simple DNPH sampler. *the Annual meeting of the Society of Indoor Environment, Japan.* (Tokyo), pp. 136-139. (Japanese).

Shinohara, N., Mizukoshi, A. & Yanagisawa, Y. (2004). Identification of responsible volatile chemicals that induce hypersensitive reactions to multiple chemical sensitivity patients. *Journal of Exposure Analysis and Environmental Epidemiology* 14: 84-91.

Shinohara, N., Fujii, M., Yamasaki, A. & Yanagisawa, Y. (2007). Passive Flux Sampler for Measurement of Formaldehyde Emission Rates. *Atmospheric Environment* 41: 4018-4028.

Shinohara N., Kajiwara T., Ohnishi M., Kodama K. & Yanagisawa Y. (2008). Passive Emission Colorimetric Sensor (PECS) for Measuring Emission Rates of Formaldehyde based on an Enzymatic Reaction and Reflectance Photometry. *Environmental Science and Technology* 42(12): 4472-4477.

Shinohara, N., Kataoka, T., Takamine K., Gamo, M. (2011). Distribution and variability of the 24-h average air exchange rates and interzonal flow rates in 26 Japanese residences over 5 seasons. *Atmospheric Environment* 45(21): 3548-3552.

Tateno H., Ebana,T, Yamamoto M., Urashima Y., Kozuka S., Mukaihara N. & Fujita K. (1999). Concentration of Aldehydes and Ketones In Room Air at Sapporo City (part 1), *Annual report of Sapporo City Institute of Public Health*, 26: 54-58.

Tichenor, B.A. (1989). Indoor Air Sources: Using Small Environmental Test Chambers to Characterize Organic Emissions from Indoor Materials and Products, EPA-600 8-89-074.

Tokyo Metropolitan Government Bureau of Public Health (2002). Results of survey of indoor volatile organic compounds in 2001.

Tokyo Metropolitan Institute of Public Health (2002). Situation of Indoor air pollution due to chemical substances - Formaldehyde and volatile organic compounds.

Uhde, E., Borgschulte, A. & Salthammer, T. (1998). Characterization of the field and laboratory emission cell -- flec: flow field and air velocities. *Atmospheric Environment* 32: 773-781.

WHO (World Health Organization). (1999). Air Quality Guidelines for Europe, WHO Regional Publications European Series, Regional Office for Europe, Copenhagen.

Wolkoff, P., Clausen, P.A., Nielsen, P.A., Gustafsson, H., Jonsson, B. & Rasmusen, E. (1991). Field and Laboratory Emission Cell: FLEC. *Healthy buildings '91, ASHRAE*, 160-165.

18

Comparison of Indoor and Outdoor Bioaerosols in Poultry Farming

Elżbieta Lonc and Kinga Plewa
Department of Microbial Ecology and Environmental Protection, Institute of Genetics and Microbiology, Wrocław University, Poland

1. Introduction

Intensive poultry production, implying large densities of animals in small areas, is a significant source of air pollution which may constitute a considerable health hazard to the birds, farmers and those living in the proximity of the farm (Lonc & Plewa, 2009). On the other hand, the spread of bioaerosols on the outside of animal housing may result in local or even more extensive environmental pollution (Bakutis et al., 2004).

Under commercial production the airborne particles will contain a mixture of biological material from a range of sources. The chickens produce large amounts of dust as a result of epithelial desquamation, as well as from feed, manure, faeces and litter (Matković et al., 2009). This dust consists of a variety of airborne particles of biological origin, i.e. bacteria, fungi, endotoxins (lipopolysaccharide, LPS) of Gram-negative bacteria, 1.3-beta-glucan of fungi, fungal spores and mycelium fragments. Hence, a more descriptive term for these airborne particles is bioaerosol in which the microorganisms can occur either as liquid droplets or as dry particles [Dutkiewicz, 1987; Matković et al., 2009; Nevalainen, 2007]. In specific conditions, bioaerosols may show pathogenic, toxic or allergy-causing effects. The particles in a bioaerosol are generally 0.3 to 100 μm in diameter; however, the respirable size fraction of 1 to 10 μm is of primary concern. Bioaerosols, ranging in size from 1.0 to 5.0 μm, generally remain in the air, whereas larger particles are deposited on surfaces (Srikanth et al., 2008).

Bioaerosol may contain representatives of Gram-positive bacteria: *Corynebacterium, Staphyloccocus, Streptococcus, Micrococcus, Pantoea* and *Sarcina* (Siemiński, 2001). Their presence in large numbers may present a significant immunological challenge to the human respiratory system. In dust are suspended also endotoxins (lipopolysaccharide complex - LPS) associated with the outer membrane of Gram-negative pathogens, such as *Escherichia coli, Salmonella, Shigella, Pseudomonas, Neisseria* and *Haemophilus influenzae.* LPS is composed of two major parts, the hydrophobic lipid A and the hydrophilic polysaccharide part (commonly called the "O" region). Most biological effects of LPS are due to the lipid A part, however O-region plays an important role in effective colonisation of host tissues. Inhalation of organic dust contaminated by endotoxins may cause chronic bronchitis and inflammatory reaction in the lungs (Bakutis et al., 2004, Schierl et al., 2007, Pomorska et al., 2009).

As with bacteria, the fungi present in the poultry dust bioaerosols may be derived from soil, dust feed and litter, but to a lesser extent from the birds themselves. Fungi are ubiquitous in all atmospheres. In general, both outdoor and indoor atmospheres are dominated by representatives of the genera *Cladosporium, Penicillium, Aspergillus, Alternaria* and by yeasts and Mycelia sterilia.*Cladosporium* is nearly always the dominant fungus in outdoor as well as indoor atmospheres. The abundance of the other fungi varies with the season and place. In relation to outdoor environments, indoor atmospheres typically display lower diversity (Araujo & Cabral, 2010). Long-term or repeated exposure to high concentrations of airborne fungal spores is recognised as contributing to the decline in lung function and allergic diseases such as asthma and allergic alveolitis known as farmer's lung disease (Crook et al., 2008).

Literature data usually pertain to the air biopollutant concentration inside the poultry houses. Much less is known about the relationships between the indoor and outdoor biological pollution, as well as about the spreading of indoor bioaerosols in the surroundings of the farms.

The aim of the study was to assess the influence of microbiological air contamination in the intensive poultry breeding, both inside and outside farms. The comparative quantity and quality analysis concerns bacteria as well as fungi isolated from the air samples taken during two seasons.

2. Materials and methods

Seasonal sampling was conducted in the summer of 2009 and spring of 2010 in two (I and II) poultry houses on family farms located near Wrocław in Lower Silesia, Poland (Fig. 1.)

Both farms were accommodated to 18 000 and 23 000 broilers, with the density of 16-17 chicken per square meter. The broilers were kept on the rye straw deep litter in buildings equipped with mechanical ventilation (inlet and outlet ventilators), heating with a central thermogen and artificial lighting with regularly distributed bulbs.

Air samples were taken using a MAS-100 air sampler (Merck KgaA, Darmstadt, Germany) which is representative of the new generation impactor samplers and is frequently used for indoor and outdoor sampling. These instruments are based on the principles described by Andersen and aspirate air through a perforated plate, which results in impaction of particles from an airstream onto the surface of agar medium. The speed of air flow through the sampler was about 11 m/s, air volumes were 5-200 litres (depending on the expected contamination level) and the sampling rate was 100 l/min. Indoor and outdoor samples were collected in the poultry biozone during the fattening period. The biopollutants were determined on the basis of airborne bacteria and fungi. The samples for each group of bacteria and fungi were taken at the central point of poultry houses 1.3 m from the ground level. The emission level outside the farming objects was determined similarly, i.e. 1.3 m with sampling points situated 10 m, 50 m and 100 m away from the farming buildings. At the same time both humidity and temperature were measured with a termohigrometer (Label).

Microbiological studies of the air samples were used to determine the number of mesophilic bacteria, *Enterobacteriaceae* representatives, mannitol+ staphylococci, *Salmonella sp.* and mould fungi. The mesophilic bacteria were isolated with the use of TSA agar (BioMérieux). *Enterobacteriaceae* families were determined with the use of VRB medium (BioMérieux). The estimation of *Salmonella sp.* was done on SS agar (BioMérieux). Mannitol salt agar

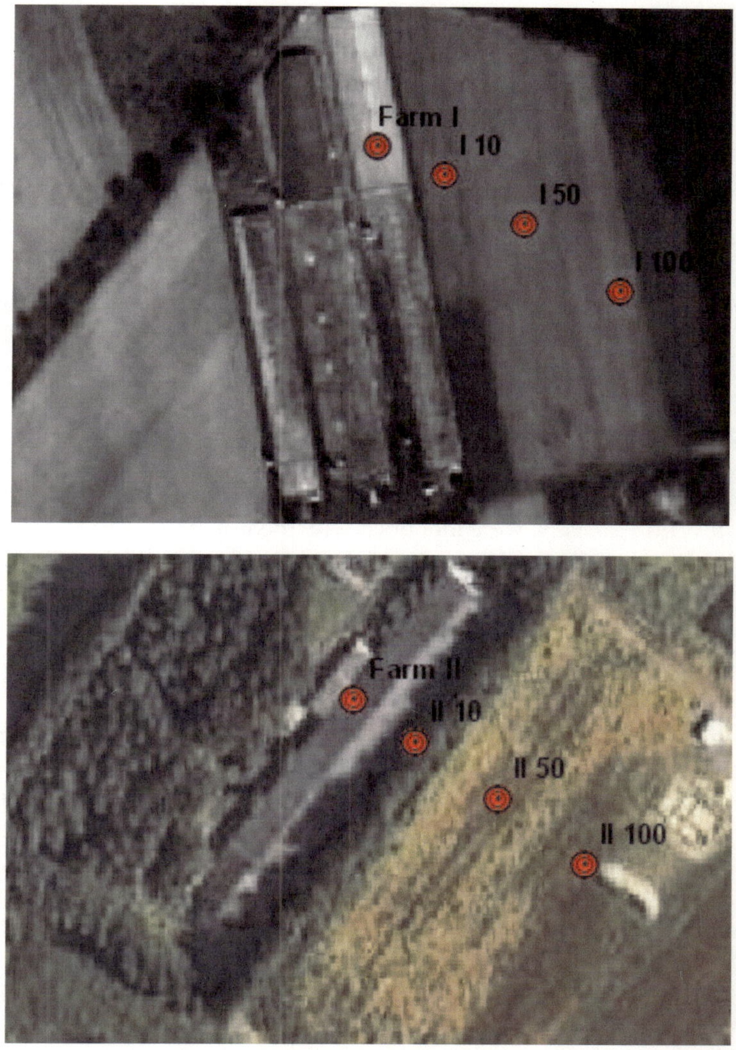

Fig. 1. Poultry houses I and II; the sampling sites outside the poultry house at the distance of 10 m, 50 m and 100 m from the farming object respectively, as well as at the center of building.

(BioMérieux) plates were inoculated for culturing and counting *staphylococci*. Mould fungi were determined with the use of Sabouraud (Merck) medium. Colonies were counted after 48 h of incubation at 37^0C for bacteria and after 5 days at 26^0C for moulds and subsequently the colony-forming units (CFU) were determined. Quantitative results were expressed in CFU/m3, i.e. colony forming units in 1 m^3 of the examined air and the total microbial count was corrected using the conversion formula devised by Feller:

$$Pr = N [1/N + 1/N-1 + 1/N-2+....+1/N-r+1]$$

where:

N = 400 (number of holes in perforated lid of the sampler)
r - number of CFU counted on Petri dish
Pr - statistically corrected total count of bacteria/moulds in tested air volume
Bacterial species were identified on the basis of gram staining, microscopic morphology, oxidase and coagulase activity, catalase test results and metabolic properties according to standard procedures described in Bergey's Manual of Determinative Bacteriology (2001). The following commercial systems were used: API 20E (BioMérieux, France) for enteric gram-negative organisms; API 20 NE (BioMérieux) for fastidious and nonfermenting gram-negative organisms; API Staph (BioMérieux) for gram-positive staphylococci, API 20C AUX (BioMérieux) for identification of yeasts, Slidex - Strepto Kit (BioMérieux) for the identification of Lancefield A,B,C,D,F et G group antigens of streptococci and Slidex Staph Plus (BioMérieux) to detect clumping factor, protein A and group-specific antigen bound to the *S. aureus*. Moulds colonies were identified on the basis of colour, texture, topography of the culture surface, smell of the colony, colour of the reverse of the colony and the presence of the diffuse pigment. Microscopic features of the fungal colonies, i.e. the presence of macroconidia and microconidia, their shape and appearance were identified later. Fungal species of the genera *Aspergillus* and *Penicilium* were identified with the use of the keys by Raper and Fennell as well as Raper et. al., while the *Fusarium* species were identified using the key by Kwaśna (1991). Other species were identified based on the "Atlas of Clinical Fungi"(2010).

3. Results. Quantitative and qualitative relationships between indoor and outdoor microflora examined in summer and spring

The studies were carried out in the summer of 2009 and in the spring of 2010, when the temperature of atmospheric air ranged between 15.2^{0}C and + 24.5^{0}C; the inside temperature in the poultry houses varied from 22^{0}C to 27^{0}C. Indoor relative air humidity was about 70-85 %, outdoor ca. 38-82%.

For both poultry houses, the indoor concentration of bacteria and moulds were always higher compared with the outdoor concentration at distance 10 m, 50 m and 100 m from the poultry houses. The number of microorganisms (as CFU/m^3) in the atmospheric air of both poultry houses ranged between 4 x 10^1– 7.2 x 10^3 for mesophilic bacteria, 0– 1.3 x 10^4 for staphylococci, 0 - 7 x 10^1 for coli group bacteria, and 2 x 10^1 - 1.3 x 10^4 for fungi (Fig. 2-5). *Salmonella sp.* were not found. On the other hand, the number of microorganisms inside both poultry houses was higher than in the surrounding area and ranged between 1.3 x 10^5– 5.2 x 10^5 for mesophilic bacteria, 1.4 x 10^5 - 2.6 x 10^5 for staphylococci, 2.0 x 10^2- 1.5 x 10^4 for coli group bacteria and 3.6 x 10^4 - 1,1 x 10^5 for fungi. *Salmonella sp.* similar like outdoor were not found.

Outside poultry house I mesophilic bacteria were the most numerous organisms in the spring and summer and formed about 55% of the local microbial community. Less numerous staphylococci and moulds constituted about 17% and 27.5%, respectively. The concentration of *Enterobacteriaceae* was fractional (0.5%). In contrast, outside poultry house II the most numerous group of bacteria were staphylococci (62%). Mesophilic bacteria and moulds constituted about 25% and 13% of the microbial community. However, air inside both poultry houses was characterized by a relatively small number of *Enterobacteriaceae*. On the other hand, mesophilic bacteria were dominant and formed about 44% (poultry house I) and 56.5% (poultry house II) of the local microbial community, whereas staphylococci constituted 40% and 27% and moulds 16% and 7% for poultry house I and II. *Salmonella sp.* was not detected in neither poultry houses.

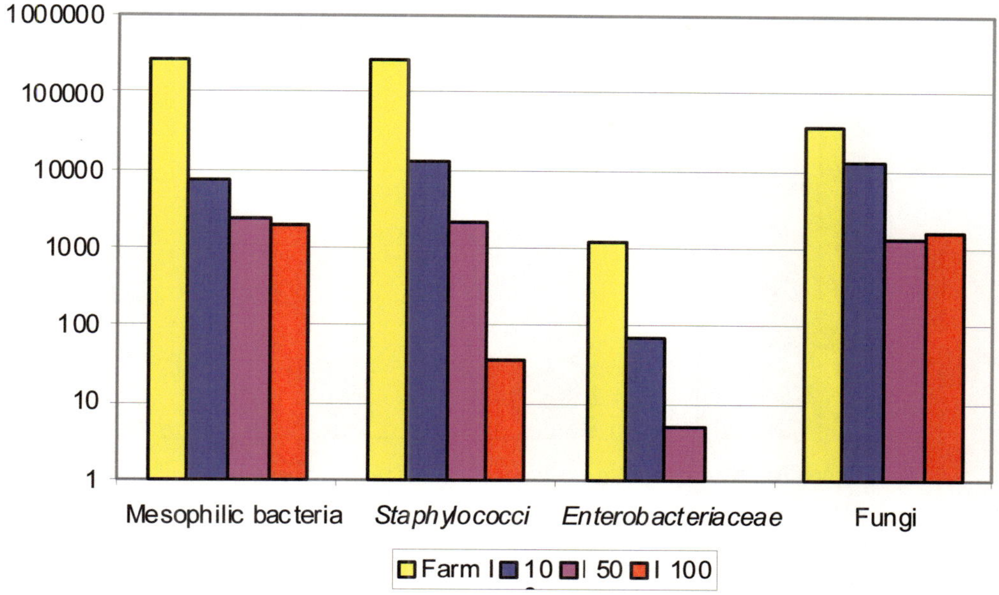

Fig. 2. Number of microorganisms in the poultry house I in summer.

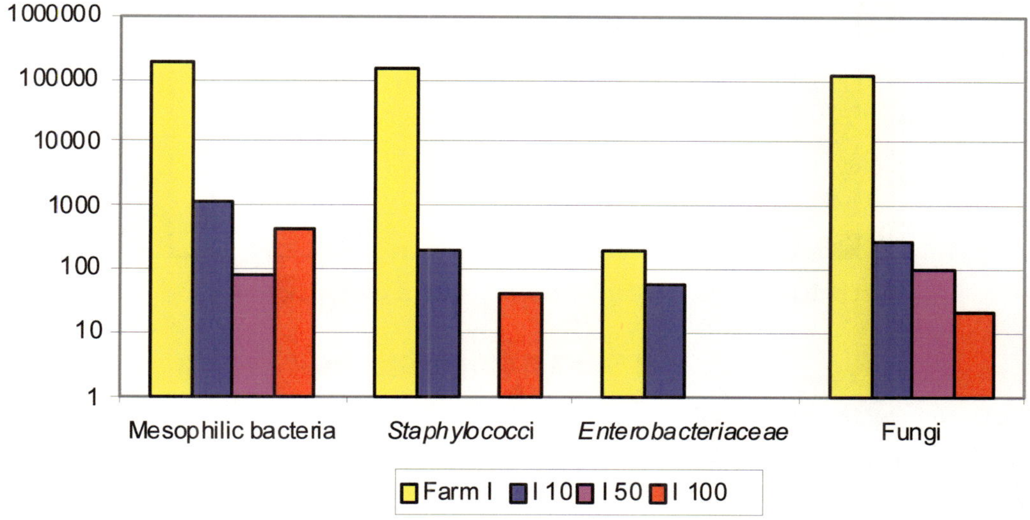

Fig. 3. Number of microorganisms in the poultry house I in spring.

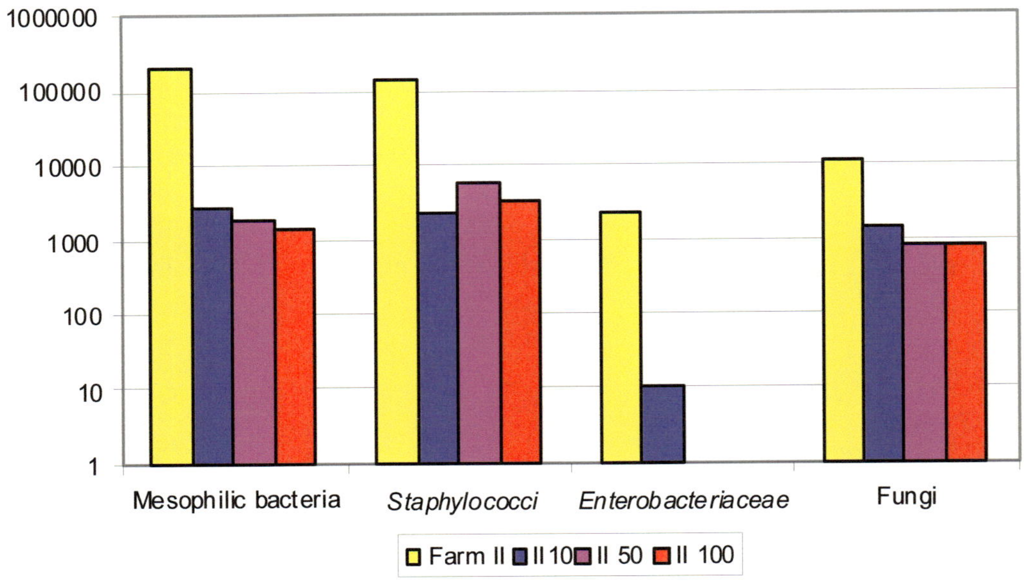

Fig. 4. Number of microorganisms in the poultry house II in summer.

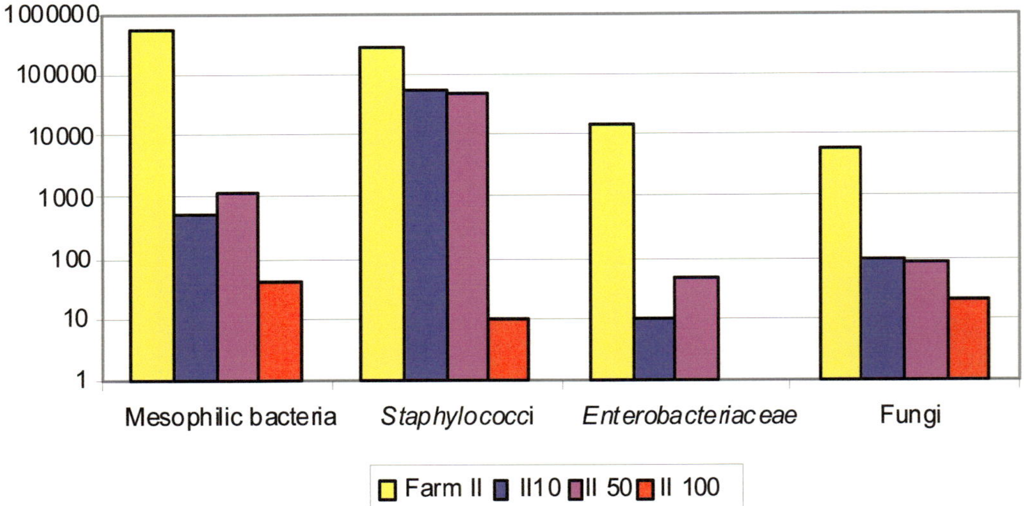

Fig. 5. Number of microorganisms in the poultry house II in spring.

The level of outdoor air contamination was evaluated in the accordance with the Polish Norm (Table 1). Contaminations by mesophilic bacteria and moulds in areas surrounding poultry house I in the summer was the highest in sampling point I 10. In relation to the Polish Norms this site was heavily polluted. On the other hand, the number of staphylococci at all sampling sites in both poultry houses (except sampling points I 50 and II 100 in the spring) indicated a high contamination. In contrast, the air in the surrounding areas could be classified as medium-contaminated at all sites around the poultry houses II in the summer and in sampling point II 50 in the spring, with mesophilic bacteria. The evaluation based on the Polish Norm revealed that none of the researched measuring sites around the poultry house II was significantly contaminated by fungal microflora.

Polish Norm	Mesophilic bacteria	*Staphylococi*	Fungi
not pollution *	< $1x10^3$	0	$3x10^3$-$5x10^3$
medium pollution **	$1x10^3$- $3x10^3$	<25	$5x10^3$-$1x10^4$
heavily pollution ***	>$3x10^3$	>25	> $1x10^4$

Table 1. Polish Norm PN-89/Z-04111/02 and PN-89/Z-04111/03 (http://www.pkn.pl).

Fifteen species of bacteria detected in the indoor air represented 10 genera *Staphylococcus (S. aureus, S. xylosus, S. saprophitycus), Micrococcus (M. sedentarius, M. luteus), Enterococcus, Streptococcus (S. mitis), Corynebacterium (C. xerosis), Pseudomonas (P. aeruginosa, P. fluorescens), Citrobacter (C. farmerii), Escherichia (E. coli), Enterobacter (E. sakazakii, E. agglomerans)* and *Proteus (P. mirabilis)* – Table. 2. Quality outdoor set consisted of 19 species representing 10 bacteria genera: *Staphylococcus (S. sciuri, S. epidermidis, S. cohnii subsp., S. lentus,S. xylosus), Micrococcus (M. lylae, M. halobius, M. luteus), Streptococcus (S. mitis), Bacillus (B. mycoides, Bacillus sp.), Pseudomonas (P. aeruginosa, P. chlororaphis), Xantomonas (X. maltophila), Shigella (S. boydii), Providencia sp., Citrobacter (C. farmeri), Enterobacter (E. agglomerans)* and *Proteus (P. mirabilis)*. For the most part, the identified bacterial species were nonpathogenic or potentially pathogenic species, with the exception of *P. aeruginosa, S. aureus, Shigella sp., E. coli, P. mirabilis* which are regarded as primarily pathogenic.

In this work we detected 30 species (16 in poultry houses and 23 in surrounding areas) representing 16 fungal genera: *Aspergillus (A. flavus* – Fig. 6*), A. niger, A terreus, A. nidulans, A. parasiticus, A. glaucus, A. clavatus* - Fig. 7*), Penicillium* – Fig. 10 *(P. chrysogenum, P. solitum, P. sticticus), Cladosporium (C. cladosporoides* – Fig. 8*), Alternaria (A. alternata* – Fig. 9*, A. tennuissima), Scopulariopsis (S. brevicaulis, S. acremonium), Fusarium* – Fig. 11 *(F. oxysporum, F. graminearum), Mucor (M. mucedo) Drechslera (D. graminae, Drechslera sp.), Verticillium sp.*, Mycelia sterilia, *Ulocladium sp., Trichoderma (T. viridae), Scedosporium sp., Candida (C. albicans, C. inconspicua, C. lambica), Rhodotorula (R. rubrum), Cryptococcus (C. laurentii)* – Table 3. The majority of these species are known as the potential respiratory allergens. The most common airborne moulds, both indoors and outdoors, were *Penicilium sp., Aspergillus sp., Cladosporium sp., Alternaria sp.,* and *Fusarium sp.* The yeast were sometimes the dominant fungus in the indoor air comparison with the outdoor air, where this group of fungi occur very sporadically.

Among fungi identified from the farm I, there distinctly dominated the species belonged to genera *Candida spp.* which constituted on average, over 69% in summer and 82.5% in spring. In comparison with the predominated yeast inside poultry houses I, in outdoor air the most frequent species were moulds *A. flavus* (80% in sampling point I 50.36% in I 10 and 52.5% in I 100) and *F. oxysporum* (26.9%, 13.5%, 16.2% in sampling point I 10, I 50, I 100, respectively). On the other hand, in the air surroundings poultry house II dominated species were *A. clavatus* (about 16%) and *A. alternata* (38.4%) in spring and *C. cladosporoides* (in summer) which constituted 68.5%. Whereas, *A. clavatus* (54.5%) and *A. flavus* (27.3%) were dominated species inside poultry house II.

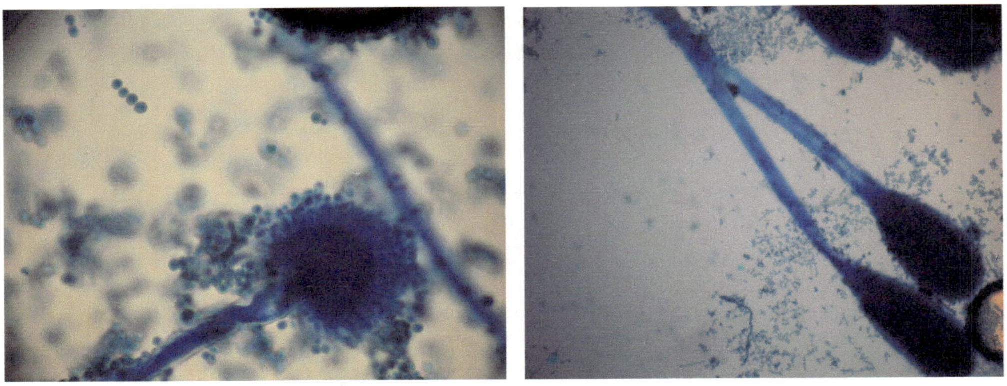

Fig. 6, 7. Conidiophores of *A. flavus* and *A. clavatus*, oryg.

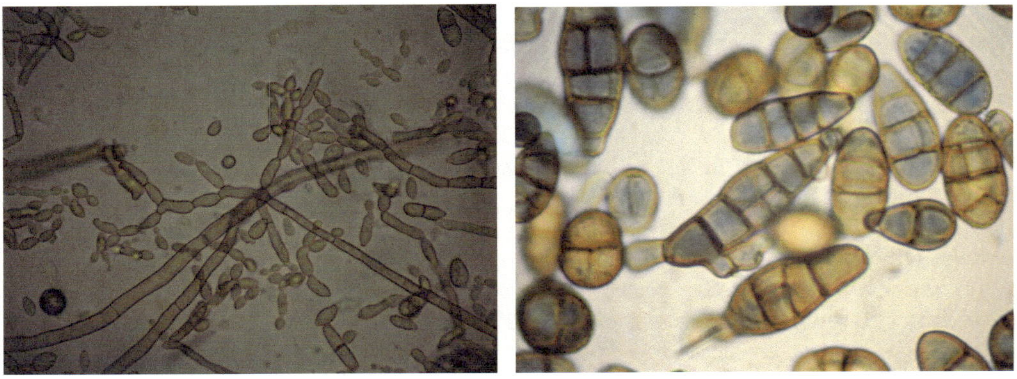

Fig. 8, 9. Conidiophores of *C. cladosporoides* and poroconidia of *A. alternata*, oryg.

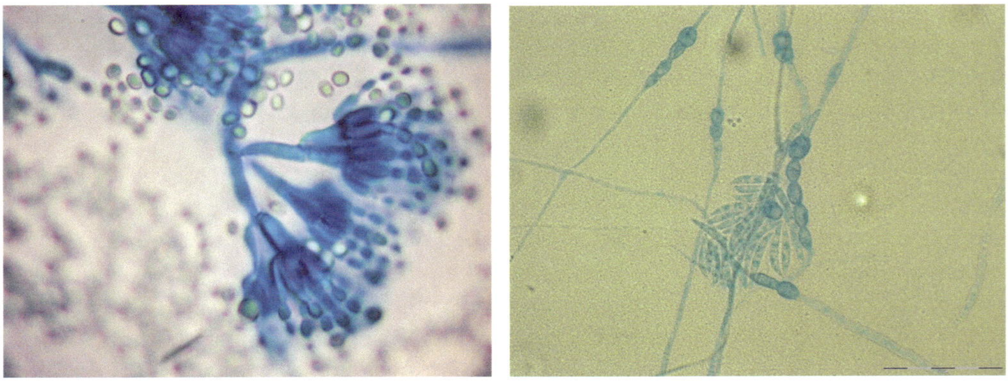

Fig. 10, 11. Conidiophores of *Penicilium sp.* and macroconidia of *Fusarium sp.*, oryg.

Genus	Species	Sampling site							
		Farm I	I 10	I 50	I 100	**Farm II**	II 10	II 50	II 100
Staphylococcus	*sciuri*		+				+		
	aureus					+	+	+	+
	epidermidis							+	
	cohnii subsp.2		+						
	lentus		+		+				
	xylosus	+	+						
	saprophitycus	+							
Micrococcus	*sedentarius*	+							
	lylae	+		+			+	+	
	halobius		+						
	luteus	+	+	+			+	+	
Enterococcus	*sp.*	+				+			
Streptococcus	*mitis*	+	+						
Bacillus	*mycoides*				+			+	
	sp.		+	+				+	
Corynebacterium	*xerosis*	+							
Psedomonas	*aeruginosa*	+	+		+				
	fluorescens	+							
	chlororaphis				+		+	+	
Xantomonas	*maltophila*				+				
Shigella	*boydii*		+						
Providencia	*sp.*		+	+					
Citrobacter	*farmerii*	+		+					
Escherichia	*coli*	+				+			
Enterobacter	*sakazakii*	+							
	agglomerans	+	+					+	
Proteus	*mirabilis*	+		+					

Table 2. Bacterial species isolated from the poultry houses I and II and from surroundings area during spring 2009 and summer 2010.

Genus	Species	Sampling site							
		Farm I	I 10	I 50	I 100	**Farm II**	II 10	II 50	II 100
Aspergillus	*flavus*	+	+	+	+	+			
	niger		+						
	terreus	+							
	glaucus		+						
	nidulans		+						
	parasiticus		+						
	clavatus					+	+	+	+
Penicilium	*solitum*	+							
	sticticus	+				+			
	chrysogenum		+		+				
Fusarium	*oxysporum*		+	+	+				
	graminearum		+	+	+				
Alternaria	*alternata*	+					+	+	+
	tennuissima					+		+	
Ulocladium	*sp.*				+				
Trichoderma	*viridae*	+	+						
Verticilium	*sp.*								+
Drechslera	*sp.*	+							
	gramineae				+				
Scopulariopsis	*brevicaulis*	+						+	+
	acremonium						+		
Cladosporium	*cladosporoides*					+	+	+	+
Mucor	*mucedo*	+	+			+	+	+	
Scedosporium	*sp.*					+	+	+	+
Mycelia	sterilia		+		+		+	+	
Rhodotorula	*rubrum*				+		+		
Candida	*albicans*	+				+			
	inconspicua	+							
	lambica							+	
Cryptococcus	*laurentii*	+				+			

Table 3. Fungal species isolated from the poultry houses I and II and from surroundings area during study period (spring 2009 and summer 2010).

4. Discussion

The literature data usually show the air biopollutant concentration inside the poultry houses. According to many studies (Agranovski et al., 2007, Radon et al., 2002, Vučemilo et al., 2006, 2007) the number of bacteria in poultry houses ranged from 10^3 to 10^{10} CFU/m^3, and the concentrations of fungi was from 2.5×10^1 to 4.9×10^6 CFU/m^3. Much less is known about the relationships between the indoor and the outdoor biological pollution. In comparison with the rate of microorganisms contamination in the poultry houses, the concentration of bacterial and fungi in the air in surrounding areas was considerable lower and did not exceed the values found inside farms. Airborne bacterial and fungi levels measured in poultry houses I and II were always higher than in adjacent areas. Therefore we can suggested that the source of microorganisms are probably the farm objects. Baykov & Stoyanov 1999 also reported higher bacterial levels inside broiler farms than in nearby areas and the average values were similar to our results, i.e. value of mean of 16020 CFU/m3 for farmhouses and range of2060 CFU/m3to 386 CFU/m3 for immediate areas (10 m and 100 m from farm object, respectively). Very high concentration of microorganisms may reflect on insufficient ventilation in relation to the number of animals kept in poultry houses.

The presence of bacteria and fungi in poultry air is a natural phenomenon. Their primary source are the animals themselves, feed and litter. Microorganisms are a constituent of solid and liquid bioaerosols. This mostly refers to saprophytes, however pathogenic microorganisms were also found in the poultry houses air. Aerial count of pathogenic bacteria and fungi depends on the health condition of animals kept in the poultry houses. In addition, microorganisms count inside poultry farms air and monitoring of its emission from this building to the adjacent environment are important parameters for the assessment of the influence of poultry houses on the environmental pollution (Matković et al., 2006). In the present study, microbiological air contamination were determined at three sites at a distance of 10 m, 50 m and 100 m from the poultry houses. The results of total microorganisms count measurements outside the both poultry houses showed it to be lower than the total bacterial and moulds count inside the poultry houses. Number of microorganisms increase at 10 m distance from the poultry houses and gradually decreased to reach the lowest value at a distance of 100 m.

Analyzing the results of the microbiological research about air pollution, it should be remembered that the results are temporary values, occurring at the moment the measurement. In connection with the physico-chemical properties of the air, the degree of contamination of the air can change diametrically within a few minutes (Donderski et al., 2005). Weather condition have a enormous influence on the count of microorganisms in the air. Temperature rise accompanied by rain scarcity can lead to a sudden increase in the concentration of microorganisms in the air. Consequently in summer with the weather conditions most friendly for the spread and development of numerous microorganisms, mesophilic bacteria, staphylococci, gram-negative bacteria and fungi were the more abundant in the air around the poultry houses than in early spring, where the temperature and humidity were lower.

Staphylococci seem to be a useful indicator bacteria (Schulz et al., 2004). Although this group of bacteria do not produce spores, they have the ability to survive in the air for a long time, which means spreading infections through the air. In the poultry houses I and II and outdoor air we observed very high numbers of potentially pathogenic staphylococci, what is really negative phenomenon. In our study the predominant species were coagulase negative. *S. aureus* and *S. saprophitycus* are pathogens for humans and the other species isolated in our studies may act as opportunistic pathogens in humans and animals. Karwowska 2005 also described the very high number of staphylococci in the air farming.

Moulds and yeast can live practically anywhere and have particularly favorable conditions inside the poultry houses. Among fungi recovered from the farm I, the species belonged to genera *Candida spp.* were dominated. This is a large group of potentially pathogenic species. They are usually an etiological factor in mycoses and less frequently, in mycoallergies. As they can produce toxins (e.g. candotoxins), the species can cause mycotoxycoses and increase microorganism sensitivity to some bacterial infections (Ejdys et al., 2009). On the other hand, in outdoor air the most frequent species were moulds *Aspergillus flavus* and *Fusarium oxysporum*. Amongst the several secondary metabolites produced by *A. flavus* are aflatoxins, the most toxic and potent carcinogenic natural compounds ever characterized. Whereas, the *F. oxysporum* is potentially producers of zearalenone, scirpentriol, NT-2 toxin, nivalenol, acetoxyscirpenediol, acetyl T-2toxin and others dangerous toxins (http://www.esgtesting.com/Portal/Documents/Toxins%20and%20fungal%20origin.pdf).

In the air surroundings poultry house II dominated species were *Aspergillus clavatus, Alternaria alternata, Cladosporium cladosporoides*. Whereas, *A. clavatus* and *A. flavus* were the most frequent species inside poultry house II. We should emphasized that *A. alternata* is one of the most common fungi associated with asthma. Not only the presence of asthma but also persistence and severity asthma have been strongly associated with sensitization and exposure to *A. alternata* (Salo et al., 2006). On the other hand, the presence of opportunistic pathogens from the genus *Aspergillus* poses a risk of invasive aspergillosis in farm workers and those living in the proximity of the farms. According to the data obtained by other authors (Soliman et al., 2009) fungi e.g. *Candida albicans, Aspergillus niger, A. nidulans, Penicilium sp.* and *Mucor sp.* were prevalent in broiler farms in Egypt. However, Romanowska-Słomka and Mirosławski 2009 described the occurrence of the moulds and yeast *Aspergillus sp., Penicillium sp., Candida sp. and Cryptococcus sp.* in poultry houses. Other investigators (Agranovski et al. 2007) isolated and identified many fungal strain, including genera: *Cladosporium, Aspergillus, Penicillium, Scopulariopsis, Fusarium, Epicoccum, Mucor, Trichophyton, Alternaria, Ulocladium, Basidiospores, Acremonium, Aureobasidium, Drechslera, Pithomyces, Chrysosporium, Geomyces and Rhizomucor* from farming areas. The presence of such fungi in farmhouses was proved by the results of this study.

The highest total *Enterobacteriacea* counts were found in indoor air and in areas nearby poultry houses I and II. In this present studies both in farms and surroundings areas *Escherichia coli, Proteus mirabilis, Shigella boydii, Citrobacter farmerii, Enterobacter agglomerans, E. sakazakii, Klebsiella pneumoniae, Providencia sp.* were identified. Different results was observed by Vučemilo et. al who found four dominating species of the *Enterobacteriaceae* family: *E. coli, Pantoea sp., Serratia plymuthica* and *Serratia marcescens*. According to Lues et. al 2007 *E. coli* and the other members of the coliforms bacteria could be a good indicators of air contamination.

5. Conclusions

The farming buildings are emitters of the considerable amounts of microbiological contaminants into the atmospheric air. This high emission of potentially pathogenic microorganisms via aerosols from animal housing facilities to the outdoor environment may constitute a considerable risk to human health and environmental pollution.

So far, in literature there are no reliable data about relationships between the indoor and the outdoor biological pollution. This study contributes to the understanding of the level concentration of bioaerosol and its composition with regard to the different distance from farms. The quantity and quality of microbial analysis shows both different bacteria genera and fungi in indoor and outdoor microbiological contamination. Comparing our own results with available literature data on the indoor and outdoor air biopollutant concentration in the poultry houses enables to understand the distribution process.

6. References

Agranovski, V.; Reponen, T.; Ristovski, Z. (2007). Survey of bioaerosol emissions from Australian poultry buildings. European Aerosol Conference. Salzburg, Abstract, 28.

Araujo, R.; Cabral, J, P. (2010). Fungal air quality in medical protected environments. In: *Air Quality*, Ashok Kumar, pp. 357- 382, Sciyo, ISBN: 978-953-307-131-2, Publisher: Sciyo.

Bakutis, B.; Monsteviliene, E.; & Januskeviciene, G. (2004). Analyses of airborne contamination with bacteria, endotoxins and dust in livestock barns and poultry houses. *Acta Veterinaria Brno*, 73, 283-289.

Baykov, B.; Stoyanov, M. (1999). Microbial air pollution caused by intensive broiler chicken breeding. *Federation of European Microbiological Societies. Microbiology ecology, 29, 389-392.*

Crook, B.; Easterbrook, A.; Stagg, S. (2008). Exposure to dust and bioaerosols in poultry farming. Summary of observations and data. Prepared by the Health and Safety Laboratory for the Health and Safety Executive.

Dehoog, S.; Guarro, J.; Gene, J.; Figureas, M.J (2008). Atlas of Clinical Fungi. Centraalbureall voor Schiielcultures/ Universitat Rovira i Virgili.

Donderski, W.; Walczak, M.; Pietrzak, M. (2005). Microbiological contamination of fair within the city of Toruń. *Polish Journal of Environmental Studies*, 14, 2, 223-230.

Dutkiewicz, J. (1987). Bacteria in farming environment. *European Journal of Respiratory diseases*, 71, 154, 71-88.

Ejdys, E.; Michalak, J.; Szewczyk, KM. (2009). Yeast-like fungi isolated from indosr air in school buildings and the surrounding outdoor air. *Acta Mycologica,* 44,1, 97-107.

Lonc, E.; Plewa, K. (2009). Microbiological air contamination in poultry houses. *Polish Journal of Environmental Studies*, 14, 4, 445-449.

Karwowska E. (2005). Microbiological air contamination in farming environment. . *Polish Journal of Environmental Studies*, 19, 1, 15-19.

Kwaśna, H.; Chełkowski, J.; Zajkowski, P. (1991). Grzyby (Mycota). Tom XXII. PAN, Warszawa Kraków, 136 ss.

Lues, J.; Theron, M.; Venter, P.; Rasephei, H. (2007). Microbial composition in bioaerosols of a high-throughput chicken-slaughtering facility. *Poultry Science,* 86, 142-149.

Pasqualotto, A. (2008). Differences in pathogenicity and clinical syndromes due to *Aspergillus fumigatus* and *Aspergillus flavus*. *Medical mycology,* 1-10.

Polish Norm (PN-89/Z-04111/02). Air purity protection. Microbiological testing. Determination number of the bacteria in the atmospheric air (emission) with sampling by aspiration and sedimentation methods.

Polish Norm (PN-89/Z-04111/03). Air purity protection. Microbiological testing. Determination number of the fungi in the atmospheric air (emission) with sampling by aspiration and sedimentation methods.

Matković, K.; Vučemilo, M.; Vinković, B.; Pavičić, Ž.; Matković, S.; Benić, M. (2009). Airborne fungi in a dairy barn with emphasis on microclimate and emission. *Veterinarski Arhiv*, 79, 3, 207-218.

Matković, K.; Vučemilo, M.; Vinković, B.; Šeol, B.; Pavičić, Ž.; Matković, S.; Tofant, A.; Matković, S. (2006). Effect of microclimate on bacterial count and airborne emission from dairy barns on the environment. *Annals of Agricultural and Environmental Medicine*, 13, 349-354.

Nevalainen, A. 2007. Bio-aerosols as exposure agents in indoor environments in relation to asthma and allergy. National Public Health Institute, Department of Environmental Health POB 95, FI-70701 Kuopio, Finland. 2007.

Pomorska, D.; Larsson, L.; Skórska, C.; Sitkowska, J.; Dutkiewicz, J. (2009). Levels of bacterial endotoxins in the samples of settled dust collected in animal houses. *Bulletin of the Veterinary Institute in Pulawy*, 53, 37-41.

Radon, K.; Danuser, B.; Iversen, M.; Monso, O.; Weber, Ch.; Hartung, J.; Palmgren, U.; Nowak, D. (2002). Air contaminants in different European farming environments. *Annals of Agricultural and Environmental Medicine*, 9, 41-48.

Romanowska-Słomka, I.; Mirosławski, J. (2009). Biological hazards in an industrial poultry farm- research results. *Bezpieczeństwo Pracy*, 7, 16-19.

Raper, K.B.; Thom, Ch.; Fennell, D.I. (1949). A manual of the Penicillia. The Williams & Wilkins Company, Baltimore, USA.

Raper K.B.; Fennell D.I. (1965). The genus Aspergillus. The Williams & Wilkins Company, Baltimore, USA.

Salo, P., Arbes, S., Sever, M., Jaramillo, R.; Cohn, R., London, S., Zeldin, D. (2006). Exposure to *Alternaria alternata* in US homes is associated with asthma symptoms. *Journal of Allergy and Clinical Immunology*, 118, 4, 892–898.

Schierl, R.; Heise, A.; Egger, U.; Schneider, F.; Eichelser, F.; Neser, S.; Nowak, D. (2007). Endotoxin concentration in modern animal houses in southern Bavaria. *Annals of Agricultural and Environmental Medicine*, 14, 1, 129-136.

Schulz, J.; Hartung, J.; Seedorf, L.; Formosa, C. (2004). Staphylococci as an indicator for bacterial emissions from a broiler house. *International Soeciety for Animal Hygiene-Sant-Maolo, 75-78.*

Soliman, S.; Sobeih, M.; Hussein, M.; Abdel-Latiff, H., Moneim, A. (2009). Seasonal epidemiological surveillance on bacterial and fungal pathogens in broiler farms in Egypt. *International Journal of Poultry Science*, 8, 8, 720-727.

Siemińki M. (2001). *Environmental health threats*, Wydawnicto Naukowe PWN, ISBN: 83-01-13561-1, Warszawa.

Srikanth, P.; Suchithra, S.; Steinberg, R. 2008. Bio-aerosols in indoor environment: composition, health effects and analysis. *Indian Journal of Medical Microbiology, 26, 4, 302-312.*

Vučemilo, M.; Vinković, B.; Matković, K. (2006). Influence of broiler age on airborne pollutant content in poultry house. *Krmiva*, 48, 3-6.

Vučemilo, M.; Matković, K.; Vinković, B.; Jakšić, S.; Granić, K.; Mas, N. (2007). The effect of animal age on air pollutant concentration in a broiler house. *Czech Journal of Animal Science*. 52, 6 170-174.

The Occurrence of Bioaerosols in the Food Preparation Areas of HIV/AIDS Hospices in Central South Africa

J. Nkhebenyane, J. F. R. Lues, P. Venter and K. Shale
School for Agriculture and Environmental Sciences,
Central University of Technology, Bloemfontein,
South Africa

1. Introduction

South Africa is amongst countries that are facing serious challenges with regard to HIV/AIDS and institutions of HIV/AIDS hospices have been introduced in many areas of the country to help with the care of patients infected by HIV. As in any domestic setting, the safety and quality of food served in a hospice depend on the kitchen design, storage conditions, and food preparation practices of the food handlers. Micro-organisms in such areas can become airborne when droplets are generated while cleaning, cooking, preparing food, speaking, coughing, sneezing or vomiting. Most residential and hospice kitchens do not normally use air-filtration systems as it is the situation in hospitals. This means that the principal factors governing the levels of airborne particles indoor are: indoor sources, outdoor particle levels, the deposition rate of particles on indoor surfaces, and the air exchange rate (Nazaroff, 2004). Exposure of building occupants to certain micro-organisms, and elevated concentrations of environmental organisms, could result in allergenic reactions, irritant responses, toxicosis, respiratory illness and other ill effects.

This is especially important in a hospice environment that accommodates patients with compromised immune systems due to infection with the human immunodeficiency virus (HIV). Tuberculosis (TB) is an archetypal example of a disease that is transmitted by airborne route. Primary pulmonary TB is caused by the inhalation of droplet nuclei carrying the causative agent, *Mycobacterium nuclei* (MTB). For hardy bacteria such as mycobacterium TB, only a single organism is needed to cause disease (Haas, 2006). TB acts synergistically with HIV and increases the risk of primary TB infection developing into the active disease by a hundred fold (Davies, 1999). The world-wide occurrence of TB is high, with approximately one third of the world's population thought to be infected with MTB (Miller, 1996). Globally, TB is estimated to cause the deaths of three million people annually, and this figure is predicted to rise to five million by the year 2050 (Davies, 1999). Nosocomial infections similar to TB are a very real problem in healthcare facilities, with approximately one in 10 patients acquiring an infection during a hospital stay (Schulgen, *et al.*, 2000).

Although most nosocomial infections are generally associated with person-to-person contact, evidence is mounting that they are mostly transmitted via aerosol route. Unlike formal healthcare facilities that generally boast air filtration systems, informal healthcare facilities like hospices have none. With patients suffering from a plethora of diseases associated with a compromised immune system, contaminated air only serves to aggravate the problem. It is therefore essential at these establishments to limit the prevalence of food-borne and airborne causative agents in the food preparation areas and through preventative measures limiting the chances for secondary infections. Therefore, the aim of this study was to quantify the microbial load of indicator microorganisms and associated environmental factors in the air (outside and inside) of a typical hospice environment. Subsequently, the relationship between environmental factors and microbial concentration was established and compared with normal breathable air in the same environment. It is expected that minimising food-borne contaminants associated with aerosols in HIV/AIDS hospices will improve the safety of food, being a considerable contributor to the food-borne contamination levels. It is envisaged that this study will contribute to the scientific knowledge of microbial contaminants associated with HIV/AIDS hospices in South Africa.

2. Materials and methods

2.1 Sample collection

Samples of breathable air were collected at ten registered hospices in two provinces in central South Africa, namely the Eastern Cape and Free State. The sampling campaigns were conducted during the southern-hemisphere winter (dry months, April-September). Samples were collected in duplicate at each hospice in the morning (before and after food preparation) and also at lunchtime (before and after food preparation), both inside and outside the hospice kitchen for both sessions.

2.2 Air sampling procedure

All microbial samples were collected 1.5 metres above the floor on 65 mm RODAC plates by means of impaction on soft agar. The (SAS) Super-90 surface air sampler (PBI International, Milan, Italy) was used for this purpose. The air sampler was calibrated at an airflow rate of 0.03 $m^3 \cdot min^{-1}$ and all detachable parts were sterilised with 70% ethanol before use and between sampling runs (Venter *et al.*, 2004). Plate count agar (PCA) was used for the isolation of total viable aerobic count (Merck, SA). Samples were then placed in a cooler box and immediately transported to the laboratory. Subsequent incubation of the plates was done at temperatures of between 25 and 37 °C for periods ranging from 24 to 72 hours. All colonies were enumerated using the positive hole correlation method and expressed as colony-forming units per cubic meter of air sampled. Subsequent replica plating was performed using a replica plating device and sterile velveteen cloth to quantify the following micro-organisms: *Staphylococcus aureus*, *Pseudomonas* spp., *Bacillus* spp., coliform and total coliform.

2.3 Facility design

Assessment of the kitchen design and setting was done by means of visual observations and note taking. Simultaneous observation of safe food handling and storage practices was also conducted. (See table 2.1)

2.4 Quantification of environmental factors

The extrinsic environmental factors capable of influencing the survival of micro-organisms, i.e. temperature (area heat stress monitor, Questemp, SA) and relative humidity (whirling psychrometer, Airflow Instrumentation, SA), were measured, as were the factors that could influence the distribution of the assessed microbiota (Chang, *et al.*, 2001), namely airflow (airflow anemometer – LCA 6000 VT, Airflow Instrumentation, SA) and airborne particle (dust) concentrations (hand-held aerosol monitor - 1005/1060, PPM Enterprises, Inc) (Venter, *et al.*, 2004). Positive and negative controls were included and all analysis and assays were repeated at least in duplicate according to Venter, *et al.*, (2004).

3. Results and discussion

3.1 Facility design

The results obtained from the technical investigations are presented in Table 1. From this, it is apparent that most hospices with the exception of a few e.g. Ons plek and Bethlehem, complied with the requirements of good preparation and handling practices of food.

Occurrence	%
Kitchen facility design	
Ceiling	60
Ventilation through natural moving air	60
Air bricks with filters	50
Food handling practices	
Cleanliness/neatness of the food handler	70
Wearing of suitable protective clothing	50
Availability of hand washing facilities	60
Storage space for hygienic storage of food	50
Availability of easy to clean refuse containers	50
Regular washing of hands before/after food preparation	60
Overall cleanliness of the kitchen	
Environment conducive for cooking/preparing food	50

*The percentages and right hand values represent the level of conformance to Regulation 918 amongst all the hospices sampled (n=10).

Table 1. Kitchen facility design and food handling practices in hospices around Central South Africa.

The lack of air filtration systems due to financial constraints, may have contributed to the presence of bio-aerosol indoors. The majority of the investigated kitchens were also not designed to provide required barriers against moisture, temperature, pests, dust and associated microbes. Therefore limited control over the quality and safety of the food stored under the noted conditions would be expected.

3.2 Influence of extrinsic factors

The extrinsic factors that influence the viability and distribution of micro-organisms that prevail in various hospice kitchens are listed in figure 1. From these results, it is evident that on average, the hospice kitchens provide an environment that would sustain microbial viability concomitant to proliferation, given that a suitable substrate and sufficient time is available. The transport and the ultimate setting of a bio aerosol are affected by its physical properties and the environmental parameters that it encounters. These physical characteristics are size, density, and shape of droplets or particles; the environmental factors include magnitude of a relative humidity and temperature, which determine the capacity to be airborne. Bioaerosols generated from suspensions undergo desiccation, whereas those generated as dusts or powders partially rehydrate. The presence of moulds as an example indicates a problem with water penetration or high humidity indoors (Goel and Goel 2009).

The persistence of micro-organisms, the presence and density of pathogens and the potential spread of microbial contamination from contaminated food in the household Kitchen have been extensively studied and re-examined. These studies indicated that domestic kitchen sites have been found to be repeatedly contaminated with a variety of bacterial contaminants, including *Listeria monocytogens* (Beumer, *et al.,* 1996), *Escherichia coli* and *Enterobacter cloacae* (Speirs, *et al.,* 1995). It is well known that dampness and other excess moisture accumulation in buildings are closely connected to observation of mould, mildew, or other microbial growth. Microbial growth has also been associated with building characteristics. In residences measures of microbial contamination have been found to be positively correlated with indoor temperature and humidity, age and size of buildings, use of wood stoves and fireplaces and absence of mechanical ventilation (Dharmage, *et al.,* 1999). From this study it became evident that the evaluated kitchens boasted levels of relative humidity of 60 ± inside as compared to the average of 40 ± outside.

The relative humidity (RH) in one of the hospices was 100% and the dominant bacterial specie was *Bacillus cereus,* therefore showing an increase associated with an increase in RH. The average temperatures were below 20 °C outside and 15 °C inside (Figure 2); hence the prevalence of *Pseudomonas aeruginosa* (Fig 1) due to their ability to survive at low temperatures (Forsythe, 2000). The average airflow for the assessed kitchen was 0.4 $m.s^{-1}$ outside compared to the average of 0.2 $m.s^{-1}$ inside. It is also interesting to note that the low airflow inside correlated with a high concentration of airborne particulates inside which was 8.04 $mg.m^{-3}$.

3.3 Airborne indicator organism presence

The presence of undesirable bio-aerosols is often associated with sick building syndrome (SBS) and building-related illnesses. Sources include furnishing and building materials, fungal contamination within wall and gaps at structural joints (Jay, 2000). Inadequacies in the building design and improper ventilation may contribute to poor indoor air quality. For purposes of this study, micro-organisms indicative of poor food manufacturing practices are defined as indicator organisms. In the formal food industry, the presence of *Escherichia coli* is indicative of faecal contamination, while the presence of *Staphylococcus aureus* points to extensive human handling, and total viable aerobic organisms is a sign of poor process hygiene. The presence of these organisms in the breathable air of the various hospice kitchens could also be attributed to the aforementioned practices, as food processing is the core business of the kitchens in this setting.

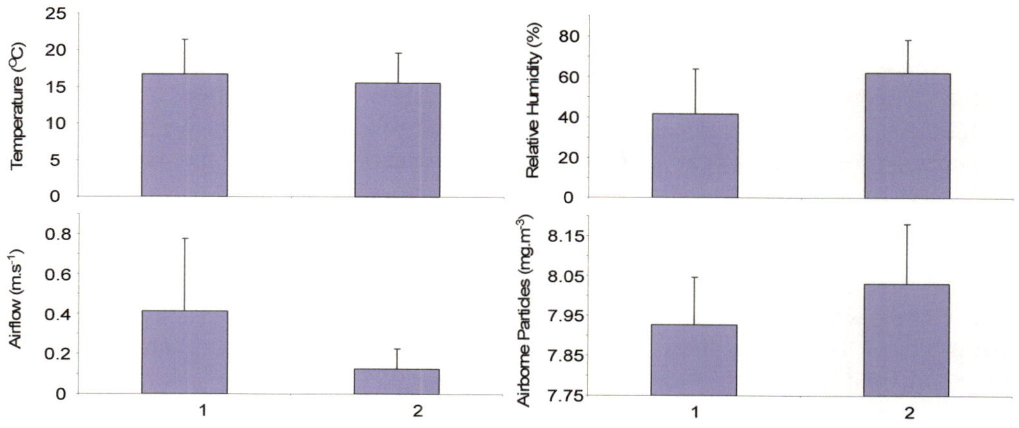

Fig. 2. The Environmental factors quantified outside (1) and within (2) hospice kitchens

In this scenario, the presence of *E. coli* could be due to faecal contaminants from the hands of food handlers, or from contaminated working surfaces and utensils. Therefore, it is of the utmost importance to observe proper personal hygiene, particularly with regard to hand-washing after visiting the toilet, in order to prevent contamination. However, three of the hospices that were investigated are without hand-washing facilities and are located in rural areas. As noted in figure 1 the average airborne particulates were 7.90 $mg.m^{-3}$ inside as compared to 8.0 $mg.m^{-3}$ outside. These results are comparable to those observed by Hargreaves *et al.*, 2003. The presence of *Bacillus spp* was also noted in the presence of these conspicuous airborne particulates which were dominant throughout the sampling period. This could be due to the fact that these are spore formers and bacteria in many cases are attached to larger airborne particles.

According to Moir *et al.*, 2002 these spores can endure a wide range of extreme environmental stresses while retaining the capacity to return to vegetative growth almost immediately once the nutrient returns to the environment. It was therefore assumed that airflow in and outside the hospice kitchens were sufficient to carry dust particles as well as different bacterial population (Figure 1). In general, the average bacterial counts varied between 1×10^1 to 1×10^2 $cfu.m^{-3}$. Compared to the literature these counts were fairly low and apart from being possible allergens they are also associated with decreased lung function, increased respiratory symptoms such as cough, shortness of breath and asthma attacks (WHO, 2002). From the observed results it is apparent that the kitchens in question boast a resident bio-aerosol population that is not significantly influenced by the noted environmental parameters. Though the source of the bio-aerosols assayed is not clear, *S. aureus* probably results from aerosols dispersed by the food handlers in the kitchens. It should also be noted that although microbial counts were low, the kitchens provided an environment conducive to microbial survival as aerosolised particles and subsequently as food contaminants. In general the kitchens had a lower temperature, increased RH, and higher airborne particle count.

4. Conclusion

Indoor air pollution is usually caused by the accumulation of contaminants from various indoor sources. The generation of pollutants within the indoor environment may come from primary sources such as fuel combustion for cooking, as well as emissions from fireplaces, stoves, cleaning products and chemicals stored in the home. It is therefore safe to assume that since all these factors were present at the study sites, they all contributed to the indoor air pollution discovered. Factors such as heating, ventilation, air-conditioning and household activities, e.g. cooking and cleaning, all play a crucial role in the wellbeing of a building's occupants. In a setting such as a hospice, where proper food storage and handling is not always possible due to lack of infrastructure, it is essential that special care is taken regarding the type of food stored and the packaging material used. Micro-organisms detected in the indoor air of the hospice kitchens included in this study could be derived from the hospice occupants, but may also emanate from the outside environment. One such example would be *Bacillus cereus,* which is a common air- and dust-borne contaminant that readily multiplies in meat products. These organisms are able to withstand unfavourable conditions such as low temperature and heat due to their ability to form spores (Whyte *et al.,* 2001). A study by Nel *et al.,* 2003, reported rapidly increasing levels of *B. cereus* when a product was exposed to poor handling and processing procedures. A hospice, where patients are provided with accommodation, food and care, would be a typical example of this setting.

From the results it can be concluded that certain food preparation and storage facilities in the hospices studied are, according to the technical data, not suitable for this purpose. However, it appeared that some of the extrinsic factors influencing microbial viability were being governed. Specific attention should be given to the upgrading of the kitchen infrastructure – for example, it would be ideal to have separate rooms for the preparation of raw and cooked food, as well as a room used only for food storage purposes. The results presented in this chapter further identified the hospice occupants as possible sources of the organisms found in the hospice kitchens and surrounding environments, since the occupants were in some cases also responsible for preparing the food, while moving continuously between the kitchen, bathroom and bedroom. In terms of residency, it would thus be ideal to separate the patients from the food preparation facilities, including the kitchen.

Companies that regularly donate food to the hospices are further cautioned to avoid donating foodstuffs that are past their sell-by date, as the inability of the assessed kitchens to control humidity fluctuations only exacerbates the problem with regard to food safety and proliferation of microbial load. It was further noted that in South Africa, unlike in more humid countries, the facility design and geographical localisation have a limited effect on the resident bio-aerosol profiles. In order to address and verify the concerns raised in this chapter, it is recommended that the ability of micro-organisms to proliferate on the foods (high-risk) provided to the hospices should be assessed and the menus adjusted in accordance to season- associated changes in the extrinsic factors that would influence microbial viability and growth. It should further be noted that the occupants of the hospices concerned have very little knowledge of proper food storage and handling practices and are to a large extent not aware of the threats posed to them by the resident microbiota. This problem could be alleviated by providing the patients and food handlers with educational training in respect of proper food safety (storage and handling).

5. Future research

Due to a lack of empirical data, aerosol transmission of influenza is often questioned and its relationship with other airborne microbiota such as bacteria and fungi still requires further research to establish their impact on food and people indoors (Blachere *et al.,* 2007).

6. References

Blachere, F.M. Lindsley, W.G., Slaven J.E., Green B.J., Anderson S.E., Chen B.T., Beezhold D.H. Bioaerosol sampling for the detection of aerosolized influenza virus. Influenza and other respiratory viruses. Vol. 1 (3), 113-120.

Beumer, R.R., Te Giffel M.C., E. Spoorenberg E. and Rombouts F.M. 1996. *Listeria* species in domestic environments. Epidemiology and Infection. 117:437-442.

Chang, C.W.; Chung, H.; Huang, C.F. and Su, H.J.J. 2001. Exposure of workers to airborne microorganisms in openair swine houses. Applied Environmental Microbiology, 67: 155-161.

Davies, 1999. The changing face of Tuberculosis: A new challenge to the developing world. Available online at: www.priory.com/cmol/TBFocus.htm.

Dharmage, S.; Bailey, M.; Raven, J.; Mitakakiss, T.; Guest, D.; Cheng, A.; Rolland, J.; Thien, F.; Abramson, M. and Haydn Walters, E. 1999. A reliable and valid home visit report for studies of asthma in young adults. Indoor Air, 9(3): 188-192.

Forsythe, S.J. 2000. *The microbiology of safe food.* In: Forsythe S.J. (eds). 1st edition, Oxford: Blackwell Science, 1-424.

Goel, M. and Goel, A. 2009. Bio-aerosols A Potential Hazard In Dental Clinic: - Composition, Health Effects And Analysis:- A Review Article. Indian Journal of Dental Sciences. Vol 1 (2): 77-82.

Haas, D. W. 2006. *Mycobacterium tuberculosis.* In: Mandell, G.L., Bennett, J.E. and Dollin, R. (eds). Principles and Practice of Infectious diseases, 5th edition, Philadelphia, PA: Churchill Livingstone, 2576-2607.

Hargreaves, M., Parappukkaran S., Morawska L., Hitchins J., He C., Gilbert D. 2003. A pilot investigation into associations between indoor airborne fungal and non-biological particle concentrations in residential houses in Brisbane, Australia. Science of the Total Environment. 312: 89-101.

Jay, M.J. 2000. Modern food microbiology. 6th edition. Chapter 9: Miscellaneous food products. Maryland: Aspen publishers.pp.163-177.

Jones, A.M., Harrison R.M. 2004. The effects of Meteorological factors on Atmospheric Bioaerosol Concentrations. Science of the Total Environment. 326:151-180.

Miller, 1996. Tuberculosis risk after exposure on aero planes. Journal of Tuberculosis and Lung disease. 77: 414-419.

Moir, A.B., Café M., Bebrama J. 2002. Spore germination. Cellular and Molecular Life Sciences, 59: 403-409.

Nazaroff, W.W. 2004. Indoor particle dynamics. Indoor Air, 14(7): 175-183.

Nel, S., Lues J.F.R., Buys E., Venter P. 2003. Bacterial populations associated with meat from the deboning room of a high throughput red meat abattoir. Meat Science . 66:667-674.

Oleske, D. and Hershow, R. 2002. Control of Transmissible Diseases in Health Care Settings. Epidemiology and the Delivery of Health Care Services. Part 2, 191-215.

Ross, M.A., Curtis L., Scheff P.A., Hryho D.O., Ramakrishma V., Wadden R.A.,Persky V.W. 2000. Association of asthma symptoms and severity with indoor bio-aerosols. Allergy. 55: 705-711.

Schulgen, G.; Kropec, A.; Kappstein, I.; Daschner, F. and Schumacher, M. 2000. Estimation of extra hospital stay attributable to nosocomial infections: Heterogeneity and timing of events. Journal of Clinical Epidemiology, 53(4): 409-417.

Speirs, J.P., Anderson A and Anderson J.G. 1995. A study of the microbial content of domestic kitchen. Journal of Environmental Health Research 5:109-122.

Toivola, M.; Alm, S.; Reponen, T.; Kolari, S. and Nevalainen, A. 2002. Personal exposures and micro-environmental concentrations of particles and bio-aerosols. Journal of Environmental Monitoring, 4: 166-174.

Venter, P.; Lues, J.F.R. and Theron, H. 2004. Quantification of bioaerosols in automated chicken egg production plants. Poultry Science, 83: 1226-1231.

Whyte, P.J., Collins D., Mcgill K., Monahan C., O'Mahony. 2001. Distribution and prevalence of airborne microorganisms in three commercial poultry processing plants. Journal of Food Protection, 64:388-391.

20

Indoor Air Quality in Primary Schools

Maria do Carmo Freitas et al.*
Instituto Tecnológico e Nuclear (ITN), URSN, Sacavém, Portugal

1. Introduction

Clean air is a basic requirement of life (World Health Organization, 2010). The Indoor Air Quality (IAQ) has been the object of several studies due to an increasing concern within the scientific community on the effects of indoor air quality upon health, especially as people tend to spend more time indoors than outdoors (Franck et al., 2011; Canha et al., 2010; WHO, 2010; Environmental Protection Agency, 2010; Saliba et al., 2009; Fraga et al., 2008; Fromme et al., 2007; Guo et al., 2004; Kosonen, 2004; Lee et al., 2002a; Lee et al., 2002b; Carrer et al., 2002; Lee et al., 2001; Li et al., 2001; Wilson & Spengler, 1996; Allen & Miguel, 1995; Jenkins et al., 1992; WHO, n.d.). The quality of air inside homes, offices, schools or other private and public buildings is an essential determinant of healthy life and people's well-being (WHO, 2010).

People can be exposed to contaminants by inhalation, ingestion and dermal contact. In the past, scientists have paid much attention to the study of exposure to outdoor air contaminants, because they have realised the seriousness of outdoor air pollution problems. However, each indoor microenvironment has unique characteristics, determined by the local outdoor air, specific building characteristics and indoor activities (Pegas et al, 2010). Indeed, hazardous substances are emitted from buildings, construction materials and indoor equipment or due to human activities indoors (WHO, 2010; Carrer et al., 2002).

Reports about buildings with air-related problems have received increasing attention since the 1970s (Spengler & Sexton, 1983; Hodgson, 1992). In an indoor environment, dust on floors and other surfaces contains minerals, metals, fibres from textiles, paper, and insulation material, particles from tobacco smoke, including polycyclic aromatic compounds (PAH's). For this reason, the indoor environment is cleaned to maintain an acceptable level of perceived cleanliness, to prevent surface degradation, to control potential risk of infection from microorganisms, and to control dust exposure in general (Wolkoff et al., 1998). All of these pollutants could cause significant damage to health globally (WHO, 2010).

---

* Nuno Canha[1], Maria Martinho[2], Marina Almeida-Silva[3], Susana Marta Almeida[3], Priscilla Pegas[4], Célia Alves[4], Casimiro Pio[4], Maria Trancoso[5], Rita Sousa[5], Filomena Mouro[5], Teresa Contreiras[6]
[1]*Instituto Tecnológico e Nuclear (ITN), URSN,Sacavém,Portugal*
[2]*United Nations, Department of Economic and Social Affairs,NY,USA*
[3]*Instituto Tecnológico e Nuclear (ITN), URSN,Sacavém,Portugal*
[4]*Universidade de Aveiro/ CESAM,Aveiro,Portugal*
[5]*Laboratório Nacional de Energia e Geologia / LAQ,Lisboa,Portugal*
[6]*Instituto Nacional de Saúde Dr Ricardo Jorge / ONSA,Lisboa,Portugal*

The IAQ in school buildings is expected to be a key role player in the assessment of the effects of the children personal exposure to air pollution as children spend at least a third of their time inside school buildings, that is, approximately seven or more hours a day in school (Almeida et al., 2010; EPA, 2010; Pegas et al., 2010; Wheeler et al., 2009; Ramachandran et al., 2005). Poor IAQ can affect scholarly performance and attendance (Daisey et al. 2003; Godoi et al. 2009). Hence, several studies about air quality in schools have recently been published (Goyal & Khare, 2009; Tippayawong et al., 2009; Fraga et al., 2008; Fromme et al., 2007; Hwang et al., 2006). Environmental asthma triggers commonly found in school buildings include respiratory viruses; cockroaches and other pests; mold resulting from excess moisture in the building; dander from animals in the classroom; and dander brought on the clothing from animals at home. Second-hand smoke and dust mites are other known environmental asthma triggers found in schools. Children with asthma may be affected by other pollutants from sources inside schools, such as unvented stoves or heaters and common products including chemicals, cleaning agents, perfumes, pesticides and sprays.

Indoor Air Quality problems in schools may be even more serious than in other categories of buildings, due to higher occupant density and insufficient outside air supply, aggravated by frequent poor construction and/or maintenance of school buildings (Pegas et al., 2010). Schools are seen as particularly likely to have environmental deficiencies because chronic shortages of funding contribute to inadequate operation and maintenance of facilities (Mendell & Heath, 2005). Previous studies showed the poor indoor environmental quality at schools may be explained by: (1) insufficient ventilation in schools, especially in winter, (2) infrequently and not thoroughly cleaned indoor surfaces, and (3) a large number of students in relation to room area and volume, with constant re-suspension of particles from room surfaces (Janssen et al., 1999).

Children constitute a sensitive group with higher risk than adults (Stranger et al., 2007a) because children are particularly vulnerable to pollutants due to their undeveloped airways (Stranger et al., 2007a; Mendell et al., 2005). Moreover, children have greater susceptibility to some environmental pollutants than adults, because they breathe higher volumes of air relative to their body weights and their tissues and organs are actively growing (Mendell & Heath, 2005). The effects of air pollution on children have been growing (Khan et al., 2007) and one of the consequences is the increase of the prevalence of allergic rhinitis (ISAAC, 1998).

The chemical and microbiological parameters required by the Portuguese Legislation for IAQ monitoring purposes are: carbon dioxide (CO_2), carbon monoxide (CO), ozone (O_3), formaldehyde (HCHO), volatiles organic compound (VOCs), bacteria and fungi (DL n.º 79/2006). Some of these parameters will be studied below.

1.1 Particulate matter

Particulate matter (PM) may be divided into two broad classes depending upon the manner by which it is introduced into atmosphere. A primary component consists of those particles released directly from their source, while a secondary component consists of those particles created in the atmosphere via chemical reactions between pollutants that were originally emitted as gases (Gilli et al., 2007; Schlesinger & Cassie, 2003; Mysliwiec & Kleeman, 2002). Indoor particle concentration depends on penetration of outdoor particles into the indoor environment and on the intensity of indoor aerosol sources (Estoková et al., 2010; Franck et al., 2011; Estoková et al., 2010). The number and behavior of inhabitants and the amount of indoor contamination sources determine temporal and spatial variations of indoor aerosol distribution. In addition, wet processes as cleaning, washing and drying increase relative

humidity which can lead to variations in particle size distribution (Estoková et al., 2010). The particles can also vary in their chemical composition (Karthikeyan & Balasubramanian, 2006).
For legislation purposes, PM is defined as "inhalable" if its aerodynamic diameter is below 10µm (PM_{10}), but there is continuing debate whether the adverse health effects of PM are associated more with small particles or not (Grigg, 2009). Inhalation of particulate material may cause prejudicial human health effects either in the short or long terms (Allen & Miguel, 1995).
Many epidemiological studies found correlations between exposure to PM (or PM components) and adverse health effects (Franck, et al., 2011; Estoková, et al., 2010; Tippayawong et al., 2009; Fang et al., 2006; Wilson & Spengler, 1996). Hazardous influence of particles is related to their penetrations and deposition into human respiratory system. Nevertheless, there is no clear agreement as to a biologically plausible mechanism, which can explain the acute mortality/morbidity, associated with PM exposure. In addition there is no consensus as to which components of PM are responsible for the excess mortality and morbidity (González-Flecha, 2004).
PM sources typically include smoking and cooking. While the school environment lacks these typical indoor PM sources, there is growing evidence of high concentrations of PM in classrooms (Stranger et al., 2007b; Janssen et al., 2001).

1.1.1 Chemical elements and water-soluble Ions

Due to inhalation exposure, the chemical composition of the particulate matter can cause toxic health effects on humans. In particular, the presence of metal substances is considered to be a significant factor of health risk. Although elemental components constitute only a small portion by mass of PM, some trace elements (e.g. Pb, As, Se, Cd, Hg, etc.) may pose a serious threat to human health, causing inflammation or DNA damage, and altering permeability by inducing production of oxygen species (OHd) in tissues (Health Effects Institute, 2002).
There have been numerous studies that have measured the concentrations of PM within indoor environments. In a study taken by the Department of Environmental Sciences, Environmental and Occupational Health Group, in the University of Wageningen in the Netherlands, with the objective to investigate the sources of high concentrations of PM_{10} particles in classrooms, they observed that the highest classroom/outdoor ratios were found for the elements from soils Si, Ca and Ti. The only measured elements that were not increased were S, Pb, Br and Cl, which are dominated by non-crustal sources. For S, Br and Pb, which are generally associated with particles <1µm, significant correlations between classroom and outdoor concentrations and between two classrooms were found (Janssen et al., 1999).
The chemical composition of particulate matter is important to gain insights into sources (Karthikeyan & Balasubramanian, 2006). Buildings can be considered to be small chemical reaction chambers embedded in the larger outdoor atmosphere with different surface to volume ratios, temperatures, and residence times, which interact with and are influenced by the outdoor (Lunden et al., 2003). Phase changes may also affect particle concentrations, and may be rapid with respect to residence times. Vapor absorption or reaction at the surfaces inside the residence may be important to the partitioning of semi-volatile constituents between the vapor and particle phases. A number of important aerosol chemical species are prime candidates for continued chemical interactions indoors, including organic carbon and ammonium nitrate (Lunden et al., 2003). Some of these chemicals were found indoors and can cause irritation of skin, respiratory system and eyes (Allen & Miguel, 1995). Different studies have shown persuasive evidence linking higher indoor NO_2 concentrations to

reduced school attendance and low ventilation rates to reduced performance (Mendell et al., 2005; Kim et al., 2007).

1.2 Volatile Organic Compounds and carbonyls

In the scientific literature, two different emissions types of Volatile Organic Compounds (VOCs) are defined: primary and secondary. The primary emissions are free (non-bound) VOCs. These generally are low molecular weight VOCs. Secondary emissions are chemically or physically bound VOCs and several of these are emitted or formed by different processes under special chemical or physical conditions (Wolkoff, 1999). VOCs are easily released into indoor air and are recognized as the major air pollutants in the indoor air (Guo et al., 2004; Viegas & Prista, 2010). One of the most important sources of VOCs are the consumer products, like wood, paint, food, cleaners, etc. Results from a study in dwellings suggest that indoor VOCs and formaldehyde may cause asthma-like symptoms (Norback et al., 1995).

Indoor air is a significant source of benzene exposure and inhalation is the main pathway of human exposure to this pollutant. Benzene is a genotoxic carcinogen in humans. There is no known exposure threshold for the risk of benzene exposure, so, it is expedient to reduce indoor exposure levels to as low as possible: no safe level of exposure can be recommended (WHO, 2010).

In schools, the most commonly measured pollutants in indoor air are formaldehyde, total VOCs, CO_2 and bioaerosols (Bayer et al., 2000).

2. Material and methods

2.1 Sampling site and schools description

This study was carried out in Lisbon, which is the largest city of Portugal. Lisbon has a population of about half a million inhabitants in 84.8 km^2 while the metropolitan area of 2870 km^2 has around 2.8 million inhabitants (Almeida et al., 2010).

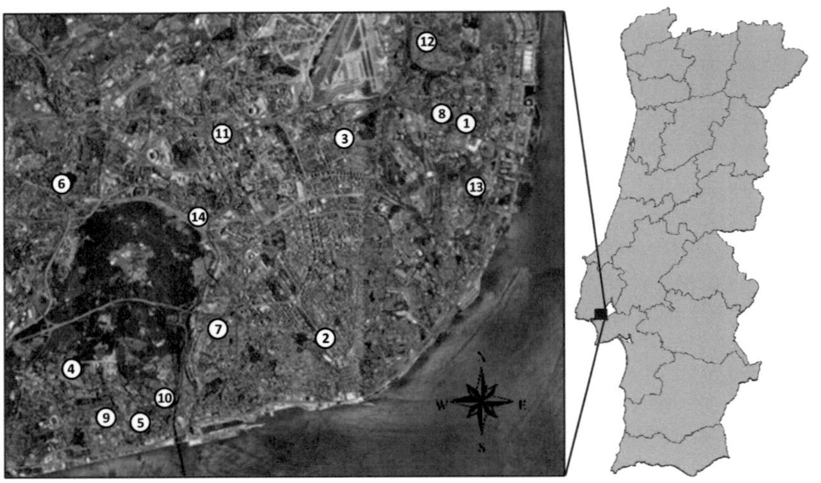

Fig. 1. Spatial distribution of the 14 primary schools in Lisbon, Portugal, studied in this work.

Data on the characteristics of classrooms and indoor air were collected in 14 primary schools in Lisbon. Figure 1 shows the location of these 14 primary schools. For each school, data

were collected in two classrooms, named for reference purposes as classroom "a" and classroom "b". The information concerning the classrooms characteristics is presented in Table 1. All schools have natural ventilation and there is no forced ventilation or air conditioning system in use (ventilation is done by opening doors and windows).
The data studied here is part of a larger study, which has been described and analysed in previous research (Almeida et al., 2011; Canha et al., 2010, 2011; Pegas et al., 2010, 2011a, 2011b).

2.2 Sampling and chemical analysis

Three campaigns for total particulate matter sampling were conducted: spring (May-June 2009, total of 34 days), autumn (October-December 2009, total of 62/68 days) and winter (January-March 2010, total of 76/78 days). Sampling of VOCs and carbonyls was performed in the same periods but only for 14 consecutive days within the studied season. Although there are results for all the campaigns and measured parameters, only the campaigns and measured parameters which have results for the two classrooms of all 14 schools were considered in this study. They are shortly described below. All the values of the parameters were normalized to the day.

2.2.1 Mass of total particulate matter (TPM)

Filters were passively exposed (Canha et al, 2011). A total of six 47-mm diameter Millipore (Isopore™) polycarbonate filters were exposed in each classroom, distributed over a tray with an area of 25 cm x 20 cm, at 120-cm high to approximate the breathing height of children inside the classrooms. Each filter was placed inside an uncovered plastic Petri dish. Filters with pore sizes of 0.4 and 0.8 μm were used. The filter loads were measured by gravimetry with a 0.1 μg sensitivity balance, in a controlled clean room (class 10,000) inside a 100 class clean hood. Filter mass before and after sampling was obtained as the average of three measurements, when observed variations were less than 5%.

2.2.2 Mass of chemical elements in TPM

The exposed Millipore-polycarbonate filters and their corresponding blank filters were irradiated at the Portuguese Research Reactor (RPI-ITN; nominal power: 1 MW) for analyses by k_0-INAA (Canha et al., 2010). Irradiation time was 5 h at a neutron flux density of 8×10^{12} cm^{-2} s^{-1}. Each sample was rolled up and put into an aluminium foil for irradiation, removed from the foil after irradiation and put in a polyethylene container for measurement. Samples were measured 7 h after 3–5 days and after 3–4 weeks, with an ORTEC® automatic sample changer, equipped with an ORTEC coaxial hyperpure germanium detector (1.90 keV resolution at 1.33 MeV; 30% relative efficiency). One Al-0.1%Au alloy disc with a thickness of 125 μm and a diameter of 0.5 cm was used as comparator for the k_0-methodology, and irradiated concurrently with the samples. A total of 4 replicates were analyzed for each type of blank filter.
The chemical elements discussed in this study are gold (Au), chromium (Cr), potassium (K), antimony (Sb), scandium (Sc), and zinc (Zn).

2.2.3 Mass of water-soluble ions in TPM

Exposed polycarbonate filters were used for the determination of water-soluble inorganic ions. For each classroom, a set of 2-4 filters were used together as a unique sample. All the polyethylene containers and other used material in the process were decontaminated and water soluble sodium and nitrate ions contents were previously determined to confirm free contamination status of the material. This step was highly crucial to avoid contaminations and biased results, due to the small mass of the samples. TPM on the samples was extracted with 25mL of distilled deionized water by ultrasonic (30 minutes) and mechanical shaking (15 hours with 350 r.p.m.). Afterwards, the mixture was filtered using a syringe filter of porosity of 0.45μm.

School	Classroom	Floor level	Students per m³	Nr Windows/ doors opened	Type of board	Floor material	Ceiling material	Heating device	Dust on surfaces	Nr Cleaning per day	View from the classroom
1	a	Ground	0.1866	2	Chalk	Brick	Slab	No	No	1	Street
	b	Ground	0.1778	2	Chalk	Brick	Slab	No	No	1	Street
2	a	Ground	0.0922	1	Chalk	Brick	Slab	Yes	Yes	1	Patio
	b	Ground	0.0922	3	Chalk	Brick	Slab	Yes	Yes	2	Patio
3	a	First	0.2334	2	Pen	Brick	Slab	Yes	Yes	1	Patio
	b	First	0.2826	0	Chalk	Brick	Slab	Yes	Yes	1	Patio
4	a	First	0.1374	2	Chalk	Wood	Slab	Yes	Yes	1	Street
	b	First	0.1522	1	Chalk	Wood	Slab	Yes	Yes	1	Street
5	a	First	0.1352	3	Chalk	Wood	Slab	Yes	Yes	1	Patio
	b	First	0.1128	3	Chalk	Wood	Slab	Yes	Yes	1	Patio
6	a	Ground	0.1250	3	Chalk	Brick	Slab	Yes	No	2	Patio
	b	First	0.1191	3	Chalk	Brick	Slab	Yes	No	2	Patio
7	a	First	0.0892	1	Chalk	Vinyl	Wood	No	Yes	1	Patio
	b	Basement	0.1126	0	Chalk	Vinyl	Wood	No	Yes	1	Street
8	a	First	0.1221	2	Chalk	Vinyl	Cork	No	Yes	2	Patio
	b	First	0.1221	2	Chalk	Vinyl	Cork	No	Yes	2	Patio
9	a	First	0.1204	3	Chalk	Brick	Slab	Yes	Yes	1	Patio
	b	First	0.1240	3	Chalk	Wood	Slab	Yes	Yes	1	Patio
10	a	First	0.0923	3	Chalk	Wood	False	Yes	Yes	1	Street
	b	First	0.1438	2	Chalk	Wood	Slab	Yes	Yes	1	Patio
11	a	Ground	0.1302	3	Chalk	Brick	Cork	Yes	Yes	2	Street
	b	Ground	0.1270	3	Chalk	Brick	Cork	Yes	Yes	2	Street
12	a	Ground	0.1324	1	Chalk	Vinyl	Slab	No	Yes	2	Street
	b	First	0.1129	1	Pen	Vinyl	Slab	No	Yes	2	Street
13	a	Ground	0.1254	2	Chalk	Brick	Slab	No	Yes	1	Patio
	b	Ground	0.1197	2	Chalk	Brick	Slab	No	Yes	1	Patio
14	a	First	0.1315	2	Chalk	Plastic	Slab	Yes	Yes	1	Patio
	b	First	0.1282	3	Chalk	Vinyl	Slab	Yes	Yes	1	Patio

Table 1. Classrooms characteristics.

The aqueous extract was analyzed by chemical suppressed ion Chromatography (Chow and Watson, 1999) - for Cl^-, NO_3^-, PO_4^{3-}, F^- and SO_4^{2-} - and Flame Atomic Absorption Spectroscopy – for Ca^+, Mg^{2+}, Na^+ and K^+.

2.2.4 VOCs & carbonyls

Volatile Organic Compounds and carbonyls were sampled in parallel using Radiello® diffusive passive tubes (cartridges codes 130 and 165, respectively) for 14 consecutive days in two replicates (Pegas et al., 2010, 2011a, 2011b). Samples were collected at a height of about 1.5 m above the classroom floor. The diffusive samplers were positioned at a distance that exceeded 1m from any window or door.

2.2.4.1 VOCs

The VOC adsorbing cartridges consisted of 60 mm length stainless steel net cylinders, with 100 mesh grid opening and 5.8 mm diameter, packed with 530±30 mg of activated charcoal with a particle size of 35–50 mesh. VOCs were extracted from the exposed samplers with 2 ml of carbon disulfide (CS_2) containing 2-fluorotoluene as an internal standard. The glass vials were shaken for approximately 30 min. The analyses of the extracts were performed by gas chromatography coupled to a flame ionisation detector (GC/FID). The equipment was calibrated before and during the sample analyses by injecting four standard solutions of all compounds identified in CS_2. The analytes in these four standard solutions were present in concentrations of 40 ng μl^{-1}, 20 ng μl^{-1}, 10 ng μl^{-1} and 5 ng μl^{-1}. Depending on the analyte, the limit of detection (LOD = 3.3 (s/S), where s is the STDEV of areas and S is the slope) ranged from 0.34 to 2.52 ng μl^{-1}.
The analyzed VOCs discussed in this study are aliphatic hydrocarbons (2-methylpentane - AC, n-hexane - AD, isooctane - AE, n-heptane - AF), aromatic hydrocarbons (benzene - AW, toluene - AY, ethylbenzene - AZ, m+p-xylene - BA, o-xylene – BC) and cyclohexane – BT.

2.2.4.2 Carbonyls

Carbonyls collected in cartridges filled with 2,4-dinitrophenylhydrazine reacted to result in the corresponding 2,4- dinitrophenylhydrazones. These were extracted with 2 ml of acetonitrile. The glass vials were shaken for approximately 30 minutes and the extract filtered through 0.45 μm disc membrane filters and injected into the high-performance liquid chromatography (HPLC) system. The carbonyl concentrations were quantified with external calibrations curves constructed from standard solutions of TO11/IP6A carbonyl–DNPH Mix. The limit of detection (LOD) ranged from 1.29 to 2.09 $\mu g\ \mu l^{-1}$.
The analyzed carbonyls studied here are alcohols (acetaldehyde – AM, methanol - AP, ethanol - AQ, isopropanol - AR) and cetones (acetone – AK).

2.3 Statistical analysis

Wilcoxon signed rank tests (Hollander & Wolfe, 1973) were used to test differences between seasonal concentrations of the studied parameters. To investigate the association between independent variables (classroom characteristics) and dependent variables (measured parameters), for each dependent variable a linear model was first applied using all the ten independent variables characterizing the classrooms. The independent variables considered are: 1) level of classroom, 2) number of students per m^3, 3) number of windows and doors opened, 4) type of board, 5) floor material, 6) ceiling material, 7) presence of heating device, 8) dusty surfaces, 9) number of cleanings per day, 10) view from classroom. The thirty-one dependent variables analysed are part of one of the following groups: 1) total particle mass, 2) chemical element mass, 3) mass of water soluble ions, 4) VOCs, 5) carbonyls.
Then, the independent variables were taken out from the model, one by one, in order to select the best model. The best model selected was the one that minimized the AIC (Akaike, 1974) and had all terms significant. This analysis was conducted in the statistics package R. All selected models have all terms significant at 5%. The multiple R-squared refers to the fraction of variance explained by the model and was calculated for all selected models.

3. Results

3.1 Seasonal variability

The seasonal variation of total particulate matter is resumed in Fig. 2. The results of the Wilcoxon signed rank tests indicated that the concentration of total particles in the air is lower in the spring than in the autumn ($p=0.001$) and in the winter ($p<0.001$). On the other hand, the tests showed no evidence to suggest a difference in the concentration of total particles in the air between the autumn and the winter ($p=0.76$).

Fig. 3 shows the box plots of Cr, K, Sb, Sc and Zn concentrations in autumn and winter in 28 classrooms of 14 schools. There is evidence to suggest that the air concentration is smaller in the winter than in the autumn for Cr ($p<0.001$), K ($p=0.03$) and Sb ($p=0.016$). On the contrary, there is no evidence supporting a difference between autumn and winter in the concentrations of Sc ($p=0.11$) and Zn ($p=0.22$).

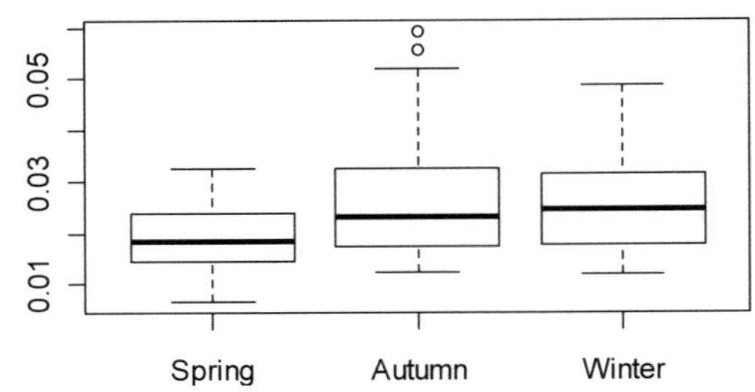

Fig. 2. Boxplot of TPM mass, in mg/day, in three seasons in 28 classrooms of 14 primary schools.

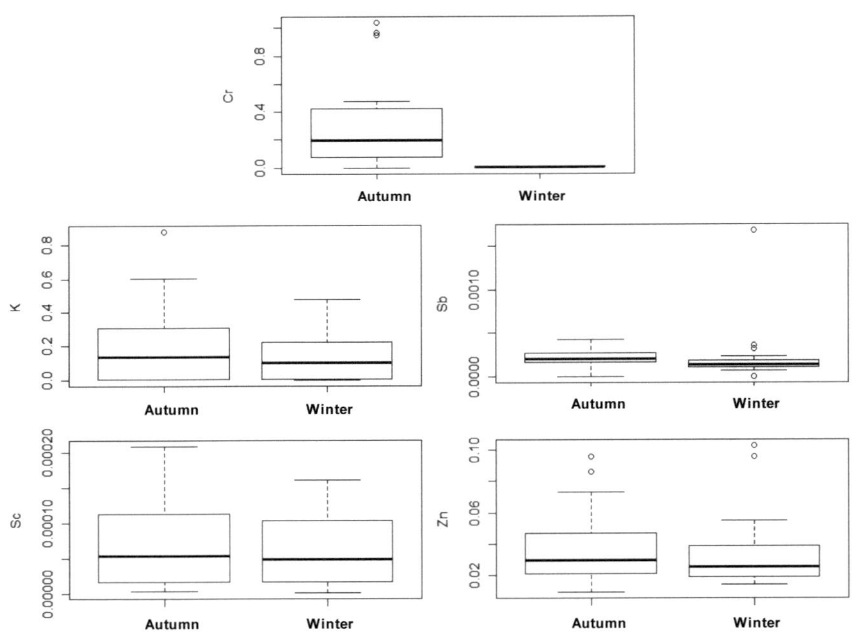

Fig. 3. Box plots of Cr, K, Sb, Sc and Zn concentrations in autumn and winter in 28 classrooms of 14 primary schools.

Figure 4 shows the seasonal variation of isooctane (AE) and acetone (AK). The statistical tests suggested that the air concentrations are larger in the winter than in the autumn for AA ($p<0.001$), AE ($p<0.001$) and AK ($p<0.001$).

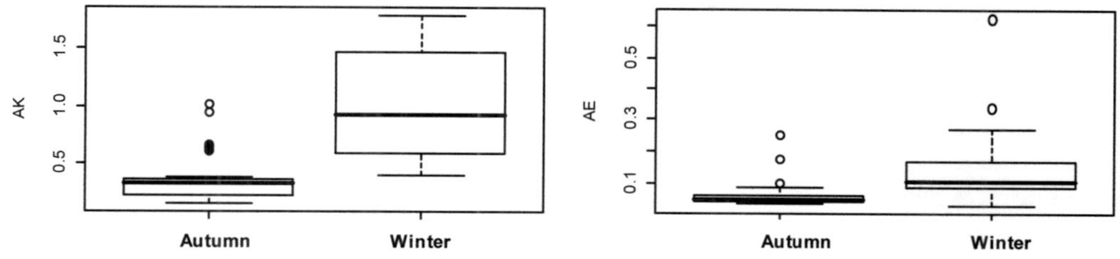

Fig. 4. Box plots of AE and AK concentrations in two seasons in 28 classrooms of 14 primary schools.

Seasonal variation of benzene (AW) and toluene (AY) are shown in Fig. 5. The test results supported that the concentration of AW in the air is lower in the spring than in the autumn ($p<0.001$). There is also evidence that the concentration is smaller in the autumn than in the winter ($p<0.001$). The results indicated no difference in the concentration of AY between the spring and the autumn ($p=0.20$), but suggested that the concentration is smaller in the spring than in winter ($p<0.001$) and also smaller in the autumn than in the winter ($p<0.001$).

3.2 Analysis of the association of the classroom characteristics and the particle mass, water soluble ions, air concentration of certain elements VOCs and carbonyls

The results obtained are summarized in Tables 2-4. The effects (i.e. regression coefficients) are shown for variables with significant effects. Figure 6 illustrates the relation of some of these variables in boxplot charts.

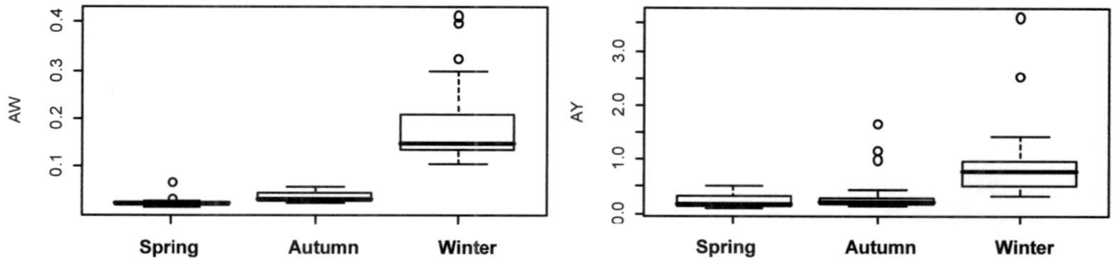

Fig. 5. Box plots of AW and AY concentrations in autumn and winter in 28 classrooms of 14 primary schools.

3.2.1 Mass of total particulate matter

In autumn and winter, 73% and 67% respectively of the variability across classrooms of the particle mass indoor is explained by the studied classroom characteristics. There are negative significant associations with the number of windows opened ($p<0.01$ in autumn; $p<0.05$ in winter) and the existence of heating device ($p<0.001$ in autumn; and $p<0.05$ in winter). Classroom facing the street - as opposed to an inner patio - are associated with lower concentrations of particle mass indoor in both autumn and winter ($p<0.001$ in autumn and $p<0.01$ in winter). The ceiling material ($p<0.001$ in autumn and $p<0.01$ in winter) has also a significant effect, with the results suggesting that wood may be associated with lower levels of particle mass indoor and false ceilings with higher levels of particle mass indoor. Regarding the particle mass in spring, none of the variables is significant at 5%.

3.2.2 Chemical elements in particulate mass

Available measurements for the chemical elements refer all to the autumn season. The classroom characteristics considered in this study explained 57% of the variability of total chromium. Significant effects were found for: (i) the ceiling material ($p<0.05$), with a positive association with wood ceilings, and (ii) the existence of a heating device ($p<0.05$) with lower Cr when devices are present.

According to the value of the multiple R^2, the floor and ceiling materials explain together 52% of the variation of the total antimony (Sb) in particle mass indoor. The significant effects of floor material ($p<0.05$) and the ceiling material ($p<0.01$) suggest lower Sb amount in classrooms with vinyl floors and slab ceilings.

For total scandium (Sc) indoor in particle mass, 57% of its variation is explained by: (i) the number of windows/doors opened ($p<0.05$), which is negatively associated to Sc, (ii) the use of whiteboard with pen ($p<0.01$), which is associated to higher Sc amount, (iii) the ceiling material ($p<0.05$), with slab and wood associated to lower levels of Sc in the classroom, and (iv) the classroom facing the street as opposed to an inner patio, the former being negatively associated to the Sc amount in the classroom ($p<0.05$).

With 55% of the variability explained, the total zinc (Zn) indoor in particle mass displays significant effects for (i) the number of students per cubic meter (positive relation, $p<0.01$), (ii) the existence of a heating device in the classroom, with a negative relation ($p<0.05$), (iii) the dust present in the classroom (negative relation, $p<0.01$), and (iv) the number of cleanings per day (negative relation, $p<0.001$).

For Au and K, the variables studied only explain 16% and 35%, respectively of their variation across classrooms. Higher concentrations of Au are associated with classrooms facing inner patios as opposed to a street ($p<0.05$). Higher concentrations of K are associated with fewer opened windows ($p<0.05$) and cork ceilings ($p<0.05$).

3.2.3 Water-soluble ions in particulate mass

All data on ions were collected in the winter season. The studied classroom characteristics appear to explain a large part of the variability across classrooms of chloride (Cl^-), magnesium (Mg^{2+}) and sodium (Na^+) ions (multiple R^2 equals 0.81, 0.77 and 0.68, respectively). On the contrary, few variation has been explained for the sulphate (SO_4^{2-}) and calcium (Ca^{2+}) ions, as the multiple R^2 are relatively low (0.18 and 0.25, respectively). This suggests that other factors, not included in this study may be responsible for the variability of these ions.

The sodium and chloride ions present significant associations with almost the same group of variables. Namely, both ions present significant associations with the floor level of the classroom ($p<0.05$) suggesting lower concentrations in the ground and 1st floors. The floor and the ceiling materials also have significant effects on these two ions with wooden floors and ceilings presenting the lowest coefficient and thus associated with lower concentrations. False ceilings are, on the contrary, associated with higher concentrations. In addition, the number of cleanings per day also has a significant negative effect (Na^+: $p<0.05$; Cl^-: $p<0.001$), with higher numbers being associated with lower concentrations of the water soluble Na^+ and Cl^- indoor. The results indicate that the use of whiteboard with pen – as opposed to blackboard with chalk

- is associated with higher levels of the soluble ion Cl^- indoor ($p<0.01$) and a larger number of windows/doors opened is associated with lower levels of Na^+ indoors.
Significant effects on water soluble Mg^{2+} and K^+ were found for exactly the same classroom characteristics. The results show significant effects with floor material (Mg^{2+}: $p<0.001$; $K+$: $p<0.01$), ceiling material (Mg^{2+}: $p<0.001$; $K+$: $p<0.05$) and number of cleanings per day (Mg^{2+}: $p<0.01$; $K+$: $p<0.05$). Higher number of cleanings as well as wood in floors and ceilings are associated with lower concentrations of Mg^{2+} and K^+. False ceilings as well as plastic and vinyl floors are associated with higher concentrations.

	Dependent variable							
Independent variables	Particle mass autumn	Particle mass winter	Au autumn	Cr autumn	K autumn	Sb autumn	Sc autumn	Zn autumn
Floor level		p<0.05						
- basement		*0*						
- ground floor		*-0.0342*						
- 1st floor		*-0.0312*						
Students/m³								0.2310**
Nr windows & doors opened	-0.0063**	-0.0050*			-0.1124*		-0.0000331*	
Whiteboard with pen (vs blackboard with chalk)							0.0001064**	
Floor material						p<0.05		
- brick floor						*0*		
- plastic floor						*0.000134*		
- vinyl floor						*-0.000122*		
- wooden floor						*-0.000063*		
Ceiling material	p<0.001	p<0.01		p<0.05	p<0.05	p<0.01	p<0.05	
- cork	*0*	*0*		*0*	*0*	*0*	*0*	
- slab	*-0.0133*	*-0.0091*		*-0.0193*	*-0.2842*	*-0.0001302*	*-0.0000769*	
- false	*0.0088*	*0.0042*		*-0.1652*	*-0.3538*	*-0.0000016*	*-0.0000093*	
- wood	*-0.0353*	*-0.0363*		*0.5571*	*-0.5319*	*0.0000750*	*-0.0001651*	
Heating device	-0.0153***	-0.0089*		-0.2163*				-0.0175*
Dust								-0.0281**
Nr cleanings per day								-0.0265***
Classroom faces street	-0.0159***	-0.0115**	-0.00056*				-0.0000460*	
Multiple R²	0.73	0.67	0.16	0.57	0.35	0.52	0.57	0.55

Table 2. Regression coefficients and their significance for particle mass and elements (significant codes: *** <0.001; ** <0.01; * <0.05).

	Dependent variable								
Independent variables	Ca^{2+} winter	Cl^{-} winter	F^{-} winter	K^{+} winter	Mg^{2+} winter	NO_3^{-} winter	Na^{+} winter	PO_4^{3-} winter	SO_4^{2-} winter
Floor level		p<0.05					p<0.05		
- basement		*0*					*0*		
- ground floor		*-0.6596*					*-0.7448*		
- 1st floor		*-0.5600*					*-0.3035*		
Students/m³									
Nr windows & doors opened							-0.1666*		
Whiteboard with pen (vs blackboard with chalk)		0.4396**	0.1064**			0.1828*		0.2052***	
Floor material		p<0.001		p<0.01	p<0.001	p<0.05	p<0.05		
- brick floor		*0*		*0*	*0*	*0*	*0*		
- plastic floor		*0.3109*		*0.0056*	*0.0459*	*0.0257*	*-0.2721*		
- vinyl floor		*0.1965*		*0.1705*	*0.0431*	*-0.1613*	*-0.1189*		
- wooden floor		*-0.3508*		*-0.1227*	*-0.0358*	*-0.1443*	*-0.5700*		
Ceiling material		p<0.01	p<0.05	p<0.05	p<0.001		p<0.05		
- cork		*0*	*0*	*0*	*0*		*0*		
- slab		*-0.2038*	*-0.0757*	*-0.0530*	*0.0183*		*-0.2732*		
- false		*0.2279*	*-0.0265*	*0.1054*	*0.0600*		*0.3312*		
- wood		-0.7294	*-0.0461*	*-0.2578*	*-0.0439*		*-1.0030*		
Heating device	-0.7883**					-0.1740**			-1.3769*
Dust									
Nr cleanings per day		-0.4039***	-0.0536*	-0.1226*	-0.0273**	-0.1469**	-0.3245*		
Classroom faces street (vs inner patio)			-0.0493**					-0.0587*	
Multiple R²	0.25	0.81	0.54	0.56	0.77	0.64	0.68	0.43	0.18

Table 3. Regression coefficients and their significance for water soluble ions (significant codes: *** <0.001; ** <0.01; * <0.05).

	Dependent variable								
Independent variables	AC winter	AD spring	AE autumn	AE winter	AF spring	AK autumn	AM spring	AP winter	AQ winter
Floor level			p<0.01			p<0.01			p<0.001
- basement			*0*			*0*			*0*
- ground floor			*-0.1111*			*-0.0400*			*-4.3574*
- 1st floor			*-0.0766*			*-0.2712*			*-4.1025*
Students/m³	7.2989***			1.4412**				6.7938***	
Nr windows & doors opened						-0.1083**			0.3988**
Whiteboard with pen (vs blackboard with chalk)									
Floor material		p<0.001			p<0.01				
- brick floor		*0*			*0*				
- plastic floor		*0.2467*			*0.5396*				
- vinyl floor		*-0.0455*			*-0.0671*				
- wooden floor		*0.0047*			*-0.0624*				
Ceiling material			p<0.001			p<0.01			
- cork			*0*			*0*			
- slab			*-0.0829*			*-0.3390*			
- false			*-0.0624*			*-0.0431*			
- wood			*-0.1451*			*-0.4950*			
Heating device		-0.0427*	-0.0561***						
Dust	-0.3884**								
Nr cleanings per day	-0.2329*						0.0919*	-0.2940*	
Classroom faces street (vs inner patio)			-0.0446**			-0.3724***			
Multiple R^2	0.69	0.71	0.80	0.25	0.43	0.70	0.21	0.52	0.66

Table 4. Regression coefficients and their significance for VOCs and carbonyls (significant codes: *** <0.001; ** <0.01; * <0.05).

	Dependent variable							
Independent variables	**AR winter**	**AW autumn**	**AW winter**	**AY autumn**	**AZ spring**	**BA spring**	**BC spring**	**BT autumn**
Floor level		p<0.01		p<0.001				p<0.01
- basement		*0*		*0*				*0*
- ground floor		*-0.0209*		*-1.0466*				*-1.3435*
- 1st floor		*-0.0213*		*-0.8763*				*-0.0700*
Students/m^3		0.0953**						
Nr windows & doors opened							0.0765*	
Whiteboard with pen (vs blackboard with chalk)			0.1659**					
Floor material	p<0.05	p<0.05			p<0.01	p<0.001	p<0.05	
- brick floor	*0*	*0*			*0*	*0*	*0*	
- plastic floor	*-10.600*	*-0.0133*			*0.8501*	*2.6104*	*0.5389*	
- vinyl floor	*-32.898*	*-0.0124*			*-0.0658*	*-0.0758*	*0.0505*	
- wooden floor	*-7.592*	*-0.0052*			*-0.0621*	*-0.0730*	*0.0299*	
Ceiling material			p<0.05	p<0.001				p<0.001
- cork			*0*	*0*				*0*
- slab			*-0.0991*	*-0.4104*				*-2.2013*
- false			*-0.1306*	*-0.0273*				*-2.3441*
- wood			*0.0764*	*0.0460*				*-3.6549*
Heating device	-35.232***	-0.0126***		-0.2995***				-1.3108**
Dust	27.212**	0.0094**	-0.1069*					
Nr cleanings per day			-0.0889*					
Classroom faces street (vs inner patio)		-0.0116***		-0.2173**				
Multiple R^2	0.53	0.82	0.53	0.92	0.46	0.78	0.40	0.69

Table 4. (cont.). Regression coefficients and their significance for VOCs and carbonyls (significant codes: *** <0.001; ** <0.01; * <0.05).

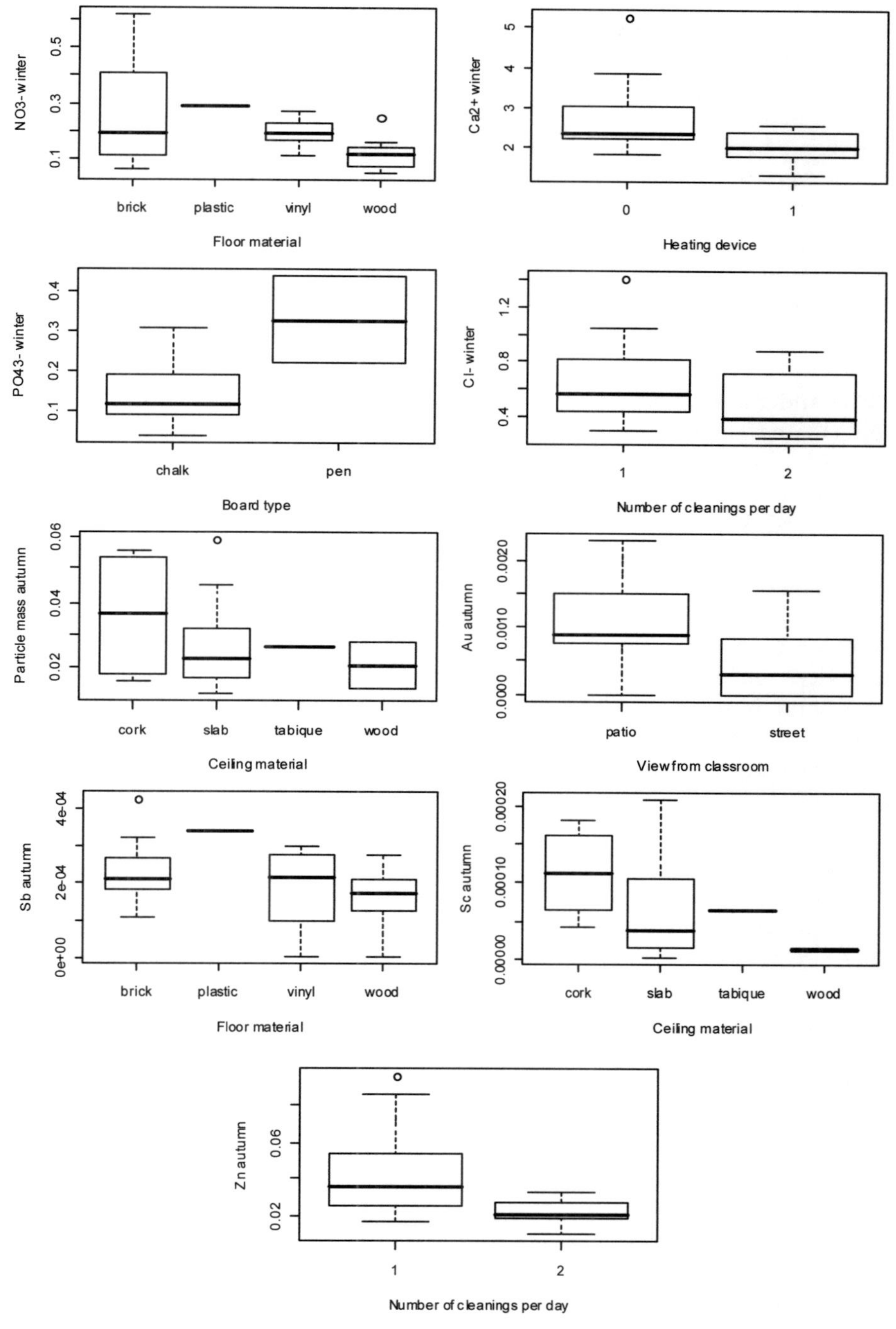

Fig. 6. Boxplot for significant parameters (selected examples).

The results for the water soluble F- indoor indicate significant effects for the use of whiteboard with pen ($p<0.01$), the ceiling material ($p<0.05$), the number of cleanings per day

($p<0.05$), and classroom facing street/inner patio ($p<0.01$). The amount of F^- seems to be lowest in classrooms with slab ceilings, facing the street, using blackboard with chalk and having more cleanings per day.

For the water soluble NO_3^- indoor, significant effects were found for the use of whiteboard with pen versus backboard with chalk ($p<0.05$), the floor material ($p<0.05$), the number of cleaning per day ($p<0.01$) and the presence of a heating device ($p<0.01$). Higher levels of this ion are associated with plastic floors, whereas vinyl and wooden floors, presence of heating device and higher number of cleanings are associated with lower concentrations.

The ion PO_4^{3-} shows significant effects for use of whiteboard with pen ($p<0.001$) and classroom facing street/inner patio ($p<0.05$). Classrooms using whiteboard with pen and facing inner patios are associated with higher concentrations of this ion.

3.2.4 VOCs and carbonyls

Toluene (AY) and isooctane (AE), both collected in autumn, present significant effects for the same variables: floor level ($p<0.001$ for AY; $p<0.01$ for AE), ceiling material ($p<0.001$), heating device ($p<0.001$) and classroom facing street/inner patio ($p<0.01$). These variables explain 92% and 80% of variability of AY and AE, respectively. For both VOCs, higher concentrations are associated with classrooms in the basement, facing inner patios or without heating devices. Classrooms with wooden ceilings are associated with higher levels of AY while classrooms with cork ceilings are associated with higher levels of AE. Lower concentrations of AY and AE are associated with classrooms on the ground floor, with heating devices, facing the street. Classrooms with slab ceilings are associated with lower levels of AY and those with wooden ceilings are associated with lower levels of AE.

No significant effects were found for the spring and winter measurements of AY and the autumn measurement of AE.

Benzene (AW) was measured in spring, autumn and winter, but only the autumn and winter measurements show significant effects with variables considered in this study, which explained 82% and 53%, respectively, of the variation of those measurements. For the autumn measurement, significant effects were found for floor level ($p<0.01$), floor material ($p<0.05$), presence of heating device ($p<0.001$), dust in surfaces ($p<0.01$) and classroom facing the street/inner patio ($p<0.001$). In particular, the effects are positive for dust in surfaces and negative for presence of heating device and classroom facing the street. Classrooms in the basement and with brick floors are associated with higher concentration of AW in autumn.

The concentration of AW in winter was shown to be significantly larger from that in the autumn (see section 3.1) and the set of variables with significant effects is also different. In winter, the floor level, the floor material, the heating device and the classroom facing the street/inner patio are no longer significant. Instead, significant effects were found with the type of board ($p<0.01$), the ceiling material ($p<0.05$), dust ($p<0.05$) and the number of cleanings per day ($p<0.05$). Wooden ceilings, the use of whiteboard with pen, and lower number of cleanings were associated with higher concentration of AW, whereas slab and false ceilings, the use of blackboard with chalk, and higher number of cleanings were associated with lower concentrations of AW. The variable dust, which showed a positive significant effect in autumn, has on the contrary a negative significant effect in the winter.

The m+p xylene (BA) indoor was collected in spring and 78% of its variation is explained by one variable alone, the floor material ($p<0.001$). Classrooms with plastic floors are associated with higher concentrations of this VOC. The n-hexane (AD) indoor, also collected in spring, shows as well a significant effect with floor material ($p<0.001$) and classrooms with plastic floors are again associated with higher concentrations. The presence of a heating device shows too a significant effect ($p<0.05$), with classroom with heating devices associated with lower concentrations. Floor material and heating device explained 71% of the variation of this VOC.

Acetone (AK) was measured in autumn and winter but only the autumn measurements displayed significant effects with the variables studied here, namely floor level ($p<0.01$), number of windows and doors opened ($p<0.01$), ceiling material ($p<0.01$) and classroom facing the street/inner patio ($p<0.001$). Altogether, these four variables explain 70% of the variation of AK in autumn. Higher floors and larger number of windows/doors opened are associated with lower concentrations. The ceiling materials associated with lower concentrations are slab and wood, and those with higher are false ceilings and cork ceilings. Classrooms facing the street are associated with lower concentrations of AK.

Indoor 2-methylpentane (AC) in winter displayed a positive significant effect for the number of students per m^3 ($p<0.001$) and negative significant effects for the number of cleanings per day ($p<0.05$) and for dust ($p<0.01$). These three variables explained 69% of variation of AC.

Cychlohexane (BT), collected in autumn, is significantly associated to floor level ($p<0.01$), ceiling material ($p<0.001$) and existence of heating device ($p<0.01$), which explain 69% of variation of BT. The ground floor is associated with lower concentrations and the basement with higher concentrations; cork ceilings and classrooms without heating devices are associated with higher concentrations.

The model selected for ethanol (AQ) indoor presents two variables with significant effects explaining 66% of the variation of this carbonyl: the floor level ($p<0.001$) - the basement is associated with higher concentrations - and the number of windows opened ($p<0.01$) with higher ethanol indoor associated with larger numbers of opened windows/doors.

The model selected for isopropanol (AR) indoor explains 53% of its variation and contains three variables with significant effects: floor material ($p<0.05$) - vinyl associated to lower concentrations and brick with higher concentrations -, heating device ($p<0.001$) – presence of device associated with lower concentrations – and the existence of dust overall ($p<0.01$) - associated with higher concentrations.

The methanol (AP) indoor displays a positive significant effect for the number of students per cubic meter ($p<0.001$) and a negative significant effect for the number of cleanings per day ($p<0.05$). The two variables explain 52% of the variation of AP.

For all other VOCs and carbonyls, the multiple R^2 is less than 50% and the selected models contain at most two variables with significant effects. It may be worth noting the positive significant effect for students per cubic meter for AE in winter. The floor material shows significant effects in the models for AZ, AF and BC (all collected in spring).

4. Discussion and conclusions

In this study, models were applied to several components of the air to investigate associations with classrooms characteristics. Some patterns emerged across these analyses:

- Classrooms facing a street seem to have lower air concentrations of several components than those facing an inner patio. This could be linked to ventilation issues as inner patios may generate less air movement and consequent accumulation of some components. Classrooms facing the inner patios are associated with higher concentration of Au, Sc, PO_4^{3-}, F^-, isooctane - AE (autumn), acetone - AK, benzene - AW (autumn) and toluene - AY, as well as TPM mass with less particle mass in the autumn and winter.

- Classrooms with higher number of windows/doors opened were associated with less particle mass, K, Sc, acetone - AK and Na^+ in the air, possibly due to increased ventilation. However, a larger number of opened windows/doors was also associated with more o-xylene - BC and ethanol - AQ, which suggests outdoor sources for these two components.
- Crowded classrooms seem to lead to increased concentrations of several components. The density of students per m^3 was found to be positively associated with the concentrations of Zn, 2-methylpentane - AC, methanol - AP, isooctane - AE (winter) and benzene - AW (autumn).
- Classrooms located in basements seem to suffer from accumulation of several components, perhaps due to lack of ventilation. The results indicated that the air of the classrooms in the basement tended to have more particle mass, cyclohexane - BT, ethanol - AQ, isooctane - AE, acetone - AK, benzene - AW (autumn), toluene - AY, Na^+ and Cl^-.
- Cleanings appear to contribute to a decrease in several air components, but to an increase of others. It is possible that some components of the cleaning products pass into the air. Classrooms with higher number of cleanings a day were associated with higher concentrations of acetaldehyde - AM but reduced concentrations of Zn, several ions (Na^+, Cl^-, K^+, NO_3^-, F^-, Mg^{2+}), 2-methylpentane - AC, methanol - AP and benzene - AW (winter).
- The results suggest that the air of dusty classrooms also favours increased concentrations of some elements, VOCs and carbonyls but is associated with lower concentrations of others; no association was found with ions. Namely, dusty classrooms were associated with lower levels of Zn, 2-methylpentane - AC, benzene - AW in winter, but higher levels of isopropanol - AR and benzene - AW in autumn. Although the presence of dust is likely to be due to less thorough cleanings, there may also be accumulation of components in the dust which would be thrown to the air by cleaning tasks.
- The presence of a heating device seems to be related to lower concentrations of a number of components, such as particle mass, Cr, Zn, Ca^{2+}, SO_4^{2-} and NO_3^-; n-hexane - AD, isooctane - AE (autumn), isopropanol - AR, benzene - AW (autumn), toluene - AY (autumn) and cyclohexane - BT. Future analyses on the type and frequency of heating devices used will be needed to reveal the mechanism underlying these associations.
- Chalk and whiteboard pens are expected to liberate distinct substances. The use of whiteboard pens was associated with higher concentrations of Sc, benzene - AW (winter), Cl^-, PO_4^{3-}, NO_3^- and F^-.
- Different construction materials appear to impact on specific elements. Overall, wood seems to lead to a reduced concentration of several elements. Wooden ceilings in particular were associated with lower concentrations of particle mass, K, Sc, cyclohexane - BT, isooctane - AE (autumn) and acetone - AK; wooden ceilings and floors were associated with lower concentrations of Na^+, Cl^-, Mg^{2+} and K^+. Plastic floors on the contrary were associated with higher concentrations of several components,

including Sb; VOCs such as n-hexane - AD, n-heptane - AF, ethylbenzene - AZ, m+p xylene - BA and o-xylene - BC; several ions, like Cl^-, Mg^{2+} and NO_3^-. These results support evidence on the emissions of hazardous substances from buildings and construction materials (WHO, 2010; Carrer et al., 2002), but must be interpreted with caution as there is only one classroom with plastic floor and one school (two classrooms) with wooden ceilings. The significant effects observed could be associated with other factors present in that particular classroom/school.

Few components in this study were measured for more than one season. The seasonal analysis, albeit limited, suggested higher concentrations in winter as compared to spring of particle mass and of two VOCs, benzene - AW and toluene - AY. Spring being the season when windows tend to be open due to higher temperatures, these results suggest that these components get trapped in classrooms for lack of ventilation.

The concentrations of isooctane - AE and acetone – AK as well as benzene - AW and toluene - AY seem to be higher in winter than in autumn. For some elements, namely Cr, K and Sb, the concentrations seem, on the contrary, to be higher in autumn than in winter.

This study suggests the importance of cleaning and ventilation practices as well as construction materials on the indoor air quality in schools. It is known for example that benzene - AW has adverse health effects. The results obtained here suggest that lower concentrations of benzene - AW may be obtained with less crowded and better ventilated classrooms, frequent cleanings and by avoiding the use of whiteboard pens.

Overall, the conclusions of this study point to the following recommendations: 1) classrooms should face streets rather than patios and should not be located in basements, 2) the density of students can affect the indoor environment and should be limited, 3) wooden materials appear to have advantages as building materials due to a lower input of contaminants. In this work, wood did not contribute to an increase of the VOCs, as reported in previous research (Norback et al., 1995). Other factors, like ventilation, cleanings and use of chalk versus whiteboard pens, can reduce or increase specific contaminants inside the classrooms.

Therefore, caution is suggested when deciding on building materials for schools and on school practices, such as cleaning and boards, as these may affect the indoor air which children will breathe for long periods of the day.

5. Acknowledgment

Financial support by Fundação para a Ciência e a Tecnologia (FCT; Portugal) through research contract PTDC/SAU-ESA/65597/2006 is gratefully acknowledged. Dr. Susana Marta Almeida thanks FCT for Ciência 2007 support. The views expressed herein are those of the author(s) and do not necessarily reflect the views of the United Nations.

6. References

Akaike, H. (1974). A new look at statistical model idemtification. *IEEE Transactions on Automatic Control,* AU-19, 716-722.

Allen, A.G. & Miguel, A.H. (1995). Indoor organic and inorganic pollutants: in-situ formation and dry deposition in southeastern Brazil. *Atmospheric Environment*, Vol.29, No.23, pp. 3519-3526, ISSN 1352-2310

Almeida, S.M.; Canha, N.; Silva, A.; Freitas, M.C.; Pegas, P.; Alves, C.; Evtyugina, M. & Pio, C.A. (2010) Children exposure to air particulate matter in indoor of Lisbon primary schools. *Atmospheric Environment*, ISSN 1352-2310 (in press; doi:10.1016/j.atmosenv.2010.11.052).

Bayer, C. W., Crow, S. & Fischer, J. (2000). *Causes of indoor air quality problems in schools. Summary of Scientific Research*, USA: Energy Division Oak Ridge National Laboratory for the U. S. Department of Energy.

Canha, N.; Freitas, M.C.; Almeida, S.M.; Almeida, M.; Ribeiro, M.; Galinha, C. & Wolterbeek, Hh.T. (2010). Indoor school environment: easy and low cost to assess inorganic pollutants. *Journal of Radioanalytical and Nuclear Chemistry*, Vol.286, No.2, pp. 495-500, ISSN 1588-2780

Canha, N.; Almeida, M.; Freitas, M.C.; Almeida, S.M. & Wolterbeek, Hh.T. (2011). Seasonal variation of total particulate matter and children respiratory diseases at Lisbon primary schools using passive methods. *Procedia Environmental Sciences*, Vol.4, pp. 170-183, ISSN 1878-0296

Carrer, P., Kotzias, D., Rameckers, E., Seppanen, O., van Bronswijk, J. & Viegi, G. (2002). *THADE project - Towards healthy air in dwellings in Europe.* European Federation of Allergy and Airways Disease Patients and Associations

Chow, J.C. & Watson, J.G. (1999). In: Landsberger, S. & Creactchman, M. (Eds.), *Elemental Analysis of Airborne Particles. Advances in Environmental, Industrial and Process Control Technologies*, Vol.1 Gordon and Breach Sciences Publishers, USA, pp. 97-137, ISBN 9056996274

Daisey, J.M., Angell, W.J. & Apte, M.G. (2003). Indoor air quality, ventilation and health symptoms in schools: an analysis of existing information. *Indoor Air*, Vol.13, No.1, pp.53–64, ISSN 1600-0668

Dales, R., Liu, L., Wheeler, A.J. & Gilbert, N. (2008). Quality of indoor residential air and health. *Canadian Medical Association Journal*, Vol.179, No.2, pp. 147-152, ISSN 1488-2329

Diário da República, Decreto-Lei n.º79/2006, de 4 de Abril. Available from <http://dre.pt/pdf1sdip/2006/04/067A00/24162468.pdf>.

Estoková, A., Stevulová, N. & Kubincová, L. (2010). Particulate matter investigation in indoor environment. *Global Nest Journal*, Vol.12, No.1, pp. 20-26.

Fang, G., Wu, Y., Chang, S., Huang, S. & Rau, J. (2006). Size distributions of ambient air particles and enrichment factor analyses of metallic elements at Taichung Harbor near the Taiwan Strait. *Atmospheric Research*, Vol.81, No.4, pp. 320-333, ISSN 0169-8095

Fraga, S., Ramos, E., Martins, A., Samúdio, M. J., Silva, G., Guedes, J., Fernandes, E. O. & Barros, H. (2008). Indoor air quality and respiratory symptoms in Porto schools. *Revista Portuguesa de Pneumologia*, Vol.14, No.4, pp. 487-507, ISSN 0873-2159

Franck, U., Herbarth, O., Roder, S., Schlink, U., Borte, M., Diez, U.,Krämer, U. & Lehmann, I. (2011). Respiratory effects of indoor particles in young children are size dependent. *Science of the Total Environment*, Vol.409, No.9, pp. 1621-1631, ISSN 0048-9697

Fromme, H., Twardella, D., Dietrich, S., Heitmann, D., Schierl, R., Liebl, B. & Rüden, H. (2007). Particulate matter in the indoor air of classrooms-exploratory results from Munich and surrounding area. *Atmospheric Environment*, Vol.41, No.4, pp. 854-866, ISSN 1352-2310

Gilli, G., Traversi, D., Rovere, R., Pignata, C. & Schilirò, T. (2007). Airborne particulate matter: Ionic species role in different Italian sites. *Environmental Research*, Vol.103, No.1, pp. 1-8, ISSN 0013-9351

Godoi, R.H.M., Avigo, D.J., Campos, V.P, Tavares, T.M., Marchi, M.R.R., Grieken, R. & Godoi, A.F.L. (2009). Indoor air quality assessment of elementary schools in Curitiba, Brazil. *Water, Air, Soil Pollution : Focus*, Vol.9, No.3-4, pp. 171–177, ISSN 1573-2940

Godwin, C., & Batterman, S. (2007). Indoor air quality in Michigan schools. *Indoor Air*, Vol.17, No. 2, pp. 109-121, ISSN 1600-0668

González-Flecha, B. (2004). Oxidant mechanisms in response to ambient air particles. *Molecular Aspects of Medicine*, Vol.25, No.1 and 2, pp. 169-182, ISSN 0098-2997

Goyal, R. G. & Khare, M. (2009). Indoor-outdoor concentrations of RSPM in classroom of a naturally ventilated school building near an urban traffic roadway. *Atmospheric Environment*, Vol.43, No.38, pp. 6026-6038, ISSN 1352-2310

Grigg, J. (2009). Particulate Matter Exposure in Children. *Proceedings of American Thoracic Society*, Vol.6, No.7, pp. 564-569, ISSN 1546-3222

Guo, H., Lee, S.C., Chan, L.Y. & Li, W.M. (2004). Risk assessment of exposure to volatile organic compounds in different indoor environments. *Environmental Research*, Vol.94, No.1, pp. 57-66, ISSN 0013-9351

Health Effects Institute (2002). HEI Perspectives, available from <http://pubs.healtheffects.org/getfile.php?u=244>

Hodgson, M. (1992). Field studies on the sick building syndrome. *Annals of the New York Academy of Sciences*, Vol.641, pp.21–36, ISSN 0077-8923

Hollander, M. & Wolfe, D.A. (1973). Nonparametric statistical methods. John Wiley & Sons.

Hwang, B., Jaakkola, J. J., Lee, Y., Lin, Y. & Guo, Y. (2006). Relation between air pollution and allergic rhinitis in Taiwanese schoolchildren. *Respiratory Research*, Vol.7, No.1, pp. 1-7, ISSN 1465-9921

ISAAC (1998). Worldwide variation in prevalence of symptoms of asthma, allergic rhinoconjunctivitis, and atopic eczema: ISAAC. *The Lancet*, Vol.351, No.9111, pp. 1225-1232, ISSN 0140-6736

Janssen, N. A., Hoek, G., Brunekreef, B. & Harssema, H. (1999). Mass concentration and elemental composition of PM10 in classrooms. *Occupational Environmental Medicine*, Vol.52, No.7, pp. 482-487, ISSN 1470-7926

Janssen, N., van Vliet, N., Aaarts, F., Harssema, H. & Brunekreef, B. (2001). Assessment of exposure to traffic related air pollution of children. *Atmospheric Environment*, Vol.35, No.22, pp. 3875–3884, ISSN 1352-2310

Jenkins, P. L., Phillips, T. J. & Mulberg, E. J. (1992). Activity patterns of californians : use of and proximity to indoor pollutants sources. *Atmospheric Environment*. Vol.26, No.12, pp.2141-2148, ISSN 1352-2310

Karthikeyan, S. & Balasubramanian, R. (2006). Determination of water-soluble inorganic and organic species in atmospheric fine particulate matter. *Microchemical Journal*, Vol.82, No.1, pp. 49-55, ISSN 1095-9149

Khan, I., Freitas, M. C., Dionísio, I. & Pacheco, A.M.G. (2007). Indoor habits of children aged 5 to years learning at the public basic schools of Lisbon city, Portugal. *Proceedings of the Ninth REHVA World Congress Clima - Well Being Indoors*, ISBN 978-952-99898-2-9

Kim, J., Elfman, L., Wieslander, G., Smedje, G. & Norback, D. (2007). Indoor molds, bacteria, microbial volatile organic compounds and plasticizers in schools - associations with asthma and respiratory symptoms in pupils. *Indoor Air*, Vol.17, No.2, pp. 153-163, ISSN 1600-0668

Kosonen, R. & Tan, F. (2004). The Effect of Perceived Indoor Air Quality on Productivity Loss. *Energy and Buildings*, Vol.36, No.10, pp. 981-986, ISSN 0378-7788

Lee, S.C., Ho, K.F., Chan, L.Y., Zielinska, B. & Chow, J.C. (2001). Polycyclic aromatic hydrocarbons (PAHs) and carbonyl compound in urban atmosphere of Hong Kong. *Atmospheric Environment*, Vol.35, No.34, pp. 5949–5960, ISSN 1352-2310

Lee, S.C., Li, W.M. & Ao, C.H. (2002). Investigation of indoor air quality at residential homes in Hong Kong—case study. *Atmospheric Environment*, Vol.36, No.2, pp. 225–237, ISSN 1352-2310

Lee, S.C., Guo, H., Li, W.M. & Chan, L.Y. (2002). Inter comparison of air pollutant concentrations in different indoor environment in Hong Kong. *Atmospheric Environment*, Vol.36, No.12, pp. 1929–1940, ISSN 1352-2310

Li, W.M., Lee, S.C. & Chan, L.Y. (2001). Indoor air quality at nine shopping malls in Hong Kong. *Science of the Total Environment*, Vol.273, No.1-3, pp. 27–40, ISSN 0048-9697

Lunden, M. M., Revzan, K.L., Fischer, M.L., Thatcher, T.L., Littlejohn, D., Hering, S. V. & Brown, N. J. (2003). The transformation of outdoor ammonium nitrate aerosols in the indoor environment. *Atmospheric Environment*. Vol.37, pp. 5633-5644, ISSN 1352-2310

Mendell, M. & Heath, G. (2005). Do indoor pollutants and thermal conditions in schools influence student performance? A critical review of the literature. *Indoor Air*, Vol.15, No.1, pp. 27-52, ISSN 1600-0668

Mysliwiec, M.J. & Kleeman, M.J. (2002). Source apportionment of secondary airborne particulate matter in a polluted atmospheric. *Environmental Science & Technology*, Vol.36, No.24, pp. 5376-5384, ISSN 0013-936X

Norback, D., Bjornsson, E., Janson, C. & Boman, G. (1995). Asthmatic symptoms and volatile organic compounds, formaldehyde and carbon dioxide in dwellings. *Occupational and Environmental Medicine*, Vol.52, No.6, pp. 388-395, ISSN 1470-7926

Pegas, P.N.; Evtyugina, M.G.; Alves, C.A.; Nunes, T.; Cerqueira, M.; Franchi, M. & Pio, C.A. (2010). Outdoor/Indoor air quality in primary schools in Lisbon: a preliminary study. *Química Nova*, Vol.33, No.5, pp. 1145-1149, ISSN 1678-7064

Pegas, P.N.; Alves, C.A.; Evtyugina, M.G.; Nunes, T.; Cerqueira, M.; Franchi, M.; Pio, C.A.; Almeida, S.M.; Cabo Verde, S. & Freitas, M.C. (2011a). Seasonal evaluation of outdoor/indoor air quality in primary schools in Lisbon. *Journal of Environmental Monitoring*, Vol. 13, pp. 657-667, ISSN 1464-0333

Pegas, P.N.; Alves, C.A.; Evtyugina, M.G.; Nunes, T.; Cerqueira, M.; Franchi, M.; Pio, C.A.; Almeida, S.M. & Freitas, M.C. (2011b). Indoor air quality in elementary schools of Lisbon in spring. *Environmental Geochemistry and Health*, ISSN 1573-2983 (in press; doi:10.1007/s10653-010-9345-3).

Ramachandran, G., Adgate, J. L., Banerjee, S., Church, T. R., Jones, D., Fredrickson, A. & Sextond, K. (2005). Indoor air quality in two urban elementary schools - measurements of airborne fungi, carpet allergens, CO_2, temperature and relative humidity. *Journal of Occupational and Environmental Hygienne*, Vol.2, No.1, pp. 553-566, ISSN 1545-9632

Saliba, N. A., Atallah, M. & Al-Kadamany, G. (2009). Levels and indoor-outdoor relatioship of PM10, and soluble inorganic ions in Beirut, Lebanon. *Atmospheric Research*, Vol.92, No.1, 131-137, ISSN 0169-8095

Schlesinger, R. B., & Cassee, F. (2003). Atmospheric secondary inorganic particulate matter: the toxicological perspective as a basics for health effects risk assessment. *Inhalation Toxicology*, Vol.15, No.3, pp. 197-235, ISSN 1091-7691

Spangler, J. D., & Sexton, K. (1983). Indoor air pollution: A public health perspective. *Science*, Vol.221, No.4605, pp.9–17, ISSN 1095-9203

Stranger, M., Potgieter-Vermaak, S. & Van Grieken, R. (2007a). Comparative overview of indoor air quality in Antwerp, Belgium. *Environment International*, Vol.33, No.6, pp. 789–797, ISSN 0160-4120

Stranger, M., Potgieter-Vermaak, S. & Van Grieken, R. (2007b). Characterization of indoor air quality in primary schools in Antwerp, Belgium. *Indoor Air*, Vol.18, No.6, pp. 454-463, ISSN 1600-0668

Tippayawong, N., Khuntong, P., Nitatwichit, C., Khunatorn, Y. & Tantakitti, C. (2009). Indoor/outdoor relationships of size-resolved particle concentrations in naturally ventilated school environments. *Building and Environment*, Vol.44, No.1, pp. 188-197, ISSN 0360-1323

Unites States Environmental Protection Agency (EPA). (2010). Managing Asthma in the School Environment - Indoor air quality tools for schools, available from <http://www.epa.gov/iaq/schools>.

Wilson, R., & Spengler, J. (1996). Particles in Our Air: Concentrations and Health Effects. Boston, Vol.25, ISBN: 978-0674240773

Wheeler, L., Buckley, R., Gerald, L. B., Merkle, S. & Morrison, T. A. (2009). Working with schools to improve pediatric asthma management. *Pediatric Asthma, Allergy & Immunology*, Vol.22, No.4, pp. 197-207, ISSN 08831874

Wolkoff, P. (1999). How to measure and evaluate volatile organic compound emissions from building products. A perspective. *The Science of the Total Environment*, Vol.227, No.2-3, pp. 197-213, ISSN 0048-9697

Wolkoff, P., Schneider, T., Kildeso, J., Degerth, R., Jaroszewski, M. & Schunk, H. (1998). Risk in cleaning: chemical and physical exposure. *The Science of the Total Environment*, Vol.215, No. 1-2, pp. 135-156, ISSN 0048-9697

World Health Organization. (n.d.). Children aged 0-4 years living in households using biomass fuels or coal as the main source of heating and cooking, available from <http://www.who.int/ceh/indicators/0_4biomassfuels.pdf>.

World Health Organization (WHO) (2010), Guidelines for indoor air quality - selected pollutants. Denmark, ISBN 978 92 890 0213 4.

Viegas, S. & Prista, J. (2010). Formaldehyde in Indoor Air: A Public Health Problem?. *WIT Transactions on Ecology and the Environment*, Vol. 136, ISSN 1743-

Part 3

Polluted Environment and Its Influence on Elderly People Health

21

Do Socio-Demographic Characteristics Modify the Association Between Air Pollution and Mortality & Morbidity?

Sabit Cakmak[1], Sara L. Martin[4], Claudia Blanco Vidal[2], Timur Gultekin[3], Vladislav Brion[4] and Maria Angelica Rubio[5]
[1]Health Canada, Ottawa, Department of Statistics,
[2]Area Descontaminacion Atmosferica,
Comisión Nacional del Medio Ambiente (CONAMA),
[3]Department of Anthropology, Ankara University,
[4]Health Canada, Ottawa, Department of Statistics
[5]Departamento de Ciencias del Ambiente, Facultad de Química y Biología,
Universidad de Santiago de Chile
Centro de Desarrollo para la Nanociencia y Nanotecnología (CEDENNA),
[1,4]Canada
[2,5]Chile
[3]Turkey

1. Introduction

Historical extreme air pollution events such as those experienced in London in the 1950s and 60s clearly demonstrated the potential of ambient air pollution to cause exacerbation of cardio-respiratory disease, manifested as pre-mature mortality and admission to hospital. In the intervening years, considerable efforts have been made to reduce pollution from the combustion of fossil fuels and industrial activity. Although these pollution mitigation strategies have been largely viewed as successful, evidence from population health studies in North America, Europe, South America, Mexico, Asia, Australia and New Zealand continues to identify ambient air quality as a population health concern (Table 1).

Reference	Data	Location	Focus	Outcomes	Subpop.
Alberdi et al., 1998	1986-1992	Madrid, Spain	TSP, SO_2	NA, R, CV	Sex, Age >65
Alberdi et al., 1998b	1986-1992	Madrid, Spain	TSP, SO_2	NA, R, CV	Sex, Age >65
Anderson et al., 1996	1987-1992	London, England	BS, SO_2, NO_2, O_3	NA, R, CV	
Bachárová et al., 1996	1987-1991	Slovak Republic	TSP, SO_2	A, NA, R, CV	
Ballester et al., 1996	1991-1993	Valencia, Spain	TSP, SO_2	NA, R, CV	Age >70

Borja-Aburto et al., 1997	1990-1992	Mexico City, Mexico	O_3, SO_2, TSP	A, NA, R, CV	Age
Borja-Aburto et al., 1998	1993-1995	Mexico City, Mexico	$PM_{2.5}$	NA, R, CV	Age >65
Boucher et al., 1996	1985-1993	Salt Lake and Utah counties, U.S.	PM_{10}	NA	
Burnett et al., 1998	1980-1994	Toronto, Canada	CO, NO_2, SO_2, TSP, $PM_{2.5}$, PM_{10}	NA, R, CV, O	Age
Burnett et al., 1998b	1980-1991	11 Canadian Cities	CO, NO_2, SO_2, O_3	NA	
Burnett et al., 2000	1986-1996	8 Canadian Cities	$PM_{2.5}$, PM_{10}, $PM_{10-2.5}$	NA	
Castillejos et al., 2000	1992-1995	Mexico City, Mexico	$PM_{2.5}$, PM_{10} $PM_{10-2.5}$	NA	
Chock et al., 2000	1989-1991	Pittsburg, Pennsylvania, U.S.	$PM_{2.5}$, PM_{10}	NA, R, CV	Age
Cifuenties et al, 2000	1988-1996	Santiago, Chile	$PM_{2.5}$, PM_{10}, CO, NO_2, SO_2, O_3	NA	
Dab et al., 1996	1987-1992	Paris, France	BS, SO_2, O_3, NO_2, PM_{13}	R morbidity and mortality	
Daniels et al., 2000	1987-1994	20 cities, U.S.	PM_{10}	A, CV	
Díaz et al., 1999	1990-1996	Madrid, Spain	TSP, SO_2, NO_2, NO_x, O_3	R, CV, Emergency hospital admission (94-96)	
Dockery et al., 1992	1985-1986	St. Louis, Illinois and Missouri; Roanne county, Tennessee	$PM_{2.5}$, PM_{10},, Aerosols	Mortality	
Fairley, 1990	1980-1986	Santa Clara County, California	PM_{10}	NA	
Fairley, 1999	1989-1996	Santa Clara County, California	$PM_{2.5}$	NA, R, CV	
Reference	Data	Location	Focus	Outcomes	Subpop.
Goldberg et al., 2000	1995-1999	Montreal, Quebec	predicted $PM_{2.5}$	NA, CV, C	Age

Gouveia& Fletcher, 2000	1991-1993	São Paulo, Brazil	$PM_{2.5}$, PM_{10}, CO, NO_2, SO_2, O_3	NA, R, CV	Socioeco. sex, age
Hales et al., 2000	1988-1993	Christchurch, New Zealand	PM_{10}, NO_x, SO_2, O_3, CO	NA, R, CV	Age >65
Gwynn et al., 2000	1988-1990	Buffalo, New York, U.S.	H^+ and SO_4^{2-} PM	R, CV and A mortality and morbidity	
Hatzakis et al., 1986	1975-1982	Athens, Greece	BS, SO_2	Mortality	
Hoek et al., 1997	1983-1991	Rotterdam, Netherlands	TSP, BS, SO_2, O_3, CO	Mortality	
Hoek et al., 2000	1986-1994	The Netherlands	PM_{10}, BS	NA, R, CV	
Hong et al., 1999	1995-1996	Inchon, South Korea	PM_{10}, SO_2,CO, O_3	NA, R, CV	
Ito et al., 1993	1965-1972	London, England	BS, $S0_2$, Acidic Aerosols	Mortality	
Ito et al., 1995	1985-1990	Cook County, Illinois and Los Angeles County, California, U.S.	PM_{10}	Mortality	
Ito et al., 1996	1985-1990	Cook County, Illinois, U.S.	PM_{10}	R, CV, C	Age, Sex, Race
Kelsall et al., 1997	1974-1988	Philadelphia, Pennsylvania, U.S.	TSP	NA, R, CV	Age
Kinney & Özkaynak, 1991	1970 - 1979	Los Angeles, County, California, U.S.	O_x, SO_4, NO_2, CO	NA, R, CV	
Kinney et al., 1995	1985-1990	Los Angeles, County, California, U.S.	PM_{10}	NA	
Klemm & Mason, 2000	1998-1999	Atlanta, Georgia, U.S.	$PM_{2.5}$	NA	Age (>65)
Kotesovec et al., 2000	1982-1994	Northern Bohemia, Czech Republic	TSP, SO_2	A, CV and C	Sex, Age
Krzyzanowski & Wojtyniak 1991/92	1977-1989	Cracow, Poland	SO_2, PM_{20}	NA, R, CV	Sex, Age
Le Tertre et al., 1998	1987-1990	Paris, France	$S0_2$	Mortality	

Lee et al., 1999	1991-1995	Seoul and Ulsan, South Korea	TSP, SO_2, O_3	NA	
Lee et al., 2000	1991-1997	7 South Korean cities	TSP, SO_2, O_3	NA	
Reference	Data	Location	Focus	Outcomes	Subpop.
Lipfert et al., 2000	1992-1995	Philadelphia, Pennsylvania	TSP	Mortality	
Lippmann et al., 2000	Various	Detroit, Michigan, U.S.	H^+ and SO_4^{2-} PM	Mortality and elderly morbidity	Age
Lyon et al., 1995	1985-1992	Utah County, U.S.	PM_{10}	NA, R, CV, O	Age
Machenbach et al., 1993	1979-1987	The Netherlands	$S0_2$	Mortality	
Mar et al., 2000	1995-1997	Phoenix, Arizona, U.S.	$PM_{2.5}$, PM_{10}, $PM_{10-2.5}$	NA, R, CV	
Michelozzi et al., 1998	1992-1995	Rome, Italy	PM_{10}, SO_2, O_3, NO_2, CO	Mortality	
Moolgavak, 2000	1987-1995	3 U.S. Counties	PM_{10}, CO, O_3	NA, R, CV	
Moolgavakar et al., 1995	1974–1984	Steubenville, Ohio, U.S.	TSP, SO_2	NA	
Moolgavakar et al., 1995b	1973-1988	Philadelphia, Pennsylvania, U.S.	TSP, SO_2,O_3	NA	
Morgan et al., 1998	1989-1993	Sydney, Australia	PM, NO_2, O_3	NA, R, CV	
Ostro, 1995	1980-1986	California, U.S.	$PM_{2.5}$	NA, R, CV	
Ostro et al., 1996	1989-1991	Santiago, Chile	PM_{10}	NA, R, CV	Age >65
Ostro et al., 1999	1989-1992	Coachella Valley, California, U.S.	PM_{10}	NA, R, CV	
Ostro et al., 1999b	1992-1995	Bangkok, Thailand	PM_{10}	R, CV	Age
Ostro et al., 2000	1989-1998	Coachella Valley, California, U.S.	PM_{10}	NA, R, CV	
Peters et al., 2000	1982-1991	Coal districts, Czech Republic;Bavarian districts, Germany	TSP, SO_2, $PM_{2.5}$, PM_{10}	NA, R(Czech Republic only), CV	
Pope et al., 1992	1985-1989	Utah County	PM_{10}	NA, R, CV, O	
Pope et al., 1996	1985-1989	Utah County	PM_{10}	NA, R, CV, O	

Pope et al., 1999	1985-1995	Wasatch Front, Utah	PM_{10}	NA, R, CV, O	
Rahlenbeck & Kahl, 1996	1981-1989	East Berlin, Germany	TSP, SO_2	NA	
Rossi et al., 1999	1980-1989	Milan, Italy	TSP, SO_2, NO_2, PM_{13}	NA, R, CV	
Saldiva et al., 1995	1990-1991	São Paulo, Brazil	PM_{10}	NA	
Samet et al., 1998	1973-1980	Philadelphia, Pennsylvania	TSP, SO_2	NA	
Reference	Data	Location	Focus	Outcomes	Subpop.
Samet et al., 2000	1987-1994	20 cities, U.S.	PM_{10}	NA, R, CV	
Schwartz & Dockery, 1992	1974–1984	Steubenville, Ohio	TSP, SO_2	NA	
Schwartz & Dockery, 1996	1973-1980	Philadelphia, Pennsylvania	TSP, SO_2	NA, R, CV	Age
Schwartz et al., 1990	1958-1972	London, England	BS, SO_2	Non-traumatic	
Schwartz, 1991	1973-1982	Detroit, Michigan, U.S.	TSP	NA	
Schwartz, 1993	1985-1988	Birmingham, Alabama, U.S.	PM_{10}	NA	
Schwartz, 1994	1977 - 1982	Cincinnati, Ohio, U.S.	TSP	A, R, CV	Age >65
Schwartz, 2000	1986-1993	10 cities, U.S.	PM_{10}	Mortality	Socioeco.
Schwartz, 2000b	1986-1993	10 cities, U.S.	PM_{10}	Mortality	Age >65
Schwartz, 2000c	1979-1986	Boston, Massachusetts, U.S.	$PM_{2.5}$	A, R, CV	
Schwartz, 2000d	1974-1988	Philadelphia, Pennsylvania	TSP and SO2	NA	
Simpson et al., 1997	1987-1993	Brisbane, Australia	PM_{10}, SO_2, O_3	NA, R, CV	Age >65
Simpson et al., 2000	1991-1996	Melbourne, Australia	$PM_{2.5}$, PM_{10}	NA, R, CV	Age
Smith et al., 1999	Various	Alabama & Illinois, U.S.	PM_{10}	Mortality	Age >65
Spix & Wichmann, 1996	1976-1985	Köln, Germany	TSP, SO_2, NO_2	Mortality	
Spix et al., 1993	1980-1989	Erfurt, Germany	TSP, SO_2	Mortality	

Styer et al., 1995	1985-1990	Utah, U.S.	PM_{10}	NA	Age, Sex, Race
Sunyer et al., 1996	1985-1991	Barcelona, Spain	BS, NO_2, SO_2, O_3	NA, R, CV	Age >70
Szafraniec et al., 1997	1993-1996	Kraków, Poland	SO_2, PM_{10}	NA, CV	Sex
Tobias & Campbell, 1999	1991-1995	Barcelona, Spain	BS	Mortality	
Touloumi et al., 1994	1984-1988	Athens, Greece	BS, CO, SO_2	Mortality	
Touloumi et al., 1996	1987-1991	Athens, Greece	BS, CO, SO_2	Mortality	
Touloumi et al., 1997	Various	6 European Cities	NO_2, O_3	Mortality	
Vigotti et al., 1996	1980-1989	Milan, Italy	TSP, SO_2	Respiratory morbidity	
Reference	Data	Location	Focus	Outcomes	Subpop.
Wichmann et al., 2000	1991-2002	Erfurt, Germany	CO, NO_2, SO_2, O_3, PM_{10}	Mortality	
Wietlishbach et al., 1996	1984-1989	Zurich, Basle and Geneva, Switerland	TSP, CO, NO_2, SO_2, O_3	NA, R, CV	Age >65
Wojtyniak & Piekarski, 1996	Various	Cracow, Lodz, Poznan and Wroclaw, Poland	SO_2, BS	NA, R, CV, D	
Wordley et al., 1997	1992-1994	Brimingham, U.K.	PM_{10}	R,CV morbidity	
X. Xu et al., 1994	1989	Dongchen and Xichen, Beijing, China	TSP, SO_2	NA, R, CV, C	
Z. Y. Xu et al., 2000	1992	Shenyang, China	TSP, SO_2	NA, R, CV, C, O	
Zanobetti & Schwartz, 2000	1986-1993	4 U.S. cities	PM_{10}	NA	Sex, Race, Edu.
Zmirou et al., 1996	1985-1990	Lyon, France	$S0_2$, NO_2, O_3, PM_{13}	NA, R, CV, D	

Table 1. Selected references examining air quality and health outcomes around the world with information on the years in which data was collected, as well as the location, the compounds, the health outcomes and subpopulations studied. In the compound column BS indicates black smoke and TSP indicates total suspended particulates. Cause of death categories studied in each paper were coded as A (accidental), NA (Non-accidental), R (respiratory including lung and chronic obstructive pulmonary disease), CV (cardiovascular or circulatory diseases), C (cancer), D (digestive system) and O (other).

Previous work that has found increases in morbidity and mortality are associated with both ambient air pollution and low socio-economic status (Dockery & Pop, 2002; Brunekreef & Holgate, 2002; Bascom et al., 1996; Hahn et al., 1996; Carr et al., 1992, Chen et al., 2001).
However, the literature regarding the effect of age, gender, and social status is conflicting with some studies documenting increased susceptibility studies (Cifuentes et al., 1999; Wojtyniak & Wysocki, 1989; Health Effects Institute[HEI], 2000; Pope, 2000) and others finding little or no effect (Gouveia & Fletcher, 2000; Samet et al., 2000; Zanobetti et al., 2000). A variety of factors have been implicated in the increased susceptibility to air pollution among the socially disadvantaged including, higher pollutant levels in living or working areas, increased cigarette smoking, fewer dietary fruits and vegetables, and reduced access to medical care (O'Neill et al., 2003, Sexton et al. 1993). However, identification of subgroups which are more susceptible to the effects of air pollution is important for three reasons: 1) developing targeted intervention programs; 2) determining whether the air pollution-health effects found in one region can be extrapolated to other geographic regions; 3) setting effective air pollution policies that reduce risk for the entire population. This study investigates whether age, gender and an indicator of social status - educational attainment - modify the effect of particulate air pollution on mortality.

2. Methods

2.1 Air pollution data

Daily air pollution data for the nine communities (communas) that make up the Conception Region (Fig. 1.), Tomé, Penco, Talcahuano, Hualpén, Concepción, San Pedro de la Paz, Chiguayante, Lota, and Coronel, were obtained from monitoring stations located within each of the centers (Fig. 2.). We obtained information for the period from 1 January 2000 to 31 December 2009, although some stations had information for only a subset of these dates. The information collected was the average concentration of particulate matter with mass median aerodynamic diameter less than 10 microns (PM_{10}) over 24 hour periods

2.2 Mortality and sociodemographic data

The daily number of non-accidental deaths (ICD-9 <800) in the study areas were obtained from the Instituto Nacional de Estadisticas, the official source of statistical data in Chile from 1 January 2000 to 31 December 2009 for all nine areas. The daily number of hospitalizations were obtained for five of the areas under study: Tomé, Talcahuano, Concepción, , Lota, and Coronel for the period of January 1 2006 to December 31 2007. Age, gender, and individual educational attainment data were obtained from the Departamento de Estadísticas e Información en Salud (DEIS).

2.3 Statistical medhods

We used time series analyses and assumed both a Poisson distribution and that there was a linear association between ambient air pollution and mortality or morbidity on a logarithmic scale (Rupprecht et al., 1995).
Natural splines were created for air pollution concentrations on the day of study with one knot for each of 15, 30, 60, 90, 120, 180, and 365 days of observation. We then selected the model with the number of knots that either minimized the Akaike Information Criteria

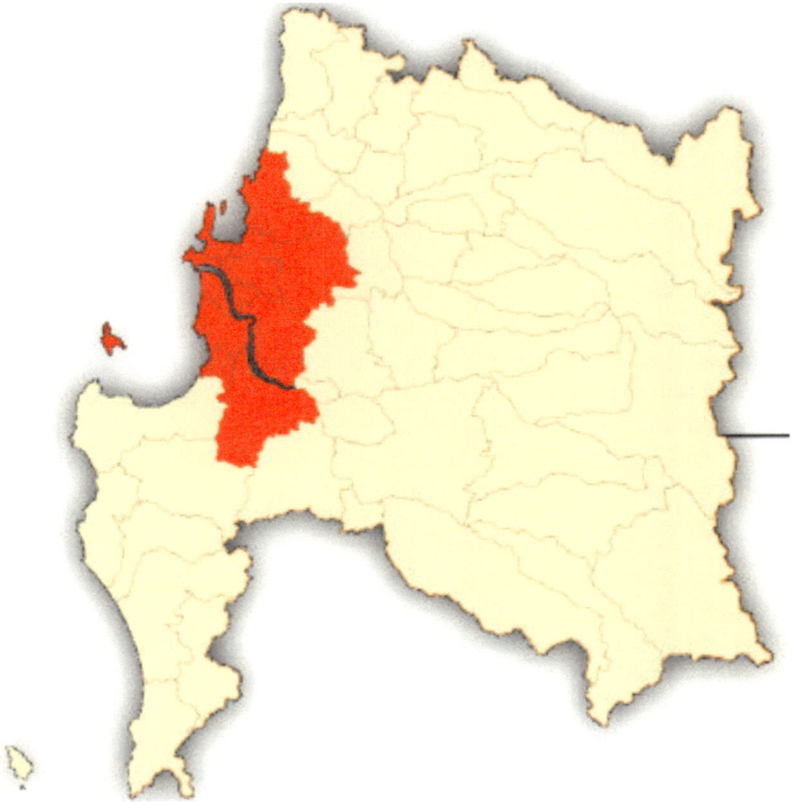

Fig. 1. Map of Chile. The red area on the map has been declared a non-attainment zone because of failure to maintain daily PM_{10} concentrations below a standard threshold. The area includes nine communities with a population of 1 million inhabitants.

(AIC), a measure of model prediction, or maximized the evidence that the model residuals did not display any type of structure, including serial correlation, using Bartlett's test (Lindstrom & Bates, 1990; Priestly, 1981). We plotted model residuals against time and found neither a pattern nor a significant correlation between air pollution and time. Once we had selected the optimal model for time, we assessed the value of including terms for the twenty-four hour means of temperature, humidity, and barometric pressure. The best meteorological predictors of death were temperature and humidity while humidex (Metererological Service of Canada, 2000), a composite measure of temperature and humidity, was the best meteorological predictor of morbidity. We considered temperature and humidex readings on the day of death and the day prior to death and accounted for non-linear associations with death by using natural spline functions. Indicator functions for the day-of-the-week were also included. The association between air pollutants and death was tested at lags of zero to seven days and results were presented for the lags which maximized the effect size. Results from each urban center were pooled using a random effects model.

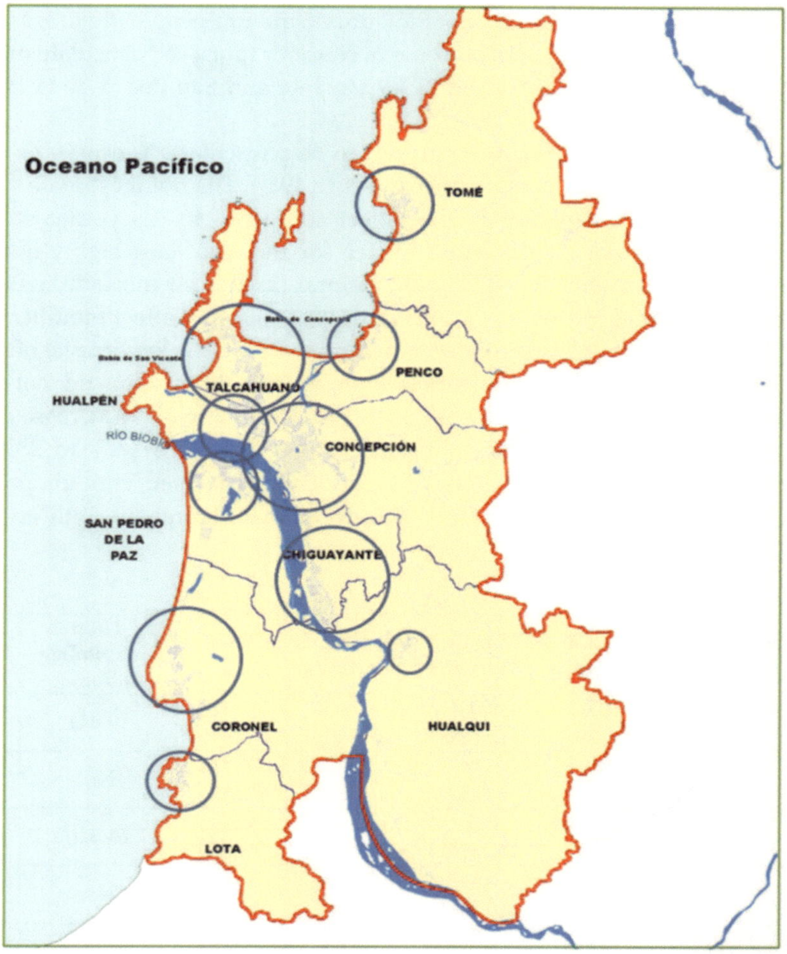

Fig. 2. Detailed Map of Chile. The locations of ten metropolitan areas highlighted in circles

Here we present the increase in relative risk (RR) of mortality or morbidity with 95% confidence intervals for an increase in PM_{10} concentration equal to the interquartile range of the pollutant's concentration over the period of study. The interquartile range includes the middle fifty-percent of the exposure data and provides a realistic estimate of the day-to-day changes in the pollutant's concentration. The interquartile range is a nonparametric measure of the data's spread and, as such, is not influenced by skewed data, extreme values or outliers which are unstable and infrequently seen. A random effects model was used to pool the estimates of relative risk following a DerSimonian- Laird test for homogeneity among estimates.

3. Results

Regional population sizes varied by over fourfold from 49,923 in Penco to 224,212 in Conception (Table 2). The number of daily deaths varied by four to fivefold between

Conception and Penco. In the population of about one million people, there was an average of 15 deaths per day. The twenty-four hour mean concentrations of particulate matter varied by about 50% - 60% between regions with Chiguayante and San Pedro de la Paz reaching the greatest concentrations of PM_{10} (Table 2).

Risk of mortality from cardiac disease appeared to be particularly sensitive to increases in air pollution with an estimated increase of 26% (7% to 49%). The point estimate for mortality relative risk was somewhat greater in the oldest compared to the youngest age group, however, the effect was not significantly greater for those at least eighty-five years old compared to less than sixty-five ($p > 0.05$). The point estimates for mortality risk from PM_{10} were similar for males and females ($p > 0.05$) indicating a lack of effect modification by sex. The effect of PM_{10} on mortality was greatest among those with the lower level of educational attainment. An interquartile increase in pollutants among those who did not complete a college or university degree was associated with a 16.8% (3% to 33%) increase in mortality whereas among college and university graduates there was 13% (-1% to 28%) increase, which was not statistically significant. The risk of death associated with air pollution was particularly high among the elderly with low educational attainment with an increase of 19% (3% to 35%).

	Population 100,000s	Total Mortality	Cardiac Mortality	Respiratory Mortality	PM_{10} (μg/m³)	Total Hospitalization	Temperature
Tomé	5.47	0.935 (0.964)	0.081 (0.288)	0.285 (0.539)	47.613 (45.975)	12.441	12.592 (4.388)
Penco	4.99	0.681 (0.819)	0.067 (0.262)	0.175 (0.423)	56.118 (49.525)	NA	12.592 (4.388)
Talcahuano	17.13	3.010 (1.832)	0.264 (0.526)	0.791 (0.921)	50.030 (28.060)	61.760	13.355 (5.871)
Hualpén	8.8	1.272 (1.131)	0.113 (0.343)	0.346 (0.578)	34.645 (19.025)	NA	13.355 (5.871)
Concepción	22.42	3.487 (1.939)	0.321 (0.570)	1.006 (1.002)	41.734 (23.350)	101.414	13.355 (5.871)
San Pedro	8.92	0.975 (1.006)	0.070 (0.265)	0.269 (0.524)	56.118 (49.525)	NA	13.355 (5.871)
Chiguayante	9.98	1.042 (1.022)	0.091 (0.298)	0.302 (0.544)	56.118 (49.525)	NA	12.852 (3.101)
Lota	4.89	1.126 (1.077)	0.100 (0.320)	0.293 (0.544)	49.778 (31.325)	15.047	12.852 (3.101)
Coronel	10.31	1.344 (1.173)	0.129 (0.365)	0.358 (0.610)	52.148 (29.500)	22.280	12.852 (3.101)

Table 2. Population size, mean daily total mortality, 24-hour mean daily air pollution levels and 24-hour mean weather for nine urban centers in Chile from January 2000 to December 2009. Mean daily total mortality rates and 24 hour mean weather variables are accompanied by their standard deviation, while the interquartile range is reported for the concentration of PM_{10}.

When regions were pooled, an interquartile increase in concentration of PM_{10} was associated with a 5.5% (0.3% to 11%) increased risk of death from all causes (Table 3).

		Relative Risk
Mortality	All Causes	1.055 (1.003, 1.109)
	Cardiac	1.260 (1.065, 1.490)
	Respiratory	1.041 (1.024, 1.076)
Sex	Male	1.043 (1.020, 1.085)
	Female	1.061 (1.024, 1.099)
Age	< 64	1.053 (1.013, 1.096)
	65 - 74	1.048 (1.007, 1.089)
	85 +	1.061 (1.016, 1.107)
Education	< College	1.168 (1.029, 1.325)
	> College	1.130 (0.998, 1.280)
Ages > 85 & lowest educational strata		1.190 (1.031, 1.349)

Table 3. Increase in relative risk of mortality by age group, sex, educational attainment, associated with an interquartile increase in PM_{10} adjusted for long-term trends, day-of-the-week, and temperature and humidity for nine urban centers in Chile from January 2000 to December 2009.

The risk of hospitalization from all causes and from respiratory disease showed no evidence of effect modification by age or sex with an increase in air pollution (Table 4). However, risk of hospitalization from cardiac disease was greatest among those 85 years old and greater, with an increase of 23% (6% to 44%) among the elderly versus 3% (-3% to 10%) among those less than 64 years of age; but, similar to risk of hospitalization from all cause and respiratory disease, cardiac disease showed no effect modification by sex.

		All Cause RR	Cardiac RR	Respiratory RR
Age	**All**	1.032 (1.011 to 1.053)	1.029 (0.983 to 1.077)	1.056 (1.005 to 1.111)
	< 64	1.037 (1.017 to 1.059)	1.033 (0.974 to 1.097)	1.067 (1.014 to 1.123)
	65 to 74	1.034 (0.996 to 1.074)	1.089 (1.006 to 1.178)	1.071 (0.945 to 1.214)
	75 to 84	1.036 (0.991 to 1.084)	1.050 (0.969 to 1.137)	1.119 (1.003 to 1.249)
	> 85	1.048 (0.977 to 1.124)	1.232 (1.058 to 1.435)	1.081 (0.946 to 1.235)
Sex	**All**	1.032 (1.011 to 1.053)	1.029 (0.983 to 1.077)	1.056 (1.005 to 1.111)
	Females	1.031(1.010 to 1.054)	0.998 (0.940 to 1.059)	1.046 (0.986 to 1.109)
	Males	1.034 (1.007 to 1.062)	1.055 (0.998 to 1.116)	1.073 (1.006 to 1.144)

Table 4. Relative Risk (RR) of hospitalization (morbidity) associated with an interquartile increase in concentrations of PM_{10} adjusted for long-term trends, day-of-the-week, and humidex for the five urban centers in Conception from January 1 2006 to December 31 2007.

4. Discussion

Although progress has been made steadily over time at reducing ambient concentrations of particulate matter (PM_{10}) (Fig.3), the results of this work suggests that there remains a risk to human health from exposure to this pollutant.The burden of mortality and morbidity due to increases particulate matter (PM_{10}) in the short-terms has the greatest influence on the health of those who are elderly with low educational attainment and those with cardiac disease. In general, effect modification was observed by age and by education but not by sex and effect modification was less pronounced for morbidity data than for mortality data. Air quality guidelines that seek to protect the entire population, including high risk subgroups, should consider the greater sensitivity of those who are elderly, have lower educational attainment or suffer from cardiac disease.

4.1 Effect modification by age and educational attainment

Age significantly modified the effect of cardiac morbidity for the five Chilean communities studied here. Modification by age was less pronounced for all cause mortality, all cause morbidity and respiratory morbidity. Similarly, we observed little modification by educational attainment for total mortality. However, we did find that the combination of old age and low educational attainment resulted in elevated risk from air borne particulate matter.

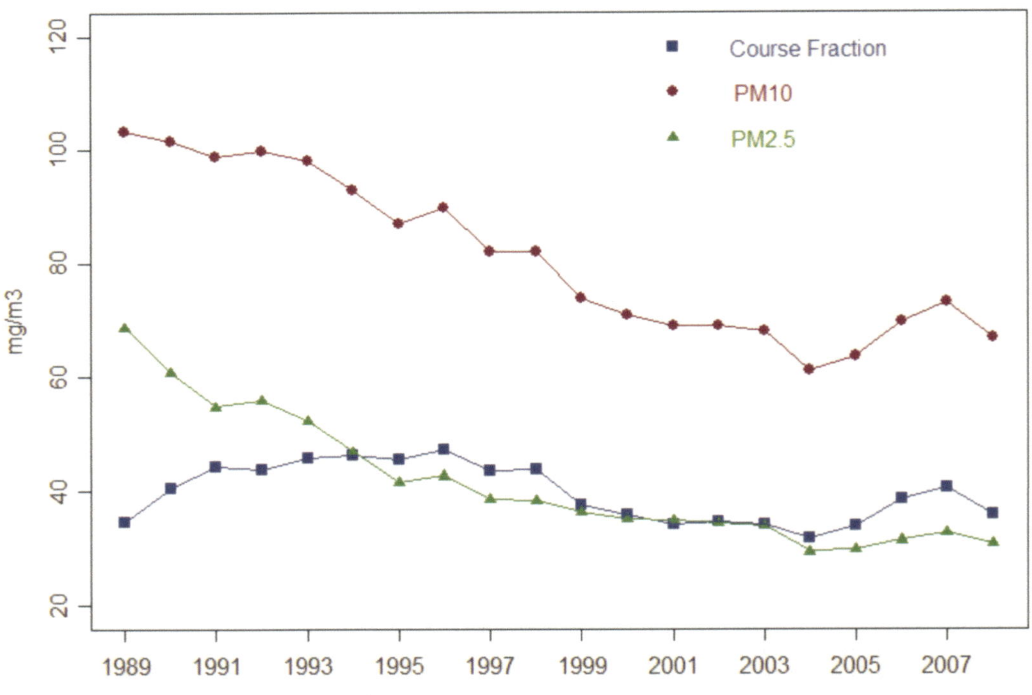

Fig. 3. Air pollution levels over time for all nine centres combined.

Previous work has reported modification of the effect of air pollutants by age (Bell et al., 2005; Pope, 2000; Pope et al., 2002; Spix et al., 1998; Zanobetti et al., 2000). For example, previous work indicated that compared to those under sixty-five years of age, Chileans eighty five years and older were observed to be more than twice as likely to die from acute increases in PM_{10}, and over 50% more likely to die from increases in ozone and SO_2 (Camak et al., 2009). Similarly, Bell et al. (2008) reported increased mortality effects in the elderly from ozone in The National Morbidity Mortality and Air Pollution Study of 98 U.S cities (Bell & Dominici, 2008) and Filleul et al. (2004) reported a greater effect of air pollution mortality in those over sixty-five years old in France, though these effects were not statistical significant (Filleul et al., 2004).

Previous work has also reported effect modification by educational attainment and other indicators of social status (Bell et al., 2008; Forastiere et al., 2009; Dales, 2002; O'Neil et al., 2008; Ou et al., 2008; Prescott & Vestbo, 1999; Zanobetti et al., 2000). For example, in the Harvard Six-Cities and American Cancer Society cohort studies, there was an increased risk of mortality from long-term exposure to particulate matter among those with lower educational attainment (Health Effects Institute, 2000; Pope et al., 2002; Villeneuve et al., 2002). Similarly, in Hamilton, Canada, the non-accidental mortality risk estimates associated with sulphur dioxide and coefficient of haze were greater in areas of the city with lower educational attainment as well as greater employment in manufacturing (Jerrett et al. 2004). However, this finding is far from consistent: no relation to level of education was found in a study of mortality risk estimates from gaseous and particulate air pollution in Hong Kong (Ou et al., 2008); no effect modification by education was found among urban Americans from 98 communities for ozone levels (Bell & Dominici, 2008); and neither a time-series study of 20 U.S (Samet et al., 2000) cities nor one focusing on Vancouver, Canada found social status modified the effect of air pollution on mortality (Villeneuve et al., 2003). Furthermore, a study of São Paulo, Brazil the authors reported that a monotonically increasing effects of air pollution with increasing education (Gouvenia & Fletcher, 2000). This type of conflicting results lead the authors of a systematic review of the Medline database up to May 2006 to state that because of inconsistent findings in both long-term and short-term exposure studies "Current evidence does not yet justify a definitive conclusion that socioeconomic characteristics modify the effects of air pollution on mortality" (Laurent et al., 2009). Nevertheless, here we report that in combination with old age, risk increases with lower educational attainment.

4.2 The influence of social status

There are many possible reasons why one might expect lower socioeconomic position to increase susceptibility to the deleterious effects of air pollution including: increased exposure to the air pollutants of interest, increased exposure to co-pollutants from occupational dusts and fumes and cigarette smoke, fewer dietary fruits and vegetables, and reduced access to medical care and medicines (O'Neill et al., 2003; Sexton et al., 1993; Spix et al., 1998). Unfortunately, information on these variables was not available. However, because the overall effect size is based on the association between daily changes in air pollution and daily changes in mortality or morbidity, these other variables would only confound the overall pollution-illness association if they change day-to-day which is unlikely (Bell et al., 2005). It is possible that these variables differ between the educational groups and may partly account for the between-group estimates of effect found here.

5. Conclusion

We found that the burden of all cause mortality and cardiac morbidity due to increased particulate air pollution is disproportionately experienced by the elderly who have low educational attainment. These findings suggest that the determination of air quality guidelines designed to protect the general population may be insufficient to protect this vulnerable subgroup.

6. Acknowledgments

The authors would like to thank Dra. Danuta Rajs Grzebien of the Departamento de Estadísticas e Información de Salud, Ministerio de Salud for providing morbidity data, and Roberto Martínez González and Joyce Vera Bascour from the Secretaría Regional Ministerial del Medio Ambiente Region Metropolitana for providing data and comments.

7. References

Dockery DW, Pope CA.Outdoor Particulates. *Environmental Epidemiology Oxford University Press*, New York. 2002;119-166.

Brunekreef B, Holgate ST. Air pollution and health. *Lancet* 2002;360:1233-1242.

Bascom R., Bromberg PA, Costa DA, Devlin R, Dockery DW, Frampton MW, Lambert W, Samet JM, Speizer FE, Utell M. Health effects of outdoor air pollution. *Am J Respir Crit Care Med* 1996;153:3-50.

Hahn RA, Eaker ED, Barker ND, Teutsch SM, Sosniak WK, Krieger N. Poverty and death in the United States. *Int J Health Serv* 1996; 26:673-690

Carr W, Zeitel L, Weiss K. Variations in asthma hospitalizations and deaths in New York City. *Am J Public Health* 1992; 82(59):65

Chen Y, Dales R, Krewski D. Asthma and the risk of hospitalization in Canada : the role of socioeconomic and demographic factors. *Chest* 2001; 119:708-713.

Cifuentes L, Vega J, Lave L. Daily mortality by cause and socio-economic status in Santiago, Chile 1988-1996. *Epidemiology* 1999; 10:S45

Wojtyniak B, Wysocki M. Chronic airways disease in Poland. Recent trends. *Chest* 1989; 96(3):324S-328S

Health Effects Institute. Reanalysis of the Harvard Six Cities Study and the American Cancer Society Study of Particulate Air Pollution and Mortality. 2000;1-285.

Pope CA, III. Epidemiology of fine particulate air pollution and human health: biologic mechanisms and who's at risk? *Environ Health Perspect* 2000;108(4):713-723.

Gouveia N, Fletcher T. Time Series analysis of air pollution and mortality: effects by cause, age and socioeconomic status. *J Epidemiol Community Health* 2000;54:750-755.

Samet JM, Dominici F, Curriero FC, Coursac I, Zeger SL. Fine Particulate Air Pollution and Mortality in 20 U.S. Cities 1987-1994. *N Eng J Med* 2000;343:1742-1749.

Zanobetti A, Schwartz J, Gold D. Are there sensitive subgroups for the effects of airborne particles? *Environ Health Perspect* 2000;108(9):841-845.

O'Neill, MS, Jerrett M, Kawachi I, Levy JI, Cohen AJ, Gouveia N, Wilkinson P, Fletcher T, Cifuentes L, Schwartz, J, Workshop on Air Pollution and Socioeconomic Conditions. Health, Wealth, and Air Pollution: Advancing Theory and Methods. *Environ Health Perspect* 2003;111:1861-1870.

Sexton K, Gong Jr. H, Bailar JC III, Ford JG, Gold DR, Lambert WE, Utell MJ. Air pollution health risks: do class and race matter? *Toxicology and Industrial Health* 1993;9:843-878.

Rupprecht G, Patashnick H, Beeson DE, Green RN, Meyer MD. A new automated monitor for the measurement of particulate carbon in the atmosphere. In: Particulate Matter: Health and Regulatory Issues. Proceedings of an International Specialty Conference, April 1995, Pittsburgh, PA, *Air and Waste Management Publications* Pittsburgh, PA, 1995;309-319

Lindstrom ML, Bates DM. Nonlinear mixed effects models for repeated measures data. *Biometrics* 1990;46(3):673-687).

Priestly MB. *Spectral Analysis of Time Series Academic Press, San Diego* 1981. Meteorological Service of Canada. 2002. http://www.mscsmc.ec.gc.ca/cd/brochures/humidity_e.cfm

Pope CA, III, Burnett RT, Thun MJ, Calle EE, Krewski D, Ito K, Thurston GD, Lung Cancer, Cardiopulmonary Mortality, and Long-term Exposure to Fine Particulate Air Pollution. *JAMA* 2002;287:1132-1141.

Spix C, Anderson HR, Schwartz J, Vigotti MA, Letertre A, Vonk JM, Touloumi F, Balducci T, Piekarski L, Bacharova A, Tobias A, Ponka, Katsouyanni K. Short-term effects of air pollution on hospital admissions of respiratory diseases in Europe: a quantitative summary of APHEA study results. *Arch Environ Health* 1998;53:54-64.

Bell ML, Dominici F, Samet JM. A meta-analysis of time-series studies of ozone and mortality with comparison to the national morbidity, mortality, and air pollution study. *Epidemiology* 2005;16:425-426.

Cakmak S, Dales RE, Blanco Vidal C. Air Pollution and Mortality in Chile: susceptibility among the elderly. *Environ Health Perspect* 2009;115:524-527.

Bell ML, Dominici F. Effect modification by community characteristics on the short-term effects of ozone exposure and mortality in 98 US communities. *Am J Epidemiol* 2008;167:986-997.

Filleul L, Le Tertre A, Baldi I, and Tessier JF. Difference in the relation between daily mortality and air pollution among elderly and all-ages populations in southwest France. *Environ Res* 2004;94:249-253.

Ou CQ. Hedley AJ. Chung RY. Thach TQ. Chau YK. Chan KP. Yang L. Ho SY. Wong CM. Lam TH. Socioeconomic disparities in air pollution-associated mortality. *Environmental Research* 2008 Jan:107[2], 237-244.

Forastiere F, Stafoggia M., Tasco C, Picciotto S, Agabati N, Cesaroni G, and Perucci CA Socioeconomic status, particulate air pollution, and daily mortality: differential exposure or differential susceptibility. 2009;50[3], 208-216.

Prescott E, Vestbo J. Socioeconomic status and chronic obstructive pulmonary disease. *Thorax* 1999;54:737-741.

Dales RE, Choi B, Chen Y, Tang M. Influence of family income on hospital visits for asthma among Canadian school children. *Thorax* 2002;57:513-517.

O'Neill MS, Bell ML, Ranjit N, C LA, Loomis D, Gouveia N, Borja-Aburto VH, Air Pollution and Mortality in Latin America: The Role of Education. *Epidemiology*. 2008; 19(6): 810-819).

Villeneuve PJ, Goldberg M.S., Krewski D, Burnett RT, Chen Y. Fine particulate air pollution and all-cause mortality within the Harvard Six-Cities Study: variations in risk by period of exposure. *Ann Epidemiol* 2002;12:568-576.

Jerrett M. Burnett RT. Brook J. Kanaroglou P. Giovis C. Finkelstein N. Hutchison B. Do socioeconomic characteristics modify the short term association between air pollution and mortality? Evidence from a zonal time series in Hamilton, Canada. *J Epidemiol Community Health* 2004:58:31-40.

Villeneuve PG, Burnett RT, Shid Y, Krewski D,, Goldberg MS, Hertzmang C, Chend Y, Brook J. A time-series study of air pollution, socioeconomic status, and mortality in Vancouver, Canada. *Journal of Exposure Analysis and Environmental Epidemiology* 2003; 13, 427–435. doi:10.1038/sj.jea.7500292

Laurent O, Bard D, Filleil L, Segala C. Effect of socioeconomic status on the relationship between atmospheric pollution and mortality. *Journal of Epidemiology & Community Health* 2009;61:665-675.

Klemm, R.J.; Mason, R.M. Jr. Aerosol Research and Inhalation Epidemiological Study (ARIES): Air Quality and Daily Mortality Statistical Modeling - Interim Results . *J. Air Waste Manage. Assoc.* 2000, *50*, 1433-1439.

Daniels, M.J.; Dominici, F.; Samet, J.M.; Zeger, S.L. Estimating Particulate Matter-Mortality Dose-Response Curves and Threshold Levels: An Analysis of Daily Time-Series for the 20 Largest US Cities. *Am. J. Epidemiol.* 2000, *152*, 397-406.

Samet, J.M,; Dominici, F.; Curriero, F.C; Coursac, I.; Zeger, S.L. Fine Particulate Air Pollution and Mortality in 20 U.S. Cities, 1987-1994. *N. Engl. J. Med.* 2000, 343, 1742-1749.

Schwartz, J. Assessing Confounding, Effect Modification, and Thresholds in the Association between Ambient Particles and Daily Deaths. *Environ. Health Perspect. 2000,* 108, 563-568.

Schwartz, J. The Distributed Lag between Air Pollution and Daily Deaths. *Epidemiol.* 2000, *11*, 320-326.

Smith, R.L.; Davis, J.M.; Speckman, P. Assessing the human health risk of atmospheric particles *Novartis. Found. Symp.* 1999, 220, 59-72.

Schwartz, J. Air Pollution and Daily Mortality in Birmingham, Alabama. *Am. J. Epidemiol.* 1993, *137*, 1136-1147.

Schwartz, J. Harvesting and Long Term Exposure Effects in the Relation between Air Pollution and Mortality.*Am. J. Epidemiol.* 2000, *151*, 440-448.

Gwynn, R.C.; Burnett, R.T.; Thurston, G.D. A Time-Series Analysis of Acidic Particulate Matter and Daily Mortality and Morbidity in the Buffalo, New York, Region. *Environ. Health Perspect.* 2000, *108*, 125-133.

Schwartz, J. Total Suspended Particulate Matter and Daily Mortality in Cincinnati, Ohio. *Environ. Health Perspect.* 1994, *102*, 186-189.

Ostro, B.D.; Hurley, S.; Lipsett, M.J. Air Pollution and Daily Mortality in the Coachella Valley, California: A Study of PM10 Dominated by Coarse Particles. *Environ. Res.* 1999, *81*, 231-238.

Ostro, B.D.; Broadwin, R.; Lipsett, M.J. Coarse and fine particles and daily mortality in the Coachella Valley, California: a follow-up study. *J. Expo. Anal. Environ. Epidemiol.* 2000, *10*, 412-419.

Ito, K.; Kinney, P.L.; Thurston, G.D. Variations in PM-10 Concentrations within two Metropolitan Areas and their Implications for Health Effects Analyses. *Inhal. Toxicol.* 1995, *7*, 735-745.

Ito, K.; Thurston, G.D. Daily PM10/Mortality Associations: An Investigation of At-Risk Subpopulations. *J. Expo. Anal. Environ. Epidemiol.* 1996, *6*, 79-95.

Styer, P.; McMillan, N.; Gao, F.; Davis, J.; Sacks, J. Effect of Outdoor Airborne Particulate Matter on Daily Death Counts. *Environ. Health Perspect.* 1995, *103*, 490-497.

Moolgavkar, S.H. Pollution and Daily Mortality in Three U.S. Counties. *Environ. Health Perspect.* 2000 *108*, 777-784.

Zanobetti, A.; Schwartz, J. Race, Gender, and Social Status as Modifiers of the Effects of PM10 on Mortality. *J. Occup. Environ. Med.* 2000, *42*, 469-474.

Schwartz, J. Particulate Air Pollution and Daily Mortality in Detroit. *Environ. Res.* 1991, *56*, 204-213.

Lippmann, M.; Ito, K.; Nadas, A.; Burnett, R.T. *Association of Particulate Matter Components with Daily Mortality and Morbidity in Urban Populations. Health Effects Institute Research Report Number 95*; Health Effects Institute: Cambridge, MA, 2000.

Dockery, D.W.; Schwartz, J.; Spengler, J.D. Air Pollution and Daily Mortality: Associations with Particulates and Acid Aerosols. *Environ. Res.* 1992, *59*, 362-373.

Schwartz, J.; Dockery, D.; Neas, L.M. Is Daily Mortality Associated Specifically with Fine Particles? *J. Air Waste Manage. Assoc.* 1996, *46*, 927-939.

Kinney, P.L.; Özkaynak, H. Associations of Daily Mortality and Air Pollution in Los Angeles County. *Environ. Res.* 1991, *54*, 99-120.

Kinney, P.L.; Ito, K.; Thurston, G.D. A Sensitivity Analysis of Mortality/PM-10 Associations in Los Angeles. *Inhal. Toxicol.* 1995, *7*, 59-69.

Goldberg,, M.S.; Bailar, J.C. III; Burnett, R.T.; Brook, J.R.; Tamblyn, R.; Bonvalot, Y.; Ernst, P.; Flegel, K.M.; Singh, R.K.; Valois, M.F. *Identifying Subgroups of the General Population That May Be Susceptible to Short-Term Increases in Particulate Air Pollution: A Time-Series Study in Montreal, Quebec. Health Effects Institute Research Report Number 97*; Health Effects Institute, Cambridge, MA, 2000.

Schwartz, J.; Dockery, D.W. Increased Mortality in Philadelphia Associated with Daily Air Pollution Concentrations. *Am. Rev. Respir. Dis.* 1992, *145*, 600-604.

Moolgavkar, S.H.; Luebeck, E.G.; Hall, T.A.; Anderson, E.L. Air Pollution and Daily Mortality in Philadelphia. *Epidemiol.* 1995, *6*, 476-484.

Schwartz, J. Daily deaths are associated with combustion particles rather than SO2 in Philadelphia. *Occup. Environ. Med.* 2000, *57*, 692-697.

Samet, J.; Zeger, S.; Kelsall, J.; Xu, J.; Kalkstein, L. Does Weather Confound or Modify the Association of Particulate Air Pollution with Mortality? An analysis of the Philadelphia Data, 1973-1980. *Environ. Res.* 1998, *77*, 9-19.

Kelsall, J.E.; Samet, J.M.; Zeger, S.L.; Xu, J. Air Pollution and Mortality in Philadelphia, 1974-1988. *Am. J. Epidemiol. 1997*, *46*, 750-762.

Wyzga, R.E.; Lipfert, F.W. Temperature - Pollution Interactions with Daily Mortality in Philadelphia. In *Particulate Matter: Health and Regulatory Issues, VIP-49, Proceedings of an International Specialty Conference, Pittsburgh, Pennsylvania, April 4-6, 1995,* 3-42.

Lipfert, F.W.; Morris, S.C.; Wyzga, R.E. Daily Mortality in the Philadelphia Metropolitan Area and Size-Classified Particulate Matter. *J. Air. Waste Manage. Assoc.* 2000, *50,* 1501-1513.

Mar, T.F.; Norris, G.A.; Koenig, J.Q.; Larson, T.V. Associations between Air Pollution and Mortality in Phoenix, 1995-1997. *Environ. Health Perspect.* 2000, *108,* 347-353.

Chock, D.P.; Winkler, S.L.; Chen, C. A Study of the Association between Daily Mortality and Ambient Air Pollutant Concentrations in Pittsburgh, Pennsylvania. *J. Air Waste Manage. Assoc.* 2000, *50,* 1481-1500.

Pope, C.A. III; Hill, R.W.; Villegas, G.M. Particulate Air Pollution and Daily Mortality on Utah's Wasatch Front. *Environ. Health Perspect.* 1999, *107,* 567-573.

Boucher, K.M.; Lyon, J.L.; Lillquist, D.R. Daily Mortality and Exposure to PM_{10} Air Pollution: A Comparison of Salt Lake and Utah Counties, 1985-1993. In *Proceedings of the Second Colloquium on Particulate Air Pollution and Human Health,* Park City, Utah, May 1-3, 1996; pp 4-36-4-54.

Ostro, B. Fine Particulate Air Pollution and Mortality in Two Southern California Counties. *Environ. Res.* 1995, *70,* 98-104.

Fairley, D. The Relationship of Daily Mortality to Suspended Particulates in Santa Clara County, 1980-1986. *Environ. Health Perspect.* 1990, *89,* 159-168.

Fairley, D. Daily Mortality and Air Pollution in Santa Clara County, California: 1989-1996. *Environ Health Perspect.* 1999, *107,* 637-641

Moolgavkar, S.H.; Luebeck, E.G.; Hall, T.A.; Anderson, E.L. Particulate air pollution, sulfur dioxide and daily mortality: A reanalysis of the Steubenville data. *Inhal. Toxicol.* 1995, *7,* 35-44.

Schwartz, J.; Dockery, D.W. Particulate Air Pollution and Daily Mortality in Steubenville, Ohio. *Am. J. Epidemiol.* 1992, *135,* 12-19.

Burnett, R.T.; Brook, J.R.; Cakmak, S.; Raizenne, M.; Stieb, D.; Vincent, R.; Krewski, D.; Brook, J.R.; Philips, O.; Özkaynak, H. The Association Between Ambient Carbon Monoxide Levels and Daily Mortality in Toronto, Canada. *J. Air Waste Manage. Assoc.* 1998, *48,* 689-700.

Burnett, R.T. In *National Ambient Air Quality Objectives for Ground-Level Ozone, Science Assessment Document;* Canadian Environmental Protection Act Federal - Provincial Advisory Committee Working Group on Air Quality Objectives and Guidelines; Health Canada and Environment Canada: Ottawa, 1999; pp A1-A8.

Burnett, R.T.; Cakmak, S.; Brook, J.R. The Effect of the Urban Ambient Air Pollution Mix on Daily Mortality Rates in 11 Canadian Cities. *Can. J. Public Health. 1998, 89,* 152-156

Burnett, R.T.; Brook, J.; Dann, T.; Delocla, C.; Philips, O.; Cakmak, S.; Vincent, R.; Goldberg, M.S.; Krewski, D. Association Between Particulate- and Gas-Phase Components Of Urban Air Pollution and Daily Mortality in Eight Canadian Cities. *Inhal. Toxicol.* 2000, *12 (Supplement 4),* 15-39.

Pope, C.A. III; Schwartz, J; Ransom, M.R. Daily Mortality and PM10 Pollution in Utah Valley. *Arch. Environ. Health.* 1992, *47,* 211-217.

Lyon, J.L.; Mori, M.; Gao, R. Is there a causal association between excess mortality and exposure to PM10 air pollution? Additional analyses by location, year, season and cause of death. *Inhal. Toxicol.* 1995, *7,* 603-614.

Pope, C.A. III; Kalkstein, L.S. Synoptic Weather Modeling and Estimates of the Exposure-Response Relationship between Daily Mortality and Particulate Air Pollution. *Environ. Health Perspect.1996, 104,* 414-420.

Borja-Aburto, V.H.; Loomis, D.P.; Bangdiwala, S.I.; Shy, C.M.; Rascon-Pacheco, R.A. Ozone, Suspended Particulates, and Daily Mortality in Mexico City. *Am. J. Epidemiol.* 1997, 258-268.

Borja-Aburto, V.H.; Castillejos, M.; Gold, D.R.; Bierzwinski, S.; Loomis, D. Mortality and Ambient Fine Particles in Southwest Mexico City, 1993-1995. *Environ. Health Perspect.* 1998, *106,* 849-855.

Castillejos, M.; Borja-Aburto, V.H.; Dockery, D.W.; Gold, D.R.; Loomis, D. Airborne coarse particles and mortality. *Inhal. Toxicol.* 2000, *12(S1),* 61-72.

Ostro, B.D.; Sanchez, J.M.; Aranda, C.; Eskeland, G.S. Air Pollution and Mortality: Results from a Study of Santiago, Chile. *J. Expo. Anal. Environ. Epidemiol.* 1996, *6,* 97-114.

Saldiva, P.H.; Pope, C.A. III; Schwartz, J.; Dockery, D.W.; Lichtenfels, A.J.; Salge, J.M.; Barone, I.; Bohm, G.M. Air pollution and mortality in elderly people: A time-series study in Sao Paulo, Brazil. *Arch. Environ. Health.* 1996, *50,* 159-163.

Touloumi, G.; Pocock, S.J.; Katsouyanni, K.; Trichopolous, D. Short-term effects of air pollution on daily mortality in Athens: A time-series analysis. *Int. J. Epidemiol.* 1994, *23,* 957-967.

Hatzakis, A.; Katsouyanni, K.; Kalandidi, A.; Day, N.; Trichopoulos, D. Short-term effects of air pollution on mortality in Athens. *Int. J. Epidemiol.* 1986, *15*:73-81.

Touloumi, G.; Samoli, E.; Katsouyanni, K. Daily mortality and "winter type" air pollution in Athens, Greece - a time series analysis within the APHEA project. *J. Epidemiol. Community Health. 1996, 50(suppl 1),* S47-S51.

Touloumi, G.; Katsouyanni, K.; Zmirou, D.; et al. Short-term Effects of Ambient Oxidant Exposure on Mortality: A Combined Analysis within the APHEA Project. *Am. J. Epidemiol.* 1997, *146,* 177-185.

Zmirou, D.; Schwartz, J.; Saez, M.; et al. Time-Series Analysis of Air Pollution and Cause Specific Mortality. *Epidemiol.* 1998, *9,* 495-503.

Sunyer, J.; Castellsagué, J.; Sáez, M.; Tobias, A.; Antó, J.M. Air pollution and mortality in Barcelona. *J. Epidemiol. Community Health. 1996, 50(Suppl 1),* S76-S80.

Tobias, A.; Campbell, M.J. Modelling influenza epidemics in the relation between black smoke and total mortality. A sensitivity analysis. *J. Epidemiol. Community Health. 1999, 53,* 583-584.

Wietlisbach, V.; Pope, C.A. III; Ackermann-Liebrich, U. Air pollution and daily mortality in three Swiss urban areas. *Soz. Präventivmed.* 1996, *41,* 107-115.

Wordley, J.; Walters, S.; Ayres, J.G. Short term variations in hospital admissions and mortality and particulate air pollution. *Occup. Environ. Med.* 1997, *54,* 108-116.

Bachárová, L.; Fandáková, K.; Bratinka, J.; Budinská, M.; Bachár, J.; Gudába, M. The association between air pollution and the daily number of deaths: findings from the

Slovak Republic contribution to the APHEA project. *J. Epidemiol. Community Health.* 1996, *50(Suppl 1)*, S19-S21.

Krzyzanowski, M.; Wojtyniak, B. Air pollution and daily mortality in Cracow. *Public. Health Rev.* 1991/92, *19*, 73-81.

Wojtyniak, B.; Piekarski, T. Short term effect of air pollution on mortality in Polish urban populations - what is different? *J. Epidemiol. Community Health.* 1996, *50(Suppl 1)*, S36-S41.

Szafraniec, K.; Tęcza, W.; Jedrychowski, W. Long-term and Short-term Changes in Air Pollutants and Mortality: Experience among Inhabitants in Krakow, Poland. In *Health Effects of Particulate Matter in Ambient Air: Proceedings of an International Conference,* Prague, Czech Republic, April 23-25, 1997; 196-202.

Kotesovec, F.; Skorkovsky, J.; Brynda, J.; Peters, A.; Heinrich J. Daily Mortality and Air Pollution in Northern Bohemia: Different Effects for Men and Women. *Cent. Eur. J. Public Health* 2000, *8*, 120-127.

Peters, A.; Skorkovsky, J.; Kotesovec, F.; Brynda, J.; Spix, C.; Wichmann, H.E.; Heinrich, J. Associations between Mortality and Air Pollution in Central Europe. *Environ. Health Perspect.* 2000, *108*, 283-287.

Rahlenbeck, S.I.; Kahl, H. Air pollution and mortality in East Berlin during the winters of 1981-1989. *Int. J. Epidemiol.* 1996, *25*, 1220-1226.

Spix, C.; Heinrich, J.; Dockery, D.; Schwartz, J.; Völksch, G.; Schwinkowski, K.; Cöllen, C.; Wichmann, H.E. Air pollution and daily mortality in Erfurt, East Germany, 1980-89. *Environ. Health Perspect.* 1993, *101*, 518-526.

Wichmann, H.-E.; Spix, C.; Tuch, T.; Wolke, G.; Peters, A.; Heinrich, J.; Kreyling, W.G.; Heyder, J. *Daily Mortality and Fine and Ultrafine Particles in Erfurt, Germany. Part I: Role of Particle Number and Particle Mass, Health Effects Institute Research Report Number 98*; Health Effects Institute: Cambridge, MA, 2000.

Spix, C.; Wichmann, H.E. Daily mortality and air pollutants: findings from Köln, Germany. *J Epidemiol. Community Health.* 1996, *50(suppl 1)*, 52-58.

Schwartz, J.; Marcus, A. Mortality and Air Pollution in London: A Time Series Analysis. *Am. J. Epidemiol.* 1990 *131*, 185-194.

Ito, K.; Thurston, G.D.; Hayes, C.; Lippmann, M. Associations of London, England, Daily Mortality with Particulate Matter, Sulfur Dioxide, and Acidic Aerosol Pollution. *Arch. Environ. Health.* 1993, *48*, 213-220.

Anderson, H.R.; Ponce de Leon, A.; Bland, J.M.; Bower, J.S.; Strachan, D.P. Air pollution and daily mortality in London: 1987-92. *B.M.J. 1996, 312*, 665-669.

Zmirou, D.; Barumandzadeh, T.; Balducci, F.; Ritter, P.; Laham, G.; Ghilardi, J.-P. Short term effects of air pollution on mortality in the city of Lyon, France, 1985-90. *J. Epidemiol. Community Health.1996, 50(suppl 1)*, S30-S35.

Alberdi JC, Díaz J, Montero JC, Mirón I. Daily mortality in Madrid community 1986-1992: Relationship with meteorological variables. *Eur J Epidemiol.* 1998;14:571-578.

Alberdi Odriozola, J.C.; Díaz Jiménez, J.; Montero Rubio, J.C.; Mirón Pérez, I.J.; Pajares Ortiz, M.S.; Ribera Rodrigues P. Air pollution and mortality in Madrid, Spain: a time-series analysis. *Int. Arch. Occup. Environ. Health.* 1998, *71*, 543-549.

Díaz, J.; García, R.; Ribera, P.; Alberdi, J.C.; Hernández, E.; Pajares, M.S.; Otero, A. Modeling of air pollution and its relationship with mortality and morbidity in Madrid, Spain. *Int. Arch. Occup. Environ. Health.* 1999, *72*, 366-376.

Morris, W.T. *Regression analysis of daily mortality and air pollution using real and simulated data;* Department of Trade and Industry: London, 1996.

Vigotti, M.A.; Rossi, G.; Bisanti, L.; Zanobetti, A.; Schwartz, J. Short term effects of urban air pollution on respiratory health in Milan, Italy, 1980-89. *J. Epidemiol. Community Health.* 1996, *50(suppl 1)*, S71-S75.

Rossi, G.; Vigotti, M.A.; Zanobetti, A.; Repetto, F.; Gianelle, V.; Schwartz, J. Air Pollution and Cause-Specific Mortality in Milan, Italy, 1980-1989. *Arch. Environ. Health.* 1999, *54*, 158-164.

Mackenbach, J.P.; Looman, C.W.N.; Kunst, A.E. Air pollution, lagged effects of temperature, and mortality: The Netherlands 1979-87. *J. Epidemiol.Community Health.* 1993, *47;* 121-126.

Buringh, E.; Fischer, P.; Hoek, G. Is SO_2 a causative factor for the PM-associated mortality risks in the Netherlands? *Inhal. Toxicol.* 2000, *12(S1)*, 55-60.

Hoek, G.; Brunekreef, B.; Verhoeff, A.; van Wijnen, J.; Fischer, P. Daily Mortality and Air Pollution in the Netherlands. *J. Air Waste Manage. Assoc.*2000, 50, 1380-1389.

Le Tertre, A.; Quénel, P.; Medina, S.; Le Moullec, Y.; Festy, B.; Ferry, R.; Dab, W. Modélisation des liens court terme entre la pollution atmosphérique et la santé. Un exemple: SO_2 et mortalité totale, Paris, 1987-1990. *Rev. Épidémiol. Santé Publique.* 1998, *46*, 316-328.

Dab, W.; Medina, S; Quénel, P.; et al. Short term respiratory health effects of ambient air pollution: results of the APHEA project in Paris. *J. Epidemiol. Community Health.* 1996, *50(suppl 1)*, S42-S46.

Michelozzi, P.; Forastiere, F.; Fusco, D.; Perucci, C.A.; Ostro, B.; Ancona, C.; Pallotti, G. Air pollution and daily mortality in Rome, Italy. *Occup. Environ. Med.*. 1998, *55*, 605-610.

Hoek, G.; Groot, B.; Schwartz, J.D.; Eilers, P. Effects of ambient particulate matter and ozone on daily mortality in Rotterdam, the Netherlands. *Arch. Environ. Health.* 1997, *52*, 455-463.

Ballester, F.; Corella, D.; Pérez-Hoyos, S.; Hervás, A. Air pollution and mortality in Valencia, Spain: a study using the APHEA methodology. *J. Epidemiol. Community Health.* 1996, *50*, 527-533.

Ostro, B.; Chestnut, L.; Vichit-Vadakan, N.; Laixuthai, A. The Impact of Particulate Matter on Daily Mortality in Bangkok, Thailand. *J. Air Waste Manage. Assoc. 1996, 49,* PM100-PM107.

Xu, X.; Dockery, D.W.; Gao, J.; Chen, Y. Air Pollution and Daily Mortality in Residential Areas of Beijing, China. *Arch. Environ. Health.* 1994, *49*, 216-222.

Hong .Y.-C.; Leem, J.-H.; Ha, E.-H.; Christiani, D.C. PM_{10} Exposure, Gaseous Pollutants, and Daily Mortality in Inchon, South Korea. *Environ. Health. Perspect.* 1999, *107*, 873-878.

Lee, J.-T.; Shin, D.; Chung ,Y. Air Pollution and Daily Mortality in Seoul and Ulsan, Korea. *Environ. Health Perspect.* 1999, *107*, 149-154.

Lee, J.T.; Kim, H.; Hong ,Y.C.; Kwan, H.J.; Schwartz, J.; Christiani, D.C. Air Pollution and Daily Mortality in Seven Major Cities of Korea, 1991-1997. *Environ. Res. 2000, 84,* 247-254.

Xu, Z.Y.; Yu, D.G.; Jing , L.B.; Xu, X.P. Air Pollution and Daily Mortality in Shenyang, China. *Arch. Environ. Health* 2000, *55,* 115-120.

22

Short-Term Exposure to Outdoor Pollutants and Loss of Pulmonary Function in the Elderly

Yun-Chul Hong and Jin Hee Kim
Department of Preventive Medicine,
Seoul National University College of Medicine,
Institute of Environmental Medicine,
Seoul National University Medical Research Center,
Korea

1. Introduction

The reduction of pulmonary function has come to be considered one of the most important health effects of air pollution because it not only affects individual respiratory health status but also predicts cardiovascular morbidity and mortality in the general population (1-3). Although numerous studies have provided an understanding of air pollution's general effects on pulmonary function, the length of the lag period for the effects of short-term exposure to air pollution has not been well elucidated.

In addition, most of the information about the pulmonary effects of air pollution has come from studies of children and adults, whereas pulmonary effects in the elderly are less well understood. Because of the considerable increase in the prevalence of respiratory diseases in the elderly population and this population's known susceptibility to toxic chemicals in the environment, the effect of air pollution on pulmonary function in the elderly has emerged as a serious concern in both public health and clinical medicine.

Although the diminution of pulmonary function because of exposure to air pollutants has been reported in previous studies (4-6), most of these reports were time-series or cross-sectional analyses that did not capture within-subject changes. To account for within-subject changes in pulmonary function, a longitudinal study, such as a cohort or panel study, is required. A cohort study would be more appropriate for evaluating the long-term health effects of air pollution, while a panel study is better suited for evaluating the short-term effects (7). Because each subject can be used as his or her own control in a panel study with repeated measurements, only rapidly changing covariates for each given subject have to be considered in a statistical analysis.

Therefore, we conducted a longitudinal panel study using repeated measurements to evaluate the effects of air pollutants on pulmonary function in the elderly, who are known to be especially susceptible to air pollution (8-10).

2. Methods

2.1 Subject population

The study population consisted of 560 elderly people (all 60 years old or older) living in Seoul, Korea. Up to 5 spirometric tests were performed on different days for each subject.

During each subject's first visit, demographic data and information, such as medical history, dietary habits, smoking and alcohol consumption were gathered using a questionnaire. Written informed consent was obtained from every subject; this study was approved by the institutional review board of the Seoul National University College of Medicine.

2.2 Air pollution and meteorological data

Air pollution data were collected from the Research Institute of Public Health and Environment; values from the monitoring site nearest to each subject's residence were used as the dataset for that subject's exposure to ambient pollutants. Daily average values for concentrations of particulate matter with a diameter of 10 µm or less (PM_{10}), sulfur dioxide (SO_2), nitrogen dioxide (NO_2), carbon monoxide (CO) and ozone (O_3) were computed for each site. Data on the daily average temperature (°C) and relative humidity (%) for each day of the study period were obtained from the Korean Meteorological Administration.

2.3 Spirometric measurements

Spirometric testing was conducted at each health evaluation visit according to the 2005 European Respiratory Society/American Thoracic Society recommendations. All tests were performed at the same hour of the morning by one trained technician, using a Microlab® (Sensormedic, USA) spirometer. The spirometric measurements used in our analyses were forced vital capacity (FVC), forced expiratory volume in one second (FEV_1), FEV_1 as a percentage of FVC (FEV_1/FVC), and forced expiratory flow between 25 and 75% of the FVC (FEF_{25-75}).

2.4 Statistical analysis

Linear mixed-effect models were used to estimate the effects of the air pollutants on the pulmonary function test parameters, which controlled for temperature, relative humidity, smoking, dietary habits, alcohol consumption, and individual characteristics. We treated age, sex, height, weight, dietary habits, alcohol consumption, date, temperature, relative humidity, smoking and pollutant levels as fixed effects. Participant identity was treated as a random effect in the models. We examined the ongoing effects of air pollution on lung-function parameters over a lag time of 7 days after exposure. We counted the day of the air-pollutant exposure as lag day 0; lag day 7 was therefore defined as an exposure the 7 days prior. We also evaluated the cumulative lag effects of air pollution using a lag-distribution model.

3. Results

The mean age of the participants was 70.7 years old; 26.1% were male and 73.9% were female. Subjects underwent a mean of 3.3 health examination visits out of 5 possible visits. The male participants were more likely to be smokers than the female Participants (Table 1). Table 2 presents the levels of air pollutants and the meteorological data for the time periods preceding each health examination visit. The mean levels of PM_{10}, SO_2, O_3, NO_2 and CO were 42.6 µg/m^3, 3.9 ppb, 19.2 ppb, 35.6 ppb and 0.6 ppm, respectively.

To determine the length of the effective time period for pulmonary impact, we assessed the effects of air pollutants on lung function from the day of exposure (lag day 0) through lag day 7 (Figure 1). To estimate the effects of the air pollution, we calculated the estimated values of lung function parameters assuming average values for age, sex, height, weight, smoking, dietary habits, alcohol consumption, outdoor temperature and humidity. We found that the effective time period for an air pollution-induced reduction of pulmonary function was from the day of exposure through the following 2 days. Compared to other air pollutants, O_3 did not show a significant association in reducing pulmonary function. We specifically calculated changes in pulmonary function due to exposure to air pollution within the past one day, because the calculated reduction in pulmonary function was most prominent for most air pollutants at lag day 1. Table 3 shows that the levels of PM_{10}, SO_2, NO_2 and CO were negatively associated with FEV_1/FVC and FEF_{25-75} but that O_3 levels were not significantly associated with changes in pulmonary function parameters.

	Male	Female	Total
No. of participants (%)	146 (26.1)	414 (73.9)	560 (100)
No. of visits [mean ± SE]	3.1 ± 0.1	3.4 ± 0.1	3.3 ± 0.1
Age [mean (range)]	71.4 (62-84)	70.5 (60-87)	70.7 (60-87)
Height [mean ± SE (cm)]	164.3 ± 0.4	151.3 ± 0.2	154.7 ± 0.3
Weight [mean ± SE (Kg)]	65.7 ± 0.8	57.1 ± 0.4	59.3 ± 0.4
No. of smokers (%)	64 (43.4)	5 (1.2)	67 (12.2)
Lung-function indicators:			
FVC [mean ± SE (L)]	2.86 ± 0.05	20.4 ± 0.02	2.27 ± 0.03
FEV_1 [mean ± SE (L)]	2.31 ± 0.04	1.74 ± 0.02	0.92 ± 0.02
FEV_1/FVC [mean ± SE (%)]	81.37 ± 0.64	86.70 ± 0.35	85.21 ± 0.33
FEF_{25-75} [mean ± SE (L/sec)]	2.31 ± 0.07	2.10 ± 0.04	2.16 ± 0.03

FVC: forced vital capacity; FEV_1: forced expiratory volume in one second; FEF_{25-75}: forced expiratory flow between 25% and 75% of forced vital capacity.

Table 1. Subject characteristics at first health evaluation visit

Pollutant	Number of measurements	Mean (SD)	Selected percentiles: 10th	25th	50th	75th	90th
PM_{10} (μg/m^3)	1850	42.6 (17.6)	21.9	29.3	39.7	53.1	63.0
SO_2 (ppb)	1850	3.9 (1.5)	2.4	2.7	3.4	4.5	6.0
O_3 (ppb)	1850	19.2 (8.4)	8.1	10.9	19.3	26.9	30.2
NO_2 (ppb)	1850	35.6 (9.1)	24.0	29.3	35.8	39.7	45.3
CO (ppm)	1850	0.6 (0.2)	0.4	0.5	0.6	0.7	0.9
Temperature (°C)	1915	17.3 (9.0)	4.0	10.1	19.1	25.1	27.0
Humidity (%)	1915	63.2 (12.8)	47.9	53.0	63.6	72.5	80.4

Levels of air pollutants for the health-examination day and the seven preceding days; meteorological data for the health examination day.

Table 2. Air-pollutant levels and meteorological data

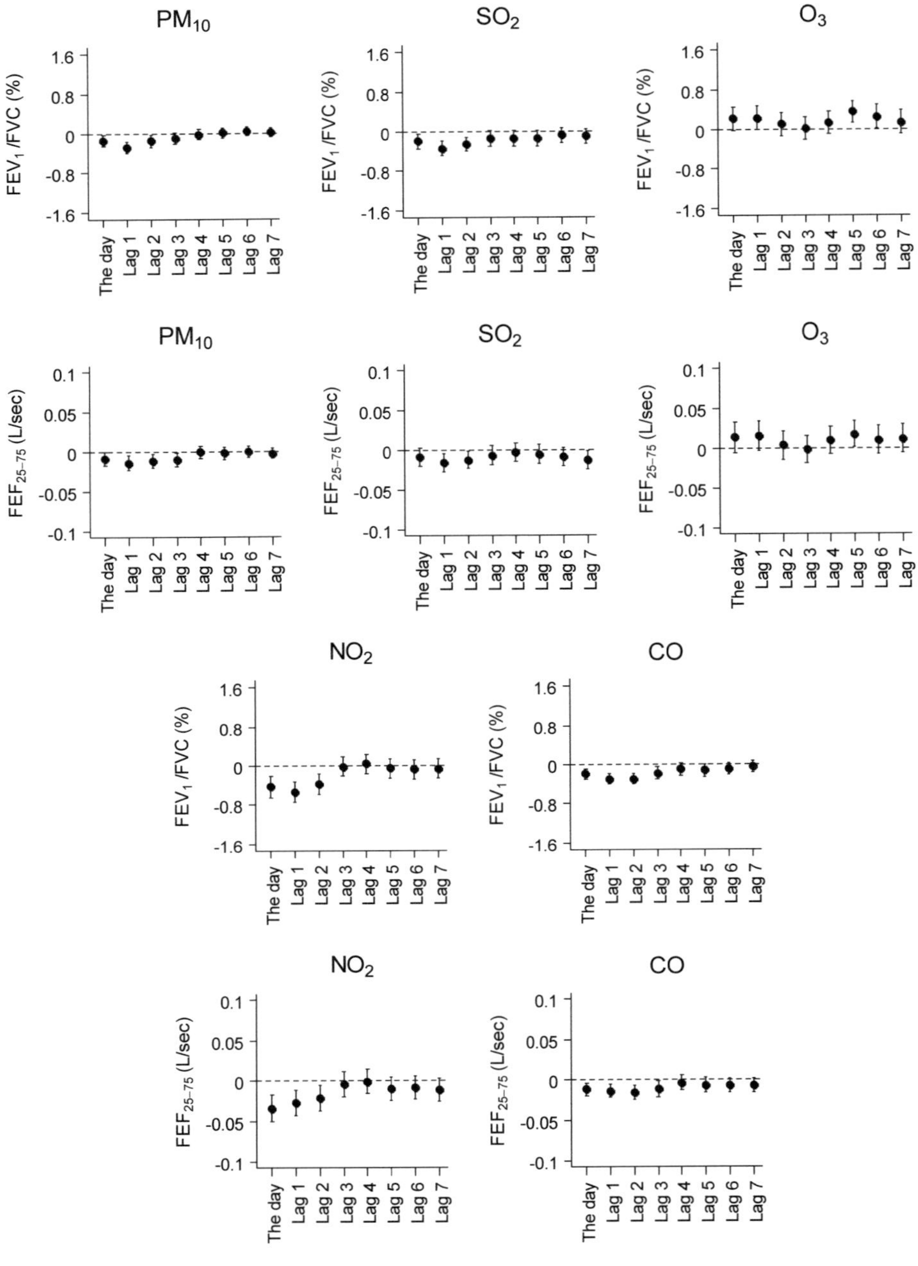

Fig. 1. The effect of PM_{10}, SO_2, O_3, NO_2, and CO on FEV_1/FVC and $FEF_{25\text{-}75}$ by single lag days. Changes in FEV_1/FVC (%) and $FEF_{25\text{-}75}$ (L/sec) were calculated per 10 $\mu g/m^3$ of change in PM_{10} levels, per 1 ppb of change in SO_2, per 10 ppb of change in O_3, per 10 ppb of change in NO_2, and per 0.1 ppm of change in CO, adjusted for age, sex, body mass index (BMI), smoking status, alcohol consumption, dietary habits, temperature and relative humidity.

Pollutant	Outcome	No.	Estimated Change	SE	p-Value	Lower 95% CI	Upper 95% CI
PM_{10}	FEV_1 (L)	1146	0.003	0.002	0.1541	-0.001	0.008
	FEV_1/FVC (%)	1146	-0.287	0.063	<0.0001	-0.410	-0.164
	FEF_{25-75} (L/sec)	1146	-0.014	0.005	0.0034	-0.023	-0.005
SO_2	FEV_1 (L)	1146	0.003	0.026	0.8972	-0.047	0.054
	FEV_1/FVC (%)	1146	-3.447	0.718	<0.0001	-4.856	-2.037
	FEF_{25-75} (L/sec)	1146	-0.157	0.055	0.0047	-0.266	-0.048
O_3	FEV_1 (L)	1146	0.004	0.004	0.3123	-0.004	0.013
	FEV_1/FVC (%)	1146	0.228	0.124	0.0671	-0.016	0.472
	FEF_{25-75} (L/sec)	1146	0.016	0.009	0.0968	-0.003	0.034
NO_2	FEV_1 (L)	1146	0.002	0.004	0.6592	-0.006	0.009
	FEV_1/FVC (%)	1146	-0.542	0.102	<0.0001	-0.743	-0.341
	FEF_{25-75} (L/sec)	1146	-0.027	0.008	0.0005	-0.043	-0.012
CO	FEV_1 (L)	1143	0.001	0.002	0.4677	-0.002	0.005
	FEV_1/FVC (%)	1143	-0.300	0.053	<0.0001	-0.403	-0.197
	FEF_{25-75} (L/sec)	1143	-0.014	0.004	0.0005	-0.022	-0.006

Change in lung-function indicators per 10 μg/m³ of change in PM_{10} levels; per 10 ppb of change in SO_2; per 10 ppb of change in O_3; per 10 ppb of change in NO_2; per 0.1 ppm of change in CO.
The effect of each air pollutant on lung function was adjusted for age, sex, body mass index (BMI), smoking status, alcohol consumption, dietary habits, temperature and relative humidity.

Table 3. The relationship between air pollutants and lung-function indicators on lag day one.

To evaluate the cumulative effect of air pollutants on pulmonary function, we performed a lag-distribution model analysis and found that a significant reduction in pulmonary function occurred when subjects had been exposed to air pollutants during the previous 2 days, as in the single-day lag model analysis (Figure 2).

3.1 Discussion

Our study demonstrates that exposure to outdoor air pollutants exerts harmful effects on lung function in the elderly and that the lag period for this effect is from the day of exposure to 2 days later.

All of these effects were observed at pollution levels within the current air-quality standard in Korea, which sets the maximum 24-hour average at 100 μg/m³ for PM_{10}, 50 ppb for SO_2, and 60 ppb for NO_2 and the maximum 8-hour average at 60 ppb for O_3 and 9 ppm for CO.

Spirometry provides a simple, convenient and reproducible measure of pulmonary function. We examined the association between exposure to ambient air pollutants and lung function test results and found statistically significant correlations between air pollutant levels of PM_{10}, NO_2, SO_2 and CO and results of FEV_1/FVC and FEF_{25-75} measurements. In contrast, FVC and FEV_1 results did not show any association with air pollutant levels. Though declines in FVC and FEV_1 have been found to be associated with occupational exposure to air pollutants, these two parameters do not change quickly during the early stages of disease (11). This stasis suggests that the primary site affected by air pollutants might be the airways, especially the small airways, rather than the pulmonary parenchyma.

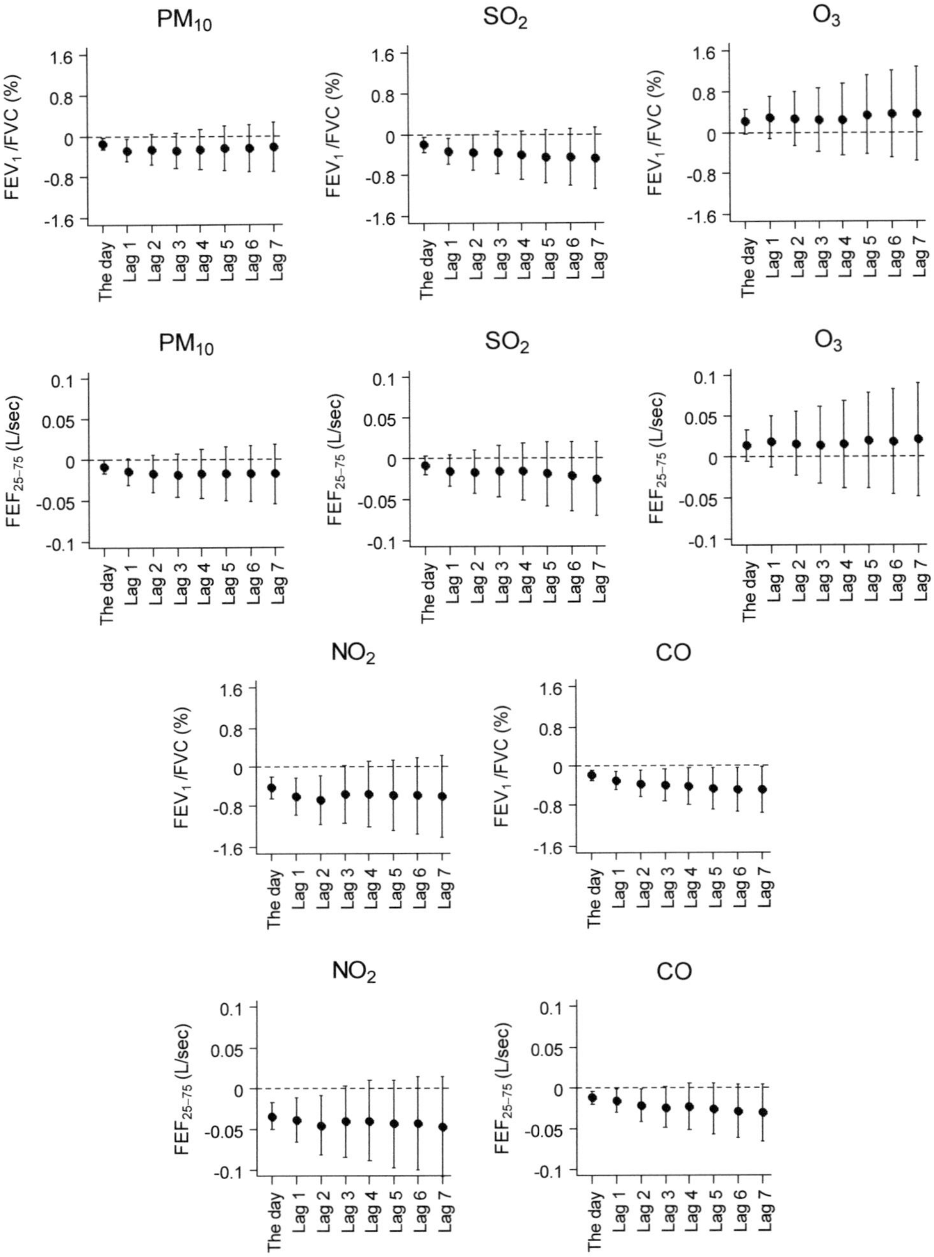

Fig. 2. The effect of PM_{10}, SO_2, O_3, NO_2, and CO on FEV_1/FVC and $FEF_{25\text{-}75}$ by distributed lag days. Changes in FEV_1/FVC (%) and $FEF_{25\text{-}75}$ (L/sec) were calculated per 10 μg/m^3 of change in PM_{10} levels, per 1 ppb of change in SO_2, per 10 ppb of change in O_3, per 10 ppb of change in NO_2, and per 0.1 ppm of change in CO, adjusted for age, sex, body mass index (BMI), smoking status, alcohol consumption, dietary habits, temperature and relative humidity.

The estimated changes for the FEV_1/FVC and FEF_{25-75} results were -0.287% and -14 ml/sec with a change in PM_{10} levels of 10 μg/m^3. An increase of 10 ppb for SO_2 reduced FEV_1/FVC results by -3.447% and FEF_{25-75} results by -157 ml/sec. An increase of 10 ppb in NO_2 reduced FEV_1/FVC by -0.542% and FEF_{25-75} by -27 ml/sec, and an increase of 100 ppb in CO reduced FEV_1/FVC by -0.300% and FEF_{25-75} by -14 ml/sec. Although these levels of reduction do not seem to be clinically significant for young adults, the impact of such air pollution on the already declining lung function of the elderly could be considerable.

The effect of air-pollution exposure on lung function is not necessarily contemporaneous (7). When we examined the pattern of lag in the relationship between air pollutants and lung function using single-lag-day and distributed-lag-day models, we found that the adverse effects of exposure to air pollutants could be detected immediately on the day of the exposure and that these effects had a lag period of 2 days except in the case of O_3, which did not show any effect during the test period. Lag structures in relationships between air pollution and respiratory health outcomes have been discussed in several studies. Goldberg et al. reported that the effect on the rate of respiratory-related deaths in persons older than 65 years was greatest following the same-day exposure (12). Braga et al. reported that respiratory deaths were affected more by exposure in the previous 1 to 2 days (13). Peters et al. reported stronger cumulative effects than the same-day effects of air pollution for asthmatic symptoms and peak expiratory flow rates (14). Our results are consistent with the short-term lag effects found in previous studies, showing that the cumulative effects of air pollution exposure on lung function were greater than the single-day lag effects, although the effect was no longer significant after lag day 2 for most of the air pollutants.

In our study, O_3 levels were not associated with changes in pulmonary function, although other pollutants were significantly associated. Estimating the effects of O_3 on lung function is challenging because of the strong correlation between O_3 levels and outdoor temperatures. However, in our results, the estimated risk level resulting from O_3 was constant, whether or not temperature was analyzed as a confounding variable.

The strengths of the present study merit further discussion. First, the panel study design, with repeated measurements on spirometric tests for each participant, provided a good opportunity to evaluate the short-term effects of the changes in air pollutant levels over time. In this longitudinal study, the subjects served as their own controls because personal characteristics could be assumed to remain constant over the study period. We used mixed-effects models to assess the effects of visit-to-visit variations in ambient air pollution on lung function to account for inter- and intra-subject variability. Individual exposure to other pollutants or other confounding factors could have biased the results if they had increased concomitantly with the measured air-pollution levels; however, this scenario is not likely.

There were also some limitations to this study. We could not completely control for those environmental factors that could have changed concomitantly with the levels of air pollutants, which could have biased the results for air-pollution effects. For example, possible environmental factors that could have confounded the results were meteorological variables, such as temperature and humidity. However, the relationships between air pollutants and pulmonary function can be significantly maintained, even after controlling for these meteorological variables. In addition, we did not measure precisely each individual's exposure level to ambient air pollutants, but we used monitoring data for the nearest site to their home. However, the misclassification of exposure levels according to the monitoring data may have contributed to a null association. Although we adjusted for other potential factors affecting lung function, such as smoking, in the statistical analyses, concomitant exposure to other pollutants, such as volatile organic chemicals or heavy metals, could also have had some impact on lung function.

In conclusion, our findings suggest that short-term exposure to air pollutants reduces lung function in the elderly for a period lasting from the day of exposure to 2 days after exposure. These results contribute to our understanding of how short-term exposure to air pollution affects lung function.

4. References

[1] Hole DJ, Watt GC, Davey-Smith G, *et al.* Impaired lung function and mortality risk in men and women: findings from the Renfrew and Paisley prospective population study. *BMJ* 1996; 313: 711-715.

[2] Mannino DM, Buist AS, Petty TL, *et al.* Lung function and mortality in the United States: data from the First National Health and Nutrition Examination Survey follow up study. *Thorax* 2003; 58: 388-393.

[3] Sircar K, Hnizdo E, Petsonk E, *et al.* Decline in lung function and mortality: implications for medical monitoring. *Occup Environ Med* 2007; 64: 461-466.

[4] Downs SH, Schindler C, Liu LJS, *et al.* Reduced Exposure to PM10 and Attenuated Age-Related Decline in Lung Function. *N Engl J Med* 2007; 357: 2338-2347.

[5] Abbey DE, Burchette RJ, Knutsen SF, *et al.* Long-term particulate and other air pollutants and lung function in nonsmokers. *Am J Respir Crit Care Med* 1998; 158: 289-298.

[6] Ackermann-Liebrich U, Leuenberger P, Schwartz J, *et al.* Lung function and long term exposure to air pollutants in Switzerland. Study on Air Pollution and Lung Diseases in Adults (SAPALDIA) Team. *Am J Respir Crit Care Med* 1997; 155: 122-129.

[7] Segala C, Fauroux B, Just J, Pascual L, Grimfeld A, Neukirch F. Short-term effect of winter air pollution on respiratory health of asthmatic children in Paris. *Eur Respir J.* 1998 Mar;11(3):677-685.

[8] Cakmak S, Dales RE, Vidal CB. Air pollution and mortality in Chile: susceptibility among the elderly. *Environ Health Perspect* 2007; 115: 524-527.

[9] Fischer P, Hoek G, Brunekreef B, *et al.* Air pollution and mortality in The Netherlands: are the elderly more at risk? *Eur Respir J Suppl.* 2003; 40: 34s-38s.

[10] Medina-Ramon M, Schwartz J. Who is more vulnerable to die from ozone air pollution? *Epidemiology* 2008; 19: 672-679.

[11] Haynes GB, Christiani DC (1993) Measures of small airways disease as predictors of chronic obstructive pulmonary disease. *Occup Med* 1993; 8: 375-395

[12] Goldberg MS, Burnett RT, Bailar JC III, *et al.* The association between daily mortality and ambient air particle pollution in Montreal, Quebec. 2. Cause-specific mortality. *Environ Res [A]* 2001; 86: 26-36

[13] Braga A, Zanobetti A, Schwartz J (2001) Structure between particulate air pollution and respiratory and cardiovascular deaths in 10 US cities. *J Occup Environ Med* 2001; 43: 927-933

[14] Peters A, Goldstein IF, Beyer U, *et al.* Acute health effects of exposure to high levels of air pollution in eastern Europe. *Am J Epidemiol* 1996; 144: 570-581

Part 4

Polluted Environment and Its Influence On Allergic Diseases

23

Aggravation of Allergic Rhinitis by Air Pollution: Demonstration by an Animal Model of Pollenosis

Takeshi Nabe and Nobuaki Mizutani
Kyoto Pharmaceutical University
Kobe Pharmaceutical University
Japan

1. Introduction

Numbers of patients suffering from allergic diseases, such as asthma, pollenosis, atopic dermatitis, etc. have been increased in industrially advanced countries. The increases are remarkable especially in urban area in such countries.

It has been generally accepted that not only genetic but also environmental factors contribute to the pathogenesis of various diseases. Allergic diseases are also caused by both factors. Genetic factors can be explained by a concept of single nucleotide polymorphism (SNP), which means that only one nucleotide mutation can make a person highly sensitive to allergic diseases. However, the recent increase in the number of allergic patients cannot be explained merely by SNP.

It has been widely indicated that environmental factors such as air pollution, improvement of hygiene, changes in foods and dwelling, etc. are closely associated with the increase in patients.

In this chapter, the relationship between air pollutants and allergic diseases in the airway tissues is Focused on. In order to demonstrate this relationship, experimental animal models of allergic asthma have been widely utilized. First, the findings obtained from animal models are summarized. Second, we have actually evaluated whether the pyrenes present in diesel exhaust particles, cigarette smoke, etc. aggravate allergic rhinitis symptoms in a pollenosis guinea pig model (Mizutani et al., 2007). The methodology of development of this model of pollenosis and the effects of pyrenes on the model are also described.

2. Air pollutants that have been demonstrated to aggravate airway allergic diseases in experimental animal models

Allergic diseases are manifested by antigen-specific IgE antibody formation, increase in Th2 cytokine (IL-4, IL-5, IL-13, etc.) production and decrease in Th1 cytokine (interferon-γ) production. In allergic airway diseases, asthma is a potentially life-threatening disorder, and thus the mechanisms underlying allergen-induced asthmatic responses have been analyzed using murine models not only by measuring levels of IgE antibody and Th2 cytokines, but also by estimating leukocyte infiltration into the lung and especially the eosinophilia, airway hyperresponsiveness to a non-specific stimulus, and airway remodeling.

Various indoor and outdoor air pollutants have been evaluated to determine whether allergic airway diseases are aggravated by exposure to pollutants. Experimental animal models of asthma especially in mice have been extensively utilized to analyze the relationships between air pollutants and disease.

2.1 Diesel exhaust particles (DEPs)

Diesel fuel combustion results in the production of DEPs. DEPs consist of an elemental carbon core with a large surface area, to which hundreds of chemicals such as pyrenes, phenanthrenes, etc. and transition metals such as zinc, aluminium, iron, etc. are attached (Peden & Reed, 2010). In human studies, it was demonstrated that intranasal instillation of DEPs increased nasal IgE antibody secretion. Furthermore, the DEP treatment increased Th2-type cytokine production in the nasal cells. Those findings strongly suggest that exposure to DEPs further aggravates patients' allergic state (Diaz-Sanchez, 1999; Riedl & Diaz-Sanchez, 2005).

In experimental animal models of allergic asthma, it has been reported that exposure to DEPs in mice resulted in enhanced allergen-induced IgE production in serum, airway Th2-type cytokine production, airway hyperresponsiveness, airway eosinophilia, etc. (Munakata, 1986; Takafuji, 1987; Fujimaki, 1994; Suzuki, 1996; Takano, 1997, 1998; Ichinose, 1998; Miyabara, 1998; Steerenberg, 1999; Kobayashi, 2000; Hashimoto, 2001; Liu, 2008). Interestingly, Takahashi et al. (2010) recently demonstrated that long-term mite antigen exposure-induced airway remodelling was also augmented by DEP exposure.

The mechanisms underlying DEP-induced aggravation of allergic responses are currently under investigation. Most studies have reported that exposure to DEPs induces production of reactive oxygen species (ROS) such as superoxide anion, hydrogen peroxide, hydroxy radical, etc., leading to cellular damage. The production of ROS may play important roles in the augmentation of antigen-induced asthmatic responses in the lung (Riedl & Diaz-Sanchez, 2005). Further analyses are required in order to understand the detailed molecular mechanisms of the effects of DEPs.

2.2 Residual oil fly ash (ROFA)

ROFA is an air pollutant produced by the combustion of fossil fuels, and contributes to total primary particulate matter emissions in the United States. ROFA is rich in water-soluble transition metals. Epidemiological and human experimental studies have attributed increased respiratory inflammation to high metal content of pollutants.

It has been demonstrated that exposure to ROFA enhances allergen-induced asthmatic responses in mice (Hamada, 1999; Goldsmith, 1999; Gavett, 1999; Arantes-Costa, 2008). Interestingly, Lambert et al. (2000) reported that water-soluble metals, either $NiSO_4$, VSO_4 or $FeSO_4$ are also capable of enhancing those asthmatic responses, indicating that the enhanced allergic responses by ROFA were mediated by soluble metal constituents. The relationships between environmental metal constituents and asthmatic responses should be further analyzed clinically and experimentally.

2.3 Cigarette smoke

Cigarette smoking has been implicated in the development of diseases in multiple organs, including cardiovascular diseases, malignancy, and respiratory disorders. Among the respiratory diseases, cigarette smoking is one of main causes of chronic obstructive pulmonary disease (COPD).

Epidemiologic studies in asthmatics have reported an association between environmental cigarette smoke (ETS) exposure and asthma symptoms. In asthmatic children, parental smoking increases levels of asthma symptoms and the frequency of asthma exacerbations (Evans, 1987; Chilmonczyk, 1993; Britton, 2005). In experimental animal models, chronic coexposure to ETS increased levels of allergen-induced airway remodelling and airway responsiveness by up-regulating the expression of chemokines (Min, 2007), suggesting that ETS is a risk factor for asthma. Other studies using animal models have also reported that exposure to ETS aggravates airway allergy (Seymour, 1997, 2003, 2005; Rumold, 2001), although there are also controversial reports (Kang, 1996; Boweles, 2005).

In contrast, the effect of mainstream or active cigarette smoking (MTS) on asthma is controversial. MTS has been associated with increased an serum level of IgE and airway hyprresponsiveness (Barbee, 1987; Mitsunobu, 2004). However, other studies in asthmatic patients have failed to find any relationship between MTS and asthma (Siroux, 2000; Vidal, 2004). Even in experimental animal models, the impact of MTS on OVA-induced asthmatic responses in mice is controversial (Robbins, 2005; Moerloose, 2005, 2006; Thatcher, 2008). Thus, the difference between the effects of ETS and MTS on asthma should be further analyzed in experimental studies.

2.4 Nanoparticles

The development of nano-technology has increased opportunities to be exposed to engineered nanomaterials present in the environment. Nanomaterials are included in industrially manufactured products such as ink, toner, cosmetics, latex, etc. However, it has been largely unclear how exposure to these nanomaterials affects human health, especially the airway tissues.

Inoue et al. (2005, 2009a, 2009b) and others (Alessandrini, 2006; de Haar, 2008) have extensively studied the effects of nanoparticles on allergen-induced asthmatic responses in mice, reporting that relatively small diameters of particles induced enhancement of allergic airway inflammation. For example, nanoparticles with a diameter of 14 nm produced more prominent allergic airway inflammation, characterized by infiltration of eosinophils and neutrophils, by an increase in epithelial goblet cell number, and by increases in levels of cytokines and chemokines in the lung than those with a diameter of 56 nm.

Further studies are required to fully understand the mechanisms underlying the aggravation of nanomaterials on the allergic airway inflammation.

2.5 Asian sand dust

Asian sand dust is a dust storm originating in the deserts of China and Mongolia, and heading toward Japan, Taiwan, Korea, etc. It has been recognized that Asian sand dust may be artificially formed by environmental deterioration such as deforestation, etc. The diameters of particles in sand dust are several to several tens of micrometers. Such coarse particles may have limited adverse effects on the respiratory organ. However, recent studies have indicated that Asian sand dust contains sulfates and nitrates (Ro, 2005) that may originate from industrial areas in China. In addition, it was reported that fungi are adsorbed to Asian sand dust (Ichinose, 2008a).

Ichinose et al. (2008b) first reported that exposure to Asian sand dust to OVA-sensitized mice enhanced allergen challenge-induced asthmatic responses including lung eosinophilia, Th2 cytokine and chemokine production in the lungs. More interestingly, they

Air pollutant	Author, publication year	Species	Allergen	Characteristic effects of pollutants on allergic responses
DEP	Muranaka et al., 1986	Mouse	OVA, JPCA	Enhancement of IgE production
	Takafuji et al., 1987	Mouse	OVA	Enhancement of IgE production
	Fujimaki et al., 1995	Mouse	OVA, JPCA	Enhancement of IL-4 production
	Suzuki et al., 1996	Mouse	Mite	Enhancement of IgE and IgG1 production
	Takano et al., 1997	Mouse	OVA	Enhancement of lung eosinophilia and Th2 cytokine production
	Takano et al., 1998	Mouse	OVA	Enhancement of AHR
	Ichinose et al., 1998	Mouse	OVA	Enhancement of lung eosinophilia, airway epithelial damage
	Miyabara et al., 1998	Mouse	OVA	Enhancement of lung eosinophilia, production of Th2 cytokines, and increase in goblet cells in the epithelium
	Steerenberg et al., 1999	Rat	Grass pollen	Enhancement of IgE and IgG1 production
	Kobayashi, 2000	Guinea pigs	OVA	Enhancement of sneezing and nasal eosinophilia
	Hashimoto et al., 2001	Guinea pigs	OVA	Enhancement of IAR and LAR, mucus hypersecretion, lung eosinophilia, and airway vascular permeability
	Liu et al., 2008	Mouse	Af	Hypermethylation of IFN gamma promotor, and hypomethylation of IL-4 promotor
	Takahashi et al., 2010	Mouse	Mite	Enhancement of airway remodelling, AHR, Th2-type airway inflammation
ROFA	Hamada et al., 1999	Mouse	OVA	Enhancement of AHR and airway inflammation
	Goldsmith et al., 1999	Mouse	OVA	Enhancement of AHR
	Gavett et al., 1999	Mouse	OVA	Enhancement of IL-4 and IL-5 production
	Lambert et al., 2000	Rat	HDM	Enhancement of IgE production, bronchoconstriction, lymphocyte proliferation, and Th2 cytokine production
	Arantes-Costa et al., 2008	Mouse	OVA	Enhancement of AHR, and airway epithelial damage
ETS	Kang et al., 1996	Guinea pig	CRa	No change in anaphylactic antibody production Reduction of antigen-induced bronchospasm
	Seymour et al., 1997	Mouse	OVA	Enhancement of IgE and IgG1 production, lung eosinophilia, Th2 cytokine production
	Rumold et	Mouse	OVA	Enhancement of IgE and IgG1 production, lung

	al., 2001			eosinophilia, Th2 cytokine production
	Seymour et al., 2003	Mouse	Af	Enhancement of AHR, eosinophilia, and Th2 cytokine production
	Boweles et al., 2005	Mouse	OVA	Neither change in AHR, IgE production nor airway inflammation
	Seymour et al., 2005	Mouse	Af	Enhancement of nitric oxide production
	Min et al., 2007	Mouse	OVA	Enhancement of AHR, airway remodelling, epithelial chemokine expression, and increase in TGF-b^{+} cells
MTS	Robbins et al., 2005	Mouse	OVA, RW	Enhancement of cytokine production Reduction of lung eosinophilia, Th2 cytokine production and AHR Neither change in IgE nor IgG1 production
	Moerloose et al., 2005	Mouse	OVA	Enhancement of airway inflammation and responsiveness
	Moerloose et al., 2006	Mouse	OVA	Enhancement of IgE production, increases in eosinophils, CD4^{+} T cells, and goblet cell in the lung No change in AHR
	Thatcher et al., 2008	Mouse	OVA	Reduction of airway eosinophilia, goblet cell metaplasia, IL-4 and IL-5 production, and IgE production
Nano Ps	Inoue et al., 2005	Mouse	OVA	Enhancement of IgE production and airway inflammation
	Alessandrini et al., 2006	Mouse	OVA	Enhancement of BAL cellularity, Th2 cytokine production, AHR, mucus production
	de Haar et al., 2008	Mouse	OVA	Enhancement of proliferation of CD4^{+} cells, cytokine production, expression of co-stimulatory molecules
	Inoue et al., 2009a	Mouse	OVA	Enhancement of IgE production and airway inflammation (by carbon nanotubes)
	Inoue et al., 2009b	Mouse	OVA	Enhancement of IgE production and airway inflammation (by latex nanomaterials)
ASD	Ichinose et al., 2008b	Mouse	OVA	Enhancement of IgE production, lung eosinophilia, goblet cell proliferation, cytokine production
	Ichinose et al., 2009	Guinea pig	JCPA	Enhancement of nasal obstruction, histamine and CysLT release in NCLF, nasal eosinophilia, and IgE production Neither change in sneezing nor nasal secretion

Table 1. Representative studies evaluating relationship between air pollutants and airway allergic responses using experimental animal models. Abbreviations: Af, Aspergillus fumigatus; AHR, airway hyperresponsiveness; ASD; Asian sand dust, BAL; bronchoalveolar lavage fluid, CRa; cockroach allergen, CysLT; cysteinyl leukotriene, DEP; diesel exhaust particles, ETS; environmental tobacco smoke, IAR; Immediate asthmatic response, IL; interleukin, JCPA; allergen of Japanese cedar pollen, LAR; late asthmatic response, MTS; mainstream cigarette smoke, Nano Ps; nano particles, NCLF; nasal cavity lavage fluid, OVA; ovalbumin, ROFA; residual oil fly ash, RW; ragweed

demonstrated that allergic rhinitis symptoms induced by Japanese cedar pollen in guinea pigs were also augmented by exposure to Asian sand dust (Ichinose, 2009).
However, the relationship between Asian sand dust and health problems remains inconclusive, and further epidemiological and experimental studies are required.

3. Aggravation of allergic rhinitis by pyrenes: Demonstration by Japanese cedar pollen-induced allergic rhinitis model of guinea pigs

Pyrenes, such as benzo(a)pyrene (BaP) and 1-nitropyrene (1-NP), which are encountered in the environment mainly in the form of air pollution, are ubiquitous environmental pollutants found in DEP and cigarette smoke (Rosenkranz, 1980; Scheepers, 1995; Bai, 1998; Ohura, 2004). Carcinogenic and mutagenic effects of BaP and 1-NP in various cell types have been well documented (Bai, 1998; el-Bayoumy, 1995; Nakanishi, 2000). In addition, exposure to BaP enhances allergen-induced IgE and Th2 cytokine productions in mice (Kanoh, 1996; Kadkohda, 2005).
As described above, analyses of the relationships between air pollutants and airway allergy have been conducted using asthmatic mouse models. Meanwhile, pollenosis is a major health problem in Japan because the proportion of people with pollenosis in this country has been estimated to be more than 30%. Although the allergic symptoms of pollenosis, such as rhinitis and conjunctivitis, are not life-threatening like the airway obstructive response in asthma, chronic nasal blockage considerably lowers the quality of life of pollenosis patients. In addition, the nasal tissue is the first organ that contacts not only allergens but also air pollutants. Furthermore, "global warming" could increase the quantity of pollen from trees; it was experimentally demonstrated that a doubling of the atmospheric CO_2 concentration significantly stimulated ragweed pollen production (Wayne, 2002), suggesting that the health problem associated with pollens may be further exacerbated in future. Thus, the exposure effects of air pollutants on pollenosis should also be thoroughly examined.
We have established an experimental allergic rhinitis model in sensitized guinea pigs, using Japanese cedar pollen as the antigen (Nabe, 1997a, 1998). This experimental model has been used to assess whether short and long-term daily treatment with pyrenes, BaP and 1-NP aggravate antigen-induced sneezing and nasal blockage (Mizutani, 2007).

3.1 Development of an allergic rhinitis model showing nasal blockage

Japanese cedar pollen is also an air pollutant in the spring in Japan, and the most prevalent pollenosis allergen in this country. Thus, we have used cedar pollen as an allergen for development of an animal model of allergic rhinitis.
To begin with, we attempted to develop an animal model of allergic rhinitis that clearly shows allergic nasal symptoms including sneezing and nasal blockage like the patients. The guinea pig has long been used as a species showing a high responder of bronchial smooth muscle to various endogenous molecules such as histamine, cysteinyl leukotirenes, etc. Thus, we and others have used guinea pigs as a model animal of allergic asthma (Hutson, 1988; Matsumoto, 1994; Nabe, 1997b). From our experience of using of this species in asthma, we also used the guinea pig to develop an experimental model of allergic rhinitis.
In a disease model that can be utilized for pharmacological examinations and analyses of pathogenesis of diseases, several important considerations arise as follows: 1) The model animal should clearly exhibit symptoms that are similar to patients with the disease and actually torment patients, 2) symptoms should be reproducibly caused by reproducible methods, 3) symptoms can be measured as quantitatively as possible.

To satisfy these points, as shown in Fig. 1 (upper panel), guinea pigs were intranasally sensitized with the pollen extract+$Al(OH)_3$, and then intranasally challenged by a quantitative inhalation of the pollen once a week for several months (Nabe, 1997a). After the respective pollen challenge periods, the allergen-specific IgE antibody level in serum was measured, sneezing frequency was counted, and the degree of nasal blockage was assessed by measuring specific airway resistance (sRaw) using a double-flow plethysmograph system.
Because a major antigen protein in Japanese cedar pollen is Cry j 1, the amount of Cry j 1-specific IgE antibody in the serum was measured until the 29th challenge. Consequently, Cry j 1-specific IgE antibody level was increased during the repeated pollen challenges (Fig. 1, lower left panel) (Nabe, 1997a, 2005). In addition, after respective pollen challenges, sneezing was induced within 1 h after a challenge (Nabe, 1998). Regarding nasal blockage, both early and late phase nasal blockage were induced with their respective peaks at 1-2 h and 4-6 h after pollen challenges. The magnitude of biphasic nasal blockage was enhanced until the 7th challenge, followed by induction of almost reproducible nasal blockage after respective pollen challenges until around 30 challenges (Nabe, 1998). Images of the time-course of sneezing, and early and late phase nasal blockage after a certain challenge period are illustrated in the lower right panel of Fig. 1.
Induction of sneezing and biphasic nasal blockage was very similar to the symptoms of allergic rhinitis in pollenosis patients. Although nasal secretion is also a characteristic sign in the patients, and could be clearly observed in the model guinea pigs, we did not attempt to quantify the secretions.

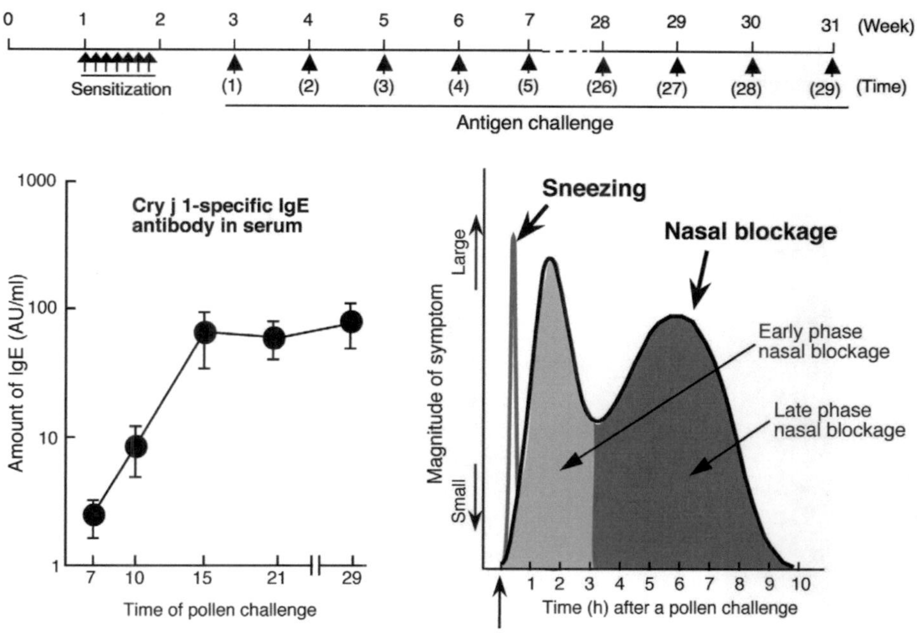

Fig. 1. Schedule for sensitization and challenge with Japanese cedar pollen in guinea pigs (upper panel), time-course change in amount of Cry j 1-specific IgE antibody in the serum during the sensitization and challenge period (lower left panel), and images of time-course changes in sneezing and nasal blockage induced after a certain period of pollen challenge. Each value in the lower left panel represents the mean±S.E. of 8 animals.

3.2 Aggravation of pollen-induced nasal blockage by BaP and 1-NP

As shown in Fig. 2 (upper panel), guinea pigs that had been sensitized with pollen extract plus $Al(OH)_3$ were repeatedly challenged with the pollen once a week. From 6 days before the first sensitization, BaP (100 µg/10 µl per nostril) or 1-NP (10 µg/10 µl per nostril) was daily administered into both nostrils (Fig. 2, upper panel). As expected, BaP aggravated both the early and late phase nasal blockage with statistical significance, and 1-NP also significantly enhanced the late phase response (Fig. 2, lower left and middle panels). In contrast, neither sneezing frequency nor the increase in Cry j 1-specific IgE antibody were affected even by long-term treatment (Fig. 2, lower right panel, and Table 2) (Mizutani, 2007).

Unexpectedly, a relatively short period (2 weeks) of treatment with BaP or 1-NP failed to significantly affect the magnitudes of early and late phase nasal blockage or the sneezing frequency (Mizutani, 2007).

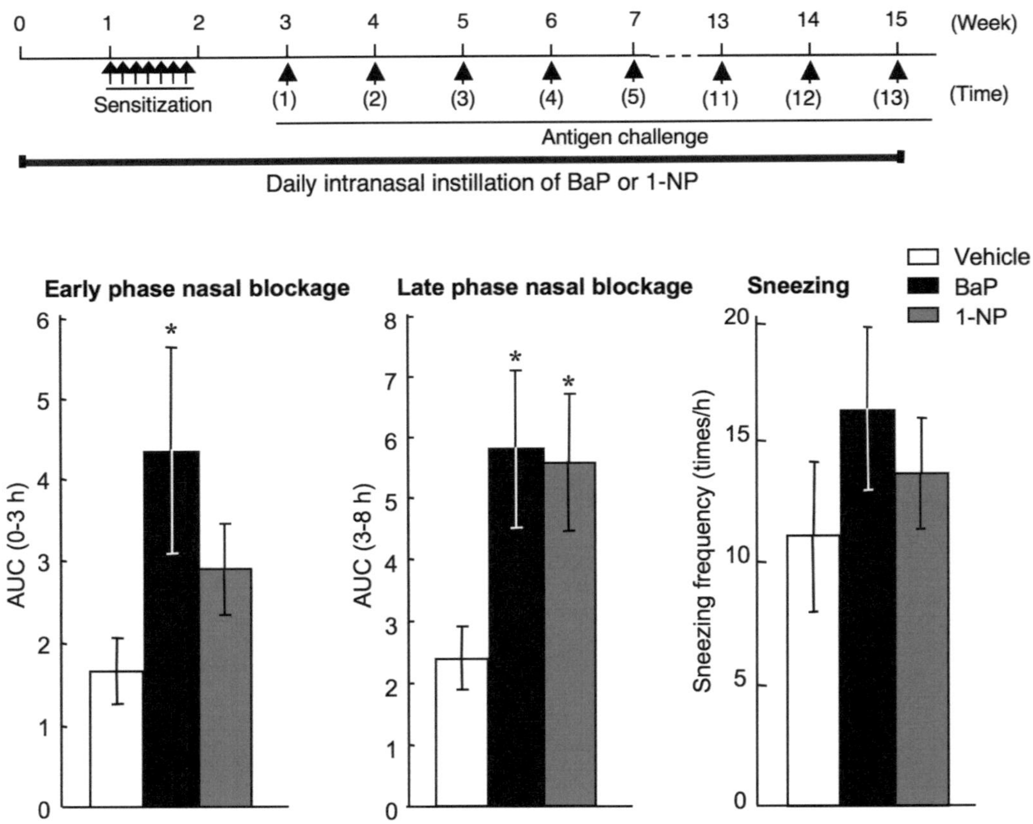

Fig. 2. Schedule for exposure to benzo(a)pyrene (BaP) or 1-nitropyrene (1-NP) during the sensitization and challenge period (upper panel), and effects of BaP and 1-NP on induction of the early and late phase nasal blockage (lower left and middle panels) and sneezing (lower right panel). Each column represents the mean±S.E. of 10 animals. AUC 0-3 h: Area under the curve for increase in sRaw in 0-3 h after the pollen challenge, AUC 3-8 h: Area under the curve for increase in sRaw in 3-8 h after the challange.

We have reported that sneezing is mediated mainly by histamine that is released from the nasal mucosal mast cells via antigen-IgE antibody reaction (Yamasaki, 2001; Fukuda, 2003). Our findings suggest that the pyrenes did not affect the antigen-IgE antibody reaction of mast cells. Meanwhile we have previously suggested that oxidative stress can be closely associated with the induction of biphasic nasal blockage (Mizutani, 2008). As other studies have demonstrated that BaP induces an increase in oxidative stress (Jeng, 2010; Gao,2011), the BaP-induced enhancement of nasal blockage may be due to increased oxidative stress. The aggravation of nasal blockage was reduced by cessation of the exposure to pyrenes in our model of pollenosis (Mizutani, 2007), indicating that avoidance of air pollutants is an appropriate method for treating the allergy.

	Amount of IgE (AU/ml)
Vehicle	45.3±19.5
BaP	49.1±22.0
1-NP	32.9±11.5

Table 2. Effects of benzo(a)pyrene (BaP) and 1-nitropyrene (1-NP) on the increase in Cry j 1-specific IgE at the 13th pollen challenge in sensitized guinea pigs. Each value represents the mean±S.E. of 10 animals.

4. Conclusion

It has been experimentally demonstrated that air pollutants such as DEP, ROFA, cigarette smoke, nanoparticles, Asian sand dust, etc. can aggravate allergic disorders. Exposure to those environmental pollutants in genetically allergic persons could synergistically aggravate their allergic symptoms. In future, both epidemiological and experimental analyses of the relationships between all candidate pollutants and allergic diseases are further required.

5. References

Alessandrini, F.; Schulz, H.; Takenaka, S.; Lentner, B.; Karg, E.; Behrendt, H. & Jakob, T. (2006). Effects of Ultrafine Carbon Particle Inhalation on Allergic Inflammation of the Lung. *The Journal of Allergy and Clinical Immunology*, Vol.117, No.4 (April 2006), pp. 824-830, ISSN 0091-6749

Arantes-Costa, F. M.; Lopes, F. D.; Toledo, A. C.; Magliarelli-Filho, P. A.; Moriya, H. T.; Carvalho-Oliveira, R.; Mauad, T.; Saldiva, P. H. & Martins, M. A. (2008). Effects of Residual Oil Fly Ash (ROFA) in Mice with Chronic Allergic Pulmonary Inflammation. *Toxicologic Pathology*, Vol.36, No.5 (May 2008), pp. 680-686, ISSN 0192-6233

Bai, F.; Nakanishi, Y.; Takayama, K.; Pei, X. H.; Tokiwa, H. & Hara, N. (1998). Ki-Ras Mutation and Cell Proliferation of Lung Lesions Induced by 1-Nitropyrene in A/J

Mice. *Molecular Carcinogenesis*, Vol.22, No.4 (August 1998), pp. 258-264, ISSN 0899-1987

Barbee, R. A.; Halonen, M.; Kaltenborn, W.; Lebowitz, M. & Burrows, B. (1987). A Longitudinal Study of Serum IgE in a Community Cohort: Correlations with Age, Sex, Smoking, and Atopic Status. *The Journal of Allergy and Clinical Immunology*, Vol.79, No.6 (June 1987), pp. 919-927, ISSN 0091-6749

Bowles, K.; Horohov, D.; Paulsen, D.; Leblanc, C.; Littlefield-Chabaud, M.; Ahlert, T.; Ahlert, K.; Pourciau, S. & Penn, A. (2005). Exposure of Adult Mice to Environmental Tobacco Smoke Fails to Enhance the Immune Response to Inhaled Antigen. *Inhalation Toxicology*, Vol.17, No.1 (January 2005), pp. 43-51, ISSN 0895-8378

Britton, J. (2005). Passive Smoking and Asthma Exacerbation. *Thorax*, Vol.60, No.10 (October 2005), pp. 794-795, ISSN 0040-6376

Chilmonczyk, B. A.; Salmun, L. M.; Megathlin, K. N.; Neveux, L. M.; Palomaki, G. E.; Knight, G. J.; Pulkkinen, A. J. & Haddow, J. E. (1993). Association Between Exposure to Environmental Tobacco Smoke and Exacerbations of Asthma in Children. *The New England Journal of Medicine*, Vol.328, No.23 (June 1993), pp. 1665-1669, ISSN 0028-4793

de Haar, C.; Kool, M.; Hassing, I.; Bol, M.; Lambrecht, B. N. & Pieters, R. (2008). Lung Dendritic Cells are Stimulated by Ultrafine Particles and Play a Key Role in Particle Adjuvant Activity. *The Journal of Allergy and Clinical Immunology*, Vol.121, No.5 (May 2008), pp. 1246-1254, ISSN 0091-6749

Diaz-Sanchez, D.; Garcia, M. P.; Wang, M.; Jyrala, M. & Saxon, A. (1999). Nasal Challenge with Diesel Exhaust Particles Can Induce Sensitization to a Neoallergen in the Human Mucosa. *The Journal of Allergy and Clinical Immunology*, Vol.104, No.6, (December 1999), pp. 1183-1188, ISSN 0091-6749

el-Bayoumy, K.; Chae, Y. H.; Upadhyaya, P.; Rivenson, A.; Kurtzke, C.; Reddy, B. & Hecht, S. S. (1995). Comparative Tumorigenicity of Benzo[a]pyrene, 1-Nitropyrene and 2-Amino-1-methyl-6-phenylimidazo[4,5-b]pyridine Administered by Gavage to Female CD Rats. *Carcinogenesis*, Vol.16, No.2 (February 1995), pp. 431-434, ISSN 0143-3334

Evans, D.; Levison, M. J.; Feldman, C. H.; Clark, N. M.; Wasilewski, Y.; Levin, B. & Mellins, R. B. (1987). The Impact of Passive Smoking on Emergency Room Visits of Urban Children with Asthma. *The American Review of Respiratory Disease*, Vol.135, No.3 (March 1987), pp. 567-572, ISSN 0003-0805

Fujimaki, H.; Saneyoshi, K.; Nohara, O.; Shiraishi, F. & Imai, T. (1995). Intranasal Instillation of Diesel Exhaust Particulates and Antigen in Mice Modulated Cytokine Productions in Cervical Lymph Node Cells. *International Archives of Allergy and Immunology*, Vol.108, No.3 (November 1995), pp. 268-273, ISSN 1018-2438

Fukuda, S.; Midoro, K.; Gyoten, M.; Kawano, Y.; Ashida, Y.; Nabe, T.; Kohno, S. & Nagaya, H. (2003). Effects of TAK-427 on Acute Nasal Symptoms and Nasal Obstruction in Guinea Pig Model of Experimental Allergic Rhinitis. *European Journal of Pharmacology*, Vol.476, No.3 (August 2003), pp. 239-247, ISSN 0014-2999

Gao, M.; Li, Y.; Long, J.; Shah, W.; Fu, L.; Lai, B. & Wang, Y. (2011). Induction of Oxidative Stress and DNA Damage in Cervix in Acute Treatment with Benzo[a]pyrene. *Mutation Research*. Vol.719, No.1-2 (February 2011), pp. 52-59, ISSN 0027-5107

Gavett, S. H.; Madison, S. L.; Stevens, M. A. & Costa, D. L. (1999). Residual Oil Fly Ash Amplifies Allergic Cytokines, Airway Responsiveness, and Inflammation in Mice. *American Journal of Respiratory and Critical Care Medicine*, Vol.160, No.6 (December 1999), pp. 1897-1904, ISSN 1073-449X

Goldsmith, C. A.; Hamada, K.; Ning, Y.; Qin, G.; Catalano, P.; Krishna Murthy, G. G.; Lawrence, J. & Kobzik, L. (1999). Effects of Environmental Aerosols on Airway Hyperresponsiveness in a Murine Model of Asthma. *Inhalation Toxicology*, Vol.11, No.11 (November 1999), pp. 981-998, ISSN 0895-8378

Hamada, K.; Goldsmith, C. A. & Kobzik, L. (1999). Increased Airway Hyperresponsiveness and Inflammation in a Juvenile Mouse Model of Asthma Exposed to Air-Pollutant Aerosol. *Journal of Toxicology and Environmental Health*. Part A, Vol.58, No.3 (October 1999), pp. 129-143, ISSN 1528-7394

Hashimoto, K.; Ishii, Y.; Uchida, Y.; Kimura, T.; Masuyama, K.; Morishima, Y.; Hirano, K.; Nomura, A.; Sakamoto, T.; Takano, H.; Sagai, M. & Sekizawa, K. (2001). Exposure to Diesel Exhaust Exacerbates Allergen-Induced Airway Responses in Guinea Pigs. *American Journal of Respiratory and Critical Care Medicine*, Vol.164, No.10 Pt 1 (November 2001), pp. 1957-1963, ISSN 1073-449X

Hutson, P. A.; Church, M. K.; Clay, T. P.; Miller, P. & Holgate, S. T. (1988). Early and Late-Phase Bronchoconstriction After Allergen Challenge of Nonanesthetized Guinea Pigs. I. The Association of Disordered Airway Physiology to Leukocyte Infiltration. *The American Review of Respiratory Disease*, Vol.137, No.3 (March 1988), pp. 548-557, ISSN 0003-0805

Ichinose, T.; Takano, H.; Miyabara, Y. & Sagai, M. (1998). Long-Term Exposure to Diesel Exhaust Enhances Antigen-Induced Eosinophilic Inflammation and Epithelial Damage in the Murine Airway. *Toxicological Sciences*, Vol.44, No.1 (July 1998), pp. 70-79. ISSN 1096-6080

Ichinose, T.; Yoshida, S.; Hiyoshi, K.; Sadakane, K.; Takano, H.; Nishikawa, M.; Mori, I.; Yanagisawa, R.; Kawazato, H.; Yasuda, A. & Shibamoto, T. (2008a). The Effects of Microbial Materials Adhered to Asian Sand Dust on Allergic Lung Inflammation. *Archives of Environmental Contamination and Toxicology*, Vol.55, No.3 (October 2008), pp. 348-357, ISSN 0090-4341

Ichinose, T.; Yoshida, S.; Sadakane, K.; Takano, H.; Yanagisawa, R.; Inoue, K.; Nishikawa, M.; Mori, I.; Kawazato, H.; Yasuda, A. & Shibamoto, T. (2008b). Effects of Asian Sand Dust, Arizona Sand Dust, Amorphous Silica and Aluminum Oxide on Allergic Inflammation in the Murine Lung. *Inhalation Toxicology*, Vol.20, No.7, (May 2008), pp. 685-694, ISSN 0895-8378

Ichinose, T.; Hiyoshi, K.; Yoshida, S.; Takano, H.; Inoue, K.; Nishikawa, M.; Mori, I.; Kawazato, H.; Yasuda, A. & Shibamoto, T. (2009). Asian Sand Dust Aggravates Allergic Rhinitis in Guinea Pigs Induced by Japanese Cedar Pollen. *Inhalation Toxicology*, Vol.21, No.12 (October 2009), pp. 985-993, ISSN 0895-8378

Inoue, K.; Takano, H.; Yanagisawa, R.; Sakurai, M.; Ichinose, T.; Sadakane, K. & Yoshikawa, T. (2005). Effects of Nano Particles on Antigen-related Airway Inflammation in Mice. *Respiratory Research*, Vol.6, (September 2005), pp. 106, ISSN 1465-9921

Inoue, K.; Koike, E.; Yanagisawa, R.; Hirano, S.; Nishikawa, M. & Takano, H. (2009a). Effects of Multi-walled Carbon Nanotubes on a Murine Allergic Airway Inflammation Model. *Toxicology and Applied Pharmacology*, Vol.237, No.3 (June 2009), pp. 306-316, ISSN 0041-008X

Inoue, K.; Takano, H.; Yanagisawa, R.; Koike, E. & Shimada, A. (2009b). Size Effects of Latex Nanomaterials on Lung Inflammation in Mice. *Toxicology and Applied Pharmacology*, Vol.234, No.1 (January 2009), pp. 68-76, ISSN 0041-008X

Jeng, H. A.; Pan, C. H.; Diawara, N.; Chang-Chien, G. P.; Lin, W. Y.; Huang, C. T.; Ho, C. K. & Wu, M. T. (2010). Polycyclic Aromatic Hydrocarbon-Induced Oxidative Stress and Lipid Peroxidation in Relation to Immunological Alteration. *Occupational and Environmental Medicine*, (December 2010), ISSN 1351-0711

Kadkhoda, K.; Pourfathollah, A. A.; Pourpak, Z. & Kazemnejad, A. (2005). The Cumulative Activity of Benzo(a)pyrene on Systemic Immune Responses with Mite Allergen Extract After Intranasal Instillation and Ex Vivo Response to Ovalbumin in Mice. *Toxicology Letters*, Vol.157, No.1 (May 2005), pp. 31-39, ISSN 0378-4274

Kang, B. C.; Zhou, K.; Lai, Y. L. & Hong, C. B. (1996). Experimental Asthma Developed by Room Air Contamination with Cockroach Allergen. *International Archives of Allergy and Immunology*, Vol.111. No.3 (November 1996), pp. 299-306, ISSN 1018-2438

Kanoh, T.; Suzuki, T.; Ishimori, M.; Ikeda, S.; Ohasawa, M.; Ohkuni, H. & Tunetoshi, Y. (1996). Adjuvant Activities of Pyrene, Anthracene, Fluoranthene and Benzo(a)pyrene in Production of Anti-IgE Antibody to Japanese Cedar Pollen Allergen in Mice. *Journal of Clinical & Laboratory Immunology*, Vol.48, No.4 (1996), pp. 133-147, ISSN 0141-2760

Kobayashi, T. (2000). Exposure to Diesel Exhaust Aggravates Nasal Allergic Reaction in Guinea Pigs. *American Journal of Respiratory and Critical Care Medicine*, Vol.162, No.2 Pt 1 (August 2000), pp. 352-356. ISSN 1073-449X

Lambert, A. L.; Dong, W.; Selgrade, M. K. & Gilmour, M. I. (2000). Enhanced Allergic Sensitization by Residual Oil Fly Ash Particles Is Mediated by Soluble Metal Constituents. *Toxicology and Applied Pharmacology*, Vol.165, No.1 (May 2000), pp. 84-93, ISSN 0041-008X

Liu, J.; Ballaney, M.; Al-alem, U.; Quan, C.; Jin, X.; Perera, F.; Chen, L. C. & Miller, R. L. (2008). Combined Inhaled Diesel Exhaust Particles and Allergen Exposure Alter Methylation of T Helper Genes and IgE Production in Vivo. *Toxicological Sciences*, Vol.102, No.1 (March 2008), pp. 76-81. ISSN 1096-6080

Matsumoto, T.; Ashida, Y. & Tsukuda, R. (1994). Pharmacological Modulation of Immediate and Late Airway Response and Leukocyte Infiltration in the Guinea Pig. *The Journal of Pharmacology and Experimental Therapeutics*, Vol.269, No.3 (June 1994), pp. 1236-1244, ISSN 0022-3565

Min, M. G.; Song, D. J.; Miller, M.; Cho, J. Y.; McElwain, S.; Ferguson, P. & Broide, D. H. (2007). Coexposure to Environmental Tobacco Smoke Increases Levels of Allergen-induced Airway Remodeling in Mice. *The Journal of Immunology*, Vol.178, No.8 (April 2007), pp. 5321-5328, ISSN 0022-1767

Mitsunobu, F.; Ashida, K.; Hosaki, Y.; Tsugeno, H.; Okamoto, M.; Nishida, N.; Nagata, T.; Tanizaki, Y. & Tanimoto, M. (2004). Influence of Long-term Cigarette Smoking on Immunoglobulin E-Mediated Allergy, Pulmonary Function, and High-Resolution Computed Tomography Lung Densitometry in Elderly Patients with Asthma. *Clinical and Experimental Allergy*, Vol.34, No.1 (January 2004), pp. 59-64, ISSN 0954-7894

Miyabara, Y.; Ichinose, T.; Takano, H.; Lim, H. B. & Sagai, M. (1998). Effects of Diesel Exhaust on Allergic Airway Inflammation in Mice. *The Journal of Allergy and Clinical Immunology*, Vol.102, No.5 (November 1998), pp. 805-812, ISSN 0091-6749

Mizutani, N.; Nabe, T.; Ohtani, Y.; Han, H. Y.; Fujii, M.; Yoshino, S.; Hirayama, T. & Kohno, S. (2007). Polycyclic Aromatic Hydrocarbons Aggravate Antigen-Induced Nasal Blockage in Experimental Allergic Rhinitis. *Journal of Pharmacological Sciences*, Vol.105, No.3, (November 2007), pp. 291-297, ISSN 1347-8613

Mizutani, N.; Nabe, T.; Fujii, M.; Yoshino, S. & Kohno, S. (2008). Involvement of Peroxynitrite in Pollen-Induced Nasal Blockage in Guinea Pigs. *European Journal of Pharmacology*, Vol.582, No.1-3 (March 2008), pp. 139-144, ISSN 0014-2999

Moerloose, K. B.; Pauwels, R. A. & Joos, G. F. (2005). Short-term Cigarette Smoke Exposure Enhances Allergic Airway Inflammation in Mice. *American Journal of Respiratory and Critical Care Medicine*, Vol.172, No.2 (July 2005), pp. 168-172, ISSN 1073-449X

Moerloose, K. B.; Robays, L. J.; Maes, T.; Brusselle, G. G.; Tournoy, K. G. & Joos, G. F. (2006). Cigarette Smoke Exposure Facilitates Allergic Sensitization in Mice. *Respiratory Research*, Vol.7, (March 2006), pp. 49, ISSN 1465-9921

Muranaka, M.; Suzuki, S.; Koizumi, K.; Takafuji, S.; Miyamoto, T.; Ikemori, R. & Tokiwa, H. (1986). Adjuvant Activity of Diesel-Exhaust Particulates for The Production of IgE Antibody in Mice. *The Journal of Allergy and Clinical Immunology*, Vol.77, No.4 (April 1986), pp. 616-623, ISSN 0091-6749

Nabe, T.; Shimizu, K.; Mizutani, N.; Saeki, Y.; Yamamura, H.; Takenaka, H. & Kohno, S. (1997a). A New Model of Experimental Allergic Rhinitis Using Japanese Cedar Pollen in Guinea Pigs. *Japanese Journal of Pharmacology*, Vol.75, No.3 (November 1997), pp. 243-251, ISSN 0021-5198

Nabe, T.; Shinoda, N.; Yamada, M.; Sekioka, T.; Saeki, Y.; Yamamura, H. & Kohno, S. (1997b). Repeated Antigen Inhalation-Induced Reproducible Early and Late Asthma in Guinea Pigs. *Japanese Journal of Pharmacology*, Vol.75, No.1 (September 1997), pp. 65-75, ISSN 0021-5198

Nabe, T.; Mizutani, N.; Shimizu, K.; Takenaka, H. & Kohno, S. (1998). Development of Pollen-induced Allergic Rhinitis with Early and Late Phase Nasal Blockage in Guinea Pigs. *Inflammation Research*, Vol.47, No.9 (September 1998), pp. 369-374, ISSN 1023-3830

Nabe, T.; Kubota, K.; Terada, T.; Takenaka, H. & Kohno, S. (2005). Effect of Oral Immunotherapy on Nasal Blockage in Experimental Allergic Rhinitis. *Journal of Pharmacological Sciences*, Vol.98, No.4 (August 2005), pp. 380-387, ISSN 1347-8613

Nakanishi, Y.; Pei, X. H.; Takayama, K.; Bai, F.; Izumi, M.; Kimotsuki, K.; Inoue, K.; Minami, T.; Wataya, H. & Hara, N. (2000). Polycyclic Aromatic Hydrocarbon Carcinogens Increase Ubiquitination of p21 Protein After the Stabilization of p53 and the Expression of p21. *American Journal of Respiratory Cell and Molecular Biology*, Vol.22, No.6 (June 2000), pp. 747-754, ISSN 1044-1549

Ohura, T.; Amagai, T.; Fusaya, M. & Matsushita, H. (2004). Polycyclic Aromatic Hydrocarbons in Indoor and Outdoor Environments and Factors Affecting Their Concentrations. *Environmental Science & Technology*, Vol.38, No.1 (January 2004), pp. 77-83, ISSN 0013-936X

Peden, D. & Reed, C. E. (2010). Environmental and Occupational Allergies. *The Journal of Allergy and Clinical Immunology*, Vol.125, No.2 Suppl.2, (February 2010), pp. S150-S160, ISSN 0091-6749

Riedl, M. & Diaz-Sanchez, D. (2005). Biology of Diesel Exhaust Effects on Respiratory Function. *The Journal of Allergy and Clinical Immunology*, Vol.115, No.2 (February 2005), pp. 221-228, ISSN 0091-6749

Ro, CU.; Hwang, H.; Kim, H.; Chun, Y. & Van, Grieken. R. (2005). Single-particle Characterization of Four "Asian Dust" Samples Collected in Korea, Using Low-Z Particle Electron Probe X-ray Microanalysis. *Environmental Science & Technology*, Vol.39. No.6 (March 2005), pp. 1409-1419, ISSN 0013-936X

Robbins, C. S.; Pouladi, M. A.; Fattouh, R.; Dawe, D. E.; Vujicic, N.; Richards, C. D.; Jordana, M.; Inman, M. D. & Stampfli, M. R. (2005). Mainstream Cigarette Smoke Exposure Attenuates Airway Immune Inflammatory Responses to Surrogate and Common Environmental Allergens in Mice, Despite Evidence of Increased Systemic Sensitization. *The Journal of Immunology*, Vol.175, No.5 (September 2005), pp. 2834-2842, ISSN 0022-1767

Rosenkranz, H. S.; McCoy, E. C.; Sanders, D. R.; Butler, M.; Kiriazides, D. K. & Mermelstein, R. (1980). Nitropyrenes: Isolation, Identificaton, and Reduction of Mutagenic Impurities in Carbon Black and Toners. *Science*, Vol.209. No.4460 (August 1980), pp. 1039-1043, ISSN 0036-8075

Rumold, R.; Jyrala, M. & Diaz-Sanchez, D. (2001). Secondhand Smoke Induces Allergic Sensitization in Mice. *The Journal of Immunology*, Vol.167, No.8 (October 2001), pp. 4765-4770, ISSN 0022-1767

Scheepers, P. T.; Martens, M. H.; Velders, D. D.; Fijneman, P.; van Kerkhoven, M.; Noordhoek, J. & Bos, R. P. (1995). 1-Nitropyrene as a Marker for the Mutagenicity of Diesel Exhaust-derived Particulate Matter in Workplace Atmospheres. *Environmental and Molecular Mutagenesis*, Vol.25, No.2 (1995), pp. 134-147, ISSN 0893-6692

Seymour, B. W.; Pinkerton, K. E.; Friebertshauser, K. E.; Coffman, R. L. & Gershwin, L. J. (1997). Second-hand Smoke Is an Adjuvant for T Helper-2 Responses in a Murine Model of Allergy. *The Journal of Immunology*, Vol.159, No.12 (December 1997), pp. 6169-6175, ISSN 0022-1767

Seymour, B. W.; Schelegle, E. S.; Pinkerton, K. E.; Friebertshauser, K. E.; Peake, J. L.; Kurup, V. P.; Coffman, R. L. & Gershwin, L. J. (2003). Second-hand Smoke Increases Bronchial Hyperreactivity and Eosinophilia in a Murine Model of Allergic

Aspergillosis. *Clinical and Developmental Immunology*, Vol.10, No.1 (March 2003), pp. 35-42, ISSN 1740-2522

Seymour, B. W.; Peake, J. L.; Pinkerton, K. E.; Kurup, V. P. & Gershwin, L. J. (2005). Second-hand Smoke Increases Nitric Oxide and Alters the IgE Response in a Murine Model of Allergic Aspergillosis. *Clinical and Developmental Immunology*, Vol.12, No.2 (June 2005), pp. 113-124, ISSN 1740-2522

Siroux, V.; Pin, I.; Oryszczyn, M. P.; Le Moual, N. & Kauffmann, F. (2000). Relationships of Active Smoking to Asthma and Asthma Severity in the EGEA Study. Epidemiological Study on the Genetics and Environment of Asthma. *The European Respiratory Journal*, Vol.15, No.3 (March 2000), pp. 470-477, ISSN 0903-1936

Steerenberg, P. A.; Dormans, J. A.; van Doorn, C. C.; Middendorp, S.; Vos, J. G. & van Loveren, H. (1999). A Pollen Model in the Rat for Testing Adjuvant Activity of Air Pollution Components. *Inhalation Toxicology*, Vol.11, No.12 (December 1999), pp. 1109-1122, ISSN 0895-8378

Suzuki, T.; Kanoh, T.; Ishimori, M.; Ikeda, S. & Ohkuni, H. (1996). Adjuvant Activity of Diesel Exhaust Particulates (DEP) in Production of Anti-IgE and Anti-IgG1 Antibodies to Mite Allergen in Mice. *Journal of Clinical & Laboratory Immunology*, Vol.48, No.5 (1996), pp. 187-199. ISSN 0141-2760

Takafuji, S.; Suzuki, S.; Koizumi, K.; Tadokoro, K.; Miyamoto, T.; Ikemori, R. & Muranaka, M. (1987). Diesel-Exhaust Particulates Inoculated by the Intranasal Route Have an Adjuvant Activity for IgE Production in Mice. *The Journal of Allergy and Clinical Immunology*, Vol.79, No.4 (April 1987), pp. 639-645, ISSN 0091-6749

Takahashi, G.; Tanaka, H.; Wakahara, K.; Nasu, R.; Hashimoto, M.; Miyoshi, K.; Takano, H.; Yamashita, H.; Inagaki, N. & Nagai, H. (2010). Effect of Diesel Exhaust Particles on House Dust Mite-Induced Airway Eosinophilic Inflammation and Remodeling in Mice. *Journal of Pharmacological Sciences*, Vol.112, No.2 (February 2010), pp. 192-202, ISSN 1347-8613

Takano, H.; Yoshikawa, T.; Ichinose, T.; Miyabara, Y.; Imaoka, K. & Sagai, M. (1997). Diesel Exhaust Particles Enhance Antigen-Induced Airway Inflammation and Local Cytokine Expression in Mice. *American Journal of Respiratory and Critical Care Medicine*, Vol.156, No.1 (July 1997), pp. 36-42. ISSN 1073-449X

Takano, H.; Ichinose, T.; Miyabara, Y.; Yoshikawa, T. & Sagai, M. (1998). Diesel Exhaust Particles Enhance Airway Responsiveness Following Allergen Exposure in Mice. *Immunopharmacology and Immunotoxicology*, Vol.20, No.2 (May 1998), pp. 329-336. ISSN 0892-3973

Thatcher, T. H.; Benson, R. P.; Phipps, R. P. & Sime, P. J. (2008). High-Dose But Not Low-Dose Mainstream Cigarette Smoke Suppresses Allergic Airway Inflammation by Inhibiting T Cell Function. *American Journal of Physiology, Lung Cellular and Molecular Physiology*, Vol.295, No.3 (September 2008), pp. L412-L421, ISSN 1040-0605

Vidal, C.; Boquete, O.; Gude, F.; Rey, J.; Meijide, L. M.; Fernández-Merino, M. C. & González-Quintela, A. (2004). High Prevalence of Storage Mite Sensitization in a General Adult Population. *Allergy*, Vol.59, No.4 (April 2004), pp. 401-405, ISSN 0105-4538

Wayne, P.; Foster, S.; Connolly, J.; Bazzaz, F. & Epstein, P. (2002). Production of Allergenic Pollen by Ragweed (*Ambrosia artemisiifolia L.*) is Increased in CO_2-Enriched Atmospheres. *Annals of Allergy, Asthma & Immunology*, Vol.88, No.3 (March 2002), pp. 279-282, ISSN 1081-1206

Yamasaki, M.; Sasaki, K.; Mizutani, N.; Nabe, T.; Sakura, Y.; Matsumoto, T.; Ashida, Y. & Kohno, S. (2001). Pharmacological Characterization of the Leukocyte Kinetics After Intranasal Antigen Challenge in a Guinea Pig Model of Allergic Rhinitis. *Inflammation Research*, Vol.50, No.9 (September 2001), pp. 474-482, ISSN 1023-3830

24

The Impact of Asthma and Allergic Diseases on Schoolchildren: Are They at Increased Risk of Absenteeism and Poor School Performance?

Abdulbari Bener
Dept. of Epidemiology and Medical Statistics, Hamad Medical Corporation
Dept. of Public Health, Weill Cornell Medical College
State of Qatar

1. Introduction

1.1 Asthma and allergic diseases in children

Asthma is the most common chronic illness of childhood in both developed and developing countries and there is a wide concensus that asthma and allergies have become more prevalent among children (Robertson et al., 2004). Among children, higher prevalence rates of asthma have been found in industrialized western countries than in developing countries in Asia and Africa (Beasley et al., 2000). In some western countries, the prevalence of asthma and allergies has reached alarming proportions, affecting more than one-third of the children within the general population (Khaldi et al., 2005). It appears that differences in asthma prevalence between population groups are due to differential exposure to environmental factors: genetic variations alone could not account for the risk in the prevalence of disease over a few decades. Allergen exposure in early life appears to correlate with sensitization and expression of asthma and atopy. Lifestyle factors including diet and ambient air pollution may be disease modifiers (Shapiro & Stout, 2002).
Air pollution has a positive and significant effect on asthma exacerbation. A cohort study on asthma and exposure to ozone reported that pollution has been associated with new onset asthma as well as other respiratory diseases (McConnell et al., 2002). Urban atmospheric pollution has a well known impact on acute and chronic respiratory disease. The United Nations estimated that over 600 million people in urban areas worldwide were exposed to dangerous levels of traffic generated air pollutants (Cacciola et al., 2002). There is substantial epidemiological evidence indicating a link between respiratory and cardiovascular morbidity and outdoor air pollution levels (Bener et al., 2009).

1.2 Magnitude of asthma and allergic diseases

A recent study on asthma reported a high prevalence of asthma among Qatari children(Janahi et al., 2006). The rapid growth and changing environmental and social conditions in the State of Qatar affected the prevalence of allergic diseases in Qatar. Exposure to air pollution has been considered to be one of the leading factors in public health problems in oil-rich developing countries. In Qatar, air pollution originates mostly from motor vehicle exhaust fumes and industry fumes. As a result, concentrations of CO, NO_2, O_3 and airborne particles are generally high. Air pollution in Qatar has been a contributing factor for the high prevalence of asthma and related allergic diseases. Air pollution is a worldwide problem related to densely populated urban areas and to heavily industrialized regions.

1.3 School failures a problem

Asthma is the most common chronic illness among school children and an important cause of school absenteeism and reduced participation in sports and other activities (Maziak et al., 2003). Asthma is the principal cause of school absences due to chronic disease in childhood accounting for 20% of school days lost among elementary and high school students. Education is one of the main foundations for the child's development and also for national human resource development. Chronic illness may lead to school failure by increasing school absence during exacerbations. The characteristics of school failure in Qatar has been studied and found that asthma is one of the leading causes of school absence. Recent studies investigated the relationship between school absenteeism, presence of asthma and air pollution.

2. Methods

2.1 Sampling design

The study included schoolchildren and adolescents in the age group 6 – 18 years, studying in the primary, preparatory and secondary levels in government and private schools in the State of Qatar. This study consists of an amalgamation of three cross-sectional studies conducted among school students on the prevalence of asthma and allergic diseases and their impact on school attendance in children. The first cross sectional study covered 3283 school children aged 6-14 years to determine the prevalence of asthma and allergic diseases among this age group. The second cross sectional study included 31,400 Qatari school children aged 6-12 years to investigate the school absenteeism as a result of asthma and wheezing. The third was a prospective cross sectional study that assessed the factors contributing to school failure among school children studying in grade 1 to 12. Students were recruited from the schools situated in both urban and semi-urban areas of Qatar.

All three studies used a multi-stage stratified random sampling technique which ensured that the school children were selected randomly. The list of names of schools in urban and semi-urban areas was obtained from the Supreme Council for Education and Higher Education. A total of 151,050 students are studying in primary, preparatory and secondary schools. There are 299 schools, of which 152 are boys and 147 for girls located in 21 different districts. During the first stage, one school from each of these 5 districts was selected randomly, thus overcoming the so called 'cluster effect'. Similarly, the classrooms and schoolchildren were selected in the second and third stages using the same simple random sampling procedure. Approval for the study was obtained from the Medical Ethics Committee of the Hamad General Hospital, Hamad Medical Corporation.

2.2 Data collection

Data collection of the three studies was during the years 2003 to 2008. The screening survey for asthma was carried out in the selected schools to represent the entire State of Qatar. The survey instrument was tested on 125 students and thus validated the questionnaire. All schools have a policy of recording illnesses including asthma and their personal details which were captured by school health nurses. We have used the School Health Registry for obtaining the students information and school absenteeism due to asthma and wheezing. An approval was obtained from the Regional Directors of Education and from individual school principals at all selected schools. Again we had a double confirmation on the data obtained on asthmatic children by using the modified version of the International Study of Asthma and Allergies in Childhood [ISAAC] questionnaire (Vichyanond et al., 1998) and another questionnaire (Bener et al., 1994a). A written consent form was obtained from the parents of each child, after giving an explanation of the aims and nature of the studies. The questionnaires with a letter of explanation in Arabic were distributed to the parents of these children and lived in either urban or semi-urban areas of Qatar.

2.3 Data collection instrument

The International Study of Asthma and Allergies in Childhood (ISAAC) questionnaires included the questions related to asthma and allergic rhinitis. The questions concerning the diagnosis of asthma were "Has the child ever been diagnosed as having asthma by a doctor?", and "has the child ever needed treatment or hospital admission due to asthma?" The diagnosis of Allergic rhinitis was based on questions such as: Has your child ever had a problem with frequent sneezing or prolonged blocked nose during the last six months when he/she did not have a cold or flu? The questions concerning the diagnosis of persistent eczema were as follows: Has your child ever had a dry and itchy red rash for at least 6 months?

2.4 Statistical analysis

Student's t-test (two tailed) was used to determine the significance of any difference between two continuous variables. Chi-square and Fisher exact test were performed to ascertain the association between two or more categorical variables. The level $p<0.05$ was considered as the cut-off value for significance.

3. Discussion

3.1 Prevalence of asthma and allergic diseases

Asthma is the single most prevalent cause of childhood disability. The children with asthma are poorer in health, limited in daily activities and experience more visits to health care professionals and hospitalizations. Despite advances in the understanding of asthma's pathophysiology, there have been increases in the prevalence, morbidity and mortality of children with asthma during the last 2 decades (Mannino et al, 2002). There have been relatively few studies on the relationship between asthma and school absenteeism and performance. Asthma and allergic diseases are the most common childhood chronic disease and continues to be a major cause of morbidity and health service use in Qatar. The most internationally accepted and validated methodology for measuring asthma prevalence in children is through school sampling using the International Study of Asthma and Allergies in Childhood (ISAAC) survey. The screening survey for asthma and allergic diseases is important because asthma prevalence seems to be increasing in rapidly developing urban communities.

In a population based sample of 3283 school children in the age group 6 – 14 years in Qatar, a high prevalence rate of diagnosed asthma (19.8%), allergic rhinitis (30.5%) and pulmonary infection (11.9%) was observed (Janahi et al., 2006). On the whole, the prevalence of asthma decreased with age, while the prevalence of pulmonary infection and throat infection increased with age. There were significant differences in the male-female prevalence rates of asthma and allergic rhinitis in all of the 3 age groups; 6-8 years, 9-11 years and 12-14 years. Prevalence rate of asthma was significantly higher in males (25.6%) than that of the females (13.4%) (p<0.001). Allergic rhinitis was significantly higher in boys of 6 – 8 years compared to girls in the same age group (41.3% vs. 29.3%; p<0.001). The overall prevalence of throat infection (46.8% vs. 38.3%), pulmonary infection (15.9% vs. 7.5%) and allergic rhinitis (33.2% vs. 27.6%) were found to be significantly higher among males than females (p<0.001). (Table 1)

Variables	Number of children											
	6-8 n=1390			9-11 n=1497			12-14 n=396			Overall n=3283		
	n(%)			n(%)			n(%)			n(%)		
	Male N=690	Female N=700	Total N=1390	Male N=808	Female N=689	Total N=1497	Male N=165	Female N=152	Total N=317	Male N=1663	Female N=1541	Total N=3204
Asthma	212 (30.7)***	93 (13.3)	305 (21.9)	177 (21.9)***	94 (13.6)	271 (18.1)	50 (22.9)*	23 (12.9)	73 (18.4)	439 (25.6)***	210 (13.4)	649 (19.8)
Eczema	155 (22.5)	160 (22.9)	315 (22.7)	159 (19.7)	153 (22.2)	312 (20.8)	72 (33.0)*	39 (21.9)	111 (28.0)	386 (22.5)	352 (22.5)	738 (22.5)
Allergic rhinitis	285 (41.3)***	205 (29.3)	490 (35.3)	216 (26.7)	179 (26.0)	395 (26.4)	68 (31.2)	48 (27.0)	116 (29.3)	569 (33.2)***	432 (27.6)	1001 (30.5)
Throat infection	314 (45.5)**	267 (38.1)	581 (41.8)	380 (47.0)**	273 (39.6)	653 (43.6)	109 (50.0)**	60 (33.7)	169 (42.7)	803 (46.8)***	600 (38.3)	1403 (42.7)
Pulmonary infection	85 (12.3)**	48 (6.9)	133 (9.6)	152 (18.8)***	58 (8.4)	210 (14.0)	36 (16.5)**	11 (6.2)	47 (11.9)	273 (15.9)***	117 (7.5)	390 (11.9)

* p<0.05; ** p<0.01; ***p<0.001 (Difference between males and females in the group)
**** Bener et al.,2005

Table 1. Prevalence rate of bronchial asthma, eczema and allergic rhinitis and other respiratory disorders in Qatari school children 6-14 years compared by gender****

The Venn diagram shows the asthma overlapping with allergic rhinitis and eczema. 71.9% of the children who had asthma also had either allergic rhinitis or eczema. 5.1% had all three diseases. Asthma with allergic rhinitis was 11.8% and asthma with eczema was 7.5%. (Figure 1)

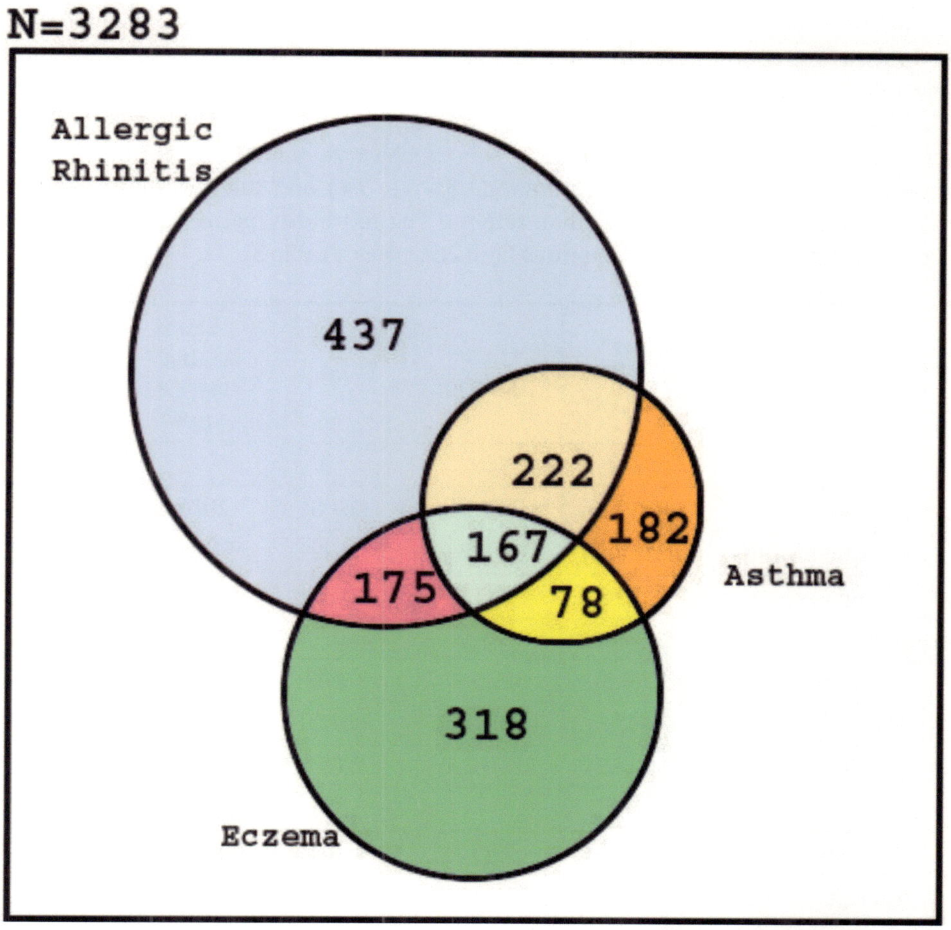

Fig. 1. Venn diagram showing the overlapping of asthma with allergic rhinitis and eczema

Another cross-sectional population based study of 31,400 primary children aged 6 -12 years revealed that 10.4% of them were reported with asthma and wheezing, with a higher frequency among boys (12.2%) than girls (8.6%) (Bener et al., 2007). (Table 2)

Variables	Boys	Girls	Total
Primary school students	n(%)	n(%)	N (%)
Number of primary school Students	16,130 (51.4%)	15,270 (48.6)	31,400 (100%)
School Registry			
Asthma and Wheezing	1,962 (12.2%)	1,308 (8.6%)	3,270 (10.4%)

*Bener et al., 2007

Table 2. Frequency of asthma, allergic rhinitis and wheezing in school children in the State of Qatar*

The comparison in prevalence of bronchial asthma and allergic rhinitis between Qatar with the neighbouring countries revealed that the prevalence of asthma (19.8%) and allergic rhinitis (30.5%) was significantly higher in school children in Qatar compared to U.A.E (13.6% & 22.9%; p<0.001) and Saudi Arabia (6.8% & 17.9%; p<0.001). These results show that allergic rhinitis is more frequent among school children than asthma in Arabian Gulf countries. The prevalence rate of asthma (11.8% vs. 9%) and allergic rhinitis (18.5% vs. 17.5%) was higher among mothers than fathers. The morbidity pattern of the asthma and allergic diseases was similar in these three Gulf countries. (Table 3)

Variable		Qatar* N=3283 n(%)	UAE** N=729	P value	Saudi Arabia*** N=3041 n(%)	P value
Child						
	Asthma	649(19.8)	99(13.6)	<0.001	207(6.8)	<0.001
	Allergic Rhinitis	1001(30.5)	167(22.9)	<0.001	544(17.9)	<0.001
	Eczema	738(22.5)	100(13.7)	<0.001	329(10.8)	<0.001
Paternal history						
	Asthma	297(9.0)	43(5.9)	0.007	137(4.5)	<0.001
	Allergic Rhinitis	575(17.5)	79(10.8)	<0.001	319(10.5)	<0.001
	Eczema	444(13.5)	76(10.4)	0.021	109(3.6)	<0.001
Maternal						
	Asthma	388(11.8)	39(5.3)	<0.001	135(4.4)	<0.001
	Allergic Rhinitis	608(18.5)	117(16.0)	NS	317(10.4)	<0.001
	Eczema	486(14.8)	64(8.8)	<0.001	114(3.7)	<0.001

*Bener et al., 2005 **Behbehani et al.,2000 *** Al-Frayh et al., 1993

Table 3. Prevalence of bronchial asthma and allergic rhinitis of school children in Qatar, UAE and Saudi Arabia

The rise in prevalence found in Gulf countries is consistent with a variety of independent studies of asthma prevalence trends conducted in the United States and other industrialized countries (Urick et al., 1996; Anderson et al., 1994). The prevalence rates of asthma in the UK (15.2%) (Doull et al., 1996) and France (14.9%) (Fontaine et al., 1999) was comparable to the rates found in the Gulf countries

The logistic regression analysis of factors involved in the etiology of asthma in our study of genetic and environmental risk factors associated with asthma showed parental asthmatic to be the significant factor after adjusting for confounding factors (Bener et al, 2005) (Table 4). In addition, our results showed that father smoking was a significant risk factor for asthma among children, which is consistent with previous reported studies (Bener et al., 1996; Jenkins et al., 1993).

Independent Variables	Relative Risk	95% Confidence Interval	p – value significance
Allergic to food	2.161	(1.641-2.846)	0.0001
Allergic to medicine	2.905	(1.736-4.861)	0.0001
Father asthmatic	2.332	(1.763-3.085)	0.0001
Mother asthmatic	1.786	(1.383-2.305)	0.0001
Sibling asthmatic	2.921	(2.368-3.603)	0.0001
Asthma in second degree relative	1.623	(1.318-1.999)	0.0001
Father smoking	1.402	(1.145-1.717)	0.001

Table 4. Genetic and environmental risk factors associated with asthma as estimated by stepwise logistic regression analysis (Bener et al., 2005).

3.2 Absenteeism among children with asthma

Numerous studies have documented that asthma is the principal cause of school absences due to chronic disease in childhood, accounting for 20% of school days lost for elementary and high school students. Few studies report difficulties for these children at school, mainly absence due to asthma and difficulties in physical education.

The studies conducted in Qatar showed a correlation between asthma and high rates of student absenteeism. Asthmatic children (34.7%) were more absent from school than the healthy peers (22.8%). Absenteeism was observed more in asthmatic children studying in primary (14.8% vs. 10%) and intermediate levels (50.3% vs. 45.8%) than the children without asthma. Among the children with asthma, Boys (55.6%) were absent more frequently than girls (44.4%). 77.5% of the children with asthma were Qatari children (Table 5).

Variable		Asthmatic Children		Non-Asthmatic Children	
		Number of Students Without Absence n=487 n(%)	Number of Absentees n=169 n (%)	Number of Students Without Absence n=2099 n(%)	Number of Absentees n=478 n(%)
Grade					
Primary (Grade 1-6)		66(13.6)	25(14.8)	529(25.2)	48(10.0)
Intermediate (Grade 7-9)		253(52.0)	85(50.3)	804(38.3)	219(45.8)
Secondary (Grade 10-12)		168(34.5)	59(34.9)	766(36.5)	211(44.1)
Gender	Boys	281(57.7)	94(55.6)	1182(56.3)	264(55.2)
	Girls	206(42.3)	75(44.4)	917(43.7)	214(44.8)
Nationality	Qatari	384(78.9)	131(77.5)	1446(68.9)	327(68.4)
	Non-Qatari	103(21.1)	38(22.5)	653(31.1)	151(31.6)

Table 5. Distribution of students absent from the school according to asthma status (Bener et al., 2007).

Our study on the impact of asthma and air pollution on school attendance of primary school children revealed that a good proportion of the primary children were absent from school because of asthma and wheezing in the studied academic year (Bener et al., 2007). A majority of the asthmatic children were absent for 1-5 days (29%), followed by 6 - 10 days (23%). Similarly, 26.7% of the total children with allergic rhinitis were absent for 1-5 days and 6 - 10 days (26.1%). There was a statistically significant difference between asthmatic and wheezing students in number of days absent from the school (p<0.0001). (Table 6)

Allergic disease	Number of days absent from school						
	None	1-5	6-10	11-15	16-20	>20	Total
Asthma	583	605	479	177	160	79	2083
Wheezing Children	280	262	234	79	60	21	936
Allergic Rhinitis	704	668	651	230	182	63	2498
Total	1567	1535	1364	486	402	163	5517

P<0.001 (very highly statistically significant)

Table 6. Number of days absent from school due to asthma, wheezing and allergic rhinitis among the primary school children during the academic year, 2003-2004 (Bener et al., 2007).

Most absenteeism occurred during the spring/summer season for both boys (45%) and girls (47%), followed by autumn for boys (33%) and girls (36%). Girls were more absent from asthma and allergic diseases during autumn (36% vs. 33%), and spring/summer (47% vs. 45%) when compared with boys. (Table 7)

Seasons	Boys Frequency of absent (%)	Girls Frequency of absent (%)	Total
Autumn	532(33%)	327(36%)	859
Winter	355(22%)	163(17%)	508
Spring/Summer	724(45%)	425(47%)	1149
Total	1611(100%)	905(100%)	1255

P = 0.036 (Statistically significant)

Table 7. Number of Days absent from school due to asthma and wheezing by season (Bener et al. 2007).

Absenteeism was reported more frequently among asthmatic children (34.7%) in Qatar compared to non-asthmatic children (22.8%). Most studies confirmed our findings and demonstrated that students with asthma miss more school days than students without asthma (Milton et al., 2004). The majority of the asthmatic children in Qatar were absent for 1 – 5 days which is similar to a study done in Rochester, Minnesota which found that public school children with asthma had 2 excess days of absenteeism per year compared to their healthy peers (Silverstein et al., 2001). In the UAE, the number of days absent from school ranged from none to more than twenty days in the academic year and the median absence was 6 days in the diagnosed asthmatic group and 5 days among wheezing children (Bener et al., 1994b). Similarly in Saudi Arabia school absenteeism was higher among asthmatic children (13.6 days/year), while it was lower among their non-asthmatic counterparts (3.7 days) (Al-Dawood et al., 2002). A cross sectional study conducted in the USA, demonstrated that children with asthma averaged 7.6 school days absent compared with 2.5 days in the non-asthmatic group (Fowler et al., 1992). The Centers for Disease Control and Prevention documented that in the USA, asthma accounted for almost 13 million missed school days and 2.5% of all outpatient visits for children younger than 18 years in 2004. (Akinbami et al, 2006).

In Qatar, 50.3% of the absenteeism was observed in asthmatic children studying in intermediate level (aged 12 – 14 years). In the United Arab Emirates, 57% of asthmatic children aged 6-9 years missed at least 1 day of school compared with 42% in 10-14 year old similar children (Bener et al., 1994b). It is possible that increased absenteeism in younger asthmatic children due to the fact that asthma exacerbations are more severe in younger children. But in Qatar, more absenteeism was reported among older children. In contrast, a study of Los Angeles Inner City schools found that younger known asthmatic students missed school more than older ones (Bonilla et al; 2005). Five-year-old children with asthma missed about twice as much school as 10 to 11 year old children with asthma. All these studies show that asthmatic children have more absenteeism days than non-asthmatic ones.

3.3 Asthma and school performance

Children with asthma may be at risk for decreased school performance for a number of reasons including increased absenteeism, iatrogenic effects of asthma medication, teachers' or parents' perception that the child is too vulnerable to participate in school activities. An assessment of school performance of asthmatic children compared with non-asthmatic children was done in table 8. The data showed that school performance of asthmatic children was poor and they were scholastically backward. Nearly half of the asthmatic children had learning disabilities (42.3%) and poor in doing homework (50.1%). Asthmatic children had poor school performance; they were disturbance to other students (44.4%), trouble maker at school (25.1%) and had a tendency to runaway from school (15.4%).

Children with asthma are conceivably at risk for decreased school functioning and it could be due to acute exacerbation of the disease, asthma medication, poor medical management of the disease and increased absenteeism. The studied children with asthma were more likely to have activity limitations than non asthmatic children.(Table 8)

School absences due to asthma has been found more harmful academically because prolonged absences from school may contribute significantly to negative school performance. It was found from the results that children with asthma were often confronted with educational difficulties and disruption resulting from frequent absences. The National Maternal and Infant Health Survey documented that children with asthma were at 1.7 times greater risk for a learning disability (Fowler et al., 1992).

School performance	Asthmatic	Non-Asthmatic	*P-Value*
	n(%) n=487	n(%) n=2099	
Student hates school	131(26.9)	703(33.5)	0.344
Students hates certain subjects	309(63.4)	1352(64.4)	0.899
Students hates certain teachers	188(38.6)	728(34.7)	0.600
Students hates school system	113(23.2)	479(22.8)	0.959
Doesn't do homework	244(50.1)	886(42.2)	0.292
Runaway from school	75(15.4)	246(11.7)	0.447
Trouble maker at school	122(25.1)	359(17.1)	0.167
Learning disabilities	206(42.3)	684(32.6)	0.171
Side talks in the class room/disturb other students	216(44.4)	791(37.7)	0.370

Table 8. Assessment of school performance among school children in Qatar according to asthma status (Bener et al., 2007).

3.4 Asthma and academic performance

Education is one of the most important aspects of human resources development. Every child should have the opportunity to achieve his or her academic potential. But, it was noticed that the studied asthmatic children were more likely to have poor academic results than those without asthma. More than half of the asthmatic children had poor examination scores; poor (34.5%) and average (31.4%) with a significant difference compared with healthy peers ($p<0.001$). Similar patterns were observed among children with allergic rhinitis, wheezing and allergic diseases. Children with allergic rhinitis (35.4%), wheezing (31.9%), and allergic diseases (30.6%) scored poor grade in their examinations. More than half of the asthmatic children were significantly below average in their academic performance compared to those without asthma ($p<0.001$). These results showed that school performance and examination scores were both influenced by the asthma incidence and the effectiveness of the management of the asthma. (Table 9).

Similar to the results on academic performance of asthmatic children in Qatar, Fowler et al (1992) noted a greater likelihood of grade failure among children with asthma compared with healthy children in a population based sample of American children in grades 1 to 12. The study observed negative correlations between absenteeism from asthma and academic performance.

Variables	Academic performance					P-Value
	Total n(%)	Poor n(%)	Average n(%)	Good n (%)	Very Good n (%)	
Asthmatic						
Yes	487 (100)	168 (34.5)	153 (31.4)	112 (23.0)	54 (11.0)	<0.001
No	2099 (99.9)	171 (8.1)	529 (25.2)	807 (38.4)	592 (28.2)	
Allergic rhinitis						
Yes	659 (100)	233 (35.4)	189 (28.7)	161 (24.4)	76 (11.5)	<0.001
No	1927 (100)	149 (8.0)	493 (25.6)	742 (38.5)	543 (28.2)	
Wheezing						
Yes	216 (99.9)	69 (31.9)	67 (31.0)	51 (23.6)	29 (13.4)	<0.001
No	2370 (100)	196 (8.3)	615 (25.9)	906 (38.2)	653 (27.6)	
Allergic Diseases						
Yes	294 (100)	90 (30.6)	89 (30.3)	73 (24.8)	42 (14.3)	<0.001
No	2292 (100)	183 (8.0)	593 (25.9)	885 (38.6)	631 (27.5)	

Table 9. Assessment of academic performance in school children in Qatar according to asthma status (Bener et al., 2007).

3.5 Asthma and behavioral problems

Behavioral problems were more persistent among asthmatic children compared to those without asthma. This is evident from the data of the school children that most of the parents of children with asthma reported behavioral problems more than the parents of those without asthma. A good proportion of the parents of asthmatic children compared to parents of non-asthmatic children, indicated that their children had behavioral problems like anxiety (65.3% vs. 42.8%), exam fear (77% vs. 70.1%), shyness (44.1% vs. 29.3%), anger (50.1% vs. 34.7%), violent behaviour (19.3% vs. 9.6%) and fights among peers (32.6% vs. 21.3%). (Table 10)

Similar to our study findings on the behavioural problems of school children with asthma, Halterman et al (2006) indicated that those children with persistent asthma scored worse on peer interactions and task orientation and were more likely to exhibit shy and anxious behaviors compared with non-asthmatic children. Mcquaid et al (2001) reported that associations between asthma and reading problems, grade repetition, learning disabilities and behavioral problems were observed in asthmatic children.

Behavioural Problems	Studied school children		P-Value
	Asthmatic n=487 n(%)	Non-Asthmatic n=2099 n(%)	
Anxiety	318(65.3)	898(42.8)	0.002
Fear	197(40.5)	798(38.0)	0.745
Exam fear	375(77.0)	1471(70.1)	0.310
Shy	215(44.1)	615(29.3)	0.031
Day dream	131(26.9)	434(20.7)	0.306
Jealousy	131(26.9)	277(13.2)	0.010
Anger	244(50.1)	728(34.7)	0.034
Stealing	75(15.4)	183(8.7)	0.127
Selfish	37(7.6)	145(6.9)	0.832
Cheating	84(17.2)	277(13.2)	0.420
Violent behaviour	94(19.3)	202(9.6)	0.038
Low self esteem	215(44.1)	665(31.7)	0.076
Bad peers	103(21.1)	497(23.7)	0.692
Fights among peers	159(32.6)	447(21.3)	0.068

Table 10. Assessment of behavioral problems among the studied school children in Qatar according to asthma status (Bener et al, 2007).

3.6 Asthma and air pollution

Academic performance can be affected by pollution through four mechanisms: absenteeism due to asthma caused by pollution, attention problems in school due to asthma caused by pollution, fatigue in doing school work due to asthma caused by pollution and negative effect of pollution on brain development (Bener et al., 2007).

The cross sectional study among 31,400 primary school students aged 6-12 years in Qatar confirmed that there was a seasonal influence of asthma and wheezing on school attendance among students in spring/summer and autumn seasons and air pollution was very high during that period. It was noted from the figure that the measured pollutants peaked the highest in spring and summer season and asthma adversely affected school attendance rates during that time. (Figure 2)

These results support the fact that air pollution has an impact on asthma. This is in agreement with other studies of two populations of Australian (Peat et al., 1987) and United Arab Emirates (Bener et al., 1994b) that high prevalence of asthma was found in primary school children during spring/summer seasons which led to more absenteeism from school.

Air pollution has been associated with a number of detrimental health effects for children especially respiratory diseases. A study evaluating the impact of air pollution on respiratory diseases showed that there was an association between increasing air pollutant levels and patients admitted for respiratory diseases (Bener et al., 2009). The data showed that as the concentrations of NO_2 and O_3, increased, there was an increase in the number of admissions from respiratory diseases. Ozone had a statistically significant effect on both upper respiratory and lower respiratory illness rates. This shows a positive association between air pollution and respiratory diseases (Table 11).

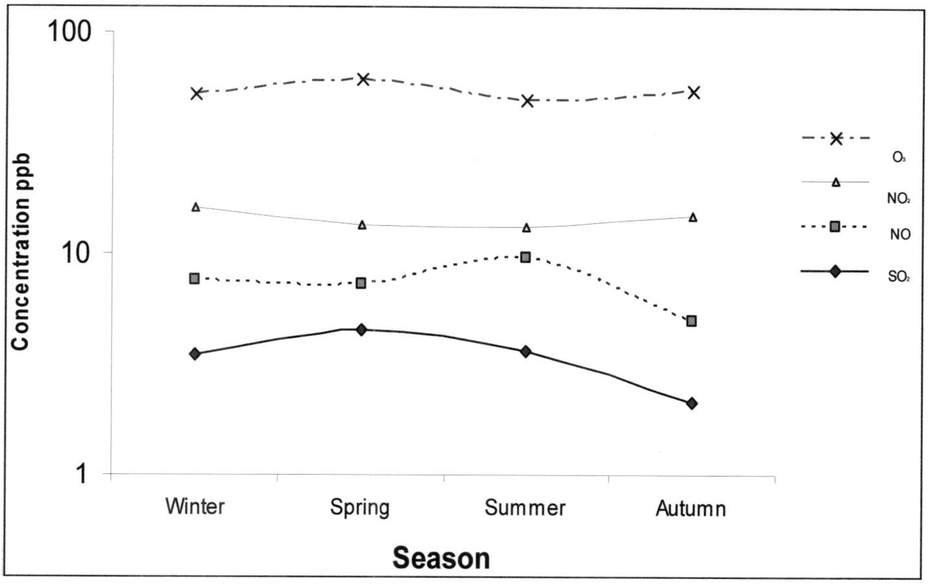

Fig. 2. Seasonal average of SO_2, NO, NO_2, and O_3 in the polluted areas, State of Qatar during the years 2003 to 2004 (Bener et al., 2007).

Variables	Yearly average			
	2002	2003	2004	2005
Air pollutants				
CO	1.070	1.050	1.13	1.19
NO_2	0.027	0.030	0.032	0.033
NO	0.013	0.015	0.028	0.029
O_3	0.028	0.025	0.027	0.029
$S0_2$	0.004	0.004	0.005	0.006
PM_{10}	91.00	99.00	105.00	111.00
Hospital Admissions				
Respiratory diseases	4.428	5.121	5.064	5.300
Cardiovascular diseases	3.419	3.368	3.400	3.914
Ischemic Heart diseases	5.218	5.359	5.247	5.599

Table 11. The trend in concentration of air pollutants and the number of daily admissions from respiratory and cardiovascular diseases, 2002 - 2005 (Bener et al., 2009).

Ozone is found in outdoor air when sunlight provides sufficient photochemical energy to drive reactions of oxygen with a number of gaseous pollutants. McConnell et al. (2002) stated in his study that children who lived in high ozone areas and play sports outdoors were more likely to be diagnosed with asthma than those who did not play sports. In the low ozone areas, there was no difference in asthma rates between children who played sports and those who did not. This shows that the extra exposure to ozone in the ozone areas causes either the onset of asthma or the earlier onset of asthma among children.

Source and Nation	Sample Size and age group	Prevalence	Days of Absence/year.
MIDDLE EAST REGION STUDIES			
Bener et al. 1994b (United Arab Emirates)	1910 school students Aged 6-14.	6.7% School Health Records. 2% Survey	6 days/yr median (diagnosed asthma) 5 days/yr median (wheezing - undiagnosed asthma).
Al-Ghamdy et al. 2000 (Saudi Arabia)	• 606 children Aged 0-13 years. • Recruited from pediatric clinics and hospitals.	Not Reported	Missing between 1-3 weeks of school/year: • 6% for mild asthma • 23% for moderate asthma • 39% for severe asthma.
Al-Dawood 2002 (Saudi Arabia)	• 1482 male school students • Aged 6-15years.	9.5%	13.6 days - students without previous physician diagnosis. 3.7 days - students with physician diagnosed asthma.
Bener et al. 2007 (Qatar)	• 31,400 school students. (national sample) • Aged 6-12years	10.4%	8.02 days / year.
Shohat et al. 2005 (Israel)	• 10,057 school students. (national sample) • Aged 13-14 years	7%	7.3 - 9.8 days / year.
ASIA-PACIFIC REGION STUDIES			
Lai et al. 2003 (Asia-Pacific Region)	• 108,000 households (Parents) in • 8 major cities of China, Hong Kong, Korea, Malaysia, Philippines, Singapore, Taiwan,and Vietnam.	Not reported.	Absence from school because of asthma was reported by 36.5% of parents.

Source and Nation	Sample Size and age group	Prevalence	Days of Absence/year.
Lim et al. 2003 (Singapore)	1,744 School Teachers	8.9%	• 5.1days/month • Range: 4-14days/ month.
EUROPEAN STUDIES			
Doull et al. 1996 (United Kingdom)	• 4830 parents of children gistered with 95 general practitioners • Aged 7-9years.	15.2%	• 7.2% had missed >5 days / year for asthma. • 0.9% had missed >20 days / year.
Fontaine et al. 1999 (France)	• 1707 students 6th grade • 1 French region.	14.9%	• 4.5% had 3 wheezing episodes/week • 18.5% of students with asthma missed days within past year.
NORTH AMERICAN STUDIES			
Newacheck and Halfon 2000 (USA)	• 62,171 children • Aged under 18 years	14.2%	9.7 days/year.
Silverstein et al. 2001 (USA)	• 184; Case-control (92 cases, 92 controls). • 5-12years	14.3%	8.95 days/year
Moonie et al. 2006 (USA)	• 9014 students • Aged 5-17.	9.7%	Mean 9.2 days/year
Mellinger-Birdsong et al. 2003 (USA)	• 2700 children • Aged 0-17 years	10.5%	• Mean 6.1days/year. • 54% missed school because of asthma.

Table 12. Key Published Articles that address Asthma and Absence from School

Most of the published articles revealed a high prevalence of asthma in their countries and there was an association between school absenteeism and asthma episodes.Children with asthma were at particular risk for academic difficulties. It is essential that asthmatic symptoms should be analyzed scientifically to discover its underlying cause and find a remedy. For school aged children, untreated asthma can lead to excessive school absences and inability to maximize their learning experiences when they are at school. Although teachers generally have accepting attitudes toward students with asthma, their knowledge about asthma is low and they do not feel adequately prepared to assist children with the management of asthma in the classroom. It is important to assist schools to manage students with asthma and minimize symptoms of asthma by optimizing the school environment. The American College of Allergists reported that school performance among a significant proportion of children with asthma is affected adversely by the schools approach to their medical condition (Richards et al., 1986). It was reported that a considerable reduction in school absenteeism can be achieved with appropriate prophylaxis and treatment (Bener et al., 1994).

In conclusion, the study findings revealed the following:

1. Asthma is a chronic childhood disease and it is a common cause of absenteeism from school among students.
2. Children with asthma experienced recurring episodes of absenteeism and this pattern may be contributing to decreased school performance.
3. Air pollution has an impact on asthma which results in significant school absenteeism among students.
4. These studies indicate that children with persistent asthma symptoms may be the necessary target of intervention to reduce absenteeism and improve school performance.

4. Acknowledgement

This work was supported by the Hamad Medical Corporation, MRC, Research Protocol No. 7083/07. The author would like to thank the Hamad Medical Corporation for their help and ethical approval.

5. References

Akinbami L, Centers for Disease Control and Prevention, National Center for Health Statistics, The State of Childhood Asthma, US, 1980-2005, Adv Data, 2006;38:1-24.

Al-Ghamdy YS, Al-Haddad NS, Abdelgadir MH, Qureshi NA, Saleh MA, Khalil MM. Socio-clinical profile of children with asthma in Al-Majmaah health province. Saudi Med J. 2000; 21(9):847-851.

Al-Frayh A, Bener A, Al-Jawadi TQ. Prevalence of asthma among Saudi schoolchildren-Saudi Medical J: 1993; 13: 521-524.

Anderson HR, Butland BK, Strachan DP. Trends in prevalence and severity of childhood asthma, BMJ, 1994;308:1600-1604.

Al-Dawood KM. Schoolboys with bronchial asthma in Al-Khobar City, Saudi Arabia: are they at increased risk of school absenteeism? J Asthma, 2002;39:413-420.

Beasley R, Crane J, Lai CK, Pearce N. Prevalence and etiology of asthma, J Allergy Clin Immunol, 2000;105:466-472.

Behbehani BA, Abal A, Syabbalo NC, Abd Azeem A, Shareef E, Al-Momen J. Prevalence of asthma, allergic rhinitis and eczema in 13-14 year old children in Kuwait: an ISAAC study. International Study of Asthma and Allergies in Children. Ann Allergy Asthma Immunol 2000; 85: 58-63.

Bonnilla S, Kehl S, Kwong KYC, Morphew T, Kachru R, Jones CA. School absenteeism in children with Asthma in a Los Angeles Inner City School, The Journal of Pediatrics, 2005;147:802-806.

Bener A, Janahi I, Sabbah A. Genetics and environmental risk factors associated with asthma in schoolchildren, European Annals of Allergy & Clinical Immunology 2005; 37(5): 163-168.

Bener A, Shanks NJ, Kamal M. Impact of asthma and air pollution on school attendance of primary school children: are they at increased risk of school absenteeism? Journal of Asthma 2007; 44(4):249-252.

Bener A, Abdulrazzaq YM, Debuse P, Al-Mutawaa J. Prevalence of asthma among Emirates schoolchildren. European Journal of Epidemiology 1994a; 10:271-278.

Bener A, Abdulrazzaq YM, Dubuse P, Abdin AH. Asthma and wheezing as the cause of school absence. J Asthma, 1994b; 31: 93-98.

Bener A, Abdulrazzaq YM, Al Mutawwa J, Debuse P. Genetics and environmental factors associated with asthma. Human Biology, 1996; 68: 405-414.

Bener A, Dogan M, Ehlayel MS, Shanks NJ, Sabbah A. The impact of air pollution on hospital admission for respiratory and cardiovascular diseases in an oil & gas-rich country. European Annals of Allergy and Clinical Immunology. 2009; 41(3): 80-84.

Doull IJ, Williams AA, Freezer NJ, Holgate ST. Descriptive study of cough, wheeze and school absence in childhood. Thorax. 1996;51(6):630-631.

Fowler MG, Davenport MG, Garg R, School functioning of US children with asthma, Pediatrics, 1992;90:939-944.

Fontaine V, Deniaud F, Lefort F, Lecoutour X, Brun J. Epidemiology of childhood asthma in the department of Calvados. Rev Pneumol Clin. 1999; 55:5-11.

Halterman J, Conn K, Forbes-Jones E, Fagnano M, Hightower A, Szilagyi P. Behavioural problems among Inner City children with Asthma: Findings from a community based sample, Pediatrics, 2006;117:e192-e199.

Janahi IA, Bener A, Bush A. Prevalence of asthma among Qatari schoolchildren: International study of asthma and allergies in childhood ISAAC Qatar. Paed Pulmon 2006; 41: 80-86.

Jenkins MA, Hoper JL, Flander LB. The association between childhood asthma and atopy and parental asthma, hay fever and smoking. *Pediatr Perinatal Epidemiol.* 1993; 7:67-76.

Khaldi F, Fakhfakh R, Mattoussi N, Ben Ali B, Zouari S, Khemiri M. Prevalence and severity of asthma, allergic rhinoconjunctivitis and atopic eczema in "Grand Tunis" schoolchildren: ISAAC. Tunis Med. 2005;83: 269-273.

Lai CK, De Guia TS, Kim YY, Kuo SH, Mukhopadhyay A, Soriano JB, Trung PL, Zhong NS, Zainudin N, Zainudin BMZ. Asthma control in the Asia-Pacific region: the Asthma insights and reality in Asia-Pacific study. J Allergy Clin Immunol. 2003; 111(2):263-268.

Lim DL, Tan TN, Quek CM, Wang XS, Shek LP, Lee BW, Goh DY. An evaluation of asthma morbidity in Singaporean schoolchildren--a teachers' survey. Asian Pac J Allergy Immunol. 2003; 21(2):71-74.

Moonie SA, Sterling DA, Figgs L, Castro M. Asthma Status and Severity Affects Missed School Days. J of Sch. Health. 2006; 76(1):18-24.

Mellinger-Birdsong AK, Powell KE, Latridis T, Bason J. Prevalence and impact of asthma in children, Georgia, 2000. Am J Prev Med. 2003; 24(3):242-248.

Maziak W, Behrens T, Brasky TM, Duhme H, Rzehak P, Weiland SK. Keil U. Are asthma and allergies in children and adolescents increasing? Results from ISAAC phase I and phase III surveys in Munster, Germany. Allergy 2003; 58:572-579.

McConnell R, Berhane K, Gilliland F, Molitor J, Thomas D, Lurmann F, Avol E, Ganderman W, Peters J. Asthma in exercising children exposed to ozone: a cohort study, Lancet 2002;359:386-391.

Mcquaid LE, Kopel SJ, Nassais JH. Behavioural adjustment I children with asthma: A meta analysis Development and Behavioural Pediatrics, 2001:22(6):430-439.

Mannino D, Homa D, Akinbami L, Moorman JE, Gwynn C, Redd SC. Surveillance for asthma - US, 1980 – 1999, MMWR CDC Surveillance summary, MMWR Morb Mortal Wkly Rep., 2002;51:1-13.

Milton B, Whitehead M, Holland P, Hamilton V. The Social and Economic consequences of childhood asthma across the life course: A systematic review, Child Care, Health and Development, 2004;30:711-728.

Newacheck PW, Halfon N. Prevalence, impact, and trends in childhood disability due to asthma. Arch Pediatr Adolesc Med. 2000; 154(3):287-293.

Peat JK, Britton WJ, Salome CM, Woolcock AJ. Bronchial hyperresponsiveness in two populations of Australian schoolchildren. II. Relative importance of associated factors. Clin Allergy. 1987;17: 283-300.

Robertson CF, Roberts MF, Kappers JH. Asthma prevalence in Melbourne schoolchildren: have we reached the peak? MJA 2004; 180: 273-276.

Richards W. Allergy, asthma and school problems, J Sch Health, 1986;56(4):151-152

Shohat T, Graif Y, Garty BZ, Livne I, Green MS. The child with asthma at school: results from a national asthma survey among schoolchildren in Israel. J Adolesc Health 2005;37(4):275-280.

Silverstein M, Mair J, Katusic S, Wollan P, O'Connell E, Yunginger J. School attendance and school performance: a population-based study of children with asthma. J Pediatr. 2001;139:278-283.

Shapiro GG, Stout JN, Childhood asthma in the US; Urban issues, Pediatr Pulmonol, 2002;33(1):47-55

The International Study of Asthma and Allergies in Childhood (ISAAC) Steering Committee. Worldwide variations in the prevalence of asthma symptoms: The International Study of Asthma and Allergies in Childhood (ISAAC). Eur Respir J, 1998; 12: 315-335.

Ulrik CS, Backer V, Hesse B, Dirksen A. Risk factors for development of asthma in children and adolescents: findings from a longitudinal population study, Respir Med. 1996;90:623-630.

Vichyanond P, Jirapongsananuruk O, Visitsuntorn N, Tuchinda M. Prevalence of asthma, rhinitis and eczema in children from the Bangkok area using the ISAAC (International Study of Asthma and Allergy in Children), J Med Assoc Thai. 1998; 81(3): 175-184..

25

The Effects of Air Pollution on Cellular Material Release, Allergenicity and Allergens Proteins of Three Ornamental Plants

Farkhondeh Rezanejad[1] and Ahmad Majd[2]
[1]*Department of Biology, Shahid Bahounar University, Kerman,*
[2]*Department of Biology, Tarbiat Moallem University, Tehran,*
[1,2]*Iran*

1. Introduction

The term allergy, coined by von Pirquet in 1906, is used to define the series of events which occurs when an antigen, which is not harmful in itself, causes an immune response, leading to symptoms and disease in genetically predisposed individuals. An antigen that induces the allergic response is called an allergen (Shaikh, 2001). The allergic response manifested on exposure to a harmless allergen is the result of a complex orchestrated interaction of various immune cells and immunoglobulins. Allergy and asthma are a spectrum of diseases based on various genetic and physiologic mechanisms (Shaikh, 2001). The changes in life style and environment have results in a sufficiently large increase in the number of patients with disease to constitute a social problem. Asthma is a complex syndrome with many clinical phenotypes. Common to all is chronic inflammation with reversible airway obstruction and airway hyperresponsiveness (AHR). The most prevalent form of asthma is atopic asthma which is initiated by the exposure to (inhaled) allergens and resultant allergen-specific immune responses (Shin et al., 2009). Asthma is characterized by inflammatory changes of the airways, in which inflammatory cells such as lymphocytes. Neutrophils and eosinophils and a number of cytokines including leukotrienes released from these cells participate in the late asthmatic reaction. Among inflammatory cells, activated lymphocytes and eosinophils play an important role in induction and persistence of the reaction (Walker et al., 1991). The results are consistent with the data showing enhanced production of LTC 4 by activated eosinophils during antigen challenge.

The transfer of pollen grains, the structures housing the male gametes of plants, from floral anther to stigma is the critical reproductive event among higher plants. Like any other plant cells, pollen grains contain many different types of proteins, which are located in major domains: in the cytoplasm and at the surface of exine and intine. These molecules are strategically sited to participate as the male partner in intercellular recognition reactions with the female stigma (Knox & Suphiohlu, 1996; Dickinson et al., 2000). Once pollen grains are placed on stigma or on artificial medium (or mucosal membrane), they release cellular material containing proteins and glycoprotein. These materials from pollen that contribute in interaction pollen-stigma can function as allergens, environment molecules interacting with the human immune system to elicit an allergic response in susceptible individual.

Pollen allergy is the most common form of seasonal respiratory allergic disease in most of countries.

Henry Hyde Salter was the first to report that air pollution was implicated in respiratory allergy. In his book "On asthma: its pathology and treatment" published in London in 1860, with great intuition he listed "Impure air, animal emanations, hay fever and foods" among the various causes of asthma (D'amato, 2002, as cited in Salter, 1869). He also described asthma as being "Paroxysmal dyspnea of a peculiar character, generally periodic with healthy respiration between attacks". Nearly 50 years latter, William Lioyd postulated that hay fever was a result of urbanization and agricultural changes (D'amato, 2002, as cited in Lloyd, 1907). Pollen allergy is one of the models most frequently used to study the interrelationship between air pollution and allergic respiratory allergy (D'Amato, 2002).

1.1 Allergies: Genetic and environment

The term 'allergy' refers to a grouping of symptoms that affects different body systems. The allergic patient may experience symptoms in only one, or several body systems. People may experience allergies that are due to a wide array of antigens (triggering substances), such as foods, pollen, environmental particles, animal dander, dust mites, cigarette smoke, ingredients in soaps, newsprint, latex and almost anything else that a person may come into contact with. Although many of the antigens that provoke allergic reactions are proteins, many non-protein components can illicit allergic reactions, such as toluene diisocyanate found in dry cleaning fluid. The following is a grouping of symptoms that are commonly associated with different body systems. Respiratory symptoms: stuffy/runny nose, sneezing, coughing, watery eyes, wheezing, recurring ear infections, tickling or sore throat, asthma. Integumentary symptoms: swelling of hands and feet, itchy, dry, red scaling skin patches, dark circles under the eyes, swollen tongue. Digestive symptoms: bloating, flatulence, diarrhea, constipation, weight loss or gain, burning anal and underarm rash, abdominal discomfort (Wayne et al., 2002).

Allergic reactions are initiated by the immune system's over response to substances it deems as distinct from itself. Although well tolerated by most people, in the allergic person contact with the offending substance (antigen), is the basis of the hypersensitivity reaction. Immunoglobulins are specific antibodies that have the responsibility of tracking down and destroying antigens that are recognized by the body. There are five different classes of antibodies, IgE, IgA, IgG, IgM, and IgD. Each of these specifically attacks different categories of antigens. Every antibody is 'antigen specific', and is programmed to react to a specific kind of invader. In the case of allergies, these antibodies become overzealous, and begin to recognize substances that are usually benign, as if they were dangerous invaders. Once an antibody recognizes a suspected antigen, it attaches to it and forms an 'antigen-antibody' complex. This complex initiates the release of histamines and other chemicals that lead to inflammation, the common theme to all hypersensitivity reactions (allergies). The inflammatory response causes the release of chemical mediators, vasodilation, increased vascular permeability, edema and tissue damage. Allergic reactions can range from a trivial annoyance such as an itchy rash and runny nose, to a fatal incident (Wayne et al., 2002). There are four different classes of allergic reactions: Type I (immediate hypersensitivity reactions), Type II (cytotoxic reactions), Type III (immune complex mediated reactions) and Type IV (cell dependent reactions). Type I reactions occur almost immediately after exposure to an antigen, and range from a temporary outbreak of hives, skin rash, headache,

GI symptoms, rhinitis, and asthma-like symptoms, to fatal anaphylactic shock characterized by difficulty breathing, closing of the throat, decreased blood pressure, tachycardia, seizures and loss of consciousness. The symptoms can be local or systemic, depending on the port of entry of the antigen. IgE immunoglobulins are widely believed to be responsible for Type I reactions. However, recent studies report that IgG, previously thought to only be involved with delayed reactions, may also be involved in the initiation of Type I reactions. This evidence supports complementary health care practitioners, who have been regularly testing patients for both IgE and IgG mediated reactions for decades, although most conventional physicians still disregard IgG testing. Type II- Type IV reactions are referred to as delayed reactions, since they can occur 24- 72 hours after encountering the offending substance. They involve IgG, and to some degree IgM, although many allergic reactions do not involve any antigen-antibody complex, but are due to the direct release of histamines and other inflammatory compounds by mast cells and other white blood cells (Wayne et al., 2002). Pollinosis occurs in 10–20% of European inhabitants. Type I immunological reaction, dependent on the presence of specific IgE antibodies, mast cells and eosinophil cells, forms the basis of this disease (Lipiec et al., 2005, as cited in Bertel et al., 2001; Kowalski, 2000).
The ability of an individual to form an allergic response and its subsequent severity is dependent on a combination of intrinsic and extrinsic factors. Intrinsic traits such as age and genetic background have been shown to have a strong influence on the development and severity of allergic disease. In addition, a multitude of experimental and epidemiological studies have demonstrated that environmental factors such as infections, air pollution, and indoor allergens may affect the symptoms of established allergic disease. Less is known about specific environmental factors leading to primary allergic sensitization in humans, i.e., the initial formation of Ag-specific IgE following Ag exposure (Riedl et al, 2005). Cookson et al (1989) noted the linkage of a specific chromosome region to allergic phenotype the 11q13 gene locus. Cytokine gene cluster at 5q is a large genetic region spanning a gamut of DNA and contains numerous genes influencing the atopy phenotype. Researchers have analyzed a mouse chromosomal segment homologous to human chromosome 5 locus exhibiting a T cell and airway phenotype regulator (Shaikh, 2001). The interaction between genetic and environmental factors is generally accepted to cause individuals to be sensitized with environmental allergens and to suffer from allergic diseases. However, it is believed that recent changes in the environment have contributed to the increase more significantly than genetic factors, since it seems unlikely that genes would change over one or two generations. Thus, it is a central issue to reveal what environmental factor(s) cause such high prevalence and to find strategies to prevent their development. As environmental factors that influence the susceptibility to the development of asthma in predisposed individuals, the Global Strategy for Asthma Management and Prevention lists indoor and outdoor allergens, occupational sensitizers, air pollution, respiratory infection, parasitic infections, socioeconomic status, family size and obesity (Kawai et al., 2007). Human allergic responses to the pollen of certain plant species (hay fever, allergenic rhinitis, pollinosis) is a serious environmental health issue (Wayne et al., 2002).

1.1.1 Air pollution

Air pollution is a major and growing environmental health problem worldwide. The World Health Organization [WHO] considers that air pollution is damaging the resources that are needed for the long term sustainable development of the planet (Chan-Yeung, 2000; as cited in WHO, 1999). This growth is largely attributable to increases in: a) the world population, b) economical activities, c) energy consumption, d) industrial activities, and e) motor vehicles (Bartra et al., 2007, as cited in Parnia & Frew, 2001). In most countries including Iran, the main source of air pollution due to particles in suspension is represented by motor vehicles particularly those that use diesel fuel. The sources of air pollution fall into three broad categories: 1- Mobile sources, which include combustion-engine vehicles such as gasoline powered cars, diesel-powered vehicles, motorcycles, and aircraft; 2- Stationary sources, which include rural sources such as agricultural production, mining, and quarrying; industrial sources such as manufacturing; and community sources such as the heating of homes and buildings, municipal waste, and incinerators; and 3- Indoor sources, which include combustion, tobacco smoking, and biological sources; and emissions from indoor materials or substances such as volatile organic compounds, asbestos, and radon (Chan-Yeung, 2000).

1.1.1.1 Suspended particulate matter and gaseous pollutants

Air pollutants are usually classified into suspended particulate matter (dusts, fumes, mists, and smokes), gaseous pollutants (gases and vapours), and odours. The most abundant components of air pollution in urban areas are nitrogen dioxide (NO2), Hydrocarbons (HC), sulphur dioxide (SO2), ozone (O3), carbon monoxide (CO) and airborne particulate matter (APM). Suspended particulate matter (PM) consists of finely divided small particulates with diameters of less than 10 μm (PM10). Suspended particulate matter comprises a wide variety of substances, which include inorganic and organic carbon (containing polycyclic aromatic hydrocarbons), acidic or neutral sulphates and nitrates, fine soil dust, residues of lead and other metals, asbestos, and other fibres. Most of these particulates are smaller than 1 μm and remain suspended for hours or days. Particles that are smaller than 2.5 μm in diameter (PM2.5) arise mainly from combustion processes, whereas larger particles are generated by grinding and other mechanical or agricultural processes (Chan-Yeung, 2000). Small particles efficiently penetrate indoors, where levels are typically 70% to 80% of outdoor levels in the absence of indoor sources (Chan-Yeung, 2000). Much research is now being carried out on diesel exhaust particles (DEPs) and their components (e.g., polycyclic aromatic hydrocarbons (PAH), since a large part of urban particulate matter originates from diesel engines. DEPs account for most airborne particulate matter (up to 90%) in the world's largest cities, and are composed of fine particles (0.1- 2.5-μm) and ultrafine (<0.1 μm) particles, although these primary DEPs can coalesce to form aggregates of varying sizes (D'Amato et al., 2010). Diesel fuel combustion results in the production of diesel exhaust particles (up to 100 times more particles than gasoline engines) and gaseous compounds such as NO2 and hydrocarbon precursors of ozone. Diesel engine use has increased in many parts of the world due to superior energy eficiency and durability. Thus, diesel exhaust particles (DEP) are a predominant and representative particulate pollutant widely used to study the effects of PM (Riedl, 2008).

1.1.2 Pollen grains

The word pollen is derived from the Greek word meaning 'fine flour'. Pollen development is an integrated process in which three elements take part: 1- The cells of the external part of the anther that are modified slightly during development. 2- The tapetum cells that differentiate during development, their content being wholly or partly reabsorbed and 3-

The microspore mother cells that under go meiosis and haploid mitosis. During development, various types of cells differentiate, with modifications in the case of tapetum and pollen that mostly involve the walls, division and differentiation (Pacini & Franchi, 1992). The transfer of pollen from floral anther to stigma is the critical reproductive event among higher plant. Like any other plant cells, pollen grains contain many different types of proteins, which are located in major domains: in the cytoplasm and at the surface of exine and intine. These molecules are strategically sited to participate as the male partner in intercellular recognition reactions with the female stigma (Rezanejad, 2009, as cited in Dickinson et al., 2000; Knox & Suphiohlu, 1996).

1.1.3 Influence of environmental pollution upon pollen allergenicity

Once pollen grains are placed on stigma or on artificial medium (or mucosal membrane), they release cellular material containing proteins and glycoprotein. These materials from pollen that contribute in interaction pollen-stigma can function as allergens, environment molecules interacting with the human immune system to elicit an allergic response in susceptible individual (Knox & Suphiohlu, 1996). Of all things that can cause an allergy, pollen is one of the most abundant and inescapable (Lokaj-Berisha et al., 2009, as cited in Shazo, 2000).

As for the health effects of air pollution in subjects living in polluted urban areas, it has been found, both in US (D'Amato, 2002; as cited in Dockery et al., 1759; Schenker, 1993) and in Europe (D'Amato, 2002; as cited in European Commission, Environmental Research Programme [UCERP], 1996) an association of daily concentrations of particulates and other components of urban air pollution (NO_2 and SO_2) and daily mortality. In this context Seaton et al. (D'Amato, 2002 as cited in Seaton et al., 1995) hypothesized that fine particulate of urban areas, penetrating deep into airways, is able to induce alveolar inflammation which is responsible for variation in blood coagulability and release of mediators which induce acute episodes of respiratory and cardiovascular diseases. Studies of Morgenstern et al. (2008) provided strong evidence for increased risk of atopic diseases and allergic sensitization when children are exposing to ambient particulate matter (Morgenstern et al., 2008). Asthma cases in China have risen an estimated 40% in the past 5 years concurrent with rapid increases in urban air pollution (Riedl, 2008, as cited in Watts, 2006).

Pollen allergy is one of the models most frequently used to study the interrelationship between air pollution and allergic respiratory allergy. Environmental pollution influences pollen allergenicity. Scientific evidence shows that pollen in heavily polluted zones expresses a larger amount of proteins described as being allergenic, compared with areas characterized by lesser pollution. The study of Cortegano et al. (2004) concluded that *Cupressus arizonica* in areas of heavy air pollution express a larger amount of Cup a 3 compared with pollen from areas with signifi cantly lower pollution levels, thus favoring sensitization of the exposed population or the appearance of respiratory allergic disease in sensitized individuals. Armentia et al. (2002) have confirmed that the protein content and biological allergenic activity of gramineous pollen specifically Lol p 5 is greater in areas of heavy air pollution. The pollen of Parietaria has also been considered in the investigation of the interaction between environmental pollution and allergenic expression. The emissions of gasoline engines without catalytic converters and of diesel engines increase the allergenic potential of Parietaria pollen compared with emissions from vehicles with catalytic converters (Bartra et al., 2007, as cited in Armentia et al., 2002; Cortegano et al., 2004). Helander et al. (1997) and Majd et al. (2004) did not observe any significant difference between protein bands of pollen grains collected from polluted and control areas (Helanderet al., 1997; Majd et al., 2004). Jilek et al. (1993) observed an increase of the major birch pollen allergen, Bet v 1, in areas where nitrogen loads are high, while Parui et al. (1998) found a decrease in Bet v 1 concentration due to air pollution (Jilek et al., 1993; Parui et al., 1998). However, studies on pollen proteins collected from polluted and unpolluted areas have shown contradictory results.

Pollen particles contain pollinic allergens. High environmental humidity conditions can subject the pollen particles to osmotic shock, resulting in the release of microparticles or paucimicronic particles that may contain allergenic proteins. The presence of these paucimicronic particles would explain the discordance occasionally observed between the appearance of respiratory allergic symptoms in a pollinic patient and the absence of actual pollen particles in the atmosphere. In the same way, through physical contact with the pollen particles, DEPs can disrupt the former, leading to the release of paucimicronic particles and transporting them by air, thus facilitating their penetration of the human airways. In vitro studies have shown that Lol p 1 and Bet v 1, which are the prevalent or majority allergens of *Lolium* and birch, respectively, bind to DEPs thanks to the absorptive capacity resulting from their physicochemical characteristics. Such "affinity" has also been demonstrated for other allergens such as Der p 1, Fel d 1 and Can f 1. Other plant-derived allergenic particles are the so-called Ubish bodies. These are spheroid structures that develop with pollen exine and are found in the anthers of many plants. These structures, measuring only a few μm in diameter, may also contain allergenic proteins. Non-biological particles in suspension, such as DEPs, act as transporters for these structures, in the same way as for other pollen-derived paucimicronic particles (Bartra et al., 2007; D'Amato et al., 2010).

Inflammatory reactions generally involve a vast array of mediators and a variety of effector cells such as mast cells, macrophages, eosinophils, platelets, and neutropb.ils. It is well recognized that eosinophils are important cells in asthma. Eosinophils release basic proteins that are cytotoxic and lipid mediators such as cysteinyl leukotrienes that cause airway obstruction and bronchial epithelial damage. In contrast, the role of the neutrophil in asthma remains relatively obscure and neutrophils have been rather neglected in studies concerning allergic diseases, although an increase in neutrophil numbers and activity was found to be correlated to airway hyperresponsiveness in asthmatic patients (Bloemen et al., 2007). Nevertheless, recent evidence suggests that neutrophils not only contribute to acute asthma exacerbations, but also are present in high numbers in the airways of patients with chronic severe asthma. Production by neutrophils of lipid mediators, reactive oxygen intermediates (ROI) and proteases such as elastase, may contribute to airway obstruction, epithelial damage and remodeling (Bloemen et al., 2007 as cited in Sampson, 2000). Laboratory studies confirm epidemiologic evidence that air pollution adversely affects lung function in asthmatics. Damage to airway mucous membranes and impaired mucociliary clearance caused by air pollution may facilitate access of inhaled allergens to the cells of the immune system, thus promoting sensitization of the airway. Consequently, a more severe immunoglobulin (Ig) E-mediated response to aeroallergens and airway inflammation could account for increasing prevalence of allergic respiratory diseases in polluted urban areas.

(D'Amato et al., 2010). Miyabara et al. (1998) reported that the mechanisms underlying allergic asthma involve numerous factors, including antibody production, chemical mediators, cytokine expression, and activation of different cells. The airway inflammation of asthma is unique in that the airway wall is infiltrated by Th2 cells, eosinophils, and mast cells. Each of these cells is thought to contribute to the physiologic changes that characterize asthma. In particular, allergen-specific IgE is believed to play a central role in the hypersensitivity reactions via mast cells. Such IgE-mediated reactions are followed by chronic inflammation leading to increased airway hyperresponsiveness. (Miyabara et al., 1998).

1.2 Animal models for asthma and air pollutioon

However, the ability to completely assess the different disease phenotypes and inherent ethical issues are limiting factors in conducting many of the required clinical studies. As a result, animal models have been developed to study the pathogenesis of the disease, including genetic factors, to define the pathogenetic pathways and suggest new therapeutic approaches (Bice et al., 2000; Shin et al., 2009). Much of the researches on the adverse effects of air pollutants, both in vivo and in vitro, have been conducted in animals. Such experimental studies are reviewed critically and the findings are compared with those in human studies. Although a majority of studies of allergic airway disease are now carried out in the mouse, the guinea pig initially was utilized as an animal model of pulmonary hypersensitivity and AHR for many decades (Shin et al., 2009 as cited in Noelpp &Noelpp-Eschenhagen, 1952). Guinea pigs were used as a histamine-induced rhinitis model, since histamine induces nasal congestion, sneezing, and rhinorrhea well in guinea pigs among small experimental animals (Kobayashi, 2000). The guinea pigs demonstrated airway constrictive responses and production of hypersensitivity antibodies including IgG1 and IgE (Ricciardolo et al., 2008). The associated pulmonary inflammatory response is consistent with asthma, composed of both eosinophils and neutrophils. The guinea pig model identified the importance of airway inflammation in the development of altered airway function (Ricciardolo et al., 2008). However, there are several disadvantages in using guinea pigs as a model of asthma. The shortage of inbred strains prevents significant investigation of the genetic effects on susceptibility to sensitization and development of allergic airway disease. In addition, major problem to the guinea pig is the predominance of IgG1 rather than IgE as the major anaphylactic antibody (Ricciardolo et al., 2008).

In Iran, the main source of outdoor air pollution due to particles in suspension is represented by heavy traffic of motor vehicles such as gasoline powered cars, diesel-powered vehicles, motorcycles, mining, industrial sources such as manufacturing, community sources such as the heating of homes and buildings, municipal waste and combustion. This survey highlights cellular material release, pollen allergenicity and study of pollen allergens in three ornamental plants of *Spartium junceum* (spanish broom), *Tagetis patula* (French Marigold) and *Lagerstroemia indica* (crepe myrtles) that have distributed widely in parks and landscapes. Also, the importance of the exposure of pollen grains to air pollutants in the induction of allergic diseases is studied.

2. Experimental methods

Pollen grains were collected randomly from plants grown in a clean (nonpolluted) area (National Botanical Garden, Paykanshahr, Tehran, 30 km far from Tehran). After sifting and drying of at room temperature, one half of pollen grains exposed to air pollutant in one area with heavy traffic (Shahid Mofateh Avenue, Tehran) during 10 days. In order to condition homogeneity, the control samples were covered with filter and placed in the vicinity of polluted ones at the same time. The type and mean of air pollutant concentrations in polluted area were reported as 0.068 ppm (SO2), 0.06 ppm (NO2), 9.7 ppm (CO), 3.1 ppm (HC) and 174 μgm^{-3} (APM). Pollen structure was studied by Scanning and Light Electron Microscopy. Pollen specimens were prepared for scanning electron microscopy observation by dusting them directly onto sticky-tape coated aluminum stubs and gold coating. Photographs were taken with a JEOL JSM 633 OF SEM. For light microscopy, Pollen grains were generally dusted onto a drop of water on a microscope slide. Specimens were viewed with an Olympus model Ah2 light microscopy connected to camera. The pollen extracts were prepared by incubating pollen grains in 0.1 M phosphate buffered saline, PBS, pH 7.4 in 15% ratio with stirring at 4–8°C for 4 h. Suspensions were centrifuged at 10 000 g for 20 minutes at 4°C and supernatants were removed. Total protein was measured by Bradford method (Bradford, 1967). Guinea pigs sensitized by injection of pollen extract on three days intervals through the intraperitoneal route with 75 µg protein, both in polluted extracts and non polluted ones. Male Hartley guinea pigs (weighing about 250- 300 g and 4 wk of age) were purchased from Pasteur institute (Karaj, Tehran). The animals were used for experiments at 5 weeks of age when they weighed about 300 to 350 g. The last injection was done subcutaneous to study skin prick test (SPT). Skin tests were read and results were recorded at 30 minutes. The definition of a positive skin test required a wheal diameter 3 mm or greater (≥ 3) than the saline control (Prakashkumar et al., 1998). At day 35, guinea pigs were sacrificed and the blood was collected by cardiac puncture. The sera of all animals were tested for IgE reaction using enzyme linked immunosorbent assay (ELISA). Proteins from samples and molecular markers were separated using SDS- PAGE (Laemmli, 1970). The unstained gels were electrotransferred to PVDF membrane for Western analysis. The membranes were incubated with the patients' sera. The IgE-binding proteins were revealed with an enzyme system using an anti-IgE peroxidase conjugate (Towbin et al., 1979). The results were analyzed using ANOVA in SPSS and Duncan's multiple range test to compare the significance ($p < 0.05$) of the treatments. Data are summarized and plotted as mean ± standard error of the mean. Five animals were used for each treatment.

3. Effect of air pollutants on pollen grains

3.1 Effect of air pollutants on structure and cellular material release in pollen grains

Pollen grains are triapertures (tricolpate) and echinate with small pores in base in *T. patula*, tricolpate with perforate sculpture in *S. junceum* and tricolporate or pseudocolpate with ornamentation of scabrate, striped-regulate, regulate –verucate and puctate depending on anther type (this species has large small anthers) and sculptures position (Figs. 1-3). Pollen sculpture and pollen coating especially in entomophilous pollen grains are resulted in adhering air pollutants to pollen surface when they are exposed to air pollutants. Studies of scanning electron microscopy showed that in pollen grains exposed to air pollutants, airborne particles accumulated on the surface of pollen and changed pollen wall structure (Figs. 1-3).

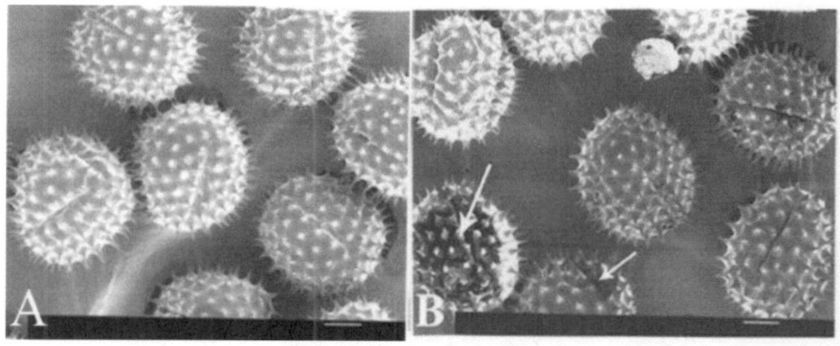

Fig. 1. A, B. Tricolpate pollen grains with echinate ornamentation in *T. patula*. A. Nonpolluted pollen, Agglomeration (arrows) of air pollutants (0.1 µm) is seen on pollen surface (B). Scale bars= respectively 50 & 10 µm.

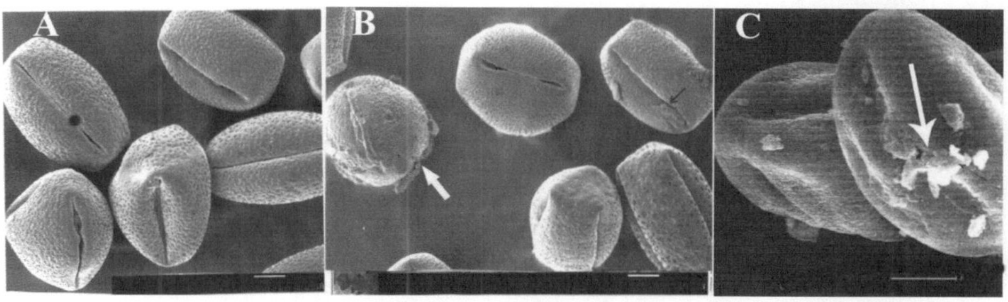

Fig. 2. A-C. Tricolpate pollen grains with perforate ornamentation in *S. junceum*. A. Nonpolluted pollen, arrows show agglomeration of air pollutants on pollen surface (B, C). Scale bars = 10 µm.

Precocious pollen germination is observed in *L. indica* as well (Fig. 3). Agglomeration of airborne particulate matter (0.1-10 µm) is resulted in thinness of pollen wall and induction of cellular material release when they are located in moist medium (Figs. 4-6). These release materials were agglomerated on the surface of pollen as well as on airborne particulate matter including DEP. Furthermore, other investigations of dust samples from highly polluted areas in Germany showed a significant degree of particle agglomeration on the surface of pollen grains (Morgenstern et al., 2008). Therefore, in vitro exposure of pollen grains to particles indicates morphological changes and increases pollen wall permeability and release of cellular matter including allergens from the pollen. In vitro exposure of pollen to gaseous pollutants (SO_2 and NO_2) under different conditions of humidity resulted in SO_2-induced, but not NO_2-induced reduction of allergen release from pollen (Behrendt et al. 1997). It is concluded that the bioavailability of pollen allergens may be modulated by air pollutants, supporting the concept of an interaction between pollen and pollutants in the atmosphere outside the organism which in turn may affect allergy-relevant phenomena. Air pollutants by attaching to the surface of pollen grains and of plant-derived paucimicronic particles, pollutants can modify the morphology of these antigen-carrying agents and alter their allergenic potential. In addition, by inducing airway inflammation, pollutants may overcome the mucosal barrier and so 'prime' allergen-induced responses. In other words airway mucosal damage and impaired mucociliary clearance induced by air pollution may facilitate the access of inhaled allergens to the cells of the immune system (D'Amato, 2002).

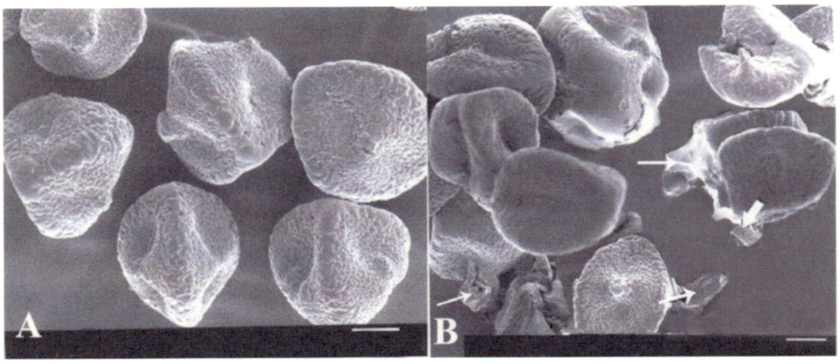

Fig. 3. A, B. tricolporate or pseudocolpate pollen grains with ornamentation of scabrate and regulate depending on anther type and pollen location in *L. indica*. Arrowhead shows agglomeration of air pollutants on pollen surface, arrow show precocious germination (B, due to air pollutants, pollen ornamentation is obscure), A. Nonpolluted pollen.

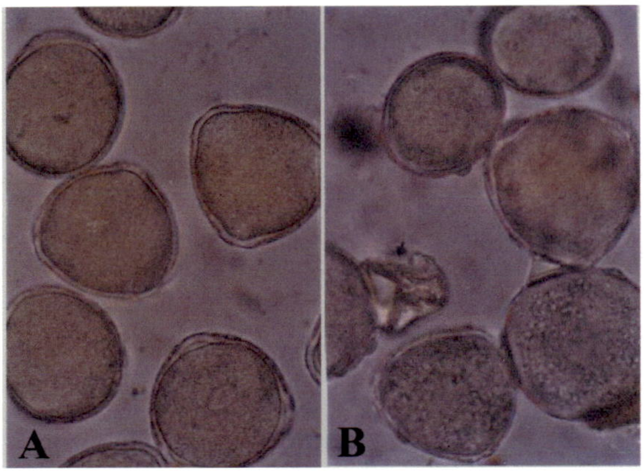

Fig. 4. A, B. Nonpolluted (A) and polluted pollen grains (B) in *S. junceum*. Thinness of exine and increase of cellular matter release in pollen exposed to air pollutants are observed.

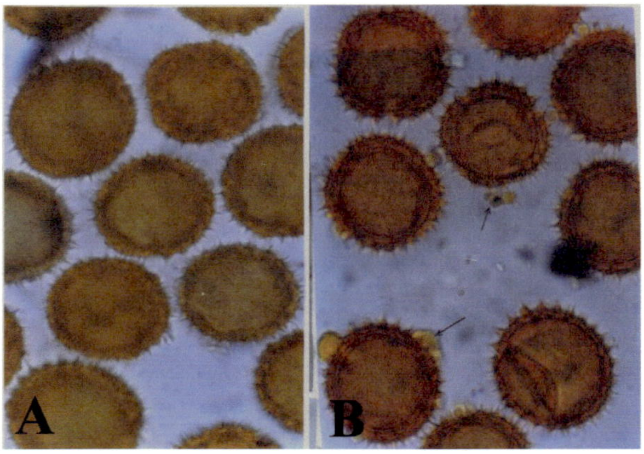

Fig. 5. A, B. Nonpolluted (A) and polluted pollen grains (B) in *T. Patula*. Increase of cellular matter release in pollen grains exposed to air pollutants is observed.

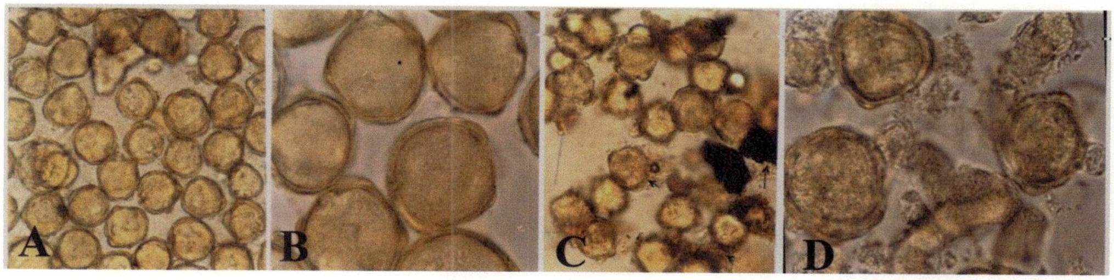

Fig. 6. A-D. Nonpolluted (A, B) and polluted pollen grains (C, D) in *L. indica*. Cellular matter release in pollen exposed to air pollutants is seen. Magnification: X100 (A, C) & X400 (B, D).

3.2 The effect of air pollution on clinical and serological tests

The results of skin tests in guinea pigs showed which pollen extracts result in a positive skin test response compared to control (buffer) ones; also the response of polluted extracts was more than nonpolluted ones (Fig. 7). Injection of polluted extracts especially in S. junceum caused the formation of wound in the place of injection so that its scar exists up to 72 hours.

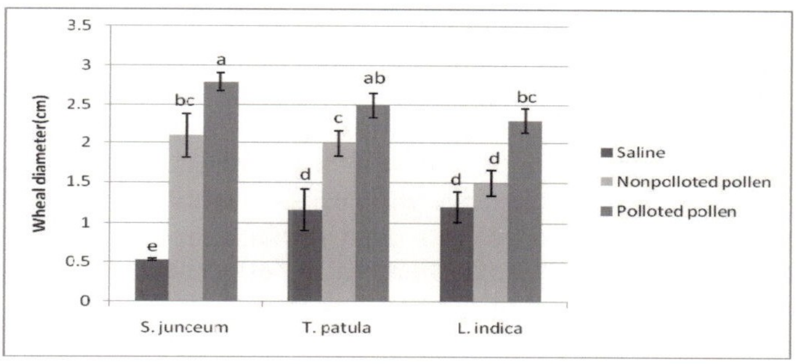

Fig. 7. Prick skin test reactivity in guinea pigs immunized with pollen extracts.

The level of IgE was higher in animals immunized and challenged with pollen extracts than control (buffer) ones. The higher level of IgE was observed in serum of animals injected with polluted pollen extract compared with nonpolluted (less polluted) ones. The induction of antibody production after DEP administration has been reported previously. For example, intranasal instillation of DEP and antigen resulted in increased levels of antigen-specific IgE in murine and human sera. Furthermore, DEP and the polyaromatic hydrocarbon fraction derived from DEP enhanced IgE production from purified human B cells in vitro (Miyabara et al., 1998, as cited in Diaz-Sanchez et al., 1994; Takafuji et al., 1987; Takenaka et al., 1995; Tsien et al., 1997). Diaz-Sanchez (1997) studied the effect of DEP on allergenecity in ragweed. He reported that DEPs can interact with aeroallergens to enhance antigen-induced responses, with the result that allergen-specific IgE levels are up to 50-fold greater in allergic patients stimulated with DEPs and allergens than in patients treated with allergen alone. Combined challenge with DEPs and ragweed allergen markedly increases the expression of human nasal ragweed-specific IgE in vivo and skews cytokine production to a type 2 helper T-cell pattern (D'Amato et al., 2010 as cited in Diaz Sanchez et al., 1997). Similarly, Kobayashi (2000) reported that the administration of DEP or exposure to DEP enhances IgE antibody production in mice and in humans (Kobayashi, 2000, as cited in Fujimaki et al., 1997 and Diaz-Sanchez et al., 1994).

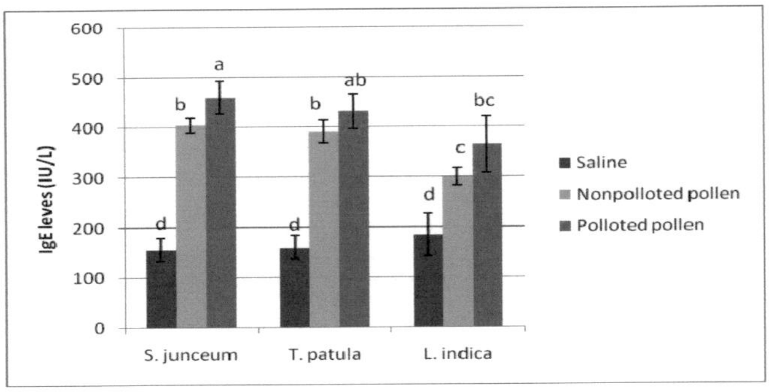

Fig. 8. ELISA reactivity of sera from guinea pigs immunized to pollen extracts.

The increase in blood eosinophils was observed in Guinae pigs sensitized with pollen extracts compared with buffer alone although in *L. indica* was not significant. This increment was higher in the extracts of pollen grains exposed to air pollutants than nonpolluted pollen extracts (Fig. 9). Any significant increase in neutrophils value was seen in animals treated with nonpolluted pollen extracts compared with buffer while their percent increase in polluted pollen extract (Fig. 10). Thus, the combination of pollen plus air pollutant is resulted in a significant increase eosinophils and neutrophils. Inflammatory reactions generally involve a vast array of mediators and a variety of effector cells such as mast cells, macrophages, eosinophils, platelets, and neutropb.ils. It is well recognized that eosinophils are important cells in asthma. Eosinophils release basic proteins that are cytotoxic and lipid mediators such as cysteinyl leukotrienes that cause airway obstruction and bronchial epithelial damage (Bloemen et al., 2007, as cited in Sampson, 2000). Kämpe et al. (2007) reported that there is an eosinophil inflammation in both the nasal and bronchial mucosa and systemically in both allergic asthma and allergic rhinitis during the pollen season. Blood eosinophilia is a common feature in patients with bronchial asthma. The role of neutrophils in mild asthma and allergic rhinitis is uncertain, whereas in severe asthma neutrophils and the neutrophil chemoattractant CXCL8 play an important role in the pathogenesis of airway inflammation. Boulay et al. (2002) also demonstrated an increase in eosinophils in induced sputum after repeated very-low dose allergen challenge in allergic rhinitis (Bloemen et al., 2007, Kämpe et al., 2007). The studies have shown that air pollutants especially Diesel exhaust particles to be able to increased total and specific IgE production, the production of cytokines inherent to Th2 cell response, eosinophilic inflammatory response, the number of peripheral blood neutrophils and platelets and histamine levels (Bartra et al., 2007). Kinhult (2003) reported migration of neutrophils from the blood into the nasal mucosa increases during the grass pollen season (Månsson et al., 2010, as cited in Kinhult, 2003). It has been often observed by many investigators that number of eosinophils and neutrophils increases in brochial alveolar lavage (BAL) fluid after challenge with allergen. Thus, it may be that lower amount of blood neutrophils in animals sensitized with nonpolluted pollen extracts is correlated to their higher value in BAL fluid, nasal alveolar lavage (NAL) fluid and Sputum. Månsson et al. (2010) reported that migration of neutrophils from the blood into the nasal mucosa increases during the grass pollen season (Månsson et al., 2010, as cited in Kinhult, 2003). This migration may be the cause of blood neutrophils decrease. The response of guinea pigs to pollen extracts of *L. indica* was low in all of reactions related to allergenecity but this response was less in nonpolluted pollen extracts. It seems this speices in not allergenetic or its allergenecity potential is low.

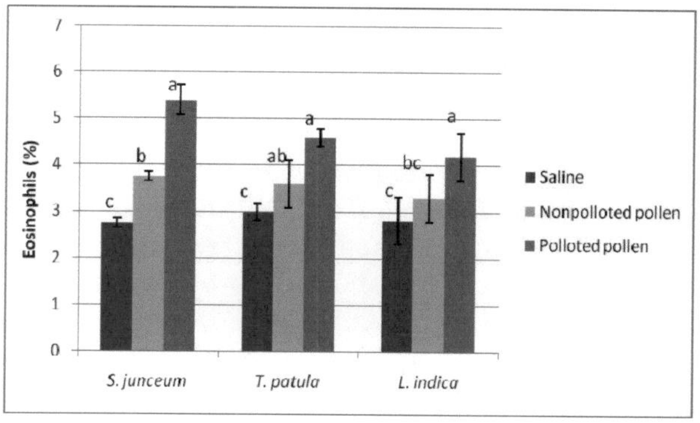

Fig. 9. Blood eosinophils in Guinae pigs immunized with nonpolluted and polluted pollen extracts.

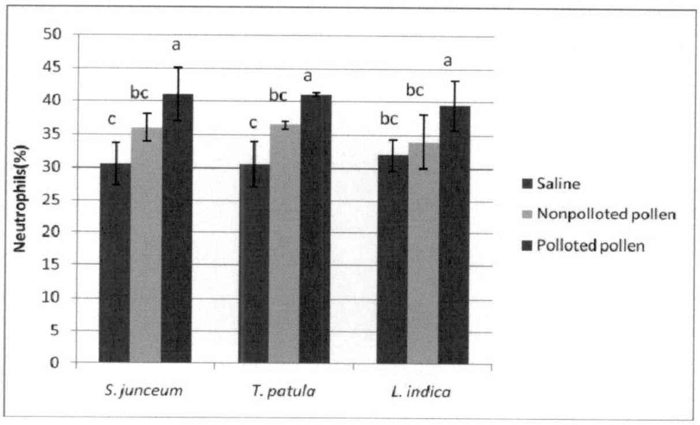

Fig. 10. Blood neutrophils in Guinae pigs immunized with nonpolluted and polluted pollen extracts.

3.3 Effect of air pollutants on total pollen protein and IgE-specific Imunoblotes

Exposure to air pollution showed no obvious difference between soluble proteins of polluted and control extracts in *S. junceum* and *T. patula*. A significant decrease of protein content was observed in pollen extracts under air pollution compared with nonpolluted ones in *T. patula* (Fig. 11).

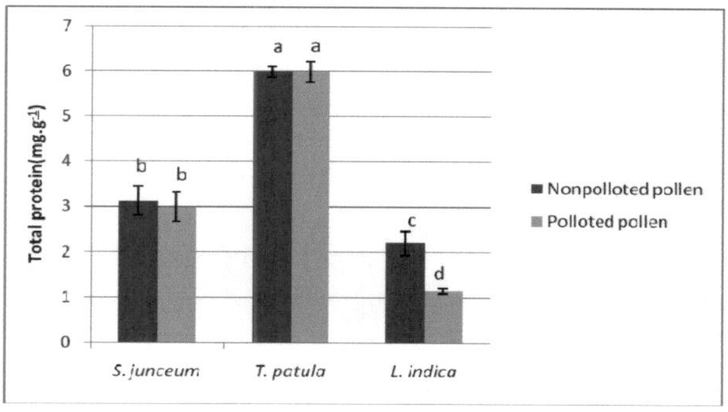

Fig. 11. Total protein content of nonpolluted and polluted pollen extracts.

Immunoblot of IgE binding to *S. junceum* pollen proteins showed that in both polluted and non polluted extracts were revealed two bands in the ranges 46-55 kDa and 35 kDa (Fig. 12). No obvious difference was observed between polluted and non polluted extracts. The Immunoblot profile of *L. indica* did not reveal any clear IgE-binding protein band, although in a few of these blots a weak band in was observed. An IgE-binding band (52-60 kDa) was observed in the immlunoblots of *T. patula* (Fig. 13). Thus, our results did not show any difference in IgE-binding bands (proteins) between polluted and non polluted pollen extracts. Also, pollen extracts of *L. indica* showed no obvious allergen. It is evident that allergenecity potential of plants is a species character and depends on genotype. Studies of effect of air pollutants on pollen proteins show contradictory results. Our results are consistent with the results of Helender et al. (1997) who observed no significant difference between the protein bands of polluted and control areas. However, studies of Behrendt et al. (1997) showed a dose-dependent shift in the intensity of IgE binding reactivity to lower molecular weight bands. In addition, Parui et al (1998) found a decrease in Bet v 1 concentration under air pollution. It is possible that the type of plant species could easily be the cause for these differences, and therefore, this matter may need to be studied further.

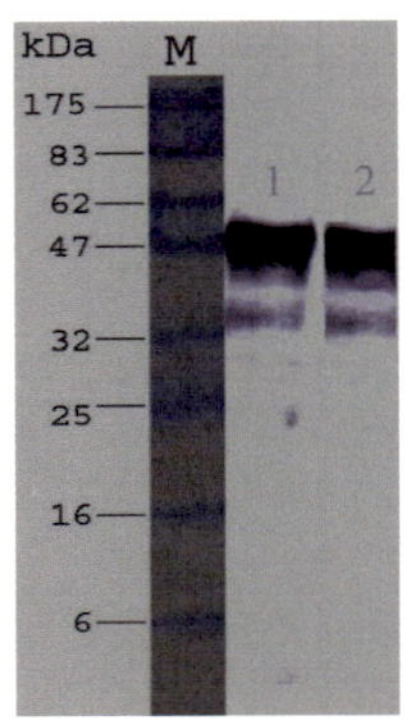

Fig. 12. Immunoblot profile of the pollen extracts in *S. junceum*. M: Marker; 1: Nonpolluted pollen extract; 2: Polluted pollen extract.

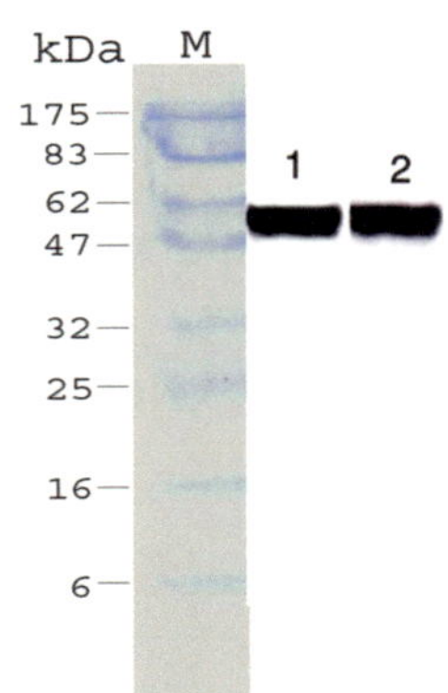

Fig. 13. Immunoblot profile of the pollen extracts in *T. patula*. M: Marker; 1: Nonpolluted pollen extract; 2: Polluted pollen extract.

4. Conclusion

There is growing evidence that air pollutants especially AMPs act as adjuvant in the immune system and lead to enhancement of allergic inflammation in predisposed animals and humans. Air pollutants may affect human B-cells and enhance IgE production by several mechanisms. Another possible mechanism of action of air pollutants on allergic responses is to act as a carrier of particles released from pollen (allergens) or derived from part of the plant such as leaf, stem and flower (for example, anther ubish bodies) allowing enhanced deposition of allergens especially pollen allergens in the lower airway. Also, allergens bound to AMP may trigger asthma attacks and AMP-binding may facilitate penetration of allergen through the airway mucosa. By attaching combination of AMP and allergen to the surface of mucosa and epithelial damage enhances epithelial permeability, stimulation of sensory nerve endings, and the release of chemical mediators. Therefore, AMP may affect both pollen wall and mucosa by increasing their permeability. Increasing pollen permeability induces cellular matter release such as allergens that in turn adheres to AMP. Induction of mucosa permeability may facilitate the access of inhaled allergens and AMP to the cells of the immune system. Furthermore, as cited by D'Amato (2002), air pollutants can modify the morphology of these antigen-carrying agents and alter their allergenic potential.

Taken together with the findings from the other researchers, living on cities with heavy traffic and industrial activities is associated with a higher risk for sensitization to pollen and other allergens. For this reason, it is suggested that government authorities could consider more carefully which plant species are used in populated areas. Species selection is also important to avoid aeroallergen from climate change mitigation tree planting and urban reforestation. Also, using of the fruits and vegetables containing polyphenols reduce damages of allergic disorders. Kishi et al. (2005) reported that a red perilla extract (luteolin being the main ingredient) and rubus suavissinmus extract (ellagitannin being the main ingredient) alleviated the symptoms of cedar pollinosis through antiallergic action (Kishi et al., 2005). Apple major polyphenol (Ap) is condensed tannin (ACT) and it is also contains such monomeric polyphenols as catechin, epicatechin, phlorizin, and chlorogenic acid. Studies on the antiallergic action of Ap have found that it suppressed the histamine release from mast cells and basophils (BRL-2H3) in rats, inhibited hyaluronidase and suppressed auricular swelling in mice. It has been reported from a clinical study that Ap alleviated the itching in atopic dermatitis patients. This phenomenon was attributed to the suppression of histamine release by ACT, the major component of apple (Kishi et al., 2005). Through analysis of the clinical evaluation of one kind of traditional remedy in patients with atopic dermatitis, flavonoids were shown to possess significant anti-allergic activity. Among the twenty kinds of flavonoids examined, fisetin, luteolin, apigenin, quercetin and kaempferol inhibited not only the release of chemical mediators but also the production of T-helper (Th)-2 type cytokines (Interleukin (IL)-4, IL-5 and IL-13) by basophils. These flavonoids inhibit expression of these cytokines through their inhibitory effect on the activation of several calcium-calmodulin dependent kinases (tanaka et al., 2003). Furthermore, air pollution control is an important character in the health of all of living organisms.

5. References

Bartra, J., Mullol, J., del Cuvillo, A., Dávila, I., Ferrer, M., Jáuregui, I., Montoro, J., Sastre. J., Valero, A. (2007). Air pollution and allergens. *Journal of Investigational Allergology and Clinical Immunology*; Vol. 17, No. 2:, (n, d.), pp. 3-8.

Cortegano I., Civantos E., Aceituno E., del Moral, A., Lopez, E., Lombardero, M., del Pozo, V., Lahoz, C. (2004). Cloning and expression of a major allergen from Cupressus arizonica pollen, Cup a 3, a PR-5 protein expressed under polluted environment. *Allergy*, Vol. 59, No., 5, (May 2004), pp. 485-490, ISSN 0105-4538.

Behrendt, H., Becker, W. M., Fritzsche, C., Sliwa-Tomczok, W., Tomczok, J., Friedrichs, K. H., Ring, J. (1997). Air Pollution and Allergy: Experimental Studies on Modulation of Allergen Release from Pollen by Air Pollutants, *International Archives of Allergy and Immunology*, Vol. 113, No. 1-3, (May-July 1997), pp. 69-74, ISBN 978-3-8055-6502-8.

Bice, D.E., Seagrave, J., Green, F. H. (2000). Animal models of asthma: potential usefulness for studying health effects of inhaled particles. Inhalation Toxicology, Vol. 12, No. 9, (September 2000), ISSN 1091-7691.

Bloemen, K., Verstraelen, s., Van Den Heuvel, R., Witters, H., Nelissen I. & Schoeters, G. (2007). The allergic cascade: Review of the most important molecules in the asthmatic lung. *Immunology Letters*. Vol. 113, (August 2007), pp. 6–18, ISSN: 0165-2478.

Bradford M. (1976). A rapid and sensitive method for the quantitation of ug quantities of protein utilizing the principle of protein-dye binding. *Analytical Biochemistry*, Vol. 72, No. 1-2, pp. 248-254. (May 1976), ISSN: 0003-2697.

Chan-Yeung M. N. W. (2000). Air pollution and health. *Hong Kong Medical Journal*. Vol. 6, No.4, pp. 390-398.

D'Amato, G. (2002). Environmental urban factors (air pollution and allergens) and the rising trends in allergic respiratory diseases. *Allergy*, Vol. 57, Suppl. 72, (November2006) pp. 30-33. ISSN 0108-1675.

D'Amato G, Cecchi L, D'Amato M, & Liccardi G. (2010). Urban air pollution and climate change as environmental risk factors of respiratory allergy. *Journal of Investigational Allergology and Clinical Immunology*; Vol. 20, No. 2:, (n, d.), pp. 95-102.

Helander, M. L., Savolainen, J. & Ahlholm, J. (1997). Effect of pollution and other environmental factors on birch pollen allergens. *Allergy*, Vol. 52, No. 12, (April 2007), 1207–1214, ISSN 0105-4538.

Jilek, A., Swoboda, I. M., Breiteneder, H., Fogy, I., Ferreira, F., Schmid, E., Heberle-Bors, E., Scheiner, O., Rumpold, H., Kraft, D., Koller, H. T. & Breitenbach, M. (1993). Biological functions, isoforms and environmental control in the Bet v 1 gene family. In: *Molecular biology and immunology of allergens*, Kraft, D. & Sehon, A. (Eds), pp. 245–271. Boca Raton, FL: CRC Press. 270: 2607-2613.

Kämpe, M., Stålenheim, G., Janson, J., Stolt, I. & Carlson, M. (2007). Systemic and local eosinophil inflammation during the birch pollen season in allergic patients with predominant rhinitis or asthma. *Clinical and Molecular Allergy*, Vol. 5, No. 4, (October 2007), pp. 1-8, ISSN: 1476-7961.

Kawai, M. Hirano, T., Higa, S., Arimitsu, J., Maruta, M., Kuwahara, Y., Ohkawara, T., Hagihara, K., T Yamadori, T., Shima, Y., Ogata, A. (2007). Flavonoids and Related Compounds as Anti-Allergic Substances. *Allergology International*, Vol. 56, No. 2 (June 2007), pp. 113-123, ISSN 1440-1592.

Kishi K., Saito M., Saito T., Kumemura M., Okamatsu H., Okita M. & Takazawa K. (2005). Clinical efficacy of apple polyphenol for treating cedar pollinsosis. *Bioscience, Biotechnology, and Biochemistry*. Vol. 69, No. 4, (n. d.), pp. 829-832, ISSN 1347-6947.

Knox, B. & Suphioglu, C. (1996). Environmental and molecular biology of pollen allergens. *Trends in Plant Science*, Vol. 1, (n. d.), pp. 156–163, ISSN: 1360-1385

Kobayashi, T. (2000). Exposure to diesel exhaust aggravates nasal allergic reaction in Guinea Pigs, *American journal of respiratory and critical care medicine*, Vol 162., No. 2 (August 2000), pp. 352–356, ISSN 1535-4970.

Laemmli, U. K. (1970). Cleavage of structural protein during the assembly of the head of bacteriophage T4. *Nature*, Vol. 227, (15 August 1970), pp. 680–685, ISSN 0028-0836.

Lipiec, A., Rapiejko, P., Samolinski, B. & Krzych, A. (2005). Correlation between conjunctival provocation test results and conjunctival symptoms in pollinosis, preliminary report. *Annals of Agricultural and Environmental Medicine*, Vol. 12, (n. d), pp. 17–20, ISSN 12321966.

Lokaj-Berisha, V., Berisha, N., Lumezi, B., Bejtullahu, G. & Ahmetaj, L. (2009). Sensitivity to pollen allergens in consecutive patients with allergic rhinitis referred to an allergy clinic in prishtina. *Macedonian Journal of Medical Sciences*, Vol. 2, No. 2, (June 2009), pp. 121-125, ISSN 1857-5773.

Majd, A., Chehregani, A., Moin, M., Gholami, M., Kohno, S., Nabe, T., & Shariatzade, M. A. (2004). The effects of air pollution on structures, proteins and allergenicity of pollen Grains. *Aerobiologia*, Vol. 20, (February 2004), pp. 111–118, ISSN 1573-3025.

Månsson, A., Bachar, O., Adner, M., Björnsson, S. & Cardell, L. O. (2010). Leukocyte phenotype changes induced by specific immunotherapy in patients with birch allergy, *Journal of Investigational Allergology and Clinical Immunology*; Vol. 20, No. 6:, (n, d.), pp. 476-483.

Miyabara, Y., Takano, H., Ichinose, T., Lim, H. B. & Saga, M. (1998). Diesel Exhaust Enhances Allergic Airway Inflammation and Hyperresponsiveness in Mice , *American journal of respiratory and critical care medicine*, Vol 157, No, 4, (April 1998), pp. 1138–1144, ISSN 1535-4970.

Morgenstern, V., Zutavern, A., Cyrys, J., Brockow, I., Koletzko, S., Kramer, U., Behrendt, H., Herbarth, O., von Berg, A., Bauer, C. P., Wichmann, H. E. & Heinrich, J. (2008). Atopic diseases, allergic sensitization, and exposure to traffic-related air pollution in children. *American journal of respiratory and critical care medicine*, Vol 177., (March 2008.), pp. 1331–1337, ISSN 1535-4970.

Pacini, E. & Franchi, G. G. (1992). Diversificatioin and evolution on the tapetum. In: *pollen and spores: Patterms of Diversification*, Blackmore S. and Barnes S. H., pp. 301- 316. Oxford university press. Oxford. U. K.., ISBN 10 019857746X.

Parui, S., Mondal A. K. & Mandal, S. (1998). Protein conten and protein skin test sensitivity of the pollen of Argemon mexicana on exposure to SO2. *Grana*, Vol. 37, (n, d), pp. 121–124, ISSN 1651-2049.

Prakashkumar, R., Mathew, P. M. & Ravindran, P. (1998). Studies on the allergenecity of nine tropical pollen allergens. *Grana*, Vol. 37, (n, d), pp. 185-188, ISSN 1651-2049.

Rezaneajd, F. (2009). Air pollution effects on structure, proteins and flavonoids in pollen grains of *Thuja orientalis* L. (Cupressaceae), *Grana*. Vol. 48, No. 3, (September 2009), pp. 205–213, ISSN 1651-2049.

Riedl, M. A., Landaw, E. M., Saxon, A., & Diaz-Sanchez, D. (2005). initial high-dose nasal allergen exposure prevents allergic sensitization to a neoantigen, *The Journal of Immunology*, Vol. 174, No. 11. pp. 7440-7445, ISSN 0022-1767.

Riedl M A. 2008. The effect of air pollution on asthma. *Current Allergy and Asthma Reports,,* Vol. 8, No. 2, (n. d), pp. 139–146, ISSN 1529-7322.

Shaikh, W. A. (2001). Genetics of asthma and allergy, In: *Allergy and Asthma,* A Tropical View. New Delhi: IJCP.

Shin, Y. S., Takeda, K., Gelfand, W. (2009). Understanding asthma using animal models. *Allergy Asthma Immunology Research,* Vol. 1, No.1, (Octobe r 2009), pp. 10-18, ISSN 2092-7363.

Tanaka, T., Higa, S., Hirano, T., Kotani, M. Matsumoto. M. Fujita, A. & Kawase, I. (2003). Flavonoids as potential anti-allergic substances. *Current Medicinal Chemistry Anti-Inflammatory & Anti-Allergy Agents,* Vol. 2, No. 1, (March 2003), pp. 57-65, ISSN: 1568-0142.

Towbin, H., Satquet, T. & Gordon, J. (1979). Electrophoretic transfer of proteins from polyacrylamide gels to nitrocellulose sheets: procedure and some applications. *Proceedings of the National Academy of Sciences.* Vol. 76, No. 9, (September 197), pp. 4350-4354.

Walker, C., Kaegi, M. K., Braun, P., et al. 1991. Activated T cells and eosinophilia in bronchoalveolar lavages from subjects with asthma correlated with disease severity. *Journal of Allergy and Clinical Immunology,* Vol. 88, N0, 6, (March 2005), pp. 935-942, ISSN: 0091-6749.

Wayne P., Foster S., Connolly J, Bazzaz F & Epstein P. 2002. Production of allergenic pollen by ragweed (Ambrosia artemisiifolia L.) is increased in CO2-enriched atmospheres, *Annals of Allergy, Asthma and* Immunology, Vol. 8, pp. 279-282.